Meeting Children's Psychosocial Needs Across the Health-Care Continuum

Meeting Children's Psychosocial Needs Across the Health-Care Continuum

SECOND EDITION

Judy A. Rollins, PhD, RN
Rosemary Bolig, PhD
and
Carmel C. Mahan, MSEd, CCLS

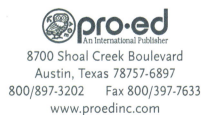

pro·ed
An International Publisher

8700 Shoal Creek Boulevard
Austin, Texas 78757-6897
800/897-3202   Fax 800/397-7633
www.proedinc.com

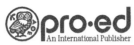

© 2018, 2005 by PRO-ED, Inc.
8700 Shoal Creek Boulevard
Austin, Texas 78757-6897
800/897-3202   Fax 800/397-7633
www.proedinc.com

Library of Congress Cataloging-in-Publication Data
Judy A. Rollins, PhD, RN, Rosemary Bolig, PhD, and Carmel C. Mahan, MSEd, CCLS.
Second edition. | Austin, Texas : PRO-ED, Inc., [2018] |
  Includes bibliographical references.
LCCN 2016056795 (print) | LCCN 2017001809 (ebook)
  | ISBN9781416410805 | ISBN 9781416410812 (ebook)
LCSH: Pediatrics—Psychological aspects. | Pediatrics—Social aspects.
  | Children—Hospital care—Psychological aspects. | Children—Hospital care—
Social aspects. | Sick children—Psychology.| Children—Diseases—Social aspects. | Child health services. | Physician and patient.
LCC RJ47.5 .R656 2017 (print) | LCC RJ47.5 (ebook) | DDC 618.92—dc23
LC record available at https://lccn.loc.gov/2016056795

Art Director: Jason Crosier
Designer: Tina Brackins
This book is designed in Janson Text and Scala Sans.

Printed in the United States of America

2 3 4 5 6 7 8 9 10 11   27 26 25 24 23 22 21 20 19 18

In memory of Rosemary Bolig, PhD, devoted friend and colleague,
passionate advocate for children and families, and pioneer
in the study of play in children's lives. (1945–2017)

Contents

Illustrations

FIGURES

TABLES

TEXT BOXES

CASE STUDIES

Preface

Throughout history, families and concerned professionals have overcome many challenges in their efforts to humanize health-care encounters for children. Many programs aimed at educating health-care professionals now include content about meeting the psychosocial needs of children and their families. Today's financially driven health-care climate, with its emphasis on managed care, threatens to undermine these accomplishments and curtail the development of new approaches.

Significant changes have occurred in health-care services for children, and the system itself remains in transition. Federal legislation, financial considerations, and societal expectations of the role of families often shift, depending on where the services take place and who provides them. In addition, not since the turn of the 20th century has the United States experienced more cultural diversity than in the last two decades, a factor that creates a whole new dynamic in children's health care.

A renewed interest in "healing" health care to complement "curing" health care has sparked attention to alternative and complementary medicine practices as well. Increasing numbers of health-care professionals and patients are bonding with the philosophy of integrative medicine and its approach of treating the whole person—mind, body, and spirit—and not just the disease. Other health-care professionals use the term *integrative health*, shifting the focus from managing disease to promoting lifelong health.

Much has transpired in children's health care since the first edition of *Meeting Children's Psychosocial Needs Across the Health-Care Continuum* was published in 2005. In this second edition, we have integrated current research and theory within the framework of this new and transitioning health-care environment.

New to this edition is the exploration of family and community issues and the impact of such issues on children's psychosocial health and well-being. For, despite the changes we experience now and will experience in the future, children in all settings will need what they have always needed: the basics, such as nurturing, predictability, adequate stimulation, interaction, a sense of control, and mastery of their environments.

The brisk pace of medical discoveries enables more children to be saved through science and technology today than ever in the past. Accompanying each new discovery, treatment, or protocol are implications for psychosocial and developmental concerns. We hope that this book will foster a commitment in the reader to keep pace with new discoveries and to consider the impact they may have, not only on children's bodies but also on their young minds and spirits.

Judy A. Rollins
Rosemary Bolig
Carmel C. Mahan

Editors and Contributors

Judy A. Rollins, PhD, RN
Rollins & Associates, Inc.
1406 28th Street NW
Washington, DC 20007
 and
Georgetown University School
    of Medicine
Department of Family Medicine
Department of Pediatrics
Washington, DC 20007
and
University of Florida
Center for Arts in Medicine
Gainesville, FL 32611

Rosemary Bolig, PhD
Child Associates
3839C Rodman Street, NW
Washington, DC 20016

Carmel C. Mahan, MSEd, CCLS
Baltimore County Public Schools
Southeast Infants and Toddlers Program
7801 E. Collingham Dr., Room 109
Baltimore, MD 21222

Elizabeth Ahmann, ScD, RN, ACC
3307 Belleview Avenue
Cheverly, MD 20785

Jessika C. Boles, PhD, CCLS
Child Life Specialist, Pediatric Critical
    Care Unit
Monroe Carell, Jr. Children's Hospital at
    Vanderbilt
Nashville, TN 37232-9002

Lynn B. Clutter, PhD, APRN, CNS, CNE
Assistant Professor of Nursing
Oxley College of Health Sciences, Room 528
University of Tulsa
800 South Tucker Drive
Tulsa, OK 74104-9700

Lois J. Pearson, MEd, CCLS
N80W15736 Rainbow Drive
Menomonee Falls, WI 53051

Teresa A. Savage, PhD, RN
University of Illinois at Chicago
College of Nursing
845 S. Damen, Room 858
Chicago, IL 60612

Mardelle McCuskey Shepley
Professor
Cornell University
3429 Martha Van Rensselaer Hall
Ithaca, NY 14853

Introduction

The past century has produced tremendous changes in the way health-care professionals view the needs of children and families. In the first half of the 20th century, it was common practice for children to be admitted to hospitals for lengthy stays with only limited family contact. Staff observed that children cried when their parents left, and because it was very time-consuming to console them, they concluded that parental visits were "disruptive" to the children. At about this time, researchers began to look at how increasing parental presence affected parents' satisfaction with their child's hospitalization. When staff observed that parental presence changed children's behavior, the research expanded to include children's reactions, preparation, length of stay, pain management, and other issues.

During this time, children were commonly "seen and not heard," and their feelings and needs were rarely discussed when family decisions were made, including decisions that involved their health care. Health-care professionals, in fear of upsetting the child, frequently counseled parents to avoid telling their child that he or she was going to the hospital. Naturally, the child was most upset when suddenly separated from the parents without explanation, changed into unfamiliar clothes, put into a strange bed, and subjected to painful and frightening tests, procedures, and surgeries.

Since the mid-1930s (Beverly, 1936), research on children's reactions to hospitalization, surgery, or other health-care encounters has demonstrated that children are vulnerable to and have adverse emotional reactions to these events that may persist over time. Findings from early studies—Edelston (1943); Levy (1945); Prugh, Staub, Sands, Kirschbaum, and Lenihan (1953); Skipper and Leonard (1968); Vaughn (1957); Vernon, Schulman, and Foley (1966); and others—consistently demonstrated such effects.

Today, lengthy hospitalizations are rare. Children undergo surgery in the outpatient setting in the morning and are home by afternoon. Advances in technology, such as monitors and other medical equipment designed for home use, have led to sophisticated home treatments that previously were delivered to children only in hospital intensive-care units. At the same time, illness and injury prevention and health promotion have brought primary care to the forefront in health care for both adults and children. In an environment of multiple health-care settings and levels of care, professionals and families concerned with humanistic health care have focused attention on smooth and seamless transitions for children as they move throughout the health-care system.

The Continuum of Care

Most children in today's health-care system experience several phases of care. These various phases are often referred to as the *continuum of care:* the progression through and between the various phases of care (Olson, 1999), which vary from child to child, depending upon diagnosis and individual needs. Although every experience is unique, each of the 10 phases has inherent psychosocial stressors for the child and family. Considering the circumstances children and families experience at each phase is helpful because circumstances, in part, dictate differences in stressors and therefore help predict their responses (see Table I.1).

Another way to view health-care services is to look at levels of care. There are three levels: primary, secondary, and tertiary. For definitions of these levels and the services provided, see Table I.2.

A child's continuum of care need not include all the phases or levels of care, and circumstances determine where the child enters the continuum. For example, a child injured playing football may enter the continuum through emergent care, receive treatment, and be sent home to recover. Another child may be diagnosed with leukemia as part of a routine health examination at the primary care provider. He or she may be sent to an outpatient specialist—a pediatric oncologist—for a complete diagnostic workup, moved to intermediate care within a hospital for initial chemotherapy, sent home with instructions to return to the oncologist at scheduled times, moved back to the hospital with fever and neutropenia, and sent home when the crisis has passed. Later, the child may again return to the hospital for intermediate care or be transferred to an intensive-care setting for a bone marrow transplant.

Managed Care

Movement along the continuum of care requires coordination. Today, managed care has become the dominant form of health care in most parts of the United States. Managed care is differentiated in several respects from the traditional academic-medicine model in which physicians are trained. Managed care's foundation is population-based medicine, which is essentially prevention. This means pooling resources to achieve a maximally fair distribution of resources. The ethic in managed care is to do what works and only what works. A different set of values guide the academic medical model: Everything that can possibly be done is done for the individual patient and continues to be done even when a situation looks futile. Another key difference involves decision making. In a managed-care medical model, the physician uses a set of regulations and guidelines to decide on a course of action and must present strong justification for doing otherwise. The academic model promotes autonomous decision making that results in huge variations in the quality of care and little in the way of effective standardized treatment, which is sometimes called "evidence-based medicine."

The Patient Protection and Affordable Care Act

On March 23, 2010, President Barack Obama signed into law the Patient Protection and Affordable Care Act (PPACA), commonly called the Affordable Care Act (ACA) or, colloquially, Obamacare. The law put in place comprehensive reforms that improve access to affordable health coverage for everyone and protect consumers from abusive insurance company practices.

Although passage of the ACA increases the number of choices available to some families, the processes for accessing these services, whether public or private, are often

Table I.1

Phases of Care and Selected Considerations	
Phase	**Selected Considerations**
1. Identification of illness or injury	Sudden or prolonged
	Part of routine health examination or traumatic
	Requires immediate attention or a slower pace
2. Urgent care	Familiar care provider in familiar surroundings or unfamiliar care provider in strange surroundings
3. Emergent care	Transported in familiar mode (family car) by family member or unfamiliar mode (ambulance, helicopter) by unfamiliar health-care providers
	Family available or unavailable
	Retained at original facility or transferred to another facility with required specialty or pediatric expertise
4. Acute-care setting within a hospital	Emergent or planned admission
	Pediatric or adult hospital
	Placed with age-mates or by diagnosis
	Family members accommodated (e.g., cot for parent at bedside) or not
5. Intensive care	Transfer planned or unplanned
	Familiar primary care provider's continued involvement or total transfer to pediatric specialty
	Family members welcome or not
6. Intermediate care	Transferred from higher level of care (intensive care, with family accustomed to close monitoring of child) or from lower level of care (outpatient facility)
	Transfer decision considered family's readiness or transfer dictated by the facility
7. Rehabilitation	Transferred to unit within present facility or transferred to a different facility
	Rehabilitation included in medical insurance benefits or not included
8. Outpatient specialty care	Occurred as part of diagnostic workup or as part of recovery and follow-up care
	Involved surgical/invasive procedures or uninvasive monitoring
	Involved preparation at home before arrival or no preparation
	Involved follow-up instructions for home care or no follow-up home care
9. Home care	Initiated with previous hospitalization or without previous hospitalization
	Included multiple care providers or a limited number of familiar care providers
10. Transition from acute to chronic illness	Expected or unexpected (e.g., occurred over time because of recurrence of health problem or natural course of disease or as a complication of illness or injury)
	Response of child and family to diagnosis and treatment focus similar from response to acute illness, or different

Note. Adapted from "Acute Illness: The Continuum of Care," by C. Olson, 1999, in M. Broome & J. Rollins (Eds.), *Core Curriculum for Nursing Care of Children and Their Families* (pp. 215–221). Pitman, NJ: Jannetti. Copyright 1999 by Jannetti. Adapted with permission.

Table I.2

Levels of Care		
Level	**Definition**	**Services**
Primary	Basic health services for medical monitoring, care of routine health problems, immunizations, and anticipatory guidance in the clinic or office setting	Health promotion and prevention Routine acute illnesses and injuries Ongoing management/monitoring of nonroutine problems Child and family education and counseling Family support and networking services Case management
Secondary	Direct services by members of an interdisciplinary team of specialized consultants, as needed, for complex and unusual health problems in a community hospital setting	Complex and specialized interdisciplinary services Child and family education and counseling Education and training for primary health-care providers Development of a service and education plan for community
Tertiary	Direct services by highly specialized members of an interdisciplinary team and specialized consultants, as needed, for complex and unusual health problems in a medical center or university health science center setting	Highly complex and specialized services by interdisciplinary team Child and family education counseling Education and training for primary health-care providers and other professionals Development of individualized hospital discharge plans Development of collaborative community service projects Research

Note. Adapted from "Chronic Conditions: The Continuum of Care," by W. Nehring, 1999, in M. Broome & J. Rollins (Eds.), *Core Curriculum for the Nursing Care of Children and Their Families* (pp. 331–341). Pitman, NJ: Jannetti. Copyright 1999 by Jannetti. Adapted with permission.

overwhelming. The ACA has many complex provisions and has set in motion a number of potential changes to established delivery systems and existing caregiving relationships. Some of the many benefits for children include health insurance availability regardless of preexisting conditions, restrictions on annual or lifetime dollar limits on benefits, essential preventive-care services without copays or cost sharing, extension of coverage to age 26 on their parents' policies, and expanded insurance for parents (Cheng, Wise, & Halfon, 2014). The law requires that all plans have a comprehensive age-appropriate child benefits package including Bright Futures and Early and Periodic Screening, Diagnosis and Treatment (EPSDT) benefits of medically necessary periodic screenings; vision, hearing, and dental services; and treatment.

The creation and implementation of marketplaces, the technical difficulties therein, and the ideological and political disagreements in states opposed to the ACA have resulted in vast differences among state plans. As of March 2016, 63% of states had expanded Medicaid in accordance with the ACA regulations (The Henry J. Kaiser

Foundation, 2016). Cheng and colleagues (2014) pointed out that even in states pushing forward with expansion, there are concerns that a lack of attention to the special needs of children could destabilize long-standing child health programs. They call for a prioritized national effort involving pediatric clinicians, state and local policy makers, and child advocates to monitor health reform's effect on children and to ensure optimal implementation.

Parents and family members can also be added to this list of advocates. They recognize that social workers, child life specialists, psychologists, and other providers of psychosocial care and services for children and families are all essential parts of comprehensive children's health care.

Children's Voices

Today, we recognize that children have strong feelings about, reactions to, and the right to full participation in events in their lives, or the lives of their family members, friends, and classmates. According to the United Nations Convention on the Rights of the Child, child participation entails the act of encouraging and enabling children to make their views known on the issues that affect them (Bellamy, 2003). In *The State of the World's Children 2003*, Bellamy disputed some of the common myths about child participation (see Table I.3).

Along the continuum of care, ethicists and other concerned professionals and parents have advocated for policies that give children a greater voice in matters that affect them. Researchers, rather than asking only parents or health-care professionals about children's experiences, now also are more likely to ask the children themselves. Research methods, such as drawing, that allow children to use more developmentally appropriate "languages" are on the rise. We have learned that children, given the proper forum, have little difficulty in expressing their points of view.

Psychosocial Care Across the Health-Care Continuum

There is now almost 90 years' worth of increasingly sophisticated research on the effects of hospitalization and other health-care experiences on children and their families. With a rapidly changing health-care environment, the health-care system for children both looks and serves children differently than it did in the recent past.

A major question, however, still remains: Are children different? Are their needs and capacities to cope with the demands of illness, treatments, and health-care environments different from those of children during the previous periods of health care? Although home care may alleviate separation, are there other new risks in treating children? Do children require less continuity of care and support from those closest to them during periods of most demand? Do children acquire or express knowledge in new ways? Are they more adaptive than we previously believed? Do the programs and policies instituted to respond to the earlier identified causes of children's upset completely mitigate the stresses faced in today's hospital, home care, and associative settings? Or are there new demands, new risks, new challenges for children and families?

Table I.3

Child Participation: Myth and Reality	
Myth	**Reality**
Child participation means choosing one child to represent children's perspectives and opinions in an adult forum.	Children are not a homogeneous group, and no one child can be expected to represent the interests of his or her peers of different ages, races, ethnicities, and gender. Children need forums of their own in which they can build skills, identify their priorities, communicate in their own way, and learn from their peers. In this way, children are better able to make their own choices as to who should represent their interests and in which ways they would like their viewpoints represented.
Child participation involves adults handing over all their power to children who are not ready to handle it.	Participation does not mean that adults simply surrender all decision-making power to children. The Convention on the Rights of the Child (CRC) is clear that children should be given more responsibility—according to their "evolving capacities" as they develop. In many cases, adults continue to make the final decision, based on the best interests of the child—but with the CRC in mind, it should be a decision informed by the views of the child. As children grow older, parents are encouraged to allow them more responsibility in making decisions that affect them—even those that may be controversial, such as custody matters following a divorce.
Children should be children, and not be forced to take on responsibilities that should be given to adults.	Children should certainly be allowed to be children, and to receive all the protection necessary to safeguard their healthy development. And no children should be forced to take on responsibilities for which they are not ready. But children's healthy development also depends upon being allowed to engage with the world, making more independent decisions, and assuming more responsibility as they become more capable. Children who encounter barriers to their participation may become frustrated or even apathetic; 18-year-olds without the experience of participation will be poorly equipped to deal with the responsibilities of democratic citizenship.
Child participation is merely a sham. A few children, usually from an elite group, are selected to speak to powerful adults who then proceed to ignore what the children have said while claiming credit for "listening" to kids.	Child participation, in many instances, has proven to be very effective. Rather than setting up an ineffectual system, it is up to all of us to devise meaningful forms of participation that benefit children and, in turn, society as a whole.
Child participation actually only involves adolescents, who are on the verge of adulthood anyway.	The public, political face of child participation is more likely to be that of an adolescent than of a 6-year-old, but it is essential to consult children of all ages about the issues that affect them. This means participation within schools and families when decisions about matters there are being discussed. At every age, children are capable of more than they are routinely given credit for—and they will usually rise to the challenges set before them if adults support their efforts.
No country in the world consults children on all the issues that affect them, and no country is likely to do so soon.	That is partly true. However, all countries that have ratified the Convention on the Rights of the Child have committed themselves to ensuring participation rights for children (e.g., the rights to freely express their views on matters that affect them and the freedom of thought, conscience, religion, association, and peaceful assembly). And almost every country can now show significant advances in setting systems and policies in place to allow children to exercise these rights.

(continues)

Table I.3 (*continued*)

Myth	Reality
Children may be consulted as a matter of form but their views never change anything.	Where children's views are sensitively solicited and sincerely understood, they often create a great deal of change: they may reveal things that adults would never have grasped independently, they can profoundly change policies or programs and, in some cases, they can protect children from future harm. The consultation of even very young children can produce remarkable results. The problem is that such careful consultation of children remains rare.
Children's refusal to participate negates their rights.	Actually, resistance itself can be an important part of participation. Whether in the give and take of the home, in the refusal to accept punishment at school, or in one's attitude towards civic engagement in the community, resistance can signal a child's or adolescent's opinion about an issue or feeling about the terms of his or her involvement. Adults should recognize resistance as a form of communication and respond to it through understanding, dialogue, and negotiation, rather than by trying to prevent it through force or persuasion. In no situation should children be forced to participate.

Note. From "The State of the World's Children," by C. Bellamy, 2003, New York, NY: UNICEF.

This second edition of *Meeting Children's Psychosocial Needs Across the Health-Care Continuum* reopens the dialogue as we look at children's health care in today's environment.

Chapter 1: Children's Hospitalization and Other Health-Care Encounters highlights the impact of a developmental approach to pediatric and family-centered care and explores interventions that may make a difference in the reactions of children, siblings, and other family members to hospitalization and other encounters with the health-care system.

Chapter 2: Preparing Children for Health-Care Encounters explores stress and coping as well as the history and theories behind various methods of preparing children for health-care encounters.

Chapter 3: Play in Children's Health-Care Settings describes play, its functions and forms, the present state of theory and research on play, and the current thinking of play researchers in health care and other contexts.

Chapter 4: The Arts in Children's Health-Care Settings discusses ways that children use the arts as tools for coping with illness and health-care experiences, describes related research findings and applications, and concludes with recommendations for individuals wishing to use the arts with children or to establish arts programming in children's health-care settings.

Chapter 5: Children and Youth With Special Health-Care Needs addresses psychosocial issues for children and youth with special health-care needs in hospitals, at home, and in the community.

Chapter 6: The Child Who Is Dying looks at the needs and concerns of the child who is dying, the impact of death at home or in the hospital within the context of palliative care, and the unique characteristics of grief for parents, siblings, grandparents, and others.

Chapter 7: Families in Children's Health-Care Settings looks at different kinds of families and explores issues that health-care professionals need to consider when working with families along the health-care continuum.

Chapter 8: The Health-Care Environment summarizes terms related to psychosocial issues, delineates the objectives of environmental psychology when applied to health-care environments, provides examples of alternative design philosophies, offers guidelines for pediatric hospitals and alternative caregiving environments, and describes more controversial dimensions of healing environments.

Chapter 9: Spiritual Issues in Children's Health-Care Settings provides an overview of spirituality, followed by theoretical and developmental aspects of spirituality and a description of spiritual care.

Chapter 10: Cultural Influences in Children's Health Care presents the dimensions of culture, the within-group complexity found among members of any given culture, and information about developing cross-cultural competence.

Chapter 11: Ethical, Moral, and Legal Issues in Children's Health Care reviews familiar ethical, moral, and legal issues; challenges conventional thinking on these issues; and raises new issues to be faced.

Chapter 12: Relationships in Children's Health-Care Settings explores the types of relationships that develop between health-care professionals and the children and families they serve, and the relationships that develop among members of the health-care team.

Chapter 13: Promoting Children's Well-Being in the Community discusses factors in the community that affect children's well-being, community services for children, and the health-care professional as an agent of change.

Meeting Children's Psychosocial Needs Across the Health-Care Continuum–Second Edition concludes with an **Epilogue** that addresses trends in children's health care, providing thought-provoking ideas for new directions in the psychosocial care of children and their families across the health-care continuum.

References

Bellamy, C. (2003). *The state of the world's children 2003*. New York, NY: UNICEF.

Beverly, B. (1936). The effects of illness upon emotional development. *Journal of Pediatrics, 8,* 533–543.

Cheng, T. L., Wise, P. H., & Halfon, N. (2014). Quality health care for children and the Afford-able Care Act: A voltage drop checklist. *Pediatrics, 134*(4), 794–802.

Edelston, H. (1943). Separation anxiety in young children: Study of hospital cases. *Genetic Psychological Monographs, 26,* 3–95.

Levy, D. (1945). Psychic trauma of operations in children. *American Journal of Diseases of Children, 7,* 69–70.

Nehring, W. (1999). Chronic conditions: The continuum of care. In M. Broome & J. Rollins (Eds.), *Core curriculum for the nursing care of children and their families* (pp. 331–341). Pitman, NJ: Jannetti.

Olson, C. (1999). Acute conditions: The continuum of care. In M. Broome & J. Rollins (Eds.), *Core curriculum for the nursing care of children and their families* (pp. 215–221). Pitman, NJ: Jannetti.

Prugh, D., Staub, E., Sands, H., Kirschbaum, R., & Lenihan, E. (1953). A study of the emotional reactions of children and families to hospitalization and illness. *American Journal of Orthopsychiatry, 23,* 70–106.

Skipper, J., & Leonard, L. (1968). Children, stress and hospitalization. *Journal of Health and Social Behavior, 9,* 275–287.

The Henry J. Kaiser Foundation. (2016). *Current status of state Medicaid expansion decisions.* Retrieved from http://kff.org/health-reform/slide/current-status-of-the-medicaid-expansion-decision/

Vaughn, G. (1957). Children in hospitals. *The Lancet, 272,* 1117–1120.

Vernon, D. T. A., Schulman, J. L., & Foley, J. M. (1966). Changes in children's behavior after hospitalization. *American Journal of Diseases of Children, 111,* 581–593.

1

Children's Hospitalization and Other Health-Care Encounters

Lois J. Pearson

Objectives

At the conclusion of this chapter, the reader will be able to:

1. Describe the course of children's development and the potential impact of hospitalization and other health-care encounters at different stages of development.
2. Indicate the various reasons for children's responses at different stages and the counterinterventions appropriate to each stage.
3. Discuss the social, economic, technological, medical, and knowledge changes that have contributed to changes in child health-care policies and practices.
4. Suggest current and future challenges to children's abilities to cope and adapt in child health-care encounters.

Those of us who have spent many years working in hospitals have come to take much for granted. We know we are kind, benevolent, capable people interested in healing, the alleviation of suffering and the prolongation of life. However, a child coming into the hospital for the first time may see us quite differently. No matter how well we do our job, we are not his parents, the hospital bed is not his own, and the world we provide is an unfamiliar and frightening one. It is a world in which children are hurt. Every body orifice may be entered and when these are exhausted we create new openings by injection, by IV, cut-down or by surgery.

—Robinson, 1972, p. 1

These words, written in 1972 in a paper titled "The Psychological Impact of Illness and Hospitalization Upon the Child—Infancy to Twelve Years," by Mary Robinson, summarized the state of health care for children at the time and challenged pediatric health-care professionals to reform caregiving to better meet the unique psychosocial needs of children and families. The challenge came at a time when current research was documenting the deleterious effects of hospitalization on children of all ages. A review of more than 200 articles in 1965 concluded that emotional distress was common both during the period of hospitalization and after discharge. Between 1963 and 1983 many additional research articles documented the prevalence of psychological upset following discharge from the hospital, including behavioral changes, increased separation anxiety, increased sleep anxiety, and increased aggression toward authority (Gaynard et al., 1990).

In addition, retrospective studies noted that children who were hospitalized as young children demonstrated adjustment difficulties as adolescents, especially children who were hospitalized for longer than 1 week or had multiple admissions before the age of 5 years (Douglas, 1975; Quinton & Rutter, 1976).

Significant changes in pediatric health care in the last three decades, especially the institution of principles of family-centered care, have affected both the way that health care is delivered to children and the psychosocial outcomes. A study in 1984 by Chess and Thomas documented that for school-age children, psychological development sometimes includes stress, but that within a supportive environment with opportunities for mastery, hospitalization can result in psychological benefits.

This chapter begins with a description of the characteristics of children in hospitals today. Next, the impact of a developmental approach to pediatric care is highlighted, and the particular interventions that may make a difference in children's reactions to hospitalization are explored, along with a brief discussion of vulnerable and resilient children. A review of parental and sibling reactions to a child's hospitalization is followed by a discussion about technology and a description of the emergency room experience. The chapter concludes with an overview of ambulatory care for children.

Characteristics of Children Hospitalized Today

According to a 2009 statistical brief from the Agency for Healthcare Research and Quality (Yu, Wier, & Elixhauser, 2011), one out of every six patients discharged from a U.S. hospital was a child younger than 17 years of age, with the majority of children being newborn infants (see Figure 1.1). The mean length of stay for children was 3.8 days, and more than 94% experienced a routine discharge, as compared to being transferred to other acute-care hospitals or other institutions, discharged to home care, or discharged against medical advice.

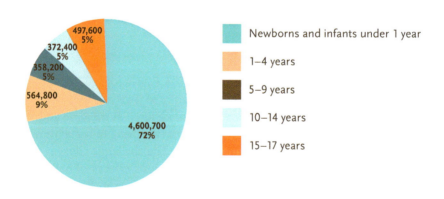

Figure 1.1. Frequency and distribution of hospital stays for children by age, 2009.

Note. AHRQ, Center for Delivery, Organization, and Markets, Healthcare Cost and Utilization Project, Kids' Inpatient Database (KID), 2009. Rates calculated using resident population for July 2009 from the U.S. Bureau of the Census. Retrieved from http://www.census.gov/popest/national/asrh/NC EST2009-sa.html.

Respiratory conditions were cited as the most frequent reason for hospital stays among non-newborns, at 23%. For the most common specific reasons for children's hospital admission, see Figure 1.2. In 2012, 12% of children had one emergency room visit in a year, while 6% of children had two or more visits (Bloom, Jones, & Freeman, 2013).

At discharge, children are less likely to receive home health-care services or long-term care than are adults. Thus, because demand for posthospital specialized care can be relatively infrequent for children, high-quality post-hospital pediatric care may be limited in many areas.

A Developmental Approach

Children's reactions to hospitalization and other health-care experiences can be best understood through the lens of psychosocial development. Erik Erikson's (1963) theory of personality development is the most widely accepted and used in pediatrics (Hockenberry & Wilson, 2014). Built on Freudian theory, Erikson's theory emphasizes a healthy personality as opposed to a pathological approach. According to Erikson, specific changes are assumed to take place during eight predictable age-related stages. Individuals face a unique conflict at each stage, which has two aspects: favorable and unfavorable (Erikson, 1959):

- Trust Versus Mistrust (birth to 1 year)
- Autonomy Versus Shame and Doubt (1 to 3 years)
- Initiative Versus Guilt (3 to 6 years)
- Industry Versus Inferiority (6 to 12 years)
- Identity Versus Role Confusion (12 to 18 years)
- Intimacy and Solidarity Versus Isolation (the 20s)
- Generativity Versus Self-Absorption (late 20s to 50s)
- Integrity Versus Despair (50s and beyond)

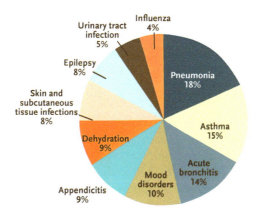

Figure 1.2. Most Common Specific Reasons for Admission to the Hospital.

Note. Adapted from AHRQ, Center for Delivery, Organization, and Markets, Healthcare Cost and Utilization Project, Kids' Inpatient Database (KID), 2009. Rates calculated using resident population for July 2009 from the U.S. Bureau of the Census and National Vital Statistics. Retrieved from http://www.census.gov/popest/national/asrh/NC-EST2009-sa.html

No core conflict is ever mastered completely. However, the individual must adequately resolve each conflict before progressing to the next stage.

Children's reactions to hospitalization at every developmental age are precipitated by stressful events. These may include separation, loss of control, bodily injury, and pain (Hockenberry & Wilson, 2014). In addition, the unfamiliarity of the hospital setting and reduced opportunities for developmentally appropriate activities contribute to the level of experienced stress. How children respond to these stressors will be influenced not only by developmental age, but also by previous experience with illness, separation, or hospitalization; innate or acquired coping skills; the seriousness of the diagnosis; and available support systems (Hockenberry & Wilson, 2014).

Although other factors affect the child's response to hospitalization, as mentioned above, a developmental approach is the most commonly used method for addressing psychosocial needs. The following sections describe concerns, responses, and interventions for children—infants through adolescents—who are hospitalized.

Infants: Newborn to 6 Months

> I was wheeled over to Julia, and got my first good look at her. I felt like I'd been drenched in ice water. She had on only the little hat and a tiny diaper. She had tubes up her nose, in her arms, and in her feet. She had electrodes on her chest, back, and sides. Her eyes were covered to protect them from the lights, which shone around the clock. She looked so frail, helpless, and so small. I started to cry and didn't stop until long after I was in my new bed. I couldn't do anything to help her, and I was so afraid that she would die. (Rapacki, 1991, p. 15)

In the United States each year, more than 300,000 infants are hospitalized in neonatal intensive care units (NICUs) (Santos, Pearce, & Stroustrup, 2015). The hospital environment can potentially affect the developmental outcomes of hospitalized children of any age. However, because very rapid brain growth and development occur at the neonatal stage, the NICU can have a profound effect on developmental outcomes (White, 2011). The NICU can expose the neonate to neurotoxic chemicals, aberrant lights, and excess sound, and confinement to the incubator-based environment can deprive the infant of the tactile stimulation so important at this stage, when children learn about their world through sensory means (Santos et al., 2015).

The hospitalization of a newborn creates a myriad of stresses for new parents. The presence of complex medical equipment in a strange and unfamiliar environment, and the reality of a very ill baby, challenge the basic parenting skills that usually focus on becoming acquainted with, feeding, and comforting a new little person. Frequently exhausted by the emotional and physical demands of labor and delivery, parents must integrate medical information at a time when they are least able to do so.

Care in the NICU is required to be family-centered as much as "infant-centered." Numerous studies have demonstrated that supporting parents in the NICU helps reduce stresses and positively affects the parent–infant relationship over time. A study by Lally and Phelps (1994) documented the importance of security, protection, and intimacy for a level of trust to develop between infant and family. When these needs are not met, infants may become depressed, develop failure to thrive, or show signs of hospitalism. (The term *hospitalism* was first used by Spitz [1945] to describe infants' inability to survive in institutional settings.)

A synthesis of research looking at the role of parenting in the NICU identified the following themes (Gibbs, Boshoff, & Stanley, 2015):

1. Relinquishing the anticipated role of parenting
2. Feeling vulnerable and powerless
3. Juggling roles and responsibilities
4. (Re) Claiming an alternative parental role
5. Navigating environmental boundaries—emotional, physical, and cultural
6. Developing partnerships with staff—constraining and enabling influences
7. Coming to know the baby
8. Adapting to parenting—life beyond the NICU

Family-centered-care principles within the neonatal intensive care unit recognize that, over time, the family has the greatest impact on a baby's health and well-being. Dr. Gretchen Lawhon states, "When two critically ill infants have the same clinical diagnosis, the one who has family present, pulling for him or her and actively participating in care, will almost always do better" (Johnson, 1995, p. 11). New NICU units are designed so that families can care for these fragile infants in individual rooms rather than in open units. Parents appreciate more privacy, more time in skin-to-skin contact with their babies, greater access to physicians, and less overstimulation from noise and lighting. The family's ability to sleep in the room with their baby is also cited as a benefit (Ortenstrand et al., 2009). For more about the NICU environment, see Chapter 8: The Health-Care Environment.

Medical advances have led to the survival of more babies; concomitantly, the intensity of psychological distress for NICU parents has increased, because premature babies and babies with low birth weights often have lifelong medical and neurodevelopmental problems (Gooding et al., 2011). Research suggests that the high numbers of invasive procedures often experienced in the NICU can contribute to long-term abnormalities in the brain's white matter and lower IQs for very preterm infants (Vinall et al., 2014). (See Text Box 1.1.)

The Newborn Individualized Developmental Care and Assessment Program (NIDCAP) was developed as a foundation for the provision of developmentally supportive care in the neonatal intensive care unit (Als & Gilkerson, 1995). The plan begins with detailed observations of infant behavior and builds on the infant's unique strategies in creating a plan of care, including the infant's autonomic, motor, and state systems. These observations help both professionals and parents to respond to the infant's many cues in providing supportive care. Research identifies significantly greater satisfaction of families cared for using the NIDCAP developmental-care program than those cared for in traditional programs (Wielenga, Smit, & Unk, 2006).

The NIDCAP framework also describes a developmental-care environment that includes

- *Consistency of caregiving*—Each infant is assigned a primary multidisciplinary care team that includes the family to create an individualized care plan;

Text Box 1.1

Aspects of Family-Centered Care and Family Support

Information/materials
Breastfeeding support
Skin-to-skin holding
Transport support
Sibling support
Photography
Palliative-care support
Parent-education seminars
Parent-to-parent support
Transition-to-home support
Bereavement support
Unlimited parental presence
Parents on rounds
Parents as faculty
Family advisory councils
NICU staff emotional support
NICU staff FCC support
Parent participants in care and decision making
Support of specific populations (rural, urban, cultural)
Family support activities (scrapbooking/crafts)

- *Structuring the infant's 24-hour day*—Cares should be clustered to respect the infant's sleep–wake cycles and to promote growth;
- *Pacing of caregiving*—The family is an integral part of caregiving as the infant begins to recognize parents' voice, touch, and feel and receives comfort and more stable physiological measures with family presence and participation;
- *Supports during transitions*—Infants often need increased support between caregiving activities and between sleep and wakeful periods;
- *Appropriate positioning*—Placing the infant in special positions for cares and rest enhances the infant's ability to seek comfort and encourages stability;
- *Individualized feeding support*—Both the method and schedule of feeding need to be based on each infant's individual needs and competencies, so that feeding is perceived as pleasurable;
- *Opportunities for skin-to-skin holding*—Kangaroo care (see Figure 1.3) encourages respiratory stability and more restful sleep for infants, which enhances critical brain development while helping parents feel less anxious and more fulfilled;
- *Collaborative care*—All exams, procedures, and tests should be planned with the infant's primary caregiver and parents present to provide comfort and lessen stress;

- *Quiet, soothing environment*—Measures like rocking chairs or recliners at the bedside for parents, homelike family spaces, and the ability to personalize the infant's bedside with family photos, soft music, clothing, and blankets help decrease family stress. Subtle lighting to reflect day/night sequencing and reduction of noise levels in special-care nurseries are also important to reduce potentially harmful stimuli; and

- *Developmental support*—The caregiving team should include developmental-care specialists as well as other disciplines to provide psychosocial care including social work, pastoral care, and child life. (Als & Gilkerson, 1995, pp. 5–6)

Research documenting the importance of developmental-care principles for newborn intensive care units has demonstrated that high-risk infants (e.g., very low birth weight, ventilated patients) have improved medical outcomes, including decreased intracranial hemorrhages, reduced severity of chronic lung disease, improved growth, and earlier discharge. Similar results are seen in healthy preterm infants, indicating that supporting and protecting the infant's developing nervous system improves brain functioning (Als et al., 1994). A 2015 study compared the two-year neurodevelopmental outcomes of 124 NICU graduates who received conventional care to those of 137 children who had received developmental care in the NICU. Children in the developmental-care group showed less psychomotor delay than did those in the conventional-care group (Kiechl-Kohlendorfer, Merkel, Neubauer, Peglow, & Griesmaier, 2015).

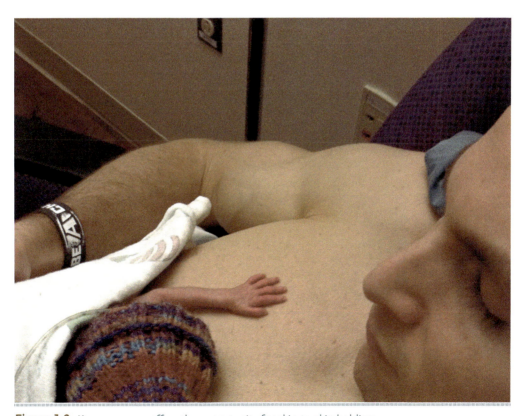

Figure 1.3. Kangaroo care offers the opportunity for skin-to-skin holding.

Support for NICU parents is equally important. To better understand the parents' experience and the role of staff, Smith, SteelFisher, Salhi, and Shen (2012) conducted interviews with 24 current or graduate NICU families. A qualitative analysis revealed five coping strategies parents used. See Table 1.1 for a list of the strategies and some of the ways staff supported them.

The March of Dimes has taken advantage of the availability of technology for support by providing March of Dimes NICU online resources (Gooding et al., 2011), where families can gain information and join online communities for NICU families. The organization also has a Share Your Story feature within the online community. Families with access to these resources consistently report higher satisfaction rates. In

Table 1.1

Parental Coping Strategies and Staff Support Interventions		
Parental Coping Styles	**Staff Support of Parental Coping Styles**	**Examples**
1. Participating in the care of their child	Facilitating participation of the parents with the infant's care	Providing informal and formalized training on providing care and opportunities to practice Providing a welcoming environment and specific encouragement to overcome anxieties about handling their child
2. Getting away from the NICU	Encouraging parents to take time away from the NICU	Emphasizing documentation of the infant's progress Demonstrating affection for the infant Addressing concerns that make parents hesitant to leave the NICU
3. Gathering information	Providing accurate, constant, clinical information	Answering and encouraging questions Recommending resources Limiting unscheduled nonemergency calls to home
4. Involvement of family and friends	Monitoring the impact of family/friends on parents	Serving as gatekeeper when needed Facilitating less intrusive visits by enforcing strict visiting rules with guests Providing information about website to provide standardized updates to friends and family, without having to interact individually
5. Engagement with other NICU parents	Arranging voluntarily activities or programs in which parents whose infants have similar medical conditions may interact	Facilitating coffee hours or scrapbooking sessions Arranging more structured relationships with graduate parents

Note. Adapted from "Coping with the Neonatal Intensive Care Unit Experience," by V. Smith, G. Steel-Fisher, C. Salhi, and L. Shen, 2012. *The Journal of Perinatal & Neonatal Nursing, 26*(4), pp. 346–350.

addition to making technology-based support available, the March of Dimes provides support staff for NICU families. The presence of a March of Dimes NICU Family Support staff member was demonstrated to ease the stress of NICU parents, who also reported higher parenting confidence (Gooding et al., 2011).

Another family-centered-care initiative is Creating Opportunities for Parent Empowerment (COPE), an evidence-based educational-behavioral program (Cope for Hope, 2015). COPE programs are available to parents who have children in the pediatric intensive care unit (PICU) or in the NICU. Results of a randomized, controlled trial with 260 families with preterm infants found that infants in the COPE program stayed an average of 3.8 fewer days in the NICU and 3.9 fewer days in total in the hospital than did comparison infants who did not have the intervention (Melnyk et al., 2006). Further, parents in units with a COPE program demonstrated greater satisfaction with and more confidence in their ability to care for a preterm infant, as well as less anxiety and fewer depression symptoms during and after their NICU stay, than parents who didn't participate in a COPE program. A more recent study confirmed previous findings regarding reduced hospital stay and also reported reduced readmission rates (Gonya, Martin, McClead, Nelin, & Shepherd, 2014). Dr. Robert White, a neonatologist, summarized his review of the NICU environment of care by saying, "We are now approaching a day when the best medical care and nurturing are not mutually exclusive concepts, and where the mother's arms are considered the optimal locus of care" (White, 2011).

Shared decision-making with informed parents able to participate in determining their infant's plan of care is an important tenet of family-centered care. New programs are emerging with a focus on prenatal care for high-risk pregnancies and babies diagnosed in utero with complex critical conditions or life-threatening anomalies. For most parents, ultrasounds are perceived as opportunities to learn the sex of their baby, while practitioners use them to assess fetal development. For one out of every 28 women, the ultrasound identifies a condition or concern that changes the entire focus of the pregnancy. The family members must now integrate the news, gather information, and discuss potential outcomes while mourning the loss of a normal pregnancy. Parents need high-level consultative care to understand available treatments and to be given realistic prognoses based on the baby's condition and information about the capabilities of neonatal development. Fetal Concerns Programs provide that level of critical support for families. Referrals to a higher-level center will provide parents with coordinated access to medical expertise in a setting that will support critical care. Parents will be offered the opportunity to meet with the neonatal team, surgeons, nurse practitioners, genetic counselors, social workers, lactation consultants, and any other health-care professionals who might interact with the family at the time of the birth. If the infant is diagnosed with a lethal condition, pregnancy choices may be supported, and if appropriate, a palliative birth plan may be determined (see Chapter 6: The Child Who is Dying). Family-centered-care principles include child life specialists if the family has children who are eagerly awaiting the birth of a little brother or sister. Tours of the hospital, including the NICU, are given, as the family may now be facing the delivery of the baby in a large birthing center far from the local hospital. Supportive family-centered care initiated during the pregnancy may then be continued throughout the birth, hospital stay, and beyond.

Older Infants: 6 Months to 1 Year

Many years later a mother recalls her child's first hospital admission:

> "I stood outside the door of the treatment room for what seemed like hours while they drew blood and started an IV. She never stopped screaming but no one would let me come in to comfort her."

The developmental needs of older infants continue to be based on the infant's ability to develop trust. Consistent, nurturing, and loving caregivers help the older infant become trusting. While the primary threat to this age group is separation anxiety (see next section), older infants are rapidly developing their own unique and engaging personalities. They control their environments and use emotional expressions such as crying and smiling to get their needs met. When these cues are missed and the infant is unable to elicit nurturing responses, a feeling of distress and decreased sense of control may increase the infant's stress levels. Additional distresses result from restriction of movement (e.g., arm or leg restraints, IVs, lab draws) and changes in rituals and routines. Maximizing parental presence and participation in cares provides the greatest protection for the older infant's successful developmental growth and minimizes the disruptive effects of hospitalization. Creating a homelike environment that includes family photos, comfort objects such as familiar blankets and stuffed animals, favorite quieting music, and opportunities for exploration and movement beyond that possible within the crib helps ensure ongoing learning for the older infant.

The primary source of stress for children from middle infancy through preschool age (ages 6 months through 3 years) is *separation anxiety*. Classic studies by Robertson (1958) and Bowlby (1960) described a series of three stages in a young child's response to separation. The initial stage, *protest*, is an active and aggressive response to the absence of the parent, and is characterized by crying, screaming, or kicking while constantly watching for signs of the parent's return. The child refuses the attention of anyone else, and seems inconsolable. The protest stage may last from several hours to as long as a week. In the next stage, *despair*, the child stops crying and appears depressed. Bowlby describes this stage as one of increasing hopelessness. The child may continue to cry intermittently but more often appears withdrawn and quiet. However, the return of the parent causes the child to once again cry vigorously. This behavior originally formed the basis for parent visiting policies in the 1950s and 1960s. The child's ability to bring his or her feelings of acute distress back to the surface was misinterpreted as "re-upsetting" the calm and complacent child who, in reality, had been in despair. The final stage, *detachment*, appears after a long period of parental absence and is characterized by the child's reinvestment in his or her surroundings and normal activity. The child copes with the pain of the parent's absence by forming superficial attachments to others, becoming increasingly self-centered, and becoming more interested in material objects (Bowlby, 1960). Although the child appears to be recovering, the parents' return is met with apathy and the child's inability to reattach. Detachment is the most serious stage, in that the adverse effects are less likely to be reversed. One of the positive outcomes of improvements in pediatric policies and increased family involvement in care is that the stage of detachment is seldom observed within the hospital setting. However, the first two stages—protest and despair—are more frequently observed, even with only brief separations from either parent.

Toddlers: 1 to 3 Years

The parent of a 22-month-old child recalls, "The part that frightened me most was when he came back from a procedure completely sedated, and a staff member commented on how 'peaceful' he looked lying there. That immediately made me think of a comment often heard at funerals. It was the defining moment of feeling so helpless when prior to that I had always been able to make things better for him. All I wanted was for him to wake up and say 'Momma.' I didn't appreciate the peacefulness of that moment. Toddlers aren't supposed to be peaceful!"

As infants grow into toddlers, hospitalization creates new challenges as developmental norms focus on increasing autonomy and goal-directed behaviors. While parental presence is still the greatest need, toddlers learn by moving, exploring, playing, and engaging in socializing activities. With limited verbal skills, egocentric toddlers make their needs known in demonstrative ways, often reacting with frustration to restrictions of movement or changes in routine. They may perceive the hospital as punishment, and if they experience pain for the first time, they may feel more confused when the parent does not rescue them from painful procedures. For this age group, the need to master experiences and gain autonomy is met through play. The presence of child life programming and opportunities to play at the bedside or in a playroom are crucial for the toddler, to ensure ongoing development (see Chapter 3: Play in Children's Health-Care Settings). While engaged in developmentally appropriate play activities, the toddler begins to master new experiences.

Often, the parents of long-stay patients miss these special moments because they cannot be at their child's bedside all day. A child life specialist at MedStar Georgetown University Hospital in Washington, DC, developed "While you were away," a project that documents a child's activities so that they can be shared with parents. The project promotes bonding (by giving the parents a positive, nonmedical thing to talk to their child about when they return) and memory-making. Children are given a poster for their room (with parental consent). Each day a child life specialist or nurse takes a photo of them playing or doing some sort of nonmedical activity. The photo is taped to the poster, along with a short description of what they were doing in the picture (see Figure 1.4). A camera, battery charger, and photo printer are kept at the nurses' station to make it easy for anyone to capture one of these moments (J. Uze, personal communication, February 19, 2016).

For toddlers, especially, it is very important to minimize the drastic differences between the hospital environment and the home environment. Activities of daily living and the home routines of bathing, eating, and playing should be respected as much as possible within the requirements of medical treatment. When toddlers experience severe restrictions and changes of routine, feelings of unpredictability and loss of control may cause them to regress to earlier, more secure developmental levels. Although this regression may appear to provide comfort to the toddler, giving up newly acquired skills is difficult and may make toddlers more susceptible to negative responses to hospitalization (Hockenberry & Wilson, 2014).

It is important to remember that because toddlers have not yet developed a sense of body image or boundaries, intrusive procedures may be highly stressful, regardless of whether the pain is actual or perceived. This age group is able to remember painful

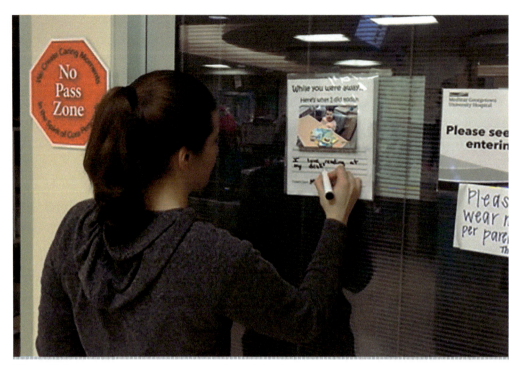

Figure 1.4. "While you were away, here's what I did today" shares moments parents might have missed.

procedures and may respond to similar tests and routines with physical resistance and uncooperativeness. Toddlers are often able to understand far more than they are able to express in words, and preparing toddlers for procedures is subsequently beneficial (see Chapter 2: Preparing Children for Health-Care Encounters). Parental participation in toddler interventions is important, both to provide security for the toddler during new experiences and to lessen a parent's anxiety by allowing the parent to engage in anticipatory coping. A prepared and less anxious parent will most likely result in a more cooperative and less frightened toddler.

Preschoolers: 4 to 5 Years

A 4-year-old bargains with the nurse, "Please don't give me a shot. I'll be good!"

Preschoolers are more secure than toddlers if they have had opportunities to develop trusting relationships through life experiences. Yet they are still very vulnerable to the stresses of hospitalization and medical care. In fact, Stanford and Thompson (1981) identified children ages 9 months through 4 years to be the most vulnerable to the negative effects of hospitalization. More independent than toddlers, preschoolers also suffer most from physical restrictions and loss of control. They may continue to view the hospital as punishment but now also engage in magical thinking: They believe that they have the ability to wish things to happen. For preschoolers, the reason for hospitalization, tests, and treatments must be concrete and hands-on. Using real equipment for preparation helps preschoolers understand and communicate. Again, play is the critical determinant for coping (see Chapter 3: Play in Children's Health-

Care Settings). Opportunities for medical play, preparation, and expressive play help the preschooler understand, as well as help adults detect a child's fears, concerns, or misconceptions. Perhaps the egocentric nature of the preschooler is most obvious when a medical person appears at the playroom door and every preschooler in the playroom responds with the certainty that he or she is the one the person is there for!

Preschoolers are particularly vulnerable to threats of bodily injury, as their concept of body integrity is not yet fully developed. Fears of mutilation are common, and their inability to understand body functioning limits their ability to understand the need to "fix" a body part through surgery. In addition, preschoolers' concept of the cause of illness is complicated by their inability to separate themselves from the external world. Therefore, they perceive that you get a cold if you go out in the cold. This understanding includes a sense of blame or responsibility, reinforcing the preschooler's feelings of having done something wrong to be deserving of punishment. Addressing these preschool misconceptions in play and preparation provides the child with increased coping skills and lessened anxiety, while enabling the child to gain support through distraction (see Chapter 2: Preparing Children for Health-Care Encounters).

Finally, in addressing the needs of the older infant, toddler, and preschool-age child, it is important to clearly establish *safe* places for children. Because the child's bed should be the ultimate "safe place," all invasive procedures should be done in a treatment room away from the child's bedside. If this need for safety isn't satisfied, a young child may not be able to sleep soundly, fearing that he or she will be approached at any moment for a painful procedure.

However, Fanurik et al. (2000) suggested that better guidelines for decisions related to the use of bedside versus treatment room need to take into account child-specific, procedural, and situational factors. In this study nurses were given a series of vignettes for children ages 3 years, 9 years, and 14 years who were scheduled for an intravenous insertion and a lumbar puncture and were surveyed about where they would want to perform each procedure. Nursing decisions considered the child's age, level of invasiveness of the procedure, child's coping skills, child's health condition, type of hospital room, child's developmental status, and parents' ability to assist their child. Although decision-making in some situations focused on medical issues, such as the stability of the patient to be moved, availability of equipment, and urgency of the procedure, other decisions revolved around psychosocial factors, such as whether moving the child to an unfamiliar space might heighten his or her anxiety level. The study did not consider levels of perceived or actual pain for the child, nor did the study attempt to define "invasiveness of procedures." Implications for this research indicate that parents and children need education about the advantages and disadvantages of each setting and should be active participants in deciding whether the bedside or treatment room should be used (Fanurik et al., 2000). They also prompt a greater awareness that what health-care professionals view as invasive or noninvasive may not be similarly defined by the child. When a decision is made to use a treatment room, the room should be designed to obscure the view of endless shelves of medical equipment and enhance coping through changes in lighting, music, or visual aids. The room should be large enough to accommodate not only the required medical staff performing the procedure but also the child's identified support person, whether that be a child life specialist or family member, or both.

The other truly safe place should be the playroom, where children can engage in play activities without the fear of intrusive examinations or procedural tasks being completed (see Chapter 3: Play in Children's Health-Care Settings). Considerations of a child's psychosocial safety need to be continually emphasized as each new group of students, residents, and staff members enters the pediatric environment.

The School-Age Child: 6 to 12 Years

They looked into my mouth and into my ears, they looked into my eyes and they touched my tummy. But they never looked at me.

—7-year-old hospitalized patient (Association for the Care of Children's Health, 1990, p. 19)

School-age children are less vulnerable to the anxieties of hospitalization because they have made many developmental achievements. They are more social, able to be separated from parents for longer periods of time, and capable of cognitive reasoning. In addition, they are able to form trusting relationships with other adults and peers (Stanford & Thompson, 1981). As concrete operational thinkers, they are able to process information and understand relationships between events and experiences.

Earlier research on school-age children's ability to tolerate parental separation was based primarily on adult recollections. Yet in later research that asked children themselves, hospitalized children ages 8 through 11 years rated "being away from my family" higher than any other fears associated with hospitalization (Hart & Bossert, 1994). This is attributed to the psychosocial challenge of hospitalization and a tendency toward regression, both of which increase the child's need to be with his or her family. Interventions to facilitate family contact are important, including easy access to phone or email, unlimited family visiting, and support services for families while they are at the hospital.

Other significant fears identified in this study included "having to stay a long time, getting a shot, having my finger stuck, and the doctor or nurse telling me something is wrong with me" (Hart & Bossert, 1994, p. 87). Anticipated responses that were not supported by research or identified by the children as stressful were concerns about missing school or fears that they might die. These results also support Erikson's stage of industry versus inferiority, and the importance of school-age children performing the normal routines and tasks of their age group. It becomes important for school-age children to know the implications of disease or treatment and hospitalization for the present and also the future, as they are able to reason and cognitively process events and consequences.

The abilities identified above help clearly define interventions to benefit the school-age child in the hospital. Activities of industry, including arts and crafts, creative writing or journaling, playing games, role-playing, socializing with other patients, and computer programming such as STARBRIGHT World, help children express feelings, master experiences by learning new skills, and cope with required procedures and treatments. Involvement in child life programming and hospital school programs is critical for school-age children because it normalizes the medical setting, provides structure and routine, and offers opportunities for peer-group interaction. Because changes in appearance and body function are also important to this age group, the hospital serves as a safe and sheltered place where children can practice new skills and gain competence and confidence with the physical changes that may result from illness or injury.

Pet therapy has been part of pediatric programming for several decades (see Figure 1.5). Generally it involves companion animals, most often dogs, visiting the hospital to brighten the spirits of hospitalized children and their families. When asked whether they like the visits, children respond positively (Goddard & Gilmer, 2015). A randomized controlled study is under way at five major pediatric hospitals to definitively study the effects of animal-assisted interventions for children with cancer (McCullough & Jenkins, 2015). Patients between the ages of 3 and 17 years in the experimental group have blood pressure and heart-rate checks before and after a 15-minute weekly visit with a therapy dog. Psychosocial and behavioral instruments are used after the visit to measure anxiety in the children and the dogs. Preliminary results show that children visited by the animals have more stable blood-pressure readings and heart rates than children in the control group, who receive standard treatment without pet therapy. Anxiety levels of both patients and parents were improved (McCullough & Jenkins, 2015). It is hoped that this groundbreaking study will increase access to therapy dogs in hospital environments, inform animal-assisted interventions best practices and standards in the context of serious pediatric illness, and improve well-being outcomes for children and families facing the challenges of cancer.

A final implication of the research of Hart and Bossert (1994) demonstrated no significant differences in the identified fears of chronically ill or acutely ill children, suggesting that prior experience or familiarity with the health-care system does not lessen children's fears. The authors attributed this finding to the fact that unknown fears are replaced by known fears. The need for preparation and supportive interventions seems to be just as great for chronically ill children who have been hospitalized before as for acutely ill children (Hart & Bossert, 1994).

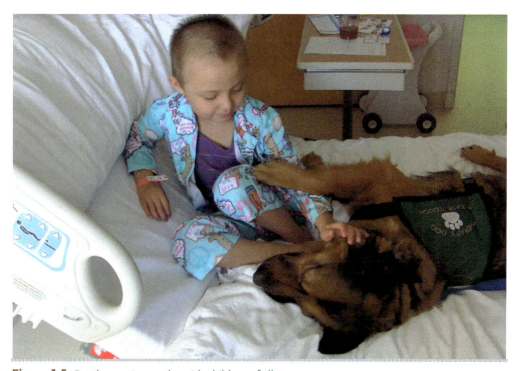

Figure 1.5. Pet therapy is popular with children of all ages.

Bossert (1994) also asked school-age children what stressful things happened to them in the hospital. From all the children's responses, interviewers identified six categories of events and examples of each as stated by the children, listed in descending order of frequency:

- *Intrusive events*—Injections, blood work, intravenous insertion, surgery, pills, nasogastric tubes, suppositories
- *Physical symptoms*—Pain, nausea, side effects of medications such as blurry vision, dizziness, burning of intravenous medication
- *Therapeutic interventions*—Physical exam by doctor, palpation of abdomen, waking after surgery, being woken up at night, dressing change, removal of stitches
- *Restricted activity*—Bed rest, holding still during X-rays, not allowed to leave unit, can't go outside
- *Separation*—Parents' leaving, missing friends or pets
- *Environment*—Cords and wires on walls that look like monsters at night, changing rooms, unpleasant or noisy roommates, impatient or "mad" doctors and nurses

In addition to the stressors they face in the hospital, preschool and school-age children, in particular, may face the challenge of homesickness. Thurber, Walton, and the Council on School Health (2007, p. 192) defined homesickness as "the distress and functional impairment caused by an actual or anticipated separation from home and attachment objects such as parents." However, according to a more recent definition that emphasizes a dual-process model—new locality adjustments as well as home-related losses—homesickness is "a 'mini-grief,' a negative emotional state primarily due to separation from home and attachment persons, characterized by longing for and preoccupation with home, and often with difficulties adjusting to the new place" (Stroebe, Schut, & Nauta, 2016, p. 350). Thus, "new place" stressors (e.g., illness, hospitalization, treatment), correlates, and consequences require a separate examination.

Thurber, Patterson, and Mount (2007) found that 88% of hospitalized children experienced some degree of homesickness, with 50% being mildly or moderately homesick. And 20% of children experienced severe homesickness with accompanying symptoms of acute depression and anxiety. Symptoms of homesickness include acute longing and preoccupying thoughts of home. One homesick child may act tearful and withdrawn, while another may be angry, irritable, or disoriented. Children with insecure attachment relationships with primary caregivers are at greater risk for homesickness. Perceived lack of control and negative attitudes about hospitalization increase the risk (Thurber, Patterson, et al., 2007). Significant differences define homesickness in the hospital and homesickness stemming from other separations that a child may experience, such as being at summer camp. Most often the child chooses or agrees to camp and is knowledgeable about the expected activities of camp, which are focused on a child's participation and enjoyment. The high anxiety levels of a child in the hospital, unexpected tests or procedures, and unfamiliar surroundings all contribute to greater severity of homesickness in the hospital setting.

Interestingly, Thurber (1999) suggested that the best way to handle homesickness is to ask children how homesick they have been feeling. This simple question helps normalize the feelings and give the child an opportunity to talk about such feelings (Thurber, Walton, et al., 2007), and it enables caregivers to begin teaching effective coping behaviors. Engaging children in enjoyable activities at the hospital is one of the most helpful coping strategies because it distracts children from thoughts of home and what they are missing. Involving children with the hospital environment in ways that enhance their commitment to it can help relieve homesickness (Rollins, 2010). For example, helping plan a holiday party or decorating the unit can provide a sense of ownership and serve to examine and address "new place" stressors in a positive way.

Parents and caregivers can apply three broad principles to help minimize the child's homesickness—providing information (see Chapter 2: Preparing Children for Health-Care Encounters), positive modeling, and coping-skills training—all of which increase a child's sense of confidence and often that of the whole family. If parents introduce the hospital experience with a positive attitude from the initial mention of the necessity of hospitalization, the child will cope in more positive ways and be at less risk for severe homesickness (Thurber, Patterson, et al. 2007).

Adolescents

If you get sick and are suddenly thrown into a situation where strange people are poking at you, asking personal questions, sticking needles into your arms, and telling you why they want to put a plastic tube into your chest, it's really overwhelming.

—Elizabeth Bonwich, age 16 (Krementz, 1989, p. 68)

Erikson conceived of the adolescent developmental stage as "identity versus role confusion," and therein lies the key to working with the hospitalized adolescent. Naturally seeking to separate from parents and family, teenagers develop a heightened dependence on peers and social groups. The hospital experience becomes threatening because it separates the teen from normal group activities, disrupts future plans, and increases insecurities about appearance and self-worth. The period of mid-adolescence, ages 14 to 18 years, is described as the most difficult time for an adolescent to be hospitalized. It is during this time when the peer group is especially important to developing self-image and independence, and doubts about sexual functioning are of greatest concern.

In addition to resulting in a loss of social support, hospitalization and illness frequently result in loss of independence and control, and adolescents may respond with feelings of anger and frustration. In general, younger adolescents are less vulnerable to these inherent risks because they have yet to develop strong emancipatory drives and more easily handle the increased dependency precipitated by the hospital experience (Stanford & Thompson, 1981). Similarly, older adolescents, having attained a confident level of independence, develop improved parent relationships and may approach the stresses of hospitalization with adult-like coping skills (Hoffman, Becker, & Gabriel, 1976).

Interventions for adolescents should focus on peer-group support. An adolescent unit that features an environment and policies specifically designed for adolescents will increase both coping and cooperation. Access to age-appropriate activities, such as video games, movies, cooking, a pool table, music, and computers, should be a feature of a teen room with programming designed exclusively for teens. Because caring for children and their families is the sole mission of children's hospitals, claiming space for such a room or even a separate ward for adolescents typically is not an issue. However, for pediatric units in a general hospital, designating a separate room for this purpose may be challenging and perhaps not a priority for hospital decision makers. Nevertheless, with an awareness of the importance of such space for meeting teenagers' psychosocial needs, health-care professionals have been very creative in capturing bits of space, for example, claiming a small seating area at the end of a corridor for teens to gather. Others have designated an area of the hospital playroom for teens only, and refer to the playroom as an "activity room" to label the space as appropriate for all ages.

Liberal visiting policies and opportunities for peer socialization require guidelines that are different from other areas of the hospital. Staff members who understand and enjoy adolescents and who possess appropriate communication skills also have a positive effect on the coping of an adolescent. Information and preparation will lessen teen fears and anxiety while enhancing anticipatory coping. The ability to listen to adolescent concerns, answer questions, and enhance decision-making should be an integral part of developmentally appropriate care.

Being in isolation is difficult for a child of any age, but it becomes especially difficult during adolescence, when peer relationships are often a central focus of everyday life and activity. According to Hart and Rollins (2011), infants under 6 months of age typically are unable to distinguish isolation from normal life and quickly adapt, as long as their physical and emotional needs are met. Separation anxiety becomes a major factor for children at ages 6 to 18 months; they become upset when parents and significant others leave the room or bedside. Toddlers have difficulty understanding the reason for isolation and can become frustrated when their sensorimotor exploration is limited. Preschoolers might feel guilty, believing isolation is punishment for something they did, and regress and become restless. School-age children are concerned over loss of control. Initially they may be angry and hostile, but later they usually exhibit one of three behavior patterns: responsibly independent, passively dependent, or manipulative. Adolescents in isolation initially might act out, regress, and display anger, denial, and hostility, while later they might respond with boredom and apathy.

Attention to privacy and confidentiality is also essential in order for adolescents to feel trusting and able to participate in their own treatment planning. Respecting wishes and honoring confidences are essential principles for building trust and acceptance. Ensuring a teen's privacy during personal cares and treatments is often an ongoing struggle within a large teaching hospital. Members of the psychosocial team may need to intervene to help adolescents feel assured that their needs will be met. Because of an adolescent's preoccupation with appearances, it may also be necessary to convey the value of personal-care needs to medical personnel. One adolescent girl remembers little about her critical illness and ICU stay except for the day when she was helped to have her hair washed! Simple touches like replacing the blankets to cover a teen after an examination may make a significant difference to an adolescent.

Hutton (2010) studied adolescents' use of ward space, looking at the ways teens created uniquely personal spaces by their arrangement of personal effects. Teens created bedside spaces that expressed their own personalities in different ways. The personal spaces provided the teens with a sense of control amidst ward rules and routines and offered an area for privacy and comfort within the social setting of a busy adolescent unit.

A relatively new concept in caring for adolescents is the establishment of a teen advisory council or committee (TAC). Initially introduced as a way to include adolescents in hospital design planning or other proposed programming, such as menu choices or teen lounge activities, the TAC proved to be a far more powerful tool for both hospitalized adolescents and staff. Given the increase in the number of adolescents with chronic illness who are living to adulthood, there is a need to involve adolescents in their illness management. Having a TAC is one way to encourage teens to meet the developmental milestones of adolescence while they learn to take greater responsibility for managing their chronic illness. Boston Children's Hospital's Teen Advisory Committee was developed after a monthly event called Teen Time proved to be highly successful (Rich, Goncalves, Guardiani, O'Donnell, & Strezelski, 2014). The group now meets monthly and includes teens and young adults with chronic illness and siblings of teens with chronic illness, all working with a multidisciplinary staff. The group has a powerful voice within the hospital and is respected and recognized by administrators. The teens working in this multidisciplinary environment began to participate more in their own care, while developing a sense of empowerment that extended beyond the hospital into their personal lives and communities (Rich et al., 2014). Ultimately the focus changed from deficits and negativity to strengths and positivity. For more about the outcomes associated with the TAC, see Table 1.2, Teen Advisory Committee: Lessons Learned.

Pediatric Intensive Care

More than 210,00 children are admitted to PICUs in North America each year (Rennick et al., 2014). Critically ill children are exposed to extreme stressors, including (a) highly invasive procedures, (b) separation from families, (c) other critically ill and dying children, (d) altered levels of consciousness, (e) elevations in light and noise levels, and (f) multiple strangers providing sophisticated caretaking procedures.

The traditional belief is that children cared for in intensive care units will have more troublesome responses than will children cared for in general pediatric wards. However, research indicates that this might not always be the case. Rennick, Johnston, Dougherty, Platt, and Ritchie (2002) compared the psychological responses of children hospitalized in a pediatric intensive care unit with those hospitalized in a general ward to identify clinically relevant factors that might be associated with psychological outcome. The researchers followed 120 children for 6 months after they were discharged from PICUs and general wards. The researchers compared groups of children based on their sense of control over their health, medical fears, post-traumatic stress, and changes in behavior, and examined relationships between children's responses and their age, the invasive procedures to which they were exposed, severity of illness, and length of hospital stay. As anticipated, the children in the PICU spent more time in the hospital. However, because children admitted to hospital wards today are much sicker than those who were hospitalized a decade ago, Rennick et al. found that the children in the general wards received just as many invasive procedures as did the children in the PICU. The primary difference was that the children in the PICU received more pain

Table 1.2

Teen Advisory Committee: Lessons Learned

Lessons Learned by Facilitators	Lessons Learned by Adolescents	Lessons Learned by Hospital Community
• Adolescents can effectively take the lead on setting and maintaining boundaries. • Structured recruitment, application, and interview processes are necessary. • One-to-one meetings between a confidential facilitator and teens are important to promote relationship building and elicit feedback about the committee. • Staff facilitators must be cognizant at all times of adolescents' developmental stage and the status of their chronic illness. • Structured routine promote predictability and cohesiveness. • Including healthy adolescent siblings enriches and deepens the group experience. • Short-term projects work best. • Multidisciplinary staff facilitators enhance discussion and promote TAC success. • Preparing hospital staff members who wish to meet with the committee is essential.	• Empowering teens to influence change promotes a greater sense of responsibility and increases their confidence. • Teens nurture and acquire qualities that exemplify the attributes of a strong, supportive leader and a responsible human being: • Punctuality and communication skills • Leadership and public-speaking skills • Teamwork skills • Advocacy and role-modeling skills • Service to the community • Compassion and empathy for others	• TAC represents the voice of all teens at the hospital. • Teens have the capacity to advise staff and providers. • Teens can function as advocates for their own needs. • TAC provides a forum for the teens' concerns to be addressed on a hospital-wide basis. • Adolescents embrace opportunities to partner and collaborate with hospital staff. • Adolescents have a strong desire to "give back" to their providers and hospital community.

Note. From "Teen Advisory Committee: Lessons Learned by Adolescents, Facilitators, and Hospital Staff," by C. Rich, A. Goncalves, M. Guardiani, E. O'Donnell, and J. Strzelecki, 2014. *Pediatric Nursing, 40*(4), p.290. Reprinted with permission of the publisher, Jannetti Publications, Inc., East Holly Avenue/Box 56, Pitman, NJ 08071-0056; (856) 256-2300; FAX (856) 589-7463; Website: www.pediatricnursing.net. For a sample copy of the journal, please contact the publisher.

medication and sedation than did the children in the general wards. The researchers found no significant differences between the groups but concluded that younger children, more severely ill children, and those who had endured more invasive procedures had significantly more medical fears, a lower sense of control over their health, and ongoing post-traumatic stress responses 6 months after discharge.

Nevertheless, research indicates that approximately 25% of children demonstrate negative psychological and behavioral responses within the first year after discharge (Colville, Kerry, & Pierce, 2008; Rennick & Rashotte, 2009). Reported responses include the following:

- Decreases in self-esteem and emotional well-being,
- Increased anxiety,
- Negative behavioral changes (e.g., sleep disturbances, social isolation),
- Delusional memories and hallucinations,
- Increased medical fears,
- Changes in friendships, and
- Psychological disorders (e.g., posttraumatic-stress disorder, major depression).

Because of continued advances in technology and surgical techniques, the composition of the PICU population has been altered such that the majority of children are now less than 6 years of age (Rennick et al., 2014). Rennick and colleagues point out that younger children remain largely excluded from psychological-outcome studies, which raises important concerns about the psychological impact of critical illness on this group of the PICU population. Young children may be excluded because they are more difficult to assess and because of a lack of instrument validation with this age group. It will be interesting to see the results of a study that is under way to assess emotional and behavioral responses following a PICU stay or ENT day surgery in children as young as 3 years, using developmentally appropriate measures (Rennick et al., 2014).

One study looked at the reactions of parents of children who had been in the PICU. Using a time frame of 8 months after discharge from the PICU, researchers interviewed parents to assess their retrospective reflections on their psychological reactions at the time of admission (Colville et al., 2009). Parents' reports focused on four themes: vivid memories of the PICU, staff communication, transitions, and the long-term impact of the experience. Memories recounted by the parents were vivid, for example, their first impressions of seeing their child in the PICU, especially the child's appearance, including machines, lines, and monitors, but also the child's physical appearance. Emotions of fear, disorientation, horror, and impotence were reported, as well as those of gratitude and relief. Some recalled the constant awareness of death, whether for their child or another child nearby (Colville et al., 2009). Parents had generally favorable reports of staff communications and interactions but observed that individual staff members had different styles of communication. Parents most appreciated the qualities of openness, patience, and approachability among staff. The transition out of the PICU and into a general ward was filled with anxiety, as the level of care decreased and parents often felt less supported. While admitting that they remained anxious about their sick child, most parents reported that the experience was positive and made them closer as a family.

Vulnerable Children

Some children, regardless of age or developmental level, have been described as psychologically vulnerable (Petrillo & Azarnoff, 1997). Despite the advances made in meeting the unique needs of children through child life, play, preparation, and family presence, these vulnerable children require individualized approaches to meet their needs. This vulnerable group may include young children and previously hospitalized children who may have misconceptions or overwhelming fears about past hospitalizations and treatments. Another subset of vulnerable children, children with emotional disturbances, tends to distort perceptions about illness or injury. Parent–child reactions may also have a role in the maladaptive behaviors of some children, especially if a parent exhibits extreme anxiety requiring the intervention of an impartial professional to correct misinformation and reduce levels of fear. Another group of especially vulnerable children includes those who have a sensory impairment, are neurologically compromised, or have developmental delays. For these children, the usual methods of preparation and coping through play or expressive arts may not be as effective, and a more individualized approach must be adapted to each child's abilities (Petrillo & Azarnoff, 1997).

One group of vulnerable children that has gained much attention in the past 10 years is children diagnosed with autism spectrum disorder (ASD). According to the Centers for Disease Control and Prevention (CDC), 1 in every 68 children is identified with ASD. That number represents a 30% increase from 2008 and a 120% increase from 2002 (CDC, 2014). Reasons for the increase in children diagnosed with ASD haven't been fully determined, but researchers believe that the greater numbers may be related to methods of identification and diagnosis and services available in communities. With the average age at diagnosis at 4.5 years, these uniquely vulnerable children will challenge the health-care system to provide sensitive and supportive family-centered care in a highly stressful medical environment (Mueller, 2015). (See Case Study.) Children with ASD are more likely to use health-care services and may have comorbidities. They are also generally hospitalized longer than other children (Lokhandwala et al., 2012). Health-care professionals are challenged to develop programming to meet the particular needs and behavioral responses of children with ASD by adapting patient routines, procedures, and policies. Assessing and recording the critical information about the child on a form (see Figure 1.6), placing it inside the child's room and medical record, and exchanging the information from shift to shift may improve the safety of hospital personnel and decrease the child and family's anxiety levels (Jolly, 2015).

Resilient Children

Despite the various risks posed by health-care experiences for many children, it is possible, as stated earlier, for some children to adapt to the experience without negative psychosocial sequelae. These children may be labeled as *resilient*. Resiliency is defined as the ability to return rapidly to a previous psychological or physiological state (Rutter, 1987). Resilient children tend to respond more quickly and appropriately to major life events, such as divorce or hospitalization, and to adapt more positively to chronic and ongoing stresses. They may cope better with the isolation and immobility required

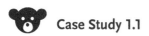 **Case Study 1.1**

A Child With Autism and His Hospital Experience

JJ, a green-eyed, blond-haired, freckle-faced 7-year-old nonverbal boy with autism, needed to be admitted to the inpatient unit for colonic washes secondary to prolonged constipation. He walked into the unit holding his mother's hand but upon arrival became agitated and stopped, looked down, and then started alternately flapping his arms and chewing on his finger. Unit hospital personnel had been informed that a child with autism was being admitted and were waiting near the entrance. Multiple staff members approached the boy all at once, talking to him, calling his name, and leaning down to try to make eye contact and direct him toward his room. When he did not respond, one staff member took his shoulders and tried to gently guide him toward the room. This caused JJ to scream loudly, shrug away from those near him, and start swinging his arms wildly. He ended up grazing one of the staff members in the face with his hand.

During this encounter, JJ's mom had been standing at his side telling the staff to please back up and not touch him. However, security was called. Once security personnel arrived, the hospital personnel and security agents decided to physically carry JJ to his room with his mom close behind them and then shut the door. JJ began banging his head on the door. His mother approached JJ in his room but appeared very distraught and was unable to comfort him. A physician was called and after confirming with JJ's mother that he had no allergies, ordered a stat dose of risperidone. Three staff members held JJ down and administered the dose of IM risperidone. JJ calmed down enough to lie on the bed, and the admission to the hospital was able to continue.

JJ remained agitated throughout the day after his initial introduction to the hospital. He continued to bite his fingers, grind his teeth, and arm-flap, and attempted to hit anyone who approached him. However, the multidisciplinary team caring for JJ contacted the autism specialist within the facility who was able to assist with the formulation of a care plan and recommended initiating medical treatment for constipation the following day. While consulting with JJ's mother, the team developed a daily picture schedule for JJ that included his normal home routine and incorporated the treatments needed during his stay. Based on recommendations from JJ's mom, the Child Life Specialist created a reward chart for JJ to help with medication compliance. She also located a game system and other activities that JJ enjoyed and could complete in his room. The nurse present on the day of admission agreed to care for JJ the next two days, the nursing management team was able to decrease the patient load to 2:1, and both the nurse and management team worked with JJ and his mom to make them as comfortable as possible. The nurse also wrote down the tips she learned from JJ's mom and passed the information on to the next shift. Although JJ had a traumatic introduction to the hospital setting, he was successfully treated and discharged after three days.

Note. From "Handle with Care: Top Ten Tips a Nurse Should Know Before Caring for a Hospitalized Child with Autism Spectrum Disorder" by A. Jolly, 2015. *Pediatric Nursing, 41*(1), pp. 11, 15. Reprinted with permission of the publisher, Jannetti Publications, Inc., East Holly Avenue/Box 56, Pitman, NJ 08071-0056; (856) 256-2300; FAX (856) 589-7463; Website: www.pediatricnursing.net. For a sample copy of the journal, please contact the publisher.

1. What causes this child to have increased anxiety? Please list common triggers.

2. What is the best method to communicate with this child?

   a. Verbal, picture, sign language, other _____

   b. Are there any special communication tools (ex: spell board) that we can obtain during your child's stay?

3. How should staff members approach the child?

4. Is the child particularly sensitive to touch, sound, smell, sight, or taste?

5. Does this child have any obsessive/restrictive behaviors?

6. How does the child demonstrate if he or she is in pain?

7. What are the child's early signs of increasing frustration and anxiety?

8. What are the best methods to comfort and de-escalate the child?

9. What are your child's strengths?

10. What is the child's home routine? We welcome you to bring in clothes, belongings, and food from home to make the child more comfortable. Please feel free to stay!

Figure 1.6. Admission assessment tool for the child with ASD.

Note. From "Handle with Care: Top Ten Tips a Nurse Should Know Before Caring for a Hospitalized Child with Autism Spectrum Disorder" by A. Jolly, 2015. *Pediatric Nursing, 41*(1), p. 15. Reprinted with permission of the publisher, Jannetti Publications, Inc., East Holly Avenue/Box 56, Pitman, NJ 08071-0056; (856) 256-2300; FAX (856) 589-7463; Website: www.pediatricnursing.net. For a sample copy of the journal, please contact the publisher.

during treatment for limited periods of time if they are able to rely on their strengths and ability to develop supportive relationships.

Protective factors that encourage resiliency in children focus on involvement in action and the ability to give directions. A resilient school-age boy who was hospitalized for many months with severe burns coped by insisting not only on removing his own dressings before each whirlpool treatment but also on doing it at his own pace. This method seemed agonizingly slow, and frustrated all the therapists, who wished to accomplish the undesirable task as quickly as possible. Yet, for the patient, it was critical to his ability to adapt to the experience and maintain some measure of control. Bolig and Weddle (1988) identified the following additional psychosocial principles that support resiliency:

1. Relating a child's actions to reactions or outcomes (e.g., "When you relax your arm, your IV runs smoothly").

2. Providing social reinforcement after, instead of before, the performance of a task.

3. Rewarding degrees of effort (e.g., how hard a child works rather than how successful he or she may be at that work, such as holding still for an IV start).
4. Encouraging extraordinary effort and tasks even under stress.
5. Modeling both the expression of feelings and self-talk.
6. Training new skills and practicing old behaviors.

Children may become more resilient if they are helped to perceive experiences constructively, are supported with policies that lessen separation from family members, and are encouraged to express their feelings (Bolig & Weddle, 1988). A summary of problems resulting from hospitalization for children of all ages and developmental stages and suggested interventions to help in coping is found in Table 1.3.

Family Reactions

The hospitalization of a child creates stress for the entire family. How a family handles the stress varies greatly depending on the family's coping abilities, past experience with an ill child and the circumstances of the hospitalization caused by the illness or injury, and whether the illness is acute or chronic.

Parents

Bossert and Hart (1999) list the sources of stress for parents during a child's acute illness:

- Child's illness
  - Diagnosis
  - Decisions about management of illness including consents for painful treatment for procedures
  - Perceived severity of the illness
- Hospital environment
  - Unfamiliar equipment, routines, policies
  - Uncertainty about parental roles and participation in cares
  - Unknown expectations of parents by staff
  - Personnel roles, number of caregivers
- Type of admission
  - Expected—with time for planning
  - Unexpected—from clinic with need to change family routines quickly
  - Emergency—most stressful because of suddenness of illness or injury
- Length of stay
- Changes in child's behavior
  - Loss of developmental milestones
  - Changes in child's emotional responses

(text continues on p. 28)

Table 1.3

Understanding Children Who Are Hospitalized: A Developmental Perspective

Age Group	Erikson	Piaget	Hospitalization-Related Issues	Possible Troublesome Responses	Interventions
Infant (0–1 years)	Trust vs. Mistrust • To get • To give in return	Sensorimotor • Exploration of physical self and environment • Object constancy • Cause and effect	Separation Lack of stimulation Pain	Failure to bond Distrust Anxiety Delayed skills development	Maximize parental involvement Maximize parental information Provide stimulation • Visual • Auditory • Tactile • Kinesthetic • Vestibular
Toddler (1–3 years)	Autonomy vs. Shame and Doubt • To hold on • To let go	Sensorimotor Preoperational (preconceptual phase) • Can hold and recall images • Increasing use of symbolization • Highly egocentric perception of world	Separation Fear of bodily injury and pain Frightening fantasies Immobility or restriction Forced regression Loss of routine and rituals	Regression (including loss of newly learned skills) Uncooperativeness Protest (verbal and physical) Despair Negativism Temper tantrums Resistance	Maximize parental involvement Maximize parental information Facilitate medical play Promote therapeutic play • Environmental exploration • Freedom within limits • Routine and ritual • Self-expression • Movement activities • Sensory stimulation games
Preschooler (3–6 years)	Initiative vs. Guilt • To make (going after) • To "make like" (playing)	Preoperational (preconceptual phase) Preoperational (intuitive phase) • Transition period between—depending solely on perception, and depending on truly logical thinking • Better able to see more than one factor at a time that influences an event	Separation Fear of loss of control, sense of own power Fear of bodily mutilation or penetration by surgery or injections, castration	Regression Anger toward primary caregiver Acting out Protest (less aggressive than toddler) Despair and detachment Physical and verbal aggression Dependency Withdrawal	Maximize parental involvement Maximize parental information Facilitate medical play Promote therapeutic play • Environmental exploration • Freedom within limits • Routine and ritual • Self-expression • Movement activities • Sensory stimulation games

(continues)

Table 1.3 *(continued)*

Age Group	Erikson	Piaget	Hospitalization-Related Issues	Possible Troublesome Responses	Interventions
School-ager (6–12 years)	Industry vs. Inferiority • To make things (completing) • To make things together	Concrete operations • Increasing ability to think logically in the physically concrete realm • Understands the meaning of series of actions, of order and sequencing	Separation Fear of loss of control Fear of loss of mastery Fear of bodily mutilation Fear of bodily injury and pain, especially intrusive procedures in genital area Fear of illness itself, disability, and death	Regression Inability to complete some tasks Uncooperativeness Withdrawal Depression Displaced anger and hostility Frustration	Maximize parental involvement Maximize parental information Encourage education and teacher involvement Facilitate medical play and information Promote therapeutic play • Skill building • Meaningful projects • Group activities • Peer support • Freedom within limits • Self-expression
Adolescent (12–18 years)	Identity and Repudiation vs. Identity Diffusion • To be oneself (or not to be) • To share being oneself	Formal operations • Deductive and abstract reasoning • Can imagine the conditions of a problem—past, present, and future—and develop hypotheses about what might logically occur under different combinations of factors	Dependence on adults Separation from family and peers Fear of bodily injury and pain Fear of loss of identity Body image and sexuality Concern about peer group status after hospitalization	Uncooperativeness Withdrawal Anxiety Depression	Encourage peer group activities Provide privacy Respect independence (choices) Encourage self-expression Address body image, sexual image, and future concerns Facilitate medical preparation Encourage education and teacher involvement Facilitate visits with peers

Note. From *From Artist to Artist-in-Residence: Preparing Artists to Work in Pediatric Healthcare Settings* (2nd ed.) (p. 24), by J. Rollins and C. Mahan, 2010, Washington, DC: Rollins & Associates. Copyright 1996 by Rollins & Associates. Reprinted with permission.

- Physical changes resulting from illness or injury including pain, altered appearance, ability to communicate, loss of mobility or strength
- Changes in routines of daily family life especially rooming in, child care arrangements, and work responsibilities (pp. 157–158)

Parents may have feelings of guilt about their role in the need for their child's hospitalization, perhaps questioning their timeliness in seeking medical care. They worry about and fear the outcome and may feel anger about the circumstances or generalized burden of the hospitalization and its impact on the whole family. If a child has been very ill at home, a parent may also feel some measure of relief that the child will now be hospitalized. Nearly all parents share a generalized feeling of anxiety.

Bossert and Hart (1999) identified a series of priorities that families use to cope with the disruption in family routine caused by hospitalization. These priorities, in order of importance, are as follows:

1. *Needs of the hospitalized child.* Most parents believe that they should be with the child as much as possible, and mothers generally spend more time in hospital than fathers. As the child's condition improves, less time may be spent at the bedside.

2. *Needs of the siblings.* Caring for the siblings at home is an area that most parents will accept outside help to manage.

3. *Work responsibilities.* Again, mothers usually take more time off from work than fathers do, and her work seems to take a lower priority than his.

4. *Home responsibilities.* Other caretakers or older siblings may help with essential tasks like preparing meals, while other home tasks may be ignored. Whether a parent rooms-in or visits, a parent's personal needs for exercise, socialization, and time with spouse may all be difficult. (p. 159).

A new understanding of the needs of the hospitalized child and the integration of family-centered care has resulted in a change of expectations for parents. Whereas, previously, parents relinquished most measures of control of their child, now they are expected to remain with their child and participate in cares (Darbyshire, 1994). Today, with all parents working in more than six out of 10 households with children (The Council of Economic Advisers, 2014), grandparents frequently help out by staying at the hospital with their grandchild during parents' working hours. (See more about grandparents in Chapter 7: Families in Children's Health-Care Settings.)

Parental presence has altered the perceived and identified needs of parents when a child is hospitalized. Parents overwhelmingly identify the need for information as critical to their coping. Not only do parents need information but they also need to receive it in understandable language and to have the opportunity to ask questions for clarification. Having this need for information filled helps a parent feel in control of what is happening in the hospital (Hallstrom, Runesson, & Elander, 2002). Parents also report that contributing their input makes them feel recognized as competent partners in the care of their child. At the same time, parents also feel vulnerable to the medical staff's moods and temperaments and may be reluctant to express frustration or criticism, fearing that it might affect their child's care.

Bossert and Hart (1999) also describe phases in parents' coping. In the initial phase of illness, parents may be passive and acquiesce to professionals' recommendations. Next, parents may enter a phase of information seeking wherein they gather information from many different professionals, analyze literature, and develop a personal understanding of the diagnosis and of management of the illness. As parents become more comfortable with the environment and information, they often become strong advocates for their child's treatment, reaffirming their roles as parents who best know their child's needs and responses.

In a study of stress appraisal and coping in 35 mothers of NICU infants, Reichman, Miller, Gordon, and Hendricks-Munoz (2000) found that 60% of the participants presented with clinically significant levels of distress and that 58% of the variance in distress could be explained by four variables. Increased distress was associated with the appraisal of uncontrollability, confrontive coping, and escape-avoidant coping. Decreased distress was associated with the coping strategy of accepting responsibility. Mothers who had greater satisfaction with their child's physician claimed to feel greater control over the situation and to function better. The authors concluded that it would be helpful if basic cognitive–behavioral strategies for anxiety reduction were taught to staff, family, and friends, and that a supportive NICU environment is essential.

Ward (2001) identified the need for parental assurance that their child was receiving the best possible care. This study of parents during their first week in the NICU acknowledged that parents frequently identified feelings of shock, anticipation, and uncertainty about the outcome for their infant. An interesting finding of the study was that fathers and mothers differed significantly in the ranking of needs. Fathers ranked assurance and information as less important than did mothers. During the first week of hospitalization, both fathers and mothers placed support needs as least important. (The author noted that the research was conducted in a setting where parent support groups were not available.)

Siblings

Although much attention is focused on the child who is the patient and on the parents' needs, brothers and sisters are also affected by a sibling's hospitalization. Siblings of a hospitalized child may experience a wide range of feelings and concerns and be forced to identify and deal with these concerns in the absence of a parent who is either physically or emotionally unavailable.

Parents may underestimate the stress that siblings feel until behavioral or physiological symptoms are noted. These may include changes in eating or sleeping patterns; the inability to concentrate in school; acting nervous, withdrawn, or angry; physically acting out with siblings or friends; and being reluctant to be away from parents. Craft (1993) identified the child's age and developmental level, the nature of the threat, the sibling–ill child relationship, the nature of the changes, the family's socioeconomic status, and available assistance and support as factors influencing sibling responses to hospitalization.

Child's Age and Developmental Level

A sibling's ability to understand and cognitively perceive events may cause children under the age of 7 years to be the most vulnerable (Craft, 1993). In a study by Knafl and Dixon (1983), the most negative reactions of siblings occurred between the ages of 4 and 11 years. The nature of the illness itself is concerning to siblings, who may worry about the outcome, fearing that their brother or sister might die. Young siblings may experience guilt, imagining that they caused the illness or injury. They may also worry about developing the same illness or injury. In one research study (Craft, 1986), 50% of siblings were fearful of getting the same illness as the hospitalized child. In addition, younger children are more vulnerable to separation from parents because of their poorly developed concept of time. Older siblings may feel guilty if a contagious illness or intentional injury is the reason for hospitalization, and they may have a perceived or actual belief that their actions had a role in the cause of the illness or injury. Older siblings also may experience more feelings of anxiety as they become increasingly able to conceptualize the impact of future outcomes. They may feel anger toward the ill sibling or toward the parents for placing more responsibilities on the older sibling at home, either in caring for other siblings or performing household tasks (Bossert & Hart, 1999).

Nature of the Threat

A sudden acute and life-threatening illness or injury creates more stress for siblings. Time elapsed since diagnosis is also a factor, as stress levels for siblings are higher with a new diagnosis of progressive illness as opposed to a previously diagnosed condition (Craft, 1993).

School-age children 8 to 12 years old whose siblings had experienced a traumatic injury in the past three months and required inpatient rehabilitation reported changes in the relationship with their sibling. This change involved realizing a closer, improved relationship with the sibling and, contrary to their normal sibling rivalry, recognizing their love for each other (Bugel, 2014). One sibling was quoted as saying, "And now that the accident happened, everything is different. We have to take care of one another. And stop fighting with one another" (Bugel, 2014, p. 182). Other changes noted by these siblings included increased involvement of other caring adults and changes in daily routines. Noteworthy to health-care professionals, siblings frequently felt left out while at the hospital and desired better communication and more information. Siblings stated a strong need for recognition and validation of their identity, and confirmation of their own importance as part of the family experience (Bugel, 2014).

Sibling–Ill Child Relationship

Siblings who have a close relationship with the hospitalized child report greater stress than those whose sibling relationships are not perceived as close. A sibling's perception of the relationship with an ill or injured brother or sister may also affect the associated feelings of guilt, anger, or anxiety. These feelings are common when a new baby is born and requires hospitalization, changing the family structure and function and the roles of other children in the family.

Nature of the Changes

Physical separation from parents and the ill sibling is a major source of stress for well siblings. They may feel physically or emotionally abandoned, interpreting these events as a loss of love, or they may feel they are being punished. The effects of separation, wespecially in younger children, may be similar to the separation anxiety described earlier in reference to the hospitalized child. In addition, changes in caregivers and routines may be difficult for well children, especially if they are cared for outside the security of their own home. Often, substitute caregivers may have different parenting styles and expectations for siblings.

Family Socioeconomic Status

Family income generally has an impact on the availability of resources and supports, an important variable for siblings. The negative effects of parental separation may be lessened if both parents are available to share the responsibilities for the ill child as well as the healthy siblings. The mother's education level and occupation also have been demonstrated to lessen siblings' anxiety (Craft, 1993). It is speculated that with more education may come an increased sensitivity to the effects of hospitalization on siblings and a greater sense of responsibility to provide support and information.

Assistance and Support

Many studies have documented the importance of including siblings in the experience of hospitalization. Siblings who are supported with developmentally appropriate explanations of the causes of illness or injury, participate by being present with the ill brother or sister, and are provided with opportunities to express their feelings demonstrate fewer adverse responses. The responsibility for supporting siblings during the hospital experience should be shared by parents and the health-care team. Perhaps the professional with the greatest ability to support siblings is the child life specialist, who possesses not only the knowledge and ability to explain causative factors in developmentally appropriate language to children but also a wealth of resources to engage siblings in expressing feelings and concerns. The ability to visit is critical, especially for younger children who have not yet reached the developmental stage of being able to think abstractly or process information cognitively (see Figure 1.7). Anytime children visit the hospital, especially within critical-care settings, developmentally appropriate preparation is essential. The use of dolls, puppets, and photographs, as well as inclusion in preadmission programming, provides important support for siblings (see Chapter 2: Preparing Children for Health-Care Encounters). If siblings are unable to visit due to distance from the hospital, similar illnesses, or other reasons, parents may encourage them to communicate through telephone calls, letters, audio- or videotapes, or more recent methods such as e-mail, texts, Skype, or FaceTime. While siblings gain a sense of inclusion by participating in creating resources at home to send to the ill child (see Figure 1.8), parents may send similar resources back home to help the well siblings cope with the separation and alternative care arrangements.

One sibling, when asked what he would want adults to know about his experience, summarized by saying, "That we're here too. Don't forget us" (Bugel, 2014, p. 182).

The Internet and Psychosocial Care

The emergence of telemedicine has had a significant impact on the practice of medicine, including diagnosis, communication, research, education—the list goes on. For

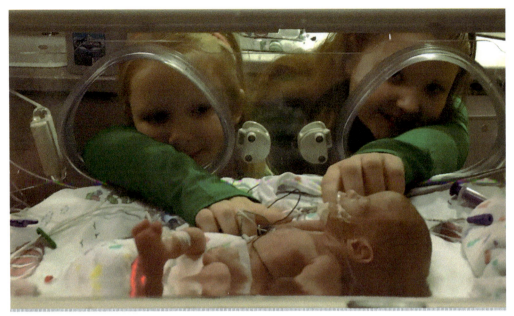

Figure 1.7. The ability to visit is especially important for young children.
Note. Photograph used with permission of Children's Hospital of Wisconsin.

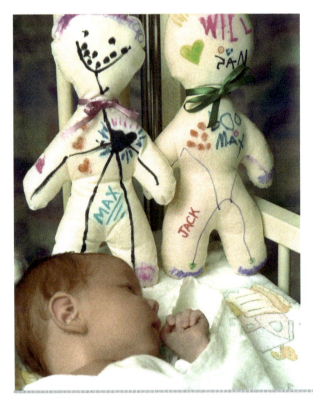

Figure 1.8. Creating a special drawing or a doll for a hospitalized brother or sister helps siblings feel included. *Note.* Photograph used with permission of Children's Hospital of Wisconsin.

families in the health-care system, the availability of the Internet and all the possibilities it provides have been similarly momentous. Instead of pagers, family members have cell phones and keep in touch wherever they are. Communication has become more timely, and loved ones are rarely out of touch with one another. The stress of waiting for word about a child's diagnosis or condition is lessened, physicians are reachable for emergencies at all hours, and separated family members are able to support one another despite distance.

Although communication is much more readily available, being able to actually *see* one another is significant. The emergence of video calling, including FaceTime and Skype, offers families the technology to not only speak with one another while separated but also to see one another, a critical advantage for the hospitalized child and family members (Nicholas, Fellner, Koller, Chow, & Brister, 2011). Parents who previously were reluctant to leave the bedside for fear of missing a doctor's bedside visit or perhaps a child's test or procedure are easily accessible. Family members with work responsibilities or those who remain at home to care for other children can be present for firsthand updates or family conferences. In cases where a newborn infant has been rushed to a high level neonatal intensive care unit hours away from the local hospital's delivery room, these systems allow a mother to see her baby and receive updates on the baby's condition in the days that she must be apart from her infant. This ability to communicate directly is significant, as recent studies have shown that the introduction of sounds like the mother's voice reduces the occurrence of cardiorespiratory events common to premature infants (Doheny, Hurwitz, Insoft, Ringer, & Lahav, 2012). Video calling may also aid in the child's development while promoting bonding when parents can't be at the hospital (Nicholas et al., 2011). One study of a neonatal unit with virtual visitation reported significantly higher satisfaction among families (Rhoads, Green, Lewis, & Rakes, 2012).

Yang and colleagues (2014) looked at the value of videoconferencing for the families of 367 children who were hospitalized for 4 days or longer. Family-Link is a videoconferencing program that uses laptops, webcams, and a secure Internet connection with Wi-Fi provided by the hospital. The families of 232 children were provided with the necessary equipment and encouraged to connect with family and friends through Family-Link, and 135 families were not offered such equipment. In the intervention group, children were provided with webcam-enabled cameras with software. Parents filled out surveys in which they assessed their child's anxiety levels before, during, and after their stay. Results demonstrated that families using Family-Link had a 37% greater reduction in anxiety levels from admission to discharge than those who didn't use it. Also, children who lived closer to the hospital and had shorter stays also benefited, with a 37% drop in anxiety levels. More than 76% of parents rated the opportunity to participate in Family-Link as "extremely important" or "important" for their child during hospitalization (Yang et al., 2014). The Family-Link system provided communication with parents and extended family members who may not have been able to visit. And the provision of laptops made the system available to those who didn't have access to FaceTime or Skype on their mobile phones or other devices (Yang et al., 2014). The study concluded that reduced stress and anxiety levels may contribute to improved patient outcomes and the higher overall well-being of hospitalized children.

Video calling has an immeasurable effect on the hospitalized child's ability to normalize his or her experience, whether simply to chat or for scheduled communication, such as school programming. For the hospitalized adolescent, the ability to text friends or family supports the important developmental need to be connected with peers.

Another area where the Internet's impact has been very significant has been in the education of hospitalized students. Although Homebound Programs and hospital school programs are available, individual students receive limited actual time with teachers, and peer interaction is typically absent. One study found that video communication, in addition to helping students make academic gains, resulted in nonacademic benefits, especially increases in self-confidence and independence, by giving students the ability to interact with peers (Fels, Waalen, Zhai, & Weiss, 2001). Moreover, students may have access to classes not generally offered at the hospital school as well as to specific teachers. Further, the availability of video-mediated communication has been associated with higher student motivation and improved communication skills (Fels et al., 2001).

The Emergency Room Experience

Children's reactions to health-care experiences and the effects of hospitalization may be exaggerated in the emergency room. The physical environment is overwhelmingly frightening, as evidenced by the presence of complex medical equipment and supplies for emergency care, as well as the procedures, from simple suturing of lacerations to the treatment of life-threatening traumatic injuries. The environment is usually busy and sometimes chaotic, with observable and heightened anxiety levels among staff, parents, and other children. The presence of police, emergency transport personnel, and other strangers not usually associated with the hospital may add to a child's sense of fear. Crowded waiting areas and the sight of other sick and injured children awaiting care may cause more anxiety for a child about to encounter his or her own medical experience, perhaps for the very first time.

Although the emergency room visit is one of the most common experiences a child and family will have with a hospital, its psychology is among the least studied and understood. Yet understanding and responding to the psychosocial aspects of an emergency are essential elements of effective care. Parents should be permitted to remain with their child in order to provide emotional support and noninvasive cares. As with other health-care experiences, a child's developmental stage predicts typical reactions and guides interventions (Brunnquell & Kohen, 1991). For example, minimizing the number of caregivers is especially important for infants and toddlers. Because restriction of movement is a major stressor for toddlers, minimizing the use of excessive restraint will be a key concern. Teaching coping strategies that encourage mastery can combat the enforced dependence the school-age child experiences. Adolescents benefit from being involved in care and decisions. Teenagers' major stressors, threats to bodily competence and future competence, can be addressed through discussions about potential psychological changes, physical responses, and long-term issues.

Brunnquell and Kohen (1991) developed a series of steps to help families in coping with emergency treatment while reducing the threatening aspects of the experience:

1. Avoid matching the emotional level of the patient and family if they are upset. Instead, respond with empathy and calmness to help the family reach a lower level of emotional arousal.

2. Assure that someone is specifically attending to emotional care, especially if the primary medical caregiver does not have time to do so, and explicitly tell the patient, family, and designated person that this task is being assigned.

3. Meet the intense information needs of patients and families. Recognize that feelings of loss of control are exacerbated by incomplete, conflicting, or delayed information.

4. Prepare patients and family members present for specific procedures as clearly as possible. Also prepare them for emergencies, such as seeing their child in distress, where the child will be going next, and how best they can support their child.

5. Take specific actions to control pain. If using anesthetics, allow sufficient time for them to take effect; many children report that they begin to feel numb only after a procedure is carried out. Also, use alternative interventions, such as relaxation or mental-imagery techniques in the emergency situation. Recognize that anxiety increases pain. (p. 246)

A study conducted in a British children's hospital identified the factors that most influenced parent satisfaction in the children's emergency department: a clear explanation of the child's diagnosis and treatment plan, allowing the parent to stay with the child at all times, rapid and adequate pain relief, and staff attitude. Parents ranked these factors as significantly more important than the time or process issues frequently targeted in administrative initiatives to improve services (Pagnamenta & Benger, 2015). Another study conducted in a children's emergency department in the United States yielded similar results. Parent satisfaction was most closely linked to communication. When parents were informed in advance about wait times or delays, parent satisfaction was not diminished (Locke, Stefano, Koster, Taylor, & Greenspan, 2011).

In a growing number of settings, the presence of a child life specialist in the emergency room has demonstrated the effectiveness in reducing children's anxiety. Heilbrunn and colleagues (2014) conducted randomized trials, giving children who were admitted to a pediatric emergency department access to child life specialists or hospital clowns and maintaining a control group. They reported that child life services reduced anxiety in children presenting with a baseline level of heightened anxiety. The reduction occurred immediately after child life intervention but was not observed in patients exposed to hospital clowning or in the control group during physician examination.

The presence of parents during procedures is also helpful for both patient and staff, provided that the parent knows what to expect and how to be supportive to increase their child's coping ability. There is a growing movement in emergency medicine and critical-care areas to permit parents to be present during resuscitation when accompanied by a staff person whose only role is to support and give information to the parent (McGahey, 2002).

Ambulatory Care

The challenges of meeting children's psychosocial needs have increased as more and more children and adolescents are treated in outpatient rather than inpatient settings. The systems for providing such care have seen a greatly increased volume of patients as well as the necessity to meet more complex medical needs. Pediatric ambulatory care must be provided in ways that (1) enhance families' strengths, (2) support the child's development, (3) promote multidisciplinary communication and cooperation, and (4) build partnerships with community-based health, early intervention, education, social services, and other human service organizations and agencies (Johnson et al., 1992).

Facilities providing ambulatory care should be designed to meet families' varied needs, including accessibility to public transportation; qualified staff, including interpreters for non–English-speaking families; and attention to a family's entrance into the clinic. Also necessary are comfortable waiting areas and well-equipped play spaces for families, who often spend many hours in outpatient settings. Research has documented that families of children who are engaged in meaningful activities express greater satisfaction with care, even in settings where lengthy waits are the norm (Locke et al., 2011). Adolescents require space that is comfortable and not located in the same waiting area as for younger children.

Educational efforts in the waiting area may be more subtle, with the availability of children's books providing children with activities but also encouraging interaction between parents and children. One pediatric hospital formed a liaison with a local used bookstore chain to place book carts in every clinic waiting area. Books on these carts were intended for children and families to take home when they left the clinic, with the hope that parents would continue to encourage reading together as a family experience.

A child's first health-care experience may be in one of the myriad urgent-care clinics springing up in neighborhoods everywhere, as parents and other caregivers seek nonurgent medical care during off-work hours when primary care facilities are frequently closed. While an adult may perceive such a visit as being convenient, a child's first impression of such a health-care experience may be completely different. The challenge is to continue to provide developmentally appropriate and psychosocially sound care for infants, children, and adolescents, regardless of the service location.

The ability to provide ambulatory care is also challenged by societal issues of poverty, drug and alcohol abuse, homelessness, and violence. An educational component of care should be provided, with resources and information readily available to families. Education for parents regarding normal growth and development must be supplemented with resources to address risk areas for each developmental stage. In addition, medical-care services may be located in community areas, such as school-based clinics and early intervention programs where children are already receiving other services. These resources should be designed to meet the needs of working families or those with limited transportation, making more services available during evenings and weekends.

Preparing children for outpatient treatment may be more challenging because professional resources to address psychosocial needs are often focused on inpatient settings. Parents may have difficulty in establishing a trusting relationship with a primary physician because of changes required by insurance providers and the consolidation of physician services into larger and larger practices as the economic demands on health care continually grow. Although the challenges of health-care economics will not be easily solved, parents should be encouraged to use clinics and physician groups that attempt to meet children's unique psychosocial as well as medical needs. The child who feels comfortable and safe in a waiting area designed especially for children may more easily adapt to being treated by more than one familiar and trusted physician. Encouraging simple medical play at home as part of usual play activities with attention to the positive aspects of medical care also may prepare children for future health-care experiences in inpatient or outpatient settings.

Conclusion

> I'm the same person I was before I got sick. I can't run or play as much as before, but I can read and sleep and do work and think—most things that everybody else does.
> —Adam Rojo, 7 years old (Krementz, 1989, p. 25)

Children in hospitals today are different than in years past. Infants are surviving earlier and longer with medical conditions that for many years had few treatment options and little hope of survival. Children of all ages are living with chronic illnesses that once were considered terminal. They may be hospitalized more often for new treatments and procedures but stay for shorter periods of time and return home with medical needs previously managed only in the inpatient setting.

In addition, injuries are now an increasing threat to children and adolescents, resulting in more hospital admissions. The result is that hospital pediatric units are now occupied by infants, children, and adolescents who are more critically ill than in the past. The one variable that has not changed is that these patients are children with emotional, developmental, educational, and socialization needs that must be met. The commitment to meet these unique psychosocial needs, in addition to increasingly complex medical needs, requires attention to all aspects of family-centered care. It also requires health-care professionals to provide not only a physical environment that is designed specifically for children and families but also a caring and nurturing environment that welcomes every child as part of a family.

Study Guide

1.   Describe the conditions for children in hospitals in the past, and discuss why and how these conditions changed.

2.   What is the *developmental* approach to pediatric care?

3.   Beyond age or developmental level, what factors influence children's responses to health-care experiences?

4.   Discuss how recent research is refuting some long-held beliefs about children's responses to health-care encounters.

5.   Use the developmental approach to describe a typical response by children in one age range to the inpatient health-care experience, and draw implications for practice.

6.   How does an *individualized care plan* help staff, children, and families in coping with health-care experiences?

7.   Explain the concept of resiliency and how it can influence children's health-care encounters. Describe methods of supporting resiliency.

8.   Recent research has identified various parental needs. Describe changes in facilities, practices, and policies that could help parents with their children's health-care experiences.

9.   With increased ambulatory and home health care, there are new issues and challenges for children and families. Cite several of these and discuss implications for health-care systems and practitioners.

10.   Consider trends in child health, disabilities, chronic illnesses, technological and medical advances, and socioeconomic factors, and then describe children's hospitalization and other health-care encounters that will occur 25 years from now.

Appendix 1.1

Resources

Organization

Association of Child Life Professionals

1820 N. Fort Myer Drive, Suite 520
Arlington, VA 22209
Phone: 800/252-4515
Fax: 571/483-4482
Email: CLCadmin@childlife.org
www.childlife.org
Represents a group of trained professionals with expertise in helping children and their families overcome life's most challenging events. Members include child life specialists, child life assistants, university educators and students, hospital administrators and staff, schoolteachers, therapeutic recreation specialists, and others in related fields.

Publications

Hart, R., & Rollins, J. (2011). *Therapeutic activities for children and teens coping with health issues.* Hoboken, NJ: John Wiley & Sons, Inc.

Features more than 200 evidence-based, age-appropriate therapeutic activities specifically designed to promote coping for children and teenagers within the health-care system. Activities target topics such as separation anxiety, self-esteem issues, body image, death, isolation, and pain.

Jolly, A. (2015). Handle with care: Top ten tips a nurse should know before caring for a hospitalized child with autism spectrum disorder. *Pediatric Nursing, 41*(1), 11–16, 22.

Provides information hospital staff should be aware of when caring for a child with ASD: the symptoms of ASD, the importance of family involvement, identifying the best way to communicate with the child, minimizing change, incorporating the child's home routine into the stay, creating a safe environment, identifying emotional disturbances, involving a multidisciplinary team of experts on admission, listening to the family, and creating a record of this information to be shared among staff members.

Video

A sick boy is able to attend school via robot and interact with students and teachers (3:55)

https://www.youtube.com/watch?v=4QBhxuE3Riw

References

Alcock, D., Goodman, J., Feldman, W., McGrath, P., Park, M., & Cappelli, M. (1985). Evaluation of child life intervention in emergency department suturing. *Pediatric Emergency Care*, *1*(3), 111–115.

Als, H., & Gilkerson, L. (1995). Developmentally supportive care in the neonatal intensive care unit. *Zero to Three*, *15*(6), 2–10.

Als, H., Lawhon, G., Duffy, F. H., McAnulty, G. C., Gibes-Grossman, R., & Blickman, J. G. (1994). Individualized developmental care for the very low birth weight preterm infant: Medical and neurofunctional effects. *Journal of American Medical Association*, *272*, 853–858.

Bloom, G., Jones, L., & Freeman, G. (2013). *Summary health statistics for U.S. children: National health interview survey, 2012.* Hyattsville MD: U.S. Department of Health & Human Services.

Bolig, R., & Weddle, K. D. (1988). Resiliency and hospitalization of children. *Children's Health Care*, *16*(4), 255–260.

Bossert, E. (1994). Stress appraisals of hospitalized school age children. *Children's Health Care*, *23*(1), 33–49.

Bossert, E. A., & Hart, D. E. (1999). Acute illness: Effects on the child's family. In M. Broome & J. Rollins (Eds.), *Core curriculum for the nursing care of children and their families* (pp. 155–164). Pitman, NJ: Jannetti.

Bowlby, J. (1960). Separation anxiety. *International Journal of Psychoanalysis*, *41*, 89–113.

Brunnquell, D., & Kohen, D. P. (1991). Emotions in pediatric emergencies: What we know, what we can do. *Children's Health Care*, *20*(4), 240–247.

Bugel, M. (2014). Experiences of school-age siblings of children with a traumatic injury: Changes, constants and needs. *Pediatric Nursing*, *40*(4), 179–186.

Centers for Disease Control. (2014). *10 things to know about new autism data.* Retrieved from http://www.cdc.gov/features/dsautismdata/

Chess, S., & Thomas, A. (1984). *Origins and evolution of behavior disorders.* New York, NY: Guilford Press.

Colville, G., Darkins, J., Hesketh, J., Bennett, V., Alcock, J., & Noyes, J. (2009). The impact on parents of a child's admission to intensive care: Integration of qualitative findings from a cross-sectional study. *Intensive and Critical Care Nursing*, *25*, 72–79.

COPE for Hope. (2015). Retrieved from http://copeforhope.com/index.php

Craft, M. J. (1986). Validation of responses reported by school-aged siblings of hospitalized children. *Children's Health Care*, *15*(1), 6–13.

Craft, M. J. (1993). Siblings of hospitalized children: Assessment and intervention. *Journal of Pediatric Nursing*, *8*(5), 289–297.

Darbyshire, P. (1994). *Living with a sick child in hospital.* London, UK: Chapman & Hall.

Doheny, L., Hurwitz, S., Insoft, R., Ringer, S., & Lahav, A. (2012). Exposure to biological maternal sounds improves cardiorespiratory regulation in extremely preterm infants. *Journal of Maternal-Fetal and Neonatal Medicine*, *25*(9), 1591–1594.

Douglas, J. W. B. (1975). Early hospital admissions and later disturbances in behavior and learning. *Developmental Medicine and Child Neurology*, *17*, 456–480.

Erikson, E. (1959). Identity and the life cycle. *Psychological Issues Monograph*. New York, NY: International Universities Press.

Erikson, E. (1963). *Childhood and society* (2nd ed.). New York, NY: Norton.

Kiechl-Kohlendorfer, U., Merkel, U., Deufert, D., Neubauer, V., Peglow, U., & Griesmaier, E. (2015). Effect of developmental care for very premature infants on neurodevelopmental outcome at 2 years of age. *Infant Behavior & Development*, *39*, 166–172.

Krebel, M., Clayton, C., & Graham, C. (1996). Child life programs in the pediatric emergency department. *Pediatric Emergency Care*, *12*(1), 13–15.

Krementz, J. (1989). *How it feels to fight for your life*. Boston, MA: Little, Brown.

Lally, R., & Phelps, P. (1994). Caring for infants and toddlers in groups: Necessary considerations for emotional, social, and cognitive development. *Zero to Three, 14*(5), 1–6.

Lazarus, R., & Folkman, S. (1984). *Stress, appraisal, and coping*. New York, NY: Springer.

Locke, R., Stefano, M., Koster, A., Taylor, B., & Greenspan, J. (2011). Optimizing patient/caregiver satisfaction through quality of communication in the pediatric emergency department. *Pediatric Emergency Care, 2*(11), 1016–1021.

Lokhandwala, T., Khana, R., & West-Strum, D. (2012). Hospitalization burden among individuals with autism. *Journal of Autism Developmental Disorders 42*(1), 95–104.

McCullough, A., & Jenkins, M. (2015). Research suggests that canine companionship helps calm children undergoing cancer treatment. *American Academy of Pediatrics*. Retrieved from https://www.aap.org/en-us/about-the-aap/aap-press-room/Pages/Research-Suggests-Canine-Companionship-Helps-Calm-Children-Undergoing-Cancer-Treatment.aspx

McGahey, P. R. (2002). Family presence during resuscitation: A focus on staff. *Critical Care Nurse, 22*(6), 29–34.

Melnyk, B., Feinstein, N., Alpert-Gillis, L., Fairbanks, E., Crean, H., Sinkin, R., . . . Gross, S. (2006). Reducing premature infants' length of stay and improving parents' mental health outcomes with the crating opportunities for parent empowerment (COPE) neonatal intensive care unit program: A randomized, controlled trial. *Pediatrics, 118*(5), e1414–e1427.

Mueller, D. (2015, April 24). *The future of autism care for children*. Retrieved from http://www.childrenshospitals.org/newsroom/childrens-hospitals-today/sprong-2015/article

Nicholas, D., Fellner, K., Koller, D., Chow, K., & Brister, L. (2011). Evaluation of videophone communication for families of hospitalized children. *Social Work in Health Care, 50*, 215–229.

Ortenstrand, A., Westrup, B., Brostrom, E., Sarman, I., Akerstrom, S., Brune, T., . . . Waldenstrom, U. (2010). The Stockholm neonatal family centered care study: Effects on length of stay and infant morbidity. *Pediatrics, 125*(2), e277. Retrieved from http://pediatrics.aappublications.org/125/e278.full.html

Pagnamenta, R., & Benger, J. R. (2008). Factors influencing parent satisfaction in a children's emergency department: Prospective questionnaire-based study. *Emergency Medicine Journal 25*, 417–419.

Petrillo, M., & Azarnoff, P. (1997). Preparation programs and new strategies. In P. Azarnoff & P. Lindquist (Eds.), *Psychological abuse of children in health care: The issues* (pp. 59–79). Tarzana, CA: Pediatric Projects.

Piaget, J. (1960). *The child's concept of the world*. Patterson, NJ: Littlefield, Adams.

Quinton, D., & Rutter, M. (1976). Early hospital admissions and later disturbances of behavior: An attempted replication of Douglas' findings. *Developmental Medicine and Child Neurology, 18*, 447–459.

Rapacki, J. D. (1991). The neonatal intensive care experience. *Children's Health Care, 20*(1), 15–18.

Reichman, S., Miller, A., Gordon, R., & Hendricks-Munoz, K. (2000). Stress appraisal and coping in mothers of NICU infants. *Children's Health Care, 29*(4), 279–293.

Rennick, J., Dougherty, G., Chambers, C., Stremier, R., Childerhose, J., Stack, D., . . . Zhang, X. (2014). Children's psychological and behavioral responses following pediatric intensive care unit hospitalization: The caring intensively study. *BMC Pediatrics, 14*, 276.

Rennick, J., Johnston, C., Dougherty, G., Platt, R., & Ritchie, J. (2002). Children's psychological responses after critical illness and exposure to invasive technology. *Journal of Developmental Behavioral Pediatrics, 23*(3), 133–144.

Rennick, J. E., & Rashotte, J. (2009). Psychological outcomes in children following pediatric intensive care unit hospitalization: A systematic review of the research. *Journal of Child Health Care, 13*, 128–149

Rhoades, S., Green, A., Lewis, S., & Rakes, L. (2012). Challenges of implementation of a web based camera system in the neonatal intensive care unit. *Neonatal Network 31*(4), 223–228.

Rich, C., Goncalves, A., Guardiani, M., O'Donnell, E., & Strzelecki, J. (2014). Teen advisory committee: Lessons earned by adolescents, facilitators, and hospital staff. *Pediatric Nursing, 40*(6), 289–296.

Robertson, J. (1958). *Young children in hospitals.* New York, NY: Basic Books.

Robinson, M. (1972, May). *The psychological impact of illness and hospitalization upon the child—Infancy to twelve years.* Paper presented to the Metropolitan Washington, DC, Association for the Care of Hospitalized Children, Washington, DC.

Rollins, J. (2010). There's no place like home for the holidays. *Pediatric Nursing, 36*(6), 283, 296.

Rollins, J., & Mahan, C. (2010). *From artist to artist-in-residence: Preparing artists to work in pediatric healthcare settings* (2nd ed.). Washington, DC: Rollins & Associates.

Rutter, M. (1987). Psychosocial resilience and protective mechanisms. American *Journal of Orthopsychiatry, 57,* 316–331.

Santos, J., Pearce, S., & Stroustrup, A. (2015). Impact of hospital-based environmental exposures on neurodevelopmental outcomes of preterm infants. *Current Opinion in Pediatrics, 27*(2), 254–260.

Smith, V., SteelFisher, G., Salhi, C., & Shen, L. (2012). Coping with the neonatal intensive care unit experience: Parents' strategies and views of staff support. *The Journal of Perinatal & Neonatal Nursing, 26*(4), 343–352.

Spitz, R. (1945). Hospitalism: An inquiry into the genesis of psychiatric conditions in early childhood. *Psychoanalytical Study of the Child, 1,* 53–74.

Stanford, G., & Thompson, R. H. (1981). *Child life in hospitals: Theory and practice.* Springfield, IL: Thomas.

Stroebe, M., Schut, H., & Nauta, M. (2016). Is homesickness a mini-grief? Development of a dual process model. *Clinical Psychological Science, 4*(2), 344–358.

The Council of Economic Advisers. (2014). *Nine facts about American families and work.* Washington, DC: The White House.

Thurber, C.A. (1999). The phenomenology of homesickness in boys. *Journal of Abnormal Child Psychology, 27,* 125–139.

Thurber, C. A., Patterson, D. R., & Mount, K. (2007). Children's adjustment to hospitalization: Is homesickness a factor? *Children's Health Care, 36*(1), 1-28.

Thurber, C. A., Walton, E., & The Council on School Health. (2007). Preventing and treating homesickness. *Pediatrics, 119*(1), 192–201.

Vinall, J., Miller, S., Bjornson, B., Fitzpatrick, K., Poskitt, K., Brant, S., . . .Grunau, R. (2014). Invasive procedures in preterm children: Brain and cognitive development at school age. *Pediatrics, 133*(3), 412–421.

Ward, K. (2001). Perceived needs of parents of critically ill infants in a neonatal intensive care unit. *Pediatric Nursing, 27*(3), 281–286.

White, R. (2011). The NICU environment of care: How we got here, where we're headed, and why. *Seminars in Perinatology 35,* 27.

Wielenga, J., Smit, B., & Unk, L. (2006). How satisfied are parents supported by NIDCAP Model of Care for their preterm infant? *Journal of Nursing Care Quarterly, 21* (1), 41–48.

Yang, N., Dharmar, M., Hojman, N., Sadorra, C., Sundberg, D., Wold, G., . . .Marcin, J. (2014). Videoconferencing to reduce stress among hospitalized children. *Pediatrics, 134*(1), 169–175.

Yu, H., Wier, L., & Elixhauser, A. (2011). *Hospital stays for children, 2009.* (HCUP Statistical Brief #118). Rockville, MD: Agency for Healthcare Research and Quality. Retrieved from http://www.hcup-us.ahrq.gov/reports/statbriefs/sb118.pdf

2 Preparing Children for Health-Care Encounters

Jessika C. Boles

Objectives

At the conclusion of this chapter, the reader will be able to:
1. Discuss the theoretical rationale behind preparing children for health-care encounters.
2. Determine evidence-based strategies for providing preparation interventions.
3. Consider the role of cognitive, social–emotional, cultural, and language development in planning preparation interventions.
4. Explore ways to incorporate technological tools into preparation interventions.
5. Describe developmentally appropriate ways to prepare children for health-care encounters.

In the previous chapter, Children's Hospitalization and Other Health-Care Encounters, a discussion of children's reactions to health-care encounters revealed that hospitalization, doctor and clinic visits, ambulatory care and emergency room visits, and home health-care encounters prove stressful for children and their families in a variety of ways. Potentially painful or invasive procedures can especially challenge a child's still-developing coping skills, which may help explain why modern theories of stress are built on studies of individuals undergoing and coping with medical procedures.

In medical settings, medical procedures are typically a significant source of stress for children (Kain & Caldwell-Andrews, 2005). Because they may also be hospitalized prior to, during, or after their surgery or procedure, children face compounded stressors from both the procedure and the hospital environment. Preparation has emerged as a psychosocial care philosophy that combines age-appropriate teaching techniques, coping-skills instruction, parental involvement, and elements of play or role rehearsal to help children know what to expect during medical events (Justus et al., 2006). Feeling knowledgeable about and prepared for health-care encounters may reduce children's distress and promote successful coping in the future.

This chapter introduces the stress and coping theories that underlie various preparation techniques used with children facing medical procedures. The importance of considering development, culture, language, and the integration of technological tools is discussed. Evidence-based recommendations are provided for planning developmentally and situationally appropriate methods of preparing children and their families to cope with stressful medical experiences.

Stress and Coping

A review of the developmental, sociological, and psychological literature reveals that the types of stressors that children and families experience can be separated into two broad working categories. First there are normative transitions, which are typically universal, anticipated, and short-term events, such as managing daily life with a busy family, tackling school assignments, or problem-solving relationship disagreements with friends (McCubbin & Patterson, 1983). The second group of stressors includes stressful life events, or "socially undesirable or negative events," such as a family member's death, the loss of a job, or even the unexpected hospitalization of a child or parent (Thoits, 2010; p. S42).

These categories, however, should be thought of as flexible heuristics because what a child finds stressful is closely related to his or her developmental level and cultural background. In addition, the knowledge and wisdom that children gain with growth, maturation, and exposure to new and varying environmental influences also change their perceptions and reactions to stressful experiences. For example, transitioning between grades in school is often an exciting experience for young children as they look forward to meeting their new teacher, seeing their classroom, and building new friendships. On the other hand, adolescents may view a new school year as a stressful experience. They may spend weeks searching for the perfect "first day of school" outfit, choosing their class schedule, or worrying about managing a growing academic load and expanding social life.

Historically, three definitional orientations have been used to study the nature and variability of stress: stimulus-oriented, response-oriented, and relational. Until the 1960s, the major stress theorists were concerned with either what constituted a stressful situation (stimulus-oriented) or the individual's physiological and psychological reactions to the stressful situation (response-oriented; Janis, 1958; Selye, 1974). Lazarus's (1966) work began to shift the emphasis of study from a stimulus–response perspective to a relational orientation. Rather than viewing a stressor and the individual's response to it as separate phenomena, Lazarus (1966) argued that they were two halves of one cyclical whole; as individuals experience an event, they react, and their reactions in turn affect their experience of the current event and perceptions of future encounters.

Today, Lazarus and Folkman's (1984) revision of the stress and coping model is the most commonly referenced source for explaining stressors, stress responses, and the role of coping in stress management. One feature that sets their theory apart is that it considers both external and internal factors in how individuals appraise, or interpret, and react to internal and external stressors. Lazarus and Folkman (1984) defined stress as the moment when the external or internal demands of experience "are appraised as taxing or exceeding the resources of the person" (p. 141). According to such a definition, any event that requires internal resources, such as thoughts and feelings, or external resources, such as assistance from others, could be viewed as stressful. Yet stress should be treated as a subjective experience, because stress begins only when an individual perceives a threat and continues only when the individual perceives his or her coping capabilities to be insufficient.

Because stress is based on individual perceptions or appraisals, stressors themselves can be quite variable. They may be social, cultural, psychological, or physiological, or involve a combination of these stimuli converging on the individual (Lazarus & Folkman, 1984). *Appraisals* are the cognitive judgments that individuals make about the demands required by an experience, as well as their beliefs about how well those demands can be managed with the resources available. In other words, an appraisal is an evaluative process that determines why and to what extent a particular transaction or series of transactions between the person and the environment is deemed stressful. These mental processes intervene between the encounter with the stressor and the resulting reaction (see Figure 2.1).

After appraising a stimulus as stressful, the individual performs a secondary appraisal to determine how the stimulus can be addressed. The individual then uses some form of cognitive or behavioral coping effort (Lazarus & Folkman, 1984). However, the individual's personal resources and constraints affect the choice of coping efforts. Constraints for children may include developmental age or limited life experiences. Efforts to cope may be focused on solving problems, acknowledging and managing emotions, expending physical effort, or moderating thought processes.

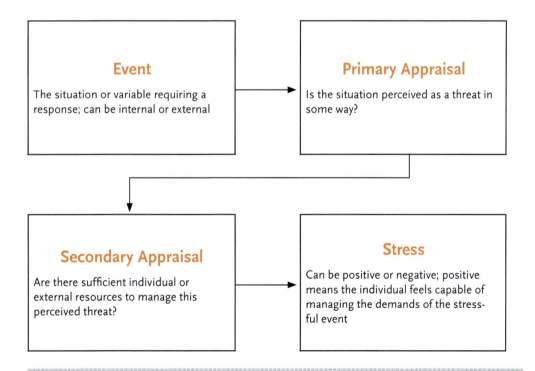

Figure 2.1. The stress and coping process.

Note. Adapted from *Stress, Appraisal, and Coping* by R. Lazarus and S. Folkman, 1984. New York, NY: Springer.

The outcome or results of these coping efforts are either adaptive or maladaptive; however, Lazarus (1981) cautioned about the criteria used to determine whether a given coping effort is adaptive or maladaptive and making such a judgment. Value systems can impinge on this designation; for example, one individual's value system may judge denial as maladaptive, yet denial may be an appropriate response for another individual or in a particular situation. Coping effort is also related to time; for example, denial may be adaptive from a short-term perspective but maladaptive in the long term. Cultural factors, as well as the individual's perspective and the function the effort serves (short or long term), must be considered when interpreting the benefits or limitations of a coping effort.

Theoretical Foundations of Preparation

Researchers found that an average of 4 million children undergo anesthesia and surgery annually in the United States (Kain & Caldwell-Andrews, 2005). Between 40% and 60% of these children will develop significant behavioral stress prior to surgery (Kain, Caldwell-Andrews, & Wang, 2002), about 50% will experience high anxiety during anesthesia induction (Davidson et al., 2006), and 16% will continue to exhibit significant behavioral changes even 30 days after surgery (Stargatt et al., 2006). Because hospitalization in itself is already stressful for many children and families (Franck et al., 2015), it understandable that an invasive and potentially painful procedure may compound a child's hospital-related distress. Noting this, health-care providers in the 1970s began to develop preparation programs for children and families to help reduce anxiety and promote effective coping with health-care encounters. It was hypothesized that preparing children and families by providing information about what to expect during a hospitalization or surgery would reduce fears about the unknown and help children and families accurately appraise potential stressors.

As preparation programs emerged, the research literature described the positive impact of such programs on children's responses to hospitalization and surgery. Several of the most widely known studies, such as those conducted by Wolfer and Visintainer (1975), Melamed and Siegel (1975), and Petrillo (1972), recommended the following key elements of effective preparation programs (Stanford & Thompson, 1981):

- conveying information to the child in a developmentally appropriate manner,
- encouraging the expression of feelings about the information or event,
- including the participation of parents or other significant family members, and
- establishing a trusting therapeutic relationship with staff members.

In one of the early studies, Vaughn (1957) described an experimental condition in which two groups of children were admitted to the hospital for strabismus repair. A control group received no intervention, while the experimental group met for 15 to 25 minutes with a psychiatrist who reassured and supported each child and provided a brief, developmentally appropriate explanation of the surgery planned for the following day. Results indicated that the control group experienced more severe and persistent emotional disturbance than did the experimental group, both during hospitalization and at 3 and 6 months following discharge.

In another classic study, Wolfer and Visintainer (1975) added "stress-point supportive care" to a preparation program that included role rehearsal, or allowing children to rehearse or enact their role during the procedure that they would experience. The intervention focused specifically on typical procedure-related stressors and then integrating a variety of techniques to prepare children for these points. Study results confirmed that the experimental group displayed less upset on both psychological and physiological measures. Participants in the experimental group who participated in the preparation program also had better posthospital adjustment scores than those in the control group. The authors came to the following conclusion:

> The exact causal sequence of this involved process is complex and unknown . . . The net effect of the preparation and supportive care can be described as stress reducing. However, the precise nature of this dynamic cognitive and affective process remains to be determined. (Wolfer & Visintainer, 1975, p. 254)

Since these formative studies, research evidence has continued to confirm the anxiety that children experience in relation to medical procedures, highlight the various benefits of preparation in these situations, and evaluate the ways in which preparation can and should be offered. In addition, scholars have explored the ways in which the child's coping style and the timing of the intervention may affect preparation provision and procedure-related anxiety. Though the majority of these studies have been conducted with children undergoing surgery, several of the major findings and implications are transferable to children facing any type of invasive or potentially painful procedure, or an unfamiliar medical experience.

According to Perry, Hooper, and Masiongale (2012), the introduction of an anesthesia mask could be one of the most stressful things a child encounters in the hospital setting. (See Figure 2.2.) Also stressful are transitions between physical hospital environments, such as the transition from a preoperative holding room to the operating room (Fortier, Del Rosario, Martin, & Kain, 2010). Children facing day-surgery procedures have described their experiences according to the following broad themes: "enduring inflicted hospital distress," "facing an unknown reality," and oscillating between "losing control" and "trying to gain control" (Weenstrom, Hallberg, & Bergh, 2008, p. 100). In short, children encounter multiple levels of stressors in the context of a procedure or surgery, including unfamiliar environments and events, a psychological (and physical) loss of control, and anesthesia itself.

Because children identify multiple sources of stress in health-care encounters, a variety of preparation techniques have been developed for both children and their parents. Despite the fact that the first preparation programs were primarily directed at children, the link between parental anxiety and children's anxiety has now been well documented (Davidson et al., 2006; Fortier et al., 2010; Li, Lopez, & Lee, 2006; Stargatt et al., 2006). High parental anxiety not only predicts higher child anxiety but also is related to decreased parental compliance with preoperative care requirements (Chahal et al., 2009) and long-term behavioral difficulties postsurgery (Stargatt et al., 2006). Furthermore, as rates of day-surgical procedures increase, parents experience an increasing burden of responsibility for their child's pre- and postoperative care, which may generate additional anxiety when compared with an inpatient stay (Li et al., 2006).

Some preparation programs have been developed specifically to target parental preparation and coping as a result of these reports. McEwen, Moorthy, Quantock,

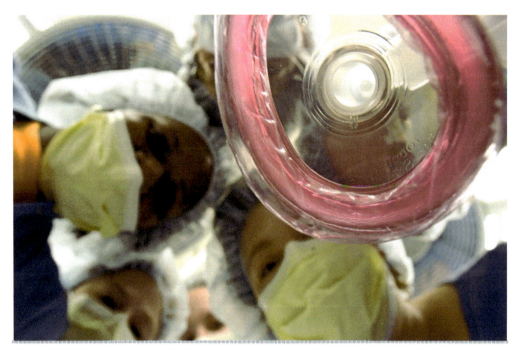

Figure 2.2. Surgery, and particularly anethesia induction, can be an unknown and frightening experience for many children.

Rose, and Kavanagh (2007) found that a brief (8-minute) video detailing the surgery experience from admission to discharge significantly reduced parental anxiety during anesthesia induction. Similarly, parents who watched a video about their role in the operating room during anesthesia induction reported feeling more confident in providing support for their child (Bailey, Bird, McGrath, & Chorney, 2015).

Other interventions have encouraged parents' involvement in providing preparation and support for their child. Some care providers have developed educational materials and programs for use in the home setting, such as a children's book and parent guide describing the surgery process (Ono, Hirabayashi, Oikawa, & Manabe, 2008), to "enable children facing surgery and their parents to learn and talk about the illness and surgery together" (p. 82). The authors found that the use of this book encouraged responsive care and strengthened parent–child relationships in the context of scheduled day surgery. Combining an educational video for children and a printed parent manual, Wakimizu, Kamagata, Kuwabara, and Kamibeppu (2009) showed that children not only gained more information about their upcoming procedure but also felt significantly less pain and anxiety at anesthesia induction.

In the Creating Opportunities for Parent Empowerment (COPE) program, educational material was delivered to mothers in audiotaped and written form, including information about children's typical responses to critical illness and the parental role in facilitating their children's adjustment (Melnyk, Small, & Carno, 2004). Mothers also received a parent–child activity workbook with three activities to perform with their children: (a) puppet play, (b) a "Jenny's Wish" book, and (c) therapeutic medical play. It was found that mothers who participated in the COPE program reported less stress and provided more support to their children during the procedure.

Other programs have provided a more family-centered approach to preparation, offering interventions that prepare both children and their parents for the medical procedure ahead. For example, many documented interventions have included parent-and-child presurgical tours (Brewer, Gleditsch, Syblik, Tietjens, & Vacik, 2006; Fincher, Shaw, & Ramelet, 2012; Li et al., 2006; Rice, Glasper, Keeton, & Spargo, 2008). These interventions have been shown to have favorable effects on both parent and child anxiety, especially in conjunction with age-appropriate explanations and demonstrations of medical equipment, such that even children as young as age 2 years and their parents experienced decreased anxiety during anesthesia induction (Kain et al., 2007). Likewise, some programs have developed novel means for providing preparatory information to children, such as through board games (Fernandes, Arriaga, & Esteves, 2014) or interactive puppet shows (Cuzzocrea et al., 2013). Even these creative means of educating children about an upcoming procedure have proved to reduce the children's anxiety related to procedures and anesthesia induction.

Using medical play, therapeutic play, or other kinds of play that involve enactment and demonstration of procedures with actual medical equipment also reduces preprocedural anxiety (Cuzzocrea et al., 2013; Li, Chan, Wong, & Lee, 2014; Li & Lopez, 2007). When provided specifically by a child life specialist, multimodal preparation including medical play, a presurgical tour, age-appropriate explanations, and role rehearsal significantly reduced both pre- and postprocedural anxiety (Brewer et al., 2006). In addition, when medical-play materials are provided for continued use at home, parents demonstrate decreased anxiety while also reinforcing their child's understanding in the comforts of the home environment (Fincher et al., 2012).

Assessment is as important as intervention when working with children in medical settings; this is an especially difficult skill. In a study that compared the ability of attending pediatric anesthesiologists, resident anesthesiologists, and mothers to predict anxiety during anesthesia induction in children from 2 to 16 years of age, researchers found that the attending pediatric anesthesiologists were the most accurate predictors (MacLaren et al., 2009). Even so, in terms of accuracy of prediction, only 47.2% of their predictions were within 1 standard deviation of the observed anxiety exhibited by the child, with 70.4% of predictions within 2 standard deviations.

As noted above, a clear predictor of children's procedure-related anxiety is parental anxiety (Fortier et al., 2010). In addition, younger children may be especially susceptible to distress in this context (Yip, Middleton, Cyna, & Carlyle, 2009), as well as those with low sociability (Fortier et al., 2010). Children who require an overnight hospital stay, endure a longer procedure, or have had numerous or difficult previous anesthesia experiences are at greater risk as well (Davidson et al., 2006; Stargatt et al., 2006). On the other hand, children who are more informed about the upcoming procedure report less anxiety (Claar, Walker, & Smith, 2002), as do those scheduled for outpatient procedures when compared with those who will require an inpatient stay (Davidson et al., 2006). The child's anxiety also transfers to recovery in the home setting, as increased anxiety is related to increased pain reporting and consumption of pain medication postsurgery (Kain, Mayes, Caldwell-Andrews, Karas, & McClain, 2006). Therefore, "preoperative teaching strategies must not only be age appropriate, but should take into consideration the child's social adaptability, cognitive ability, and temperament" (Perry et al., 2012, p. 70).

Another aspect that can help account for the range of children's responses to preparation is coping style. Although coping generally refers to "efforts to prevent or diminish threat, harm, and loss, or to reduce associated distress" (Carver & Connor-Smith, 2010, p. 684), this does not address the specific efforts employed by the individual. Originally, Lazarus and Folkman (1984) described *problem-focused* and *emotion-focused* coping. When individuals direct their efforts at the stressor, this is considered problem-focused; when efforts are directed at managing one's responses to the stressor, this is considered emotion-focused. Since then, additional dimensions of coping efforts have been highlighted, such as

- *engagement versus disengagement*—whether the individual engages with the stressor or attempts to escape the threat (Roth & Cohen, 1986),
- *accommodative*—adjusting oneself in response to the stressor (Morling & Evered, 2006), and
- *meaning-focused*—attempting to rearrange life priorities to find meaning in the stressor (Folkman, 1997).

Thus, there are a variety of ways to cope with a situation, whether applying new coping techniques and efforts to a particular source of stress or relying on previously useful efforts combined into an individual coping style.

Children learn coping strategies from infancy onward, and many strategies learned in childhood continue into adulthood. Patterns develop largely from the cultural context in which children develop, as children learn additional coping modes from parents, peers, teachers, and relatives. Culture has a significant effect on the generational transmission of coping techniques and an individual's beliefs about his or her ability to cope with stress in the immediate environment. It is important, then, when providing preparation interventions, to coach children in identifying, selecting, and modifying new and pre-existing coping strategies to apply to their impending procedures or health-care encounters.

The remaining question involves when preparation opportunities should be offered. Some have argued that preparation should be provided as soon as the surgery is scheduled, with additional information provided in the lead-up to the procedure—thereby limiting new information as the surgery date approaches (Blount, Piira, & Cohen, 2003). Others recommend beginning preparation 2 to 4 weeks before the procedure (Fernandes et al., 2014), or based on the child's age, suggesting children from age 3 to 5 years be prepared 1 to 2 days in advance, and older children, 5 to 10 days in advance (Fincher et al., 2012). On the other hand, timing may be a factor of more individualized functions than age, such as the duration and severity of the procedure, the likelihood and intensity of post-procedural discomfort, and the length of hospitalization if indicated (Jaaniste, Hayes, & van Baeyer, 2007). Children may require more advance preparation for procedures that are likely to generate higher levels of discomfort and disruption.

MacLaren and Kain (2007) offer a useful summary of the preparation literature:

When providing preparation for children, the following key elements should be included: (i) information on both procedural (what will happen) and sensory (what it will feel like; including pain) aspects of the procedure must be included; (ii) coping skills should be taught via a peer model; doll play is not sufficient; (iii) written materials alone are not the effective forms of preparation; and (iv) preparation should be provided at least 5 days in advance for children >6 years and no more than a week in advance for children <6 years. (p. 1019)

Although evidence to back these claims can be found in international medical and psychosocial journals, it is important to note that implementing empirical findings can often take 17 years or more (Morris, Wooding, & Grant, 2011). So outdated and disproven techniques can remain in circulation for just as long and thereby compromise the quality of care patients and families receive (Grimshaw, Eccles, Lavis, Hill, & Squires, 2012). Thus it is imperative that practitioners from all fields remain aware of emerging developments and their implications for policies, practices, and further research. The literature that exists today is clear that "the most effective components of preparation programs include modeling, parental involvement, child life preparation, and coping skills instruction" (Wright, Stewart, Finley, & Buffett-Jerrott, 2007, p. 70). Preparation programs that combine education, play, and therapeutic components carry great benefits for children and families when employed in developmentally appropriate ways, as discussed in more detail below.

Developmental Considerations for Preparation

Children are dynamic beings, constantly growing and changing. Their cognitive, physical, emotional, and social skills emerge at varying rates based on individual, environmental, and cultural factors. Consequently, it is important to tailor any preparation to each child according to his or her developmental level, previous experiences, and coping preferences. These may or may not correspond to chronological age, so individualized and family-centered assessments are required.

Still, there are guidelines that can help generally shape the preparation experience to meet the needs of each child. More specifically, Table 1.3: Understanding Children Who Are Hospitalized: A Developmental Perspective offers some general guidance based on children's cognitive and psychosocial development and describes the types of reactions to health-care encounters one might expect at each developmental stage. These can be helpful starting points to remember when designing a preparation intervention for a child or adolescent facing a medical experience, in combination with ongoing assessment and a flexible child-centered approach.

Cognitive Development

As discussed in Chapter 1, children's abilities to make sense of medical information increase exponentially with the passing of time and exposure to new experiences. Noting this, the complexity of the techniques used or the explanations given to prepare children for healthcare encounters should be based upon the individual child's cognitive development. Typically developing children proceed from processing information through their senses and motor responses, to understanding the symbolic connections between thought, language, and reality. As development continues, school-age children gain a more logical view of the world by using operations, and adolescents build on these foundations to explore the abstract and boundless limitations of thought and concept

(Piaget, 1967). In addition, developmental gains, such as appreciating and planning for future events, adopting and changing plans and responses, and actively monitoring one's own emotional states, are achievements that help children better prepare for recognizing and managing their stress (Jaaniste et al., 2007). This cognitive progression demands increasingly detailed explanations and more realistic teaching tools when providing preparation for older children and their parents—especially when cognitive appraisals are an integral component of the coping process.

Psychosocial Development

When taking into account Erikson's (1950) psychosocial theory, providers must recognize the competing psychological and social influences throughout childhood that contribute to how children value the relationship between themselves and the world around them. Children acquire different interests, value systems, and, therefore, coping abilities, as their development ebbs and flows through various stages: beginning with the significance of trusting a parent; continuing through normative struggles for autonomy, independence, and exploration; then transitioning to acquiring a sense of competence based on academic and social achievement; and adopting a social identity rooted in peer relationships and goals. Being mindful of these developmental "crises" can remind providers that although a procedure may be the extent of their involvement in the child's life, that single experience can compound the concurrent life stressors the child may be facing and therefore have a long-ranging developmental impact.

Cultural Development

The unique cultural communities that shape children's development encompass more than just their country of origin, primary language, or ethnicity (Rogoff, 2003). Much like Bronfenbrenner's (1979) ecological theory of human development, a child's culture consists of inter- and intrapersonal interactions with a variety of environmental contexts, from home to community, school to organizational membership, and even extending to governmental and ideological atmospheres. Given the expansiveness of culture, it is important to understand that each child and family brings its developmental background to each and every health-care encounter, which requires respectful and responsive care from providers.

Children from different cultural backgrounds may enter the health-care environment with different perceptions of medical care and will therefore identify different stressors. In a study comparing children in Nepal and children in the United States, Mahat, Scoloveno, and Cannell (2004) found that although both groups rated being poked with a needle as their primary hospital-related fear, the two groups rated additional items, such as being away from family, vomiting, or missing out on school, quite differently. More specifically, Nepalese children were more concerned about missing school and appearing ill in front of their family as compared to American children, who instead focused on personal pain or effects of illness.

In addition, preferred preparation techniques may differ across cultures. For instance, Japanese health-care providers have tried and found success in home-based preparation strategies (Wakimizu, Kamataga, Kuwabara, & Kamibeppu, 2009). The authors asserted the cultural relevance of this intervention because of the cohesive child-rearing style used in Japan, and parent beliefs that "the child should be complete-ly protected by the caregiver from all threats" (p. 394). On the other hand, in Hong Kong Chinese cultures, providing preparation in the hospital setting is the most common and culturally appropriate intervention used with children and families scheduled for medical procedures (Li & Lopez, 2007).

Children's reactions to medical procedures can also be affected by their cultural upbringing. In Japan, for instance, it was found that more than 54% of children demonstrated negative behavior changes after discharge from a day surgery procedure, which included things like separation anxiety, crying at nighttime, temper tantrums, requiring increased assistance with tasks, and other indicators of continued distress (Wakimizu, Ozeki, & Kamibeppu, 2005). Furthermore, even children who received a preprocedural therapeutic-play intervention in Hong Kong rarely reported pain after an outpatient surgery; this may be in line with Chinese children's beliefs about "obedience, social conformity, and the inhibition of self-expression" (Li et al., 2006, p. 39). On the other hand, children in Great Britain most preferred information about pain before a procedure, rating it more important than other procedure-related topics (Fortier et al., 2009).

Culture is the primary influence on a child's development and thereby an integral element to assess and consider when working with children and families in the hospital setting. In the event of an impending procedure, culture may affect the children's beliefs about the experience, preferred preparation mediums, and their associated reactions and coping skills. By remaining aware of cultural differences and being open to patient and family beliefs and preferences, preparation can be beneficial for patients and families from all backgrounds.

Language Development

When preparing children, language is another aspect of development that must be considered, because language stems from interactions between all three domains of development—cognitive, social-emotional, and physical—within the child's unique cultural context. Attention should be given not only to the words and phrasing chosen by the professional but also to the words and phrases the child chooses to use or omit when participating in a preparation intervention. Likewise, it is important to be aware of the nonverbal cues a child and family may use to communicate their thoughts and concerns.

Child life specialists and nurses generally begin offering preparation programs to children between 2½ and 3 years of age. At this age, many children are able to ask questions and participate verbally in the program, although most will learn more by manipulating and exploring objects and through visual demonstrations. As children mature, they are increasingly able to process verbal information and ask appropriate questions about it. Table 2.1 outlines some general expectations concerning language development in young children. For specific information about communicating effectively with children, see Table 2.2, Text Box 2.1, and Text Box 2.2.

A major language-related concern during preparation is the use of medical terminology with children. Many of medical terms are unfamiliar and ambiguous, even to parents. Using them may contribute to a child's fantasies or misunderstandings about what will occur, but employing accurate language can also promote the child's understanding of conversations with other providers.

Table 2.1

Sequence of Language Acquisition	
Age	**Characteristics**
Newborn	Cries as first means of oral communication
4–6 weeks	Coos
5 months	Makes monosyllabic sounds (e.g., "ba," "ga")
6–8 months	Babbles ("mamamama") Responds to own name
10 months	Uses first specific words with appropriate reference (e.g., "mama," "dada") Comprehends the word "no" and recognizes tone differences that indicate danger or upset
12 months	Uses 1–2 words other than "mama/dada" Increases vocabulary at an average of one word per week Comprehends simple one-step commands
18–20 months	Uses an average of 20 words regularly, with a much more expansive receptive vocabulary
24 months	Has a vocabulary of around 50 words Acquires one or more words per day Uses two-word sentences ("Want up") Should be able to follow simple two-step commands (e.g., "Sit down and drink your juice")
24–30 months	Uses telegraphic speech as 3–5 word sentences with subject, object, and verb (e.g., "Me want juice")
36 months	Has receptive language of about 800 words Understands simple prepositions (e.g., "Put the ball under the table") Can create sentences with increasingly accurate grammatical structures
4 years	Uses intelligible speech most of the time, with increasingly complex sentence length and structure, though with some grammatical irregularities

Note. Adapted from Berk, L. E., & Myers, A. B. (2015). *Infants and children: Prenatal through middle childhood* (8th ed.). New York, NY: Pearson Education, Inc.

When medical terminology is used, it is important that these words be paired with their more familiar or developmentally appropriate counterparts in order to scaffold the child's understanding. For example, it is helpful to explain new equipment by saying, "The IV, or tiny clear-plastic tube, is used for. . . ." Medical terms should be explained to children in language they will understand, athough this may require additional clarifications at times because of each individual child's development, culture, and previous experiences. Words or phrases that are helpful to one child may be threatening to another, but again, this is a product of developmental differences. Regardless of the child's apparent level of comprehension, opportunities for questions or clarification should always be offered on several occasions during the interaction. For an excellent commentary on choosing language, see Gaynard and colleagues (1990).

(text continues on p. 58)

Table 2.2

Age-Specific Considerations	
Age Group	**Considerations**
Infants	• Consider body language, as well as pitch, intonation, and intensity of voice. • Nonverbal behaviors work especially well for infants, with cuddling, patting, or gentle physical contact to calm them. • Avoid sudden or loud noises or speech. The actual words are not as important as the way they are spoken. • Infants are usually more at ease when upright and in visual contact with and close proximity to their parents.
Preschool and young school-age children	• Approach slowly, letting the child make the first move whenever possible. • Avoid extended eye contact until after the child is comfortable. • Position yourself at the child's eye level to help them feel more comfortable with your presence. • Children may be more responsive when they remain close to the parent, such as sitting on the parent's lap. • Be direct and concrete with young children; they are prone to intermixing fact with fantasy.
Older school-age children	• Continue using relatively simple explanations to facilitate understanding. • Children this age want concrete explanations and reasons for everything, often using knowledge seeking as a coping strategy. • Learning new things about how the body works offers an opportunity to master some aspects of the hospital experience.
Adolescents	• Be prepared to deal with a wide range of emotions and behaviors, as development varies in this age group. • Give concrete explanations that focus on the adolescent's specific concerns and match the level of detail seen in their questions and concerns. • To enhance communication, take time to discuss less-threatening topics to build rapport and help the adolescent feel comfortable expressing themselves. • Ask broad, open-ended questions before specific questions, such as "How's school?" before asking, "What is the best or worst thing about school?"

Note. Adapted from "Communicating Effectively with Young Children," by L. Clutter, C. Hess, K. Nix, J. Rollins, D. Smith, N. Stevens, and D. Wong, 1987, *Children's Nurse, 5*(4), pp. 1–3; and "Communicating Effectively with Older Children and Adolescents," by L. Clutter, C. Hess, K. Nix, J. Rollins, D. Smith, N. Stevens, and D. Wong, 1988, *Children's Nurse, 6*(1), pp. 4, 6, 8.

Text Box 2.1

General Strategies for Communicating Effectively With Children

1. Use a calm, unhurried, and confident voice.

2. Be attentive and observant to the environment around you and to the verbal and nonverbal communications that may be happening. If staff are moving quickly around in the room or the child is actively upset, focus on establishing a calming presence before trying to provide preparatory information.

3. Speak clearly, be specific, and use as few words as possible. As a general guide, use sentences with a sum of words equal to the child's age in years plus one.

4. Give children time to respond to questions. Silence can mean that they are taking a moment to find the words they need to express their thoughts and feelings, not necessarily that they are uninterested. By allowing them this extra time, you can communicate the idea that they are equally in control of the preparation interaction, which can promote trust and engagement.

5. Use play as a strategy for getting to know the child. For example, if the child has a doll or stuffed animal, you can begin by speaking to the toy and then initiate conversation with the child by asking simple questions about the toy. Or, you can enter the room with play materials, and then as the child begins to engage comfortably, transition the interaction into a preparation opportunity.

6. Listen to and observe the child at play. Often, children will express important information, such as complicated or difficult feelings or even misconceptions, through this familiar medium.

7. Look for opportunities to offer the child choices, but offer only choices that exist. For example, when a child must change into a gown, a statement such as, "I need to take your shirt off so that I can listen to your chest. Would you like me to help you take it off?" gives the child information, a choice, and some measure of control.

8. Be honest. It is better to describe how something might feel than to simply say, "It will hurt." It is also important to honestly admit when you do not know the answer to a question. Rather than answering, "I don't know," validate the child's question by saying, "That's a really good question." Then model self-advocacy skills by saying, "I think that's something your doctor would know. Should we ask her about it?"

9. Avoid expressions with dual or ambiguous meanings, such as "put to sleep" or "take your temperature." Ambiguity can not only increase the risk of miscommunication but also cause fear or anxiety (for example, "We put our dog to sleep and he died. Am I going to die?" or "Will you give my temperature back?"). Preschoolers are especially subject to these misunderstandings.

10. Avoid words that are emotionally charged; for example, replace "stick" with "slide under the skin," or "cut open" with "make a small opening."

11. State directions and suggestions in a clear and positive way, such as "You need to stay very still now."

Note. Adapted in part from "Communicating Effectively with Young Children," by L. Clutter, C. Hess, K. Nix, J. Rollins, D. Smith, N. Stevens, and D. Wong, 1987, *Children's Nurse,* 5(4), pp. 1–3; and "Communicating Effectively with Older Children and Adolescents," by L. Clutter, C. Hess, K. Nix, J. Rollins, D. Smith, N. Stevens, and D. Wong, 1998, *Children's Nurse,* 6(1), pp. 4, 6, 8.

Text Box 2.2
Communication Techniques

1. *Give children an opportunity to express their thoughts, concerns, and feelings.* Listen and respond to underlying messages rather than just verbal content. Be attentive, try not to interrupt, and avoid comments that convey disapproval or surprise.

2. *Acknowledge and validate the child's feelings.* Instead of denying them with a statement such as, "Don't be angry," say, "You sound really mad." This permits the child to accept the emotion and begin to deal with it.

3. *Match the child's affect when appropriate.* If the child is using humor and dialogue to cope, try and participate in a similar manner. However, if the child is clearly upset or angry, it would not be as appropriate to use humor. In that particular situation, it's important to match the state you would like the child to achieve by speaking calmly, modeling deep breaths, or even initiating guided imagery to promote relaxation.

4. *Avoid negative "you-messages" that often start with "you" followed by something that tends to blame, accuse, or attack the person to whom the message is directed.* Use alternatives such as:

    a. *Describe the child's situation or problem without mentioning the child.* For example, instead of saying, "You took off your bandage," say, "The bandage is off; it needs to be on."

    b. *Send "I-messages" to communicate thoughts, feelings, expectations, or beliefs without imposing blame or criticism.* For example, say, "I feel frustrated when I cannot hear what Johnny is trying to tell me because of all the noise in here."

    c. *Provide descriptive praise to point out the child's attributes or to identify your feelings about the child.* For example, after obtaining a blood sample, saying "You sat very still and told me it hurt instead of moving your arm" is more helpful than making an evaluative statement such as "You're a great patient," which may cause the child to feel doubt, denial, or fear of not measuring up at a later time. In summary, comment on the behavior, not the person.

    d. Praise the child's efforts in addition to their outcomes. Even if a child is not successful in his or her coping plan, it's important to validate the coping efforts during the procedure. Say things like, "I could really see how hard you were trying to take those deep breaths when the needle went in." By praising their effort in a specific way, it communicates that with continued effort and practice, the child may be able to change the outcome during a future procedure.

    e. *Use the third-person technique by expressing a feeling in terms of "he," "she," or "they."* This gives the child an opportunity to agree or disagree without being defensive. For example, say, "Sometimes children who are sick tell me they feel angry or sad because they cannot do what others can do." Then wait silently for a response or encourage one by saying, "I wonder if you have ever felt that way."

Note. Adapted in part from "Communicating Effectively with Young Children," by L. Clutter, C. Hess, K. Nix, J. Rollins, D. Smith, N. Stevens, and D. Wong, 1987, *Children's Nurse, 5*(4), pp. 1–3; and "Communicating Effectively with Older Children and Adolescents," by L. Clutter, C. Hess, K. Nix, J. Rollins, D. Smith, N. Stevens, and D. Wong, 1998, *Children's Nurse, 6*(1), pp. 4, 6, 8.

Overall, health-care providers must listen carefully and be sensitive to the child's use of and response to language. For example, children may interpret *shot* as involving a gun or *PICU* as "pick you." This is where attention to nonverbal cues is of great importance. Furthermore, when pairing information with play-based techniques, as discussed below, children may be better able to communicate these misconceptions, identify their fears and concerns, and express their feelings about the coming health-care encounters.

Preparing Children

Preparing children for surgery and procedures requires some knowledge of and sensitivity to the emotional and cognitive abilities of children at different ages and stages of development. An entire profession, the field of child life, was established to specifically address the psychosocial needs of children and families in health-care settings, including the need for preparation (Justus et al., 2006). Now an integral part of many interdisciplinary teams in children's health care, child life specialists are trained to assess children's developmental needs and to plan appropriate interventions, including preparation, within the context of the children's abilities, family relationships, and medical conditions (see Figure 2.3). Other individuals who may contribute to, or assume, the preparation role in a given setting include nurses, therapists, physicians, social workers, and parents. However, regardless of the position title of the person providing preparation, the most important consideration is that the information shared is in accordance with the child's developmental level.

Infants and Toddlers: Birth to 2.5 Years

Because infants and toddlers are especially sensitive to the emotional cues of their primary caregivers, preparation interventions for this age group should focus on the parents' knowledge and coping (Brewer et al., 2006). Parents often report feeling unsure about how to best support their child during a procedure or the induction of anesthesia, so preparatory information can be helpful in addressing this concern (Piira, Suguira, Champion, Donnelly, & Cole, 2005). See Case Study 2.1. When preparing infants, toddlers, and their parents for health-care encounters, include the following elements:

- **Introductions.** Introduce yourself to the parents. Attempt to engage the infant with a game of peekaboo or another game without touching or getting too close to the infant.
- **Exploration.** While explaining procedures to the parents, offer the child an opportunity to explore the medical equipment that will be used during his or her surgical experience.
- **Demonstration.** Show the baby or toddler an anesthesia mask. Model its use on yourself, then on the parents. Ask the child to imitate this behavior. Send home the mask, along with a premade surgical doll with all the tubes and bandages that the child will have. Tell the child that he or she will have what the doll has when he or she comes to the hospital. Instruct parents to reinforce the teaching at home using these materials.

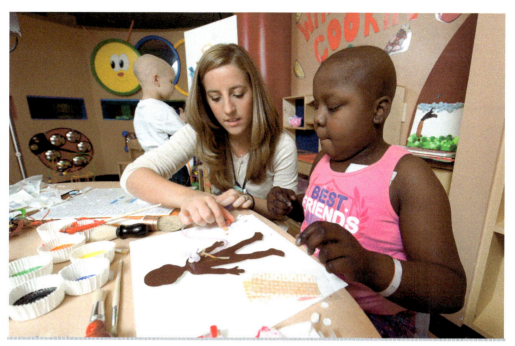

Figure 2.3. Child life specialists are trained to assess the developmental needs of children and to plan appropriate psychosocial interventions, including therapeutic play and preparation.

- **Mastery.** Show parents and the child around the environment and introduce them to the staff members. Allow the child to work the television controls, light switches, and automatic doors, with assistance, if necessary.

Preschoolers: 2.5 to 5 Years

Because this group tends to resort to magical thinking when faced with an unknown situation, preschoolers most need concrete demonstrations and opportunities to explore medical settings and equipment, typically 5 to 7 days in advance with reinforcement information provided at home (see Case Study 2.2). The following techniques can be useful with this age group:

- **Introductions.** State your name and your role on the staff (e.g., "Hi, my name is Kim. My job is to talk with children about what will happen when they come to the hospital"). Then, clearly state what will and will not occur on this occasion (e.g., "Today we will look around the hospital, talk about your surgery, and play with doctor toys. You will come back on another day for your surgery. Nothing we talk about will happen to you today"). This clarification allows the child to attend to the session without fearing what will happen next.
- **Exploration.** Next, show the child and parents where they will be on the day of surgery. Point out facilities and resources, and provide an opportunity for the child to explore the toys in the play area.
- **Explanation.** Describe admission procedures, whom the child will meet, and what will happen up until the time of surgery. Then, using dolls and medical

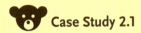 **Case Study 2.1**

Preparing an Infant for Craniofacial Surgery

Eleven-month-old Kevin was scheduled for craniofacial surgery. He arrived at the surgery center the week before surgery for a "preoperative tour" with his parents, who were very anxious. Referring physicians and nurses tend to think that such a tour is primarily for the benefit of the parents, but often the parents expect their child to gain from the experience as well.

The child life specialist encouraged Kevin to explore the toys in the play-room and the medical equipment in the preoperative area (e.g., stethoscopes, thermometers, bandages). This was followed by a demonstration of the use of the inhalation mask, and Kevin was asked to imitate the demonstration. The mask was sent home with the family so that they could rehearse that behavior for the day of surgery.

The family was then taken to the pediatric intensive care unit (PICU), where Kevin would wake up. The child life specialist demonstrated the room and bed controls, and introduced the family to some of the staff who would be caring for Kevin. She explained policies for the various areas where Kevin would be during and after surgery and gave them a handbook with additional policies and resources for families.

As she escorted the family out of the building, the child life specialist offered Kevin the opportunity to turn off lights, push the elevator buttons, and open the automatic doors. This provided Kevin with a sense of mastery over these experiences. Kevin's parents reported that they felt very reassured by the visit. The child life specialist asked them to call her if they had any additional questions or concerns.

equipment, demonstrate anesthesia induction and any new devices or equipment the child might have after the surgery (see Figure 2.4). Explain how an IV or inhalation mask works, and allow the child to insert the IV in the doll or model induction by mask with the doll. Briefly explain what the doctor will do and how it will help the child's health. Then, discuss waking in the recovery room and tell the child when he or she will be reunited with parents.

- **Visual aids.** When information is provided verbally, pair the explanation with a resource that the child can view, manipulate, or engage with through the other senses. Studies have shown that pairing narration and visualization in this way can enhance young children's memories of educational experiences (McGuigan & Salmon, 2005; Salmon, McGuigan, & Periera, 2006).
- **Appropriate choices.** Offer the child appropriate choices at every juncture. Children feel more confident when they are in control of some aspects of the procedure. Choices may include who—the child's mother or father—goes to the operating room with the child, what toys to bring to the hospital, and which movie to watch in recovery. Letting the child know the available

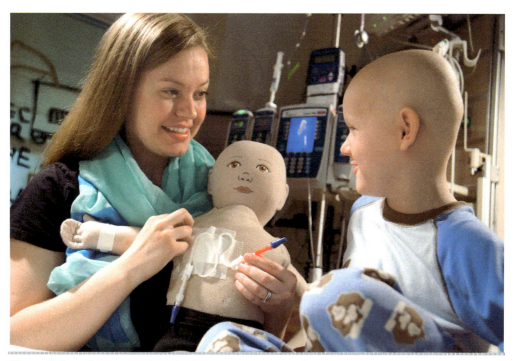

Figure 2.4. Dolls with actual medical equipment can provide realistic yet play-based visuals and demonstrations to prepare children for medical experiences.

choices in advance will give him or her positive issues to focus on; but do not offer a choice that the child does not have. This often leads to a lack of trust and diminished cooperation.

- **The child's role.** Inform the child of the "jobs" he or she needs to do related to the procedure. For example: "You will need to drink juice and eat popsicles when you come back from your surgery." This is another means of enlisting cooperation—helping children feel they are important in the process.

- **Coping strategies.** Teach the child coping strategies, such as deep breathing, singing, playing, or other forms of distraction or active coping. Enlist parents as coaches, which gives them a positive role and reduces their anxiety as well. Inform children that they may use these strategies to relieve pain or anxiety, either before or after surgery.

- **Cues.** Children may remain fearful unless they know when a task is complete. As you explain, tell the child how to know when each step is finished (e.g., "When the IV is out, the nurse will put on a bandage. That is when it will be time for you to put on your clothes and go home with your parents").

- **Questions.** Both parents and children need to feel that their questions have been answered during the preparation session. Many preschoolers are reluctant to speak to the child life specialist, nurse, or other staff member who is conducting the session. Offer the child the chance to whisper a question to the parent, who then asks the staff member. Always offer one or more ways the parent or child may contact the staff if further questions arise.

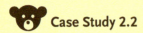 **Case Study 2.2**

Preparing a Preschooler for Surgery

Four-year-old Alex was scheduled for a tonsillectomy, adenoidectomy, and myringotomy with tubes. His mother, a single parent, had asked for books to read with him that might help them through this experience. One week before surgery, Alex came to the surgery center with his mother for preparation. He appeared shy and clung to her during introductions. The first stop was the playroom in the waiting area. Alex explored the toys and did not want to leave to proceed with the preparation. He was given a choice to drive the toy car or ride in the wagon to the next room, and he chose the car. In the preoperative area, Alex tried out the scale and the blood pressure cuff, but declined to try the thermometer. His mother tried to cajole him but was told, "Today Alex can choose not to try the thermometer. But next week, the nurse will need to measure his temperature."

The next stop was the preop playroom, where Alex and a child life specialist rehearsed what would happen to Alex, using a doll as the patient. Alex named the doll, chose a "flavor" for his anesthesia mask, and helped hold the mask to the doll's face while it fell asleep. Alex became anxious when offered an opportunity to start the doll's IV, as did his mother. After a reminder that he would be asleep, and would neither feel nor remember getting the IV, Alex decided to help. He and his mother were surprised and relieved to learn that a needle would not stay in his arm, just a tiny flexible tube. Then Alex learned that while the medicine made him stay asleep, his doctor would take out his tonsils and adenoids so that he would not get so many sore throats and also put tubes in his ears so he would get fewer earaches.

Alex saw a picture of the recovery, or "wake-up," room. He was told that when he got to the second wake-up room, his mother would be there, and that his jobs would be to drink juice and eat Popsicles and to tell his mother or a nurse whether he was hurting. He was told how he would get medicine to help stop the hurting and things he could do to help himself (e.g., watch a movie, take deep breaths, drink something cold). Lastly, he was told that when his IV was removed, he could get dressed, choose a sticker, and go home with his mother. He agreed to practice choosing a sticker the day of his preparation, which he took home along with his doll "patient." The child life specialist told him that if there was anyone at home who had not come to the preparation, Alex could use the doll to show them what he had learned. She mentioned to his mother that hearing Alex's conversation would be a way to assess how much Alex learned and that if she needed to correct any misinformation or confusion, she could do so at home or call the child life specialist for help.

School-Age Children: 6 to 11 Years

The school-age years are characterized by an increasing ability to understand rules, a concept of fairness, and cooperation with others. Children in this age group gain mastery and a sense of competence by demonstrating knowledge and skills and interacting with peers. Preparation for children in this age group (see Case Study 2.3) can include the techniques listed above and those listed below:

- **More detailed information.** Children ages 6 years and older are increasingly curious about how bodily systems work. Include an explanation of the affected organ system and how the procedure will improve the condition. Use graphics or dolls with organ systems the child can visualize or manipulate. If complex machines or equipment are used, children in this age group appreciate opportunities to explore and learn in nonthreatening and even symbolic ways, such as through demonstrations and role rehearsals (see Figure 2.5). Answer any follow-up questions, or refer the child to his or her surgeon if you do not know the answer.

- **More complex coping strategies.** School-age children may wish to use guided imagery, listen to favorite music, choose whether to watch and participate in appropriate aspects of care, or identify other ways to help them feel more control in the situation. Help them choose from among several options (e.g., "Some children like to pretend they are in a favorite place while this is happening. We can practice what that would be like. Others bring music to listen to or hold someone's hand during the difficult parts. What do you think would help you the most?").

- **More opportunities to participate in care.** Indicate those areas in which the child might like to participate during the procedure (e.g., "You may help the nurse remove the old bandage," or "You can hold the thermometer in your mouth while we measure your temperature"). Older children may be more cooperative if they feel their choices are being respected as often as possible.

- **Timing.** Tell older children about events at least a week in advance to allow them to assimilate the information and plan and rehearse their preferred

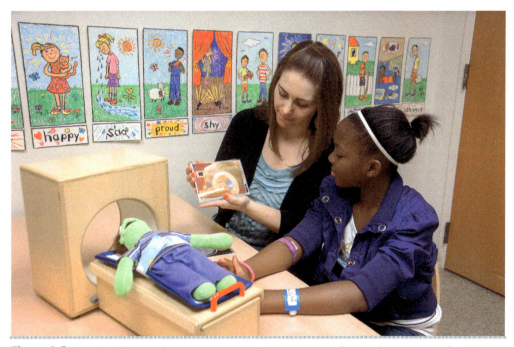

Figure 2.5. Simple dolls can play an important role in preparation for a wide age range of children, as they can be used to rehearse procedures, check for the child's understanding, and promote expression of feelings.

coping strategies. Also encourage the child and parents to inform you of any special events or plans that may conflict with the scheduled procedure. When possible, help the family advocate for adjustments to the schedule to accommodate these important and normal developmental events to promote normalcy and increased coping with the upcoming procedure.

Adolescents: 12 to 18+ Years

Adolescents face a number of physical, emotional, social, and cognitive changes that can extend well beyond the age of 18. The physical growth spurts of puberty are accompanied by an increase in hormonal activity that causes the body to become more sexually and physically mature. Along with these changes come strong emotions about developing a sense of self and purpose, or identity, fitting in socially with peers, feeling attractive to potential romantic partners, and developing close friendships. In addition, teens feel that they are maturing intellectually and should participate more in their own decision making.

A health-care encounter that involves medical tests, procedures, or surgery is perceived as a threat to many of the developmental milestones of adolescence. "Trying on" adult roles is a natural part of adolescent development, but like younger children, teens may regress when faced with a threat. However, they may simultaneously feel a need to act "tough" and "grown up" in the face of such encounters. It is not unusual for patients in this age group to act immature and frightened one minute, and cool and indifferent

 Case Study 2.3

Preparing a School-Age Child for Surgery

Kenisha, an 8-year-old girl, was scheduled for bilateral ureteral reimplants. During her preparation, she toured the surgery center and had her anesthesia and surgery explained (as happened with Alex in Case Study 2.2). At this age, children begin to fear that they will not wake up from surgery or that they will wake up during surgery and experience pain. To counter this, the child life specialist explained: "The medicine makes you stay asleep so you won't feel or remember anything about your surgery. When the surgery is done, the doctor stops giving you the medicine, and that lets you wake up."

The child life specialist used a life-size doll that opens to reveal kidneys, ureters, and bladder; the workings of the urinary tract were briefly explained. The doll was used to explain how the surgery would fix the problem and to show Kenisha how her urinary catheter would work after the surgery. Kenisha manipulated the doll's internal organs and asked questions about their function and about what would happen during surgery. She also manipulated the Foley catheter in the doll and asked why it was necessary and whether the catheter would hurt. She was reassured that it would be placed while she was asleep but was also told that she might feel a stinging sensation or pain when it was removed and during her first few voids. Kenisha elected to practice relaxation breathing to help with that part of her recovery.

the next. It is sometimes difficult for parents to help because the teen may ask for help one minute and push them away the next. Or, adolescents may invest more in the advice and opinions of their peers than in parental guidance, which attests to the important of social relationships during this developmental period.

Although the same goals for preparation remain, techniques used with younger children must be carefully modified for this age group to not only provide a beneficial intervention but also build a therapeutic relationship with the adolescent patient (see Case Study 2.4). Some of the following techniques may be especially useful for adolescents and even young adults facing a painful procedure:

- **Question list.** Encourage teens to come to the session with a list of questions they would like to ask. Normalize questions that they identify, assuring them that there is no such thing as a "dumb" or "weird" question in that situation.

- **More adult teaching tools.** Use photographs of the procedure or draw a live diagram with the teen instead of using dolls or play items. Digital representations through videos or educational apps can also be appealing to this age group.

- **Incorporation of identified support persons.** Adolescents are building more expansive social-support networks, so they may have friends, significant others, cousins, parents, or others present with them at the hospital or clinic. Taking an interest in and engaging these individuals in the preparation process can help build a trusting relationship with the teen while also ensuring that information is shared with those who can actively reinforce it at home and school.

- **Coping strategies.** Focus on coping strategies at every step of the process. Ask questions such as: "What do you think will help you with the IV?" "Do you usually look or turn away?" "Does numbing cream, listening to music, or relaxation breathing help?" Encourage teens to develop a primary and secondary coping plan that they can switch between as needed during the procedure.

- **Privacy concerns.** Be especially mindful of privacy concerns. Let teens know who will need to examine them and why. Make suggestions about how they can protect their own privacy (e.g., "If the nurse forgets to close the curtain around your bed, ask her to do so," or "Even though they want you to use the urinal, you can still go to the bathroom and close the door for more privacy"). Ask about any specific privacy concerns the teen may have. Additionally, always offer to step out of the room when an exam is being conducted to communicate that you are supportive of their desire for privacy.

- **Sensitive topics.** Although privacy is very important for this age group, it is important not to avoid sensitive or uncomfortable topics out of one's own discomfort as a provider. Adolescents and young adults often have concerns about bodily appearances, sexual functioning, long-term effects of procedures, or other topics that might be difficult to discuss. Create a comfortable environment for these kinds of conversations by saying, "Some of the other people who have had this procedure have said that it's difficult to talk about X, Y, or Z. Part of my job is to help you feel as comfortable as possible about what will happen, so I am happy to give more information about any of those things if you would like."

- **Active participation in care.** Encourage teens to actively participate in their care. Teens can choose their menus; ask what their vital signs are; help take their own vitals; and ask to see their plan of care and talk with doctors, nurses, and parents about how they can take charge of some areas. This will help them feel empowered and offer a sense of mastery, instead of encouraging a feeling of dependence.

- **Peer group contact.** Encourage teens to keep in touch with their peer group, and let the adolescent know any policies the hospital may have about using personal communication tools like smartphones, electronic tablets, or social media sites. In this age group, peer relationships are more important than ever before, and messages or visits from friends will go a long way toward facilitating a quick recovery. Feeling accepted by peers in the face of a threatening event is a major concern for adolescents, and no reassurance from adults can take the place of the experience of visiting with friends and being treated as one of the group.

Integrating Technology

According to the Joan Ganz Cooney Center at Sesame Workshop (Gutnick, Robb, Takeuchi, & Kotler, 2012), children between the ages of 5 and 9 consume an average of 5.5 hours of technological media during a typical day, whether they are playing, seeking entertainment, or working on educational activities. This includes not only watching television but also using personal electronic devices such as electronic tablets, educational video games, and other screen-based media. As high as this number may seem, it is likely to trend upward as children grow older and experience increased access to computers, smartphones, video games, and other products marketed to preteens and adolescents. Although some have warned about the detriments of the growing use of technology outlets, technology in the hospital setting can be very helpful by promoting therapeutic play and for maintaining peer relationships and even learning about health-care encounters.

Some studies have already documented the value of technological tools in helping children and families cope with procedures or surgery. For example, a noninferiority randomized trial comparing tablet-based interactive distraction (TBID) to sedation for children undergoing ambulatory surgery reported that TBID reduced perioperative anxiety, emergence delirium, and time to discharge, and increased parental satisfaction, when compared to midazolam (Seiden et al., 2014). Also, parents demonstrated decreased anxiety during their child's anesthesia induction after viewing an 8-minute video that reviewed the perioperative process (McEwen et al., 2007). Parents who received a similar video intervention in another study reported feeling greater self-efficacy while supporting their child during induction (Bailey et al., 2015).

Digital presentations of preparatory information have also shown to be preferable and helpful for children facing difficult procedures. In a study of children from 3 to 10 years of age undergoing general anesthesia for dental procedures, a digital interactive activity promoted more effective coping behavior when compared with the

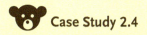 **Case Study 2.4**

Preparing a Teenager for Procedures

Danita is a 14-year-old girl who visits the hospital repeatedly for tests, procedures, and IV medications. She prepares for the outpatient days by baking cookies for the staff and patients and visiting with people she knows while waiting to be called for her procedure. Afterwards, she leaves as quickly as possible.

If her treatment requires an inpatient stay, she brings her own sheets, pillow, blanket, and seasonal decorations for her room. She chooses to make the environment as much her own as she possibly can. She also brings music, videos, and her smartphone so that she can communicate with her friends. She surrounds herself with friends and family and makes an effort to learn the names of the doctors, nurses, and staff members taking care of her.

When it is time for a procedure, she turns on her MP3 player, tunes out everything else, and copes very effectively with the experience. Her family supports her through these times, calming her with their presence and providing distracting activities to help pass the time. She has put together a very comprehensive plan for dealing with the stressors of multiple health-care encounters using a variety of coping strategies.

same information provided in a printed cartoon format (Campbell, Hosey, & McHugh, 2005). Moreover, these same coping outcomes can also be achieved remotely in the child's home with the use of technology. In Japan, children who viewed a preparatory video (accompanied by an explanatory pamphlet) in their own homes prior to a procedure gained more information and knowledge about their surgery and demonstrated less pain and anxiety at induction than children who did not receive this intervention (Wakimizu et al., 2009).

Most recently, hospitals have turned to the Internet for developing efficient, easily accessible, and comprehensive preparation programs for children and families, such as the WebTIPS program developed by Kain, Fortier, Chorney, and Mayes (2015). To evaluate the effectiveness of the WebTIPS program, Fortier and colleagues (2015) gave children scheduled for surgery and their parents 24/7 access to the online preparation website. The website consists of an animated and interactive portion for children to complete, using games and demonstrations to explain the perioperative process; the parent area of the website provides preparatory information about the sequence of events as well as coping skills to manage both their anxiety and their child's on the day of surgery. Strategically, the website also requires children and parents to work through some of the modules together, promoting parental involvement and encouraging both children and parents to practice anxiety-reducing coping skills to be used during anesthesia induction.

Parents and children in this study were given access to the website 5 days prior to surgery up until 10 days after its completion so that information could also be given about postsurgical pain at home. Upon systematic evaluation of the program, parents described the website as both helpful and useful (Fortier et al., 2015). In addition, both parents and children were less anxious during anesthesia induction when compared with children and families who did not receive the WebTIPS intervention.

Internet-based preparation programs and digital media presentations of preparatory information are a promising frontier when it comes to preparing children and families for health-care encounters. Whether through apps, games, websites, videos, or even interactive video discussions with other patients, offering preparation in a variety of formats can allow the child a sense of control and promote feelings of mastery as they decide how to engage with this new information and upcoming experience. In addition, as technological innovations flood everyday life, providing information in these ways may not only facilitate understanding but also promote coping by normalizing the child's experience of learning about a non-normative experience. Finally, digital formats may also be a developmentally appropriate way to engage children who do not respond as easily to traditional teaching techniques, such as adolescents and young adults pining for adult-like independence, or nonverbal or special needs populations, such as children with developmental disabilities or autism spectrum disorders (Shah, 2011).

Emergency Admissions or Procedures

If the preparation is for an emergency hospital admission or a procedure that was not anticipated, there may be insufficient time for the child and parent to assimilate the information presented. When there is no time at all for preparation, it is still important to focus on active coping, giving the child as much control as possible, maximizing support from parents, and helping the child and family understand what to expect from staff. This can mean modeling coping strategies, such as taking deep breaths or using guided imagery, coaching parents on ways to support their child at the bedside, and providing clarifying information about the staff in the room and the procedure being performed.

To help the child identify coping techniques, one might say, "Some children tell me it helps if they blow bubbles [or listen to music, play a game on an electronic tablet, or employ whatever distractions are available]. What do you think will help you?" An additional way to help parents support their child is to advocate for supportive positioning (Stephens, Barkey, & Hall, 1999). For example, a child seated in a parent's lap with the IV-connected arm extended flat on a table is in a much less threatening position than being held down lying supine.

Although it has not yet been systematically evaluated, the ONE VOICE (Wagers, 2013) program offers a comprehensive approach to providing support for children during any procedure, but it can be of benefit especially during emergent circumstances. The philosophy of the ONE VOICE program combines several elements deeply grounded in current empirical literature and years of interdisciplinary clinical experience; the acronym represents the following recommendations: One single voice should be heard during a procedure; Need parental involvement; Educate patient before the procedure about what is going to happen; Validate the child with words; Offer the most comfortable, nonthreatening position; Individualize your game plan; Choose appropriate distraction to be used; and, Eliminate unnecessary people not actually involved with the procedure (Wagers, 2013). Each component of the ONE VOICE approach promotes a child-centered, parent empowered, and staff-facilitated experience that supports the child while invasive medical procedures are performed (Boles, 2013).

On the other hand, when very little time is available prior to a procedure, the techniques below can be used to help promote coping even in relatively immediate and emergent situations, some of which are highlighted in Case Study 2.5.

Define Behavioral Limits

Limits can be comforting to children to let them know what to expect and what will be expected of them. For example, during an IV start, it can be helpful to say, "When it is time for the IV to go in, your job is to keep this arm very still. But you can use your other arm to squeeze your mom's hand if you'd like."

Offer Choices

Offering choices goes hand in hand with behavioral limits. As children learn where the limits lie, they can be offered choices to promote their sense of control during the experience. For example, saying, "Even though you have to stay still, you can do things like close your eyes or listen to music to help yourself. Which would you like to try?" promotes children's involvement in their care while promoting coping skills. When it comes to choices, however, it is important to remember to offer choices only where they exist; choosing not to have the procedure may not be a realistic choice, but whether to sit in Mom's lap or on the table is a choice the child may be able to make.

Negotiations

Once it is time for the procedure, it is helpful to begin on time and not allow "negotiations" for changes in rules to be used as a delaying tactic. In a child- and family-centered setting, any accommodations have presumably been made, and the only result of further delays is a power struggle that no one can win. Furthermore, this can lengthen the duration of the child's distress, which has been shown to relate to increased anxiety (Davidson et al., 2006).

Interdisciplinary Care

In situations where a procedure must take place with little advance notice, multiple professionals may be involved. For this reason, the child's anxiety may be heightened as the activity in the room increases, and the child may be uncertain about provider roles and responsibilities. Whenever possible, a child life specialist or another pediatric healthcare professional skilled in preparation and coaching should be present to help the child in coping with the procedure. This person can help explain what is happening, moderate the amount of activity in the room, and remind the child of his or her coping plan.

Honest and Accurate Information

Although one's first tendency might be to assure the child that "this won't hurt at all" or "it will be OK, I promise," as Lazarus and Folkman (1984) pointed out, cognitive appraisals are the key to successful coping with stressful experiences. Using minimizing statements, ambiguous descriptions, or incorrect information might make it difficult

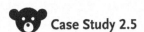 **Case Study 2.5**

Helping a Child Cope
With Emergency Procedures

Nine-year-old Georgia was admitted from the Emergency Department with suspected aseptic meningitis. She needed an IV and a lumbar puncture (LP) to rule out that diagnosis and begin proper treatment. When the child life specialist met her, Georgia had been in the treatment room for 45 minutes or more and had been through two failed IV insertion attempts. Georgia stated she was afraid of getting stuck with the needle, that it would hurt, and that she "wasn't ready."

EMLA cream* had been applied, and the child life specialist explained that it took time to work and that while they were waiting, they would do some doctor play to learn about getting an IV. She stated to Georgia, "When we're finished playing, the cream will be working, and it will be time to get your IV." They proceeded to do therapeutic medical play with a cloth doll and IV equipment. Georgia chose not to participate very actively, especially at first, but she watched everything intently. For her, the best part was seeing that what would stay in her arm was not a needle, but a soft, flexible catheter that she was allowed to touch so that she would know how it felt. She learned that she could do "the pinch test" to see if the EMLA was working so that she would not have to rely on information from anyone else, but could decide for herself how it would feel. She discussed ways she had coped in the past with unpleasant things and chose two strategies. She would count until the needle was out, and she would use her imagination to pretend to be in her own room (i.e., creative visualization).

When the time came for the IV start, Georgia decided that her mother would hold one hand, a medical student would help her hold her arm still, and the child life specialist would help coach her counting and imagery. She was quite anxious and did a lot of screeching, but she held still and counted, even though more than one IV attempt had to be made and one of them was without EMLA. She was praised by everyone in the room for doing such a great job holding still, counting, and doing her imagery, and she seemed very proud of herself. Now that the IV was in place, it was used as a vehicle for sedation for the LP.

As discussed earlier, therapeutic medical play, as well as rehearsing coping strategies for possible future procedures, can be helpful for children traumatized by difficult procedures. The focus should be on the child's ability to use the chosen strategies successfully. Children will often perform to our expectations, and if we indicate we expect them to succeed, they are much more likely to do so.

---

*EMLA cream is a thick, white cream that contains two commonly used anesthetic agents, lidocaine and prilocaine. Normally these agents need to be injected to numb the skin; however, EMLA cream is formulated to carry the agents through the skin surface to directly numb the area.

for children to accurately appraise a medical procedure and thereby experience increased difficulty managing their responses. As previous research has shown, children particularly desire comprehensive and accurate information about the procedure itself, any anticipated pain, and whether or not anesthesia will be used (Fortier et al., 2009).

Ethically, as well, we cannot reasonably ask children to cooperate with a painful or invasive procedure if we are not honest about how it will feel, how long it will take, and how they will know when it is over; this violates the ethical principle of veracity, in addition to potentially causing psychological harm. Therefore, as part of a comprehensive plan to help children and families cope more effectively with health-care encounters, honesty is paramount. Nothing else will succeed without it.

Postvention

In the worst-case scenario, a child arrives at the hospital or other health-care setting having had a traumatic emergency admission with no preparation, no coaching, and no support. In an ideal world, no child would go without preparation; however, large numbers of pediatric patients and limited staffing make this scenario a reality at times. In these situations, staff members can follow up after the procedure to offer postvention. Derived from a term used in the literature on bereavement care following a suicide (Aguirre & Slater, 2010), *postvention* refers to techniques aimed at reducing any harmful effects that may remain after a stressful event. Applied to children who have undergone medical procedures, *postvention* is often used to describe a combination of emotional support, education, expressive activities, and other opportunities for the child and parents to make sense of their experience while establishing relationships with providers involved in their care.

One helpful postvention strategy is therapeutic medical play. Offering children a doll or stuffed animal as the "patient," and medical supplies such as needles, syringes, tubing, stethoscopes, Band-Aids, and casting materials (as they may have encountered in their procedure) gives children the ability to manipulate the materials to simultaneously care for the patient and express their understanding of their experience. Integrating open-ended questions encourage verbalizations about the play (e.g., "Why does your doll need to have a surgery?," "How is your doll feeling about her surgery?") and provide an opportunity to identify and correct any medical misconceptions a child may hold. Medical play particularly offers younger children an opportunity to experience some mastery over tools that have been used on them while also promoting self-expression.

Older children and adolescents may benefit more from evaluative conversation about their procedure or surgery when asked open-ended questions, such as, "Was there anything about surgery that wasn't like what you expected?" or "How did your procedure go?" This can help them identify the appraisals they made prior to their procedure and compare them against their actual experience to shape their perceptions of future healthcare encounters. Furthermore, such information can be helpful for staff members in providing future preparation interventions for other children in this age group.

If the examples of preparation or helping children cope with procedures in Case Studies 2.1 through 2.4 seemed "how to" in nature, the example in Case Study 2.5 definitely falls into the "how *not* to" category. There were enough missed opportunities to make the situation less frightening for the child so that by the time there was an intervention, the child was almost beyond her ability to benefit. Therefore, preparation—or effectively, prevention—is potentially much more beneficial in moderating children's stress than trying to minimize damage once it has been done.

Sedation

Ways of calming children during a procedure include giving them a sedative, permitting them to have a parent present, or preparing them psychologically. In the United States, short-acting general anesthetic agents such as propofol have become increasingly common for outpatient nonsurgical procedures that children were formerly expected to tolerate without anesthesia, and sometimes even without sedation. In fact, the use of sedative premedications for children's procedures increased from 30% in 1995 to 50% in 2002 (Kain et al., 2004), and this number is likely even higher today. This rapid increase in use has been fuelled by new drugs and monitoring technology, expanded practitioner skills, the shift of procedural work to outpatient settings, and widespread acceptance of the ethical imperative to treat pain and anxiety in children (Krauss & Green, 2006).

The use of sedative agents may be only a short-term fix. Although some studies have shown that sedative premedications can be quite effective in managing children's anxiety when compared with preparation programs, Cuzzocrea and colleagues (2013) warned that this strategy "does not seem to be the best option in terms of cost and benefits over time, because it acts only on the current situation but does not help the child develop appropriate coping strategies that can help him deal with similar situations in the future" (p. 139). There may be times where sedative premedications are needed, but when indicated, preparation programs may help the child build skills that can transfer to other contexts and last across the lifespan.

Conclusion

As this chapter has revealed, children and families can learn to cope effectively with even what most would consider major stressors, including those associated with illness, surgery, and medical procedures. Just as children and families must feel prepared for health-care encounters when possible, health-care professionals should likewise be prepared to offer even young patients the developmentally appropriate and evidence-based tools that they need to cope with challenging situations. At the same time, researchers must be prepared to continue exploring techniques for best achieving these coping goals, including both pharmacological and nonpharmacological strategies, as well as ways to reduce both the number and intensity of stressors children come into contact with in health-care settings. Overall, whether facing scheduled day surgery, a potentially painful procedure, or an emergent medical encounter, children and families cope best with preparatory information, family involvement, and staff members who are responsive to their unique coping skills and preferences. These evidence-based strategies are what we all must be prepared to provide and advocate for to help children cope with health-care encounters.

Study Guide

1. Define the concepts of *stress* and *coping*.

2. Why is cognitive appraisal an important part of Lazarus and Folkman's (1984) stress and coping theory?

3. Describe the connection between parental and child anxiety in the context of medical procedures. What evidence supports the existence of such a connection?

4. What are some factors to assess when predicting a child's procedure-related distress?

5. How does culture affect a child's preparation for a surgery or procedure?

6. What are some important tips for communicating effectively with children about procedures?

7. Name two ways health-care providers can support children during an emergent procedure.

8. How can technology be used to prepare children for medical encounters?

9. What techniques would be most appropriate for preparing an adolescent for an invasive procedure?

References

Aguirre, R. T., & Slater, H. (2010). Suicide postvention as suicide prevention: Improvement and expansion in the United States. *Death Studies, 34*(6), 529–540.

Bailey, K. M., Bird, S. J., McGrath, P. J., & Chorney, J. E. (2015). Preparing parents to be present for their child's anesthesia induction: A randomized controlled trial. *Anesthesia & Analgesia, 121*(4), 1001–1010.

Berk, L. E., & Myers, A. B. (2015). *Infants and children: Prenatal through middle childhood* (8th ed.). New York, NY: Pearson Education, Inc.

Blount, R. L., Piira, T., & Cohen, L. L. (2003). Management of pediatric pain and distress due to medical procedures. In M. C. Roberts (Ed.). *Handbook of pediatric psychology* (3rd ed., pp. 216–233). New York, NY: Guilford Press.

Boles, J. C. (2013). Speaking up for children undergoing procedures: The ONE VOICE approach. *Pediatric Nursing, 39*(5), 257–259.

Brewer, S., Gleditsch, S. L., Syblik, S., Tietjens, M. E., & Vacik, H. W. (2006). Pediatric anxiety: Child life intervention in day surgery. *Journal of Pediatric Nursing, 21*(1), 13–22.

Bronfenbrenner, U. (1979). *The ecology of human development: Experiments by nature and design.* Cambridge, MA: Harvard University Press.

Campbell, C., Hosey, M. T., & McHugh, S. (2005). Facilitating coping behavior in children prior to dental general anesthesia: A randomized controlled trial. *Pediatric Anesthesia, 15,* 831–838.

Carver, C. S., & Connor-Smith, J. (2010). Personality and coping. *Annual Review of Psychology, 61,* 679–704.

Chahal N., Manlhiot, C., Colapinto, K., Van Alphen, J., McCrindle, B. W., & Rush, J. (2009). Association between parental anxiety and compliance with preoperative requirements for pediatric outpatient surgery. *Journal of Pediatric Health Care, 23,* 372–377.

Claar, R. L., Walker, L. S., & Smith, C. A. (2002). The influence of appraisals in understanding children's experiences with medical procedures. *Journal of Pediatric Psychology, 27*(7), 553–563.

Clutter, L. B., Hess, C., Nix, K. S., Ogle, M. B., Rollins, J., Smith, D., … Wong, D. (1988). Communicating effectively with older children and adolescents. *Children's Nurse, 6*(1), 4, 6, 8.

Clutter, L., Hess, C., Nix, K., Rollins, J., Smith, D., Stevens, N., & Wong, D. (1987). Communicating effectively with young children. *Children's Nurse, 5*(4), 1–3.

Cuzzocrea, F., Gugliandolo, M. C., Larcan, R., Romeo, C., Turiaco, N., & Dominici, T. (2013). A psychological preoperative program: Effects on anxiety and cooperative behaviors. *Pediatric Anesthesia, 23,* 139–143.

Davidson, A. J., Shrivastava, P. P., Jamsen, K., Huang, G. H., Czarnecki, C., Gibson, M. A., Stewart, S. A., & Stargatt, R. (2006). Risk factors for anxiety at induction of anesthesia in children: A prospective cohort study. *Pediatric Anesthesia, 16,* 919–927.

Erikson, E. (1950). *Childhood and society.* New York, NY: Norton.

Felder-Puig, R., Maksys, A., Noestlinger, C., Gadner, H., Stark, H., Pfluegler, A., & Topf, R. (2003). Using a children's book to prepare children and parents for elective ENT surgery: Results of a randomized clinical trial. *International Journal of Pediatric Otorhinolaryngology, 67*(1), 35–41.

Fernandes, S.C., Arriaga, P., & Esteves, F. (2014). Providing preoperative information for children undergoing surgery: A randomized study testing different types of educational material to reduce children's preoperative worries. *Health Education Research, 29*(6), 1058–1076.

Fincher, W., Shaw, J., & Ramelet, A. (2012). The effectiveness of a standardized preoperative preparation in reducing child and parent anxiety: A single-blind randomized controlled trial. *Journal of Clinical Nursing, 21,* 946–955.

Folkman, S. (1997). Positive psychological states and coping with severe stress. *Social Science & Medicine, 45,* 1207–1221.

Fortier, M. A., Bunzli, E., Walthall, J., Olshansky, E., Saadat, H., Santistevan, R., Mayes, L., & Kain, Z. V. (2015). Web-based tailored intervention for preparation of parents and children for outpatient surgery (WebTIPS): Formative evaluation and randomized controlled trial. *Anesthesia & Analgesia, 120*(4), 915–922.

Fortier, M. A., Chroney, J. M., Rony, R. Y., Perret-Karimi, D., Rinehart, J. B., Camiloon, F. S., & Kain, Z. N. (2009). Children's desire for preoperative information. *Anesthesia & Analgesia, 109*(4), 1085–1090.

Fortier, M. A., Del Rosario, A. M., Martin, S. R., & Kain, Z. N. (2010). Perioperative anxiety in children. *Pediatric Anesthesia, 20*, 318–322.

Franck, L. S., Wray, J., Gay, C., Dearmun, A. K., Lee, K., & Cooper, B. A. (2015). Predictors of parent post-traumatic stress symptoms after child hospitalization on general pediatric wards: A prospective cohort study. *International Journal of Nursing Studies, 52*, 20–21.

Gaynard, L., Wolfer, J., Goldberger, J., Thompson, R., Redburn, L., & Laidley, L. (1990). *Psychosocial care of children in hospitals: A clinical practice manual.* Bethesda, MD: Association for the Care of Children's Health.

Grimshaw, J. M., Eccles, M. P., Lavis, J. N., Hill, S. J., & Squires, J. E. (2012). Knowledge translation of research findings. *Implementation Science, 50*(7), 1–17.

Gutnick, A. L., Robb, M., Takeuchi, L., & Kotler, J. (2012). *Always connected: The new digital media habits of young children.* The Joan Ganz Cooney Center at Sesame Workshop. Retrieved from http://www.joanganzcooneycenter.org/upload_kits/jgcc_alwaysconnected.pdf

Jaaniste, T., Hayes, B., & van Baeyer, C. L. (2007). Providing children with information about forthcoming medical procedures: A review and synthesis. *Clinical Psychology Science and Practice, 14*, 124–143.

Janis, I. (1958). *Psychologic stress: Psychoanalytic and behavioral studies of surgical patients.* New York: Wiley.

Justus, R., Wilson, J., Walther, V., Wyles, D., Rode, D., & Lim-Sulit, N. (2006). Preparing children and families for surgery: Mount Sinai's multidisciplinary perspective. *Pediatric Nursing, 32*(1), 35–43.

Kain, Z. N., & Caldwell-Andrews, A. (2005). Preoperative psychological preparation of the child for surgery: An update. *Anesthesiology Clinics of North America, 23*, 597–614.

Kain, Z. N., Caldwell-Andrews, A. A., Krivutza, D. M., Weinberg, M. E., Wang, S-M., & Gaal, D. (2004). Trends in the practice of parental presence during induction of anesthesia and the use of pre-operative sedation premedication in the United States, 1995–2002: Results of a national follow up survey. *Pediatric Anesthesia, 98*, 1252–1259.

Kain, Z. N., Caldwell-Andrews, A. A., Mayes, L. C., Weinberg, M. E., Wang, S., McLaren, J. E., & Blount, R. L. (2007). Family-centered preparation for surgery improves perioperative outcomes in children: A randomized controlled trial. *Anesthesiology, 106*, 65–74.

Kain, Z. N., Caldwell-Andrews, A., & Wang, S. (2002). Psychological preparation of the parent and pediatric surgical patient. *Anesthesiology Clinics of North America, 20*(1), 29–44.

Kain, Z. V., Fortier, M. A. Chorney, J. M., & Mayes, L. (2015). Web-based tailored intervention for preparation of parents and children for outpatient surgery (WebTIPS): Development. *Anesthesia & Analgesia, 120*(4), 905–914.

Kain, Z. N., Mayes, L. C., Caldwell-Andrews, A. A., Karas, D. E., & McClain, B. C. (2006). Preoperative anxiety, postoperative pain, and behavioral recovery in young children undergoing surgery. *Pediatrics, 118*(2), 651–658.

Kain, Z. N., Mayes, L., Wang, S., & Hofstadter, M. B. (1999). Postoperative behavioral outcomes in children: Effects of sedative premedication. *Anesthesiology, 90*(3), 758–765.

Krauss, B., & Green, S. (2006). Procedural sedation and analgesia in children. *Lancet, 367*(9512), 766–780.

Lazarus, R. (1966). *Psychological stress and the coping process.* New York, NY: McGraw-Hill.

Lazarus, R. (1981). The costs and benefits of denial. In J. Spinetta & P. Deasy-Spitta (Eds.), *Living with childhood cancer* (pp. 50–67). St. Louis, MO: Mosby.

Lazarus, R., & Folkman, S. (1984). *Stress, appraisal, and coping.* New York, NY: Springer.

Lee, J., Lee, J., Lim, H., Son, J., Lee, J., Kim, D., & Ko, S. (2012). Cartoon distraction alleviates anxiety in children during induction of anesthesia. *Anesthesia & Analgesia, 115*(5), 1168–1173.

Li, H. C., & Lopez, V. (2007). Effectiveness and appropriateness of therapeutic play intervention in preparing children for surgery: A randomized controlled trial study. *Journal for Specialists in Pediatric Nursing, 13*(2), 63–73.

Li, H. C., Lopez, V., & Lee, T. L. (2006). Psychoeducational preparation of children for surgery: The importance of parental involvement. *Patient Education and Counseling, 65,* 34–41.

Li, W. H., Chan, S. S., Wong, E. M., & Lee, I. T. (2014). Effect of therapeutic play on pre- and post-operative anxiety and emotional responses in Hong Kong Chinese children: A randomized controlled trial. *Hong Kong Medical Journal, 20*(Suppl 7), S36-39.

MacLaren, J., & Kain, Z. N. (2007). Pediatric preoperative preparation: A call for evidence-based practice. *Pediatric Anesthesia, 17,* 1019–1020.

MacLaren, J. E., Thompson, C., Weinberg, M., Fortier, M. A., Morrison, D. E., Perret, D., & Kain, Z. N. (2009). Prediction of preoperative anxiety in children: Who is most accurate? *Anesthesia & Analgesia, 108*(6), 1777–1782.

Mahat, G., Scoloveno, M. A., & Cannell, B. (2004). Comparison of children's fears of medical experiences across two cultures. *Journal of Pediatric Health Care, 18,* 302–307.

McCubbin, H. I., & Patterson, J. M. (1983). Family transitions: Adaptation to stress. In H. I. McCubbin & C. R. Figley (Eds.), *Stress and the family: Coping with normative transitions* (Vol. 1, pp. 5–25). Oxon, England: Routledge.

McEwen, A., Moorthy, C., Quantock, C., Rose, H., & Kavanagh, R. (2007). The effect of videotaped preoperative information on parental anxiety during anesthesia induction for elective pediatric procedures. *Pediatric Anesthesia, 17,* 534–539.

McGuigan, F., & Salmon, K. (2005). Pre-event discussion and recall of a novel event: How are children best prepared? *Journal of Experimental Child Psychology, 91,* 342–366.

Melamed, B. G., & Siegel, L. J. (1975). Reduction of anxiety in children facing hospitalization by use of filmed modeling. *Journal of Consulting and Clinical Psychology, 43,* 511–521.

Melnyk, B., Small, L., & Carno, M. (2004). The effectiveness of parent-focused interventions in improving coping/mental health outcomes of critically ill children and their parents: An evidence base to guide clinical practice. *Pediatric Nursing, 30,* 143–148.

Morling, B., & Evered, S. (2006). Secondary control reviewed and defined. *Psychology Bulletin, 132,* 269–296.

Morris, Z. S., Wooding, S., & Grant, J. (2011). The answer is 17 years, what is the question: Understanding time lags in translational research. *Journal of the Royal Society of Medicine, 104*(12), 510–520.

Ono, S., Hirabayashi, Y., Oikawa, I., & Manabe, Y. (2008). Preparation of a picture book to support parents and autonomy in preschool children facing day surgery. *Pediatric Nursing, 34*(1), 82–88.

Perry, J. N., Hooper, V. D., & Masiongale, J. (2012). Reduction of preoperative anxiety in pediatric surgery patients using age-appropriate teaching interventions. *Journal of PeriAnesthesia Nursing, 27*(2), 69–81.

Petrillo, M. (1972). Preparing children and parents for hospitalization and treatment. *Pediatric Annals, 1*(3), 24–41.

Piaget, J. (1967). *Six psychological studies.* New York, NY: Random House.

Piira, T., Sugiura, T., Champion, G. D., Donnelly, N., & Cole, A. S. (2005). The role of parental presence in the context of children's medical procedures: A systemic review. *Child: Care, Health, and Development, 31,* 233–243.

Rice, M., Glasper, A., Keeton, D., & Spargo, P. (2008). The effect of a preoperative education programme on perioperative anxiety in children: An observational study. *Pediatric Anesthesia, 18,* 426–430.

Rogoff, B. (2003). *The cultural nature of human development.* New York, NY: Oxford University Press.

Roth, S., & Cohen, L. J. (1986). Approach, avoidance, and coping with stress. *American Psychologist*, *41*, 813–819.

Salmon, K., McGuigan, F., & Pereira, J. K. (2006). Brief report: Optimizing children's memory and management of an invasive medical procedure: The influence of procedural narration and distraction. *Journal of Pediatric Psychology*, *31*(5), 522–527.

Seiden, S., McMullan, S., Sequera-Ramos, L., De Olvieira, G., Roth, A., Rosenblatt, A., … Suresh, S. (2014). Tablet-based interactive distraction (TBID) vs. oral midazolam to minimize perioperative anxiety in pediatric patients: A noninferiority randomized trial. *Pediatric Anesthesia*, *24*, 1217–1223.

Selye, H. (1974). *Stress without distress.* New York, NY: The New American Library.

Shah, N. (2011). Special education pupils find learning tool in iPad applications. *Education Weekly*, *30*(22), 16-17.

Stanford, G., & Thompson, R. (1981). *Child life in hospitals: Theory and practice.* Springfield, IL: Thomas.

Stargatt, R., Davidson, A. J., Huang, G. H., Czarnecki, C., Gibson, M. A., Stewart, S. A., & Jamsen, K. (2006). A cohort study of the incidence and risk factors for negative behavior changes in children after general anesthesia. *Pediatric Anesthesia*, *16*, 846-859.

Stephens, B. K., Barkey, M. E., & Hall, H. R. (1999). Techniques to comfort children during stressful procedures. *Accident and Emergency Nursing*, *7*(4), 226–236.

Thoits, P. A. (2010). Stress and health: Major findings and policy implications. *Health and Social Behavior*, *51*(S), S41-S53.

Vaughn, G. F. (1957). Children in hospital. *The Lancet*, *272*(2), 1117–1120.

Wagers, D. (2013). *One voice.* Retrieved from http://www.onevoice4kids.com/.

Wakimizu, R., Kamagata, S., Kuwabara, T., & Kamibeppu, K. (2009). A randomized controlled trial of an at-home preparation program for Japanese preschool children: Effects on children's and caregivers' anxiety associated with surgery. *Journal of Evaluation in Clinical Practice*, *15*, 393–401.

Wakimizu, R., Ozeki, S., & Kamibeppu, K. (2005). Psychological upset and its related factors of children after leaving hospital from undergoing minor surgery. *Journal of Japan Academy of Nursing Science*, *25*(3), 75-82.

Weenstrom, B., Hallberg, L. R., & Bergh, I. (2008). Use of perioperative dialogues with children undergoing day surgery. *Journal of Advanced Nursing*, *62*(1), 96–106.

Wolfer, J. A., & Visintainer, M. A. (1975). Pediatric surgical patients' and parents' stress responses and adjustment. *Nursing Research*, *24*(4), 244–255.

Wright, K. D., Stewart, S. H., Finley, G. A., & Buffett-Jerrott, S. E. (2007). Prevention and intervention strategies to alleviate preoperative anxiety in children: A critical review. *Behavior Modification*, *31*(1), 52-79.

Yip, P., Middleton, P., Cyna, A. M., & Carlyle, A. V. (2009). Non-pharmacological interventions for assisting the induction of anesthesia in children. *Cochrane Database of Systematic Reviews*, *Jul 8*(3).

3 Play in Children's Health-Care Settings

Rosemary Bolig

Objectives

At the conclusion of this chapter, the reader will be able to:

1. Discuss the importance of play to development and coping with stress and challenges.
2. Indicate the values of play in health-care settings for children at various stages of development and with different illnesses.
3. Describe the factors that have influenced the amount and types of play facilitated in health-care settings.
4. Review current and future challenges to play and play facilitation in child health-care settings.
5. List questions for further study of play in health-care settings.

Since the earliest recognition of the negative impact of institutionalization and hospitalization on young children, play and the relationships that ensue have been among the primary prescribed antidotes. For example, in 1940 Richards & Wolff wrote:

> Through play a child grows, develops, expresses his emotions, and adjusts to his environment. Play becomes a safety valve for his hidden wishes and fears and a balance for the tensions that are a part of every growing child's life. Ill or well, the child needs play. (p. 229)

The dosage of play and the processes and procedures for ensuring its quality, however, are often debated (Turner & Brown, 2014). But those who advocate for and/or provide psychosocial care—whether in nursing, pediatric psychology, and occupational therapy contexts, or in specialized play, activities, or education programs (e.g., child life in North America)—agree that play is critical for children's expression, mastery, and learning about their experiences.

Health care and health-care settings have changed dramatically since the early recognition of the unique needs of children, including perceptions of and provisions for play in such experiences and environments. More recently—especially in its normative and unstructured forms—play appears to be less prevalent and perhaps less valued than it was in earlier efforts to ameliorate the psychosocial impacts of hospitalization and illness. The topic of play receives less attention in health-care journals, and, since the late 1980s, fewer researchers were studying play in health care or conducting basic and quantitative research on play in other contexts—until recently (Johnson, 2015b; Koller, 2008; Liddle, 2014).

However, despite the pressures for less play in school settings and the overstructuring of children's after-school time, there appears to be a reawakening to the values of play. For example, mental health has been found to be related to the quantity and quality of play—particularly unstructured or "free" play. The increased concern about the mental health of young children has raised interest in a return to less structure and academic pressure and more play (Gray, 2010).

Change is inevitable, of course, and the failure of systems and organisms to adapt results in decline if not extinction. Health-care systems and specific programs and disciplines supporting play have also changed with the demands of the times (Child Life Council, 2013, 2015; Wilson, 2014; Wilson & Chambers, 1996). In fact, in 2016 the Child Life Council changed its name to Association of Child Life Professionals to better reflect what child life specialists are and what they do. The addition of "professionals" in the organization's name makes a strong and clear statement to people outside the membership and those in traditional settings who may not understand the term *child life*.

But just as health-care professionals serving children must acknowledge that children are unique and different from adults, they must continue to articulate that play is the primary means for children to develop and to cope with life's demands. Pioneers in changing health-care practices for children and their families—researchers such as Robertson (1958) and practitioners such as Plank (1962)—fought against prevailing beliefs about children and systems of care. Now, with over 100 years of experience and research since the earliest establishment of play provisions for children in hospitals, the expanding body of knowledge about mind–body interactions, and the recognition of the bio-psychosocial model of health care (Borrell-Carrio, 2004), positions about the uniqueness of children in general, as well as children in health-care settings—and hence play—are again *in play*. Koller (2008) reasserts that play is the essence of child life practice in her review of the relevant play research, as does Liddle (2014) in her update.

Children *are* different from adults, and childhood is very brief. Experiences that *do not* occur within specific time ranges may have as much impact on the course of development as those that do occur; the manner in which experiences happen also may have short- as well as long-term effects. In many instances, an experience's effect cannot be determined for months, if not years. What appears to be a short-term gain may instead cause long-term pain. Children may be more resilient than once believed, but they also may be more vulnerable in ways that are only beginning to be understood. For example, brain research on children suggests that there are a finite number of years in which neurons must be used or connected to one another and that stress and constant threats can rewire emotion circuits: The more this aberrant pathway is used, the easier it is to trigger (Eluvathingal et al., 2006). A continual high-alert state affects cortex development, and thus children have trouble assimilating complex information such as language. An early study by Quinton and Rutter (1976), for example, found significant reading problems among children with repetitive hospitalizations, which Eluvathingal and colleagues' research may explain.

Children also bring to health care, as they do to other settings, their unique experiences and family situations—and new risks and opportunities (Halfon, Wise, & Forrest, 2014). Nevertheless, they need to be nurtured, supported, and protected from overwhelming anxiety and stimulation. They are neither more adaptive than previous generations, just because they seemingly have more to adapt to, nor are they simply "information processors" that emerging views of them may assert (Elkind, 2007). They are children who, like Kasey, a young child who child life specialist Debbie Kossoff (1996) so poignantly described in a tribute in *The Advocate*, need the reassurance and safety that play environments and facilitators provide:

> When I would appear, she would always ask to go to the playroom in her wagon. . . . At the end of her life, once we were all in the playroom, Kasey expressed an interest in creating a card using the materials I had prepared earlier for Secretary Day. Kasey always enjoyed participating in planned art projects during her hospital visits, but on this day she did not make a card for a secretary. Instead, she asked me to fill the card with love messages for her mommy, auntie, sister, uncle, daddy, and teacher and others important to her. Kasey's younger sister helped with the finishing touches by putting stickers on the card for decoration. When the cards were completed, we moved Kasey and her wagon into the middle of the room, and sat around her in a circle of love, comfort, and support and waited for the inevitable to occur (p. 29) .

Play, for Kasey, even in the last moments of her life, provided the means for solace, communicating, interpreting, and perhaps regulating events around her.

This chapter reviews what play is and is not, the functions and forms of play, the present state of theory and research on play, and the current thinking of play researchers in health care. Related contexts will be presented, as will contexts for facilitating play. We will explore multiple, interacting factors that often have very little to do with the unique nature of children or their needs, but that influence the perceived importance of play (e.g., standards movement and testing, early academic achievement). We will describe the growing body of research on play and play-based programs, especially in health-care settings, which is vital for its revival and perhaps its survival (Carlisle, 2009; Johnson, 2015a, b; Power, 2000; Thompson, 2009). Beyond this imperative for data-based information on play, and particularly for applied *evidence-based practice* in health care, there are other systems, beliefs, and attitudes toward children to consider in response to continuous challenges and demands in health care, technology, family life, and society in general. Such factors can encourage or restrict the conditions that support children's play (Frost, 2010; Nicolapoulous, 2010). Although most disciplines in pediatric health care support and use play to some degree, this chapter's focus is organized play and activities programs.

Play in Psychology, Education, and Anthropology

Play is a, if not *the*, quintessential behavior of childhood (see Figure 3.1). Since the 1920s, play has been of significant research interest and the subject of much debate.

Power (2000) reported that the research interest in play was at its height in the 1970s and waned until the late 1990s, when research interest began again. But recently, Johnson (2015a, 2015b) reported on an unprecedented public and academic interest in play—just as the amount of time children engage in play is decreasing. Various waves of research have occurred, which include determining ways to investigate play, training studies, correlational investigations of categories of play, and qualitative studies (Fein, 1997). Today, according to Johnson (2015a, p. xiii):

> Play studies assure that one can learn more about play from many different angles, rather than one vantage point. One learns and is informed by studying play using numerous tools—biological, philosophical, sociological, etc. Across disciplines one can see differences in research, methods, prescriptions and biases. Diverse disciplines sometimes complement each other in the study of play and always inform each other.

Play Perspectives

First and foremost, play is fun, joyful. Playfulness is within children's control and imagination. Therefore, it is not surprising that throughout recorded history play has been a metaphor for *freedom* and even for *power* (Sutton-Smith, 2009). Play frightens some and appears frivolous to others. Particularly in U.S. culture, play tends to be seen as diverting from, interfering with, or subverting more purposeful activity. Sometimes play is thought to decrease motivation. Play appears to be too random, too pleasurable, too self-serving to be channeled toward any important function. Play also gives control to children, making some adults feel out of control. When the lives of adults are chaotic, the adults often impose structure on children, with play often being one of the first behaviors to suffer (Alliance for Childhood, 2010).

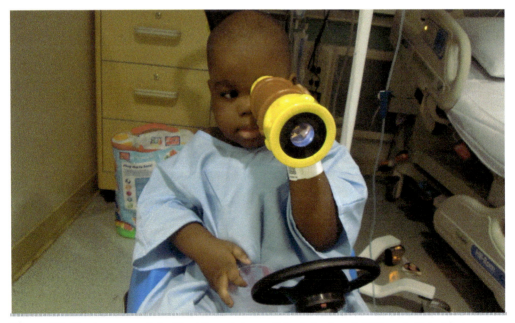

Figure 3.1. Play is an essential—if not the quintessential—behavior of childhood. *Note.* Photo courtesy of Jessica Uze.

With the changes that have occurred in the United States through demographic shifts, immigration or migration, wars, and technology, and the concurrent feelings of optimism and lack of control associated with play, it is not surprising that the belief in play's importance has often diminished in lieu of more direct means of socializing, educating, and effecting the growth and development of children. In the early part of the 20th century, for example, members of the child study movement fought back against the establishment of the highly structured Froebelian kindergarten and Montessori programs. Despite their contrast to prevailing teaching practices in their countries of origin, these methods were not as child-centered or truly play-oriented as the child study adherents would have liked. But by the rapidly changing 1960s (an out-of-control period, in the opinions of some), with the increased demand for child care, the Montessori approach was accepted, albeit adapted for this country. Behavioral theories with token economies and reinforcement schedules in education also were widely accepted in the 1960s and 1970s.

Public education systems are constantly being buffeted by these changes in perspective on how children develop and learn (Glickman, 1988). The No Child Left Behind Act and subsequent changes, including a standards-based curriculum, have had adverse effects on young children's play (Trawick-Smith, 2009). Newer legislation—the Every Student Succeeds Act (ESSA) (Camera, 2015)—has returned more control to the states and may provide for more flexibility in standards and outcomes; some forms of play may regain status (e.g., recess, socio-dramatic play).

Theory

Even the development of theory and research is not immune from societal forces. Products of their times, theorists reflect the prevailing viewpoints, values, expectations, and "knowledge" and, in turn, affect their times. Various views or paradigms have influenced not only the development of theories about human (and nonhuman) growth and development but—because play has long been recognized as a typical behavior of children—also play theory. Early theories or classical theories included explanations of play as means for discharging natural energy (Spencer, 1870/1951); renewing energy (Patrick, 1916); reliving periods of history of the human species (Hall, 1904); and practicing for adulthood (Groos, 1901).

All these early theories have had some influence on current theories about play. By the 1930s, psychoanalytic theory began to dominate views of human development, with Freud's (1952) psychosexual theory and Erikson's (1950/1963, 1972) psychosocial theory predominant in shaping the understanding of play's critical importance. By the 1960s, cognitive theory, especially the work of Piaget (1962) and Vygotsky (1978), influenced both beliefs about cognition and play's roles and the degree of centrality of adults in the learning processes.

More recent perspectives on play include concepts and theories of competence motivation, arousal-seeking, and self-regulation. For example, competence motivation theory posits that children receive satisfaction in developing competency via play, regardless of whether there are any external rewards. According to Spodek and Saracho (1988, p. 15), "play enables children to act on their environment, becoming more effective and thus receiving personal satisfaction." Arousal-seeking theory states that children need to be continually involved in information processing but that play is the way children mediate the amount of stimulation in order to achieve an optimal level of arousal. Self-regulation, in particular, is one aspect of biological theory currently under investigation (Burghart, 2005). Also, theory-of-mind research has found that pretense play is related to more complex thought (Bodrouz & Leong, 2015; Lillard et al., 2013).

The complexity of what play is may make it difficult to align these theories into a coherent or comprehensive theory-to-practice framework. However, Hendricks (2015a) has proposed a general theory of play based on the basic concept of strategies of self-realization: adaption, integration, patterns maintained, and goal attainment.

Play Themes

Throughout the years and across disciplines, play has been viewed through various lenses, with resultant perspectives that have affected the nature of scholarly inquiry as well as practice. According to Sutton-Smith (1995, pp. 279–291), these perspectives revolve around five themes:

- *Play as Progress*—Scholars in the 20th century were obsessed to demonstrate that children learn something useful from their play; although this continues today, the specific focus has shifted from physical skills, to emotional, to cognitive, depending on prevalent theories.
- *Play as Adaptation*—A curvilinear relationship has been found between play participation and general adaptation. Those children who do not get to play with others because they are too withdrawn or aggressive generally also perform poorly at school.
- *Play as Power*—Often more common among historians, sociologists, and anthropologists, this conceptualization of play concerns concepts of contest, conflict, group identity, and traditions. Psychologists, too, often deal with this in terms of intrinsic motivation, autotelia, stimulus arousal, and free choice or free will.
- *Play as Fantasy*—A relatively recent area of inquiry, play as imagination, creativity, and flexibility focuses on the importance of the individual. Imaginative play, often seen as higher order, has been found to be related to reading and other academic areas of ability.
- *The Play of Self*—Play is increasingly cited as an optimal experience or peak experience. Csikszentmihalyi (1990) describes play as the subjective experience that integrates all of learning and capacities of the individual, in much the same way that the state of "flow" does for adults. He did not however consider the ideas of play as prevention or play as healing, although they are embedded in psychodynamic theory. This orientation is increasingly being investigated with even a connection to health or wellness (Almquist, Hellnas, Stefansson, & Granlund, 2006).

Functions of Play

Play has been viewed as serving multiple, often overlapping functions, depending on the theoretical perspective or discipline (see Text Box 3.1 and Text Box 3.2). Among educators, for example, play is thought to have the functions of teaching about the world and providing experiences with symbolic possibilities. According to the National Association for the Education of Young Children (Copple & Bradekamp, 2009, p. 4):

> There are many different kinds of play . . . offering different potential benefits to children. For instance, mature dramatic play . . . contributes significantly to children's self-regulation. . . . And evidence suggests that this higher level play does not unfold substantially on its own.

A more comprehensive list of functions includes social, cultural, and emotional functions as well. Play provides a means to do the following:

- express and represent concepts and feelings
- integrate and deal with emotions
- resolve conflicts in a microsphere
- expand imagination and fantasy
- express in fantasy what is unacceptable in reality
- ingest experiences through repetition and transformation
- become empowered
- build competence

Text Box 3.1
Rethinking Children's Play

By Diane E. Levin, PhD

Has something changed in society and childhood in recent years that is affecting play? Is there really cause for concern and, if so, what can the adults who care for children do about it? Why is play important? Play is vital to most aspects of children's social, emotional, and intellectual development and academic learning. It is one of the most powerful vehicles children have for trying out and mastering new skills, concepts, and experiences. Play can help children develop the knowledge they need to connect in meaningful ways to the challenges they encounter in school—for instance, learning literacy, math, and science, as well as how to interact positively with others. Play also contributes to how children view themselves as learners. As they play, they resolve confusing and disturbing social, emotional, and intellectual issues. They come up with new solutions and ideas and experience the sense of power that comes from being in control and figuring things out on their own (something children often do not get to do in real life). This helps develop a positive attitude toward learning—about how to find interesting problems to work on and how to solve them in creative ways. Play is a dynamic and endlessly diverse process.

Note. From "Rethinking Children's Play," by Diane E. Levin, October 2004. *Our Children, 25,* 8–11. Retrieved from www.pta.org//parentinvolvement/adcouncil/oc_rethinking.asp. Copyright 1999 by Diane Levin. Reprinted with permission.

Text Box 3.2
White Paper #6: The State of Children's Play

Play, in particular, is the special manifestation of freedom in childhood. It is quite common in modern societies to regard the existence of play in childhood as an indication that childhood is proceeding naturally and that, indeed, a child is even working on growing up as he or she plays the roles of parent, teacher, banker or any of the other manifestations of older and more powerful beings. If this isn't happening, or if it is happening in ways that seem different from those of our own childhood, we may be alarmed.

Research on play has established that it has benefits for cognitive, social, and emotional development. Children who are allowed to play with certain materials show evidence of higher creativity and problem-solving ability on related tasks; children allowed to play frequently with others show higher levels of social competence; and giving children an opportunity to play symbolically with upsetting situations enables them to cope more effectively. Janet Lever, a sociologist, found more complexity in the games of boys than girls in later childhood and saw that as advantageous to their development of social and organizational skills. Lynn Barnett, a play specialist, found that preschool children anxious about the start of school who were allowed a period of free play showed decreases in distress while those who listened to stories did not.

The value of play has not been lost on educators. Some have attempted to incorporate play into the curriculum, and through "play training" have even shown the ability to increase a child's creativity and problem solving ability. But one can rightly question the remaining character of play in such situations, when adults have most of the control over the situation. Promoting the values of play without killing the essence of play brings us back to the question of structure. . . .

Note. From "White Paper #6: The State of Children's Play." Retrieved from www.academyof leisuresciences.org/alswp6.html. Copyright by Academy of Leisure Sciences. Reprinted with permission.

- encourage novel and challenging responses
- self-regulate stimuli
- promote positive effect and relaxation
- practice and prepare for a variety of roles
- communicate
- behave with flexibility
- express cultural values and beliefs symbolically
- experience peer culture and cohesion
- experience pleasure and fun
- engage in a neurological imperative

Defining Play

Although opinions differ among child practitioners as to what behaviors constitute play, increasingly most play researchers agree that some of the following criteria must be met. Play must be:

- voluntary
- internally motivated
- pleasurable, relaxed
- "as if" or pretense present
- organism- rather than object-dominated
- unique, unpredictable
- active, both motorically and cognitively

"True" play, or acts and behaviors meeting all these criteria, might be uncommon, and possible only primarily in unstructured or child-directed forms. Reviewing the literature on play in 1983, Rubin, Fein, and Vandenberg found six recurring criteria cited: (a) intrinsic motivation, (b) orientation toward means rather than ends, (c) internal rather than external locus of control, (d) noninstrumental rather than instrumental actions, (e) freedom from externally imposed rules and expectations, and (f) active engagement. However, Smith and Vollstedt (1985) found that trained observers characterize an activity as play when there is a combination of nonliterality, positive affect, and flexibility. More recently, Burghardt (2005) suggested that core behaviors (e.g., means over ends, nonfunctionality) *must* be present for play.

Alternatively, although many child practitioners often label the majority of children's behaviors as "play," *not play* is literal, with intense or neutral affect, inflexible or predictable. But studies of what children define as play have found that it involves the context in which the activity occurs. The single most important factor for kindergartners in one study was whether the activity was voluntary, or who decided on the activity and its goals (King, 1979). Among younger children (3- and 4-year-olds), play was viewed as a personal, ongoing activity (*I Play*), distinct from functional activities such as eating and napping. For first and second graders, Wing (1995) found that in addition to obligatory behavior, the effort required, involvement and evaluation from the teacher, and fun experienced were significant factors in their perception of play/not play.

Categories of Play

Among education researchers, Piaget's (1962) and Smilansky's (1968) classifications of play types have been most influential in studying play. Piaget (1962) distinguished between practice play, symbolic play, and games with rules. Smilansky (1968) elaborated by renaming practice play as "functional play," adding constructive play, naming symbolic play "dramatic," and retaining the category games with rules. Some controversy exists as to whether constructive play is indeed play because it appears to be goal-oriented or product-focused. (Adults, however, are especially likely to view this form of activity as "play.") The other types of play, according to Rubin et al. (1983), are as follows:

- *Functional play*—simple, repetitive muscle movements with or without objects
- *Dramatic play*—substitution of an imaginary situation to satisfy child's personal needs and wishes
- *Games with rules*—acceptance of prearranged rules and adjustments to these rules

More recently, additional types of play are being investigated: physical play, expressive play, manipulative play, symbolic play, dramatic play, familiarization play, games, and surrogate play (Play, in *Encyclopedia of Children's Health*, 2015). Familiarization and surrogate play appear to be of particular interest to health-care experiences and settings. Media play, likewise, is being cited and explored (White, 2012).

In several disciplines, Smilansky's (1968) categories of play have frequently been nested with Parten's (1932) categories of social participation (e.g., unoccupied, solitary, parallel, associative, cooperative), so that play is described as "functional–parallel," for example. Smilansky (1968) and Parten (1932) assumed a developmental, hierarchical sequence to their types of play. However, more recent studies have not found this; for example, constructive play remains steady throughout childhood, as does solitary play. In addition, language play and rough-and-tumble play were not considered by these early theorists and were largely ignored until recently; few of the more recently cited types of play have used this social dimension.

Content, Types, and Forms of Play

Content of play is largely the result of a transaction between children (e.g., their ages, personalities, gender, interpersonal relationships, psychological states) and the environment (e.g., people in it, space, equipment/toys, time) as well as culture (Roopnarine, 2011). *Theme* is another term used to describe play content. Gender differences, as well as age differences, influence the themes in which children most frequently engage. Boys are more likely to engage in themes and roles more distant from the house/home roles of girls, for example. Culture has a profound influence as well, with major differences in parent participation/support, especially in fantasy play (Holmes, 2013).

Types and forms of play are a result of context and content. A variety of typologies, continuums, or polarities have been used to conceptualize and juxtapose different forms of play, for example, the polarity of unstructured–structured play (Delpo & Frick, 1988) and continuum of free play to work (Bergen, 1988). Each of these approaches is an attempt to distinguish forms of play according to a number of criteria, including the degree of adult involvement, choice of objects, nature of intent of play (from adult perspectives), and types of objects, among others (White, 2015).

Research on the Effects of Play

Although specific information about the short-term effects of play exists, there is not as much research on its effect on longer-term development (Pellegrini, 2009a, 2009b; Power, 2000). Questions continue about whether play is a result of development or whether it influences development, but many believe that play both reflects and affects development. Although pretend or symbolic play, especially, has been cited as related to children's healthy development, Lillard et al. (2013) found insufficient causal evidence. There are many explanations for the difficulties in discerning the effects of play—not least of which are that play may be related to *all* aspects of development and that play may interact differently for individuals. Indirect or even sleeper effects of play's quantity and quality and its relationship to cognitive, social, emotional, and physical development may be much more difficult to discern. The lack of specifications for minimal amount or type of play required for normal or typical development or the amount required for optimal development is also an issue, as are definition and measurement (Power, 2000). Pellegrini (2011) and Brown (2014) argued that what is known, however, is what happens if there is *no* play. Children who do not play often are under extreme emotional or physical distress or have cognitive or emotional limitations. This is so even in cultures or families who do not facilitate or value play. Play has been found to be related to creativity, reading ability, and a host of other specific skills. Play seems to cause, at least in the short term, other effects, such as (a) even more play, (b) problem solving, and (c) decreased anxiety (Power, 2000).

However, qualitative and descriptive studies (Hughes, 2010; Johnson, Eberle, Hendricks, & Kuschner, 2015; Schwartzman, 1978) consistently report the following:

- Children play in every human culture, past and present.
- There are vast differences in the amount and types of play, cross-culturally and within cultures.
- Children from less technologically advanced cultures and from lower socioeconomic backgrounds engage in less complex, less frequent, and less sophisticated make-believe play.
- There are distinct differences in the play of children related to gender.
- Play frequency, complexity, and category change with age and experiences.
- Play is related to cognitive, emotional, social, and physical factors.
- Play development is predictable and orderly, yet unique to the situation and to the individual.
- Physical and psychological safety is essential for play to occur.

While the 1970s and 1980s were times of research inquiry into the influence of play in cognitive development, today there is a renewed interest in the social and emotional impact of play (Hendricks, 2015a). And, as noted earlier, there is a resurgence of interest in the academic and advocacy literature on play (Johnson, 2015a, 2015b). This resurgence may be the product of an increased availability of research funding and a growing acceptance of play's validity as a line of inquiry within various disciplines. In the past, play research, like research on love, received little widespread funding support; play researchers had difficulty in obtaining consistent funding, and play research was not always viewed as a valid scientific endeavor. One prominent play researcher recounted his early experience of being denied tenure at a research institution because of his study of play (Johnson, 2015a). In short, there have been waves of research rather than consistent lines of inquiry into the etiology and effects of this "natural" behavior of children in health care, childcare, early education, child development, or child psychology.

But perhaps the tide is changing. With the support of the Walt Disney Foundation, the Child Life Council conducted a survey of play practices in North American child life settings (Vilas, 2014), which found many details about the state of play (as well as barriers). A "play center" with videos and resources has been established as well. There are also plans for further targeted research on play in order to strengthen practice and assess short- and long-term outcomes of different forms of play. And staff skills and preparation to engage in the variety of forms of play will be investigated. The Walt Disney Foundation's support for play research in child life initiative is a commitment to developing a deeper understanding of play—especially for children in health-care contexts.

Today, researchers often view play as an integrative process, the "glue" holding together aspects of being (Hendricks, 2015b). Others are studying play's neurophysiological impact and sources, including self-regulation. Evidence indicates that when children are playing, their heart rates are lower and more variable (as opposed to during exploration, when heart rates are higher and less variable). Also, increasing evidence indicates that larger and longer-term dosages of play, in play-based early childhood education curricula, for example, have long-term positive and more enduring effects on children's self-esteem, interpersonal relationship skills, academic skills, and achievement than do directive or eclectic approaches (Carlsson-Page, McLaughlin, & Almon, 2015; Marcon, 2002; Power, 2000). Thus, while many questions about play remain unanswered, there is renewed vigor and rigor from a variety of play scholars in most disciplines.

Play in Health Care

Play—which in its "pure" form includes initiation of actions by children and control of items, symbols, and roles by children —is regarded as one of the most powerful processes by which children regulate their experiences and environments. The American Academy of Pediatrics (AAP) (2014, p. 16) has stated that "play is essential to the social, emotional, cognitive, and physical well-being of young children." Play has long been a remedy for expressing the feelings of anxiety associated with illness and hospitalization for children (Thompson, 2009). In today's health-care contexts, play, in its various types and forms, continues to be viewed as an important process for children to express their feelings and regain a sense of control and competency. Play's normalization or less structured forms have sometimes been less valued and prevalent than in years past because of changing environments and expectations. Other reasons include less time in acute settings and more intense illnesses and treatments, which make more direct instruction through preparation protocols or medical play seem essential. Therefore, there may be less emphasis on play as a normalizing experience—that is, that play is a comforting, familiar activity involving symbols and signs not related to the illness or hospitalization experience—or on its value for relationship-building (Wilson, 2014). However, a renaissance of interest in hospital play—in all its forms—is being supported by the Association of Child Life Professionals (Koller, 2008; Liddle, 2014; Vilas, 2014).

Specifically, play has an important role in primary and secondary *prevention*, enabling children to integrate experience, emotion, and cognition as experiences are occurring, so that *intervention* is less necessary. As noted above, this normative role has been less frequently cited in the professional literature, even in conceptual or theoretical articles, than in the past. Instead medical play or therapeutic play has been the focus of interest and inquiry.

Advocates and facilitators for children's psychosocial needs in health-care settings have argued cogently and emotionally for the importance of play or play opportunities for children in health-care settings. They have worked diligently to create the affective and physical environments—encompassing time, space, equipment, as well as supportive and, if possible, nonthreatening (psycho)therapeutic relationships with adults—necessary for play to occur in health-care settings (Thompson, 2009). Staff education on the needs of children and families, including the values of play and play as a diagnostic tool, has also been instituted (Po, 1992).

Rather than being concerned primarily with "user-friendly" environments or services, many hospital administrators and boards today recognize the value of providing play and play-focused programs, agreeing with the AAP statement on play programs/child life. As it further matures, the child life profession will require its own body of research and evidence, including play studies of multiple types.

Efforts to establish play-based programs flourished during the 1970s and 1980s, particularly in large teaching or children's hospitals. This period also was a time of rapid medical and surgical advances, when many life-threatening diseases or conditions became less so. Hospitals were transformed by changes in visiting policies and family participation, increased ambulatory care, and new technologies.

By the 1990s, however, expansion and growth of organized play programs slowed in the United States (Bolig, 1990). In child life and nursing services, play—especially in its unstructured forms—began to be challenged by the assertion that structured play and other interventions were more efficient and effective. Spiraling health-care costs, increased reliance on technology, and the lack of a research base for practice of play or play-program practice all interacted in undermining the support for play and organized play-based programs in health-care settings. Managed health care and ever-expanding services in same-day surgery and outpatient care greatly influenced the length of hospitalizations, thus affecting the nature of inpatient care and those using it. Care shifted to ambulatory and home-care settings. Programs and services to families in these contexts generally had not included play, until recently. Child life specialists have expanded organized play-based services in other health-related settings, such as hospice, specialized camps, schools, and funeral homes. Tonkin (2014) reported similar applications of play (and other modalities) in a wider variety of health-related settings in the United Kingdom than in the United States.

In sum, during the past 10 to 15 years, play has often been viewed as less efficient—if not less effective—than other, more direct means of informing children about impending procedures and events, or in reducing anxiety, despite the fact that there is insufficient research to support or refute either position. Some psychosocial advocates and facilitators contend that because children in hospitals are admitted for shorter periods, are sicker, and are subjected to more-intense intrusive procedures than their counterparts of just a few years ago, there is not time for children to become sufficiently acclimated to the environment or to develop the relationships with staff or other children to play, especially spontaneously. Even playing with adult modeling, interaction, or permission-giving is difficult given the constraints cited. Further, children in inpatient environments are sometimes viewed as too ill to play. (Surrogate play, a possible form of play for very ill children, has not yet been adequately studied.)

Without the necessary conditions to foster spontaneous play, facilitators often rely on more direct means of bringing children into contact with the symbols, signs, concepts, and knowledge related to their illness and procedures. Medical play—particularly in its more structured forms—appears more direct and is therefore more valued in acute-care milieus (Bolig, Yolton, & Nissen, 1991). Specific and tailored to the individual, medical play may have greater acceptance in health-care settings because it looks like a "treatment." Until recently, ambulatory settings lacked trained volunteers or professionals or consistent efforts at providing these play opportunities, and even fewer options existed for home care. This too is rapidly changing.

Perspectives on Play in Health-Care Settings

Until the 1970s and 1980s, psychoanalytic theories were used to support and explain the value and functions of play in health-care settings. These theories posit that play reduces anxiety by giving children a sense of control over the world and an acceptable way to express forbidden impulses. As in other environments, by the 1980s cognitive-developmental theories, which view play as a means to facilitate general cognitive development and consolidate previous learning while allowing for the possibility of new learning in a relaxed atmosphere, gained acceptance (Hughes, 2010). More recent theories, such as arousal modulation and neuropsychological theories, have often had a less direct influence on explanations of the value of play or specific practices in health-care settings despite an apparent obvious appeal to those with a physiological aspect to their practice. But this too is changing. Koller (2008) found nine relevant studies using physiological measures; four had been conducted after 2000. In her 2014 update, Liddle found very few additional articles with a physiological outcome. A renewed interest in play and play research creates greater incentive to frame play within the context of recent theories and research. Evidence-based practice, now an essential element of all professions, requires not only systematic assessment of effectiveness but also continuous improvement based on data (Morris, 2015).

Functions of Play in Health-Care Settings

Perspectives by various child health-care practitioners on the functions of play—that is, what play does for children—are highly variable, ranging from diversion and stimulus-reduction to mastery and internalization of control. These differing perspectives, as in other contexts, are a result of training in various disciplines, the timing of training, the types of roles engaged in "playing" with children, and institutional factors (Thompson, 2009).

Over time, however, two theories of play have dominated the thinking of a number of health-care disciplines. Psychoanalytic theory has persisted in influencing beliefs that play is *cathartic* (allowing children to express what they cannot handle rationally), and that through play children can come to master situations or come to grips with pain in reality. Piaget's (1962) cognitive theory and Vygotsky's (1978) socio-cognitive theory added other dimensions in understanding functions of play. According to Piaget (1962), play is the way younger children abstract or assimilate experiences into their existing schema or internal cognitive structures, while Vygotsky (1978) added that play is a process that advances learning.

The American Academy of Pediatrics Committee on Hospital Care (2014, p. 16), in its Child Life Policy Statement, focused on the importance of play:

> Play is an essential component of a child life program and of the child life professional's role. In addition to play's developmentally supportive benefits and as a normalizing activity for children and youth of all ages, it is particularly valuable for children who are anxious or struggling to cope with stressful circumstances. . . .Play in the health care setting is adapted to address unique needs based on developmental level, self-directed interests, medical condition and physical abilities, psychosocial vulnerabilities, and setting (e.g., bedside, playroom, clinic). Play as a therapeutic modality, including health care play or "medical play," has been found to reduce children's emotional distress and help them cope with medical experiences. (See Figure 3.2.)

Therapeutic play, a term associated with play in health-care settings, is play used to prevent psychological injury (Koller, 2008; Vilas, 2014), facilitate emotional and physical well-being (Liddle, 2014), and support continued (normative) development. Therapeutic play aims to

- meet children's ongoing developmental needs;
- help children cope with the unfamiliar hospital environment;
- increase children's understanding of their hospitalization and treatment;
- promote a sense of control, mastery, and positive self-concept;

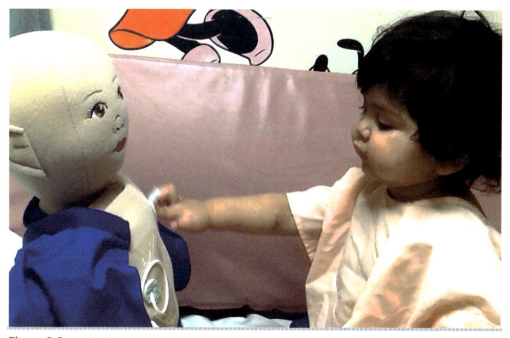

Figure 3.2. Medical play can reduce children's emotional distress and help them cope with medical experiences. *Note.* Photo courtesy of Jessica Uze.

- facilitate self-expression; and
- help children cope with separation and deprivation.

The National Association for Health Play Specialists (NAHPS) in the United Kingdom has further elaborated on the functions of play in hospitals. According to NAHPS (2015), play

- creates an environment where stress and anxiety are reduced;
- helps the child regain confidence and self-esteem;
- provides an outlet for feelings of anger and frustration;
- helps the child understand treatment and illness. Through play, children are able to effectively learn the sensory and concrete information they need to prepare for hospital procedures and treatment;
- aids in assessment and diagnosis; and
- speeds recovery and rehabilitation.

Play as therapy, however, is play to help with alleviating psychosocial injury. According to the Association for Play Therapy, Inc. (2016, p. 2), play therapy is

> the systematic use of a theoretical model to establish an interpersonal process wherein trained play therapists use the therapeutic powers of play to help clients prevent or resolve psychosocial difficulties and achieve optimal growth and development.

Thus, the primary purposes of play in health-care settings are prevention, restoration, and cure. Details regarding these purposes are found in Table 3.1.

Definitions, Types, Content, and Forms of Play in Health Care

In the professional health-care literature, play has been described in various ways—from all and any activities in which children engage to those that have the characteristics cited earlier. This lack of consensus on definition may cause few problems in practice but can cause difficulty in research design, with play defined variously and sometimes not even accurately measured. A consistent definition or description, with subtypes, would be helpful not only for researchers but also for practitioners. Having a standard for play as one process to evaluate when considering outcomes such as length of stay, type or intensity of pain medications, and other similar measures would be beneficial for understanding its particular health/physiological impact.

Types of play in health-care settings include those cited in the previous section, although again, this schema for the description of play has rarely been systematically employed. Descriptions of forms of play have, however, included normative, educative, and therapeutic play (Bolig, 1984). McCue (1988) also discussed various forms and types in health-care settings, specifically medical play. Recently, the Child Life Council's Survey of Play Practices and Innovations (Vilas, 2014) assessed 10 types of play in playrooms and six in clinics, emergency rooms, and other settings in 181 of 464 hospitals in North America (Vilas, 2014). Only medical play was listed as a type of play in all settings.

Table 3.1

Primary Purposes of Play in Health-Care Settings			
	Prevention	Restoration	Cure
Goals	To prevent deterioration, diffusion, regression	To restore after situational distress/imbalance	To cure imbalance as a result of a situation and temperament or personality problems
	To maintain internal sense of control/efficacy	To assess rapidity of return to previous state	
Population	All children	All children	Children who do not respond to restorative play or identified as having emotional problems
	Groups	Small groups	
		Individuals	
Forms of Play	Nondirective	Structured	Structured
	Unstructured	Guided	Directive
Functions of Play	To maintain a sense of control	To express feelings	To express fantasies, anxieties, and defenses through repetition and by developing a relationship with therapist through situation/objects specific to the individual
	To encourage interaction with peers in a familiar setting with objects and materials for age range and individual interests	To obtain mastery through play with objects and roles associated with health-care encounters	

Research on Play in Health-Care Settings

Research on the play of hospitalized or ill children, or in health-care settings, has recently been revitalized. Until the review of research on play in health-care settings (Koller, 2008) and the subsequent Child Life Council (2014) survey of play, most of the research, like that on play in general, was conducted in the late 1960s through the 1980s. Recently, some students in nursing, occupational therapy, child development, and related areas of study have written master's and PhD theses on play in health-care settings, and a few conceptual or theory articles. During the late 1980s through the mid-2000s, research on children's responses to health-care encounters focused on individual variation in responses to specific illnesses or disabilities. Articles have focused on the play-related concerns of specific groups of children, such as those with leukemia, receiving bone marrow transplants, or in palliative care (Gariepy & Howe, 2003; Kuntz et al., 1996). Regarding play in home care, Clark (2003) found that playful rituals or games known as *imaginal coping*—children's capacity to playfully reinterpret experiences—reduced required treatments and symptoms in home care.

A primary method of achieving the goals of health-care play and activities programs is termed *child life* in the United States (Child Life Council, 2015; Koller, 2008). Play has been studied in child life contexts or used as either a dependent or independent variable infrequently, except in more recent medical-play studies. Instead, researchers have studied play in its directive or nondirective forms within nursing care or in specific therapeutic contexts as a mediating variable. Among nursing staff, play also is viewed as the primary method of determining children's psychosocial state (Po, 1992). The general goals of these play studies have been to improve the way knowledge about impending procedures is imparted and to reduce anxiety (e.g., via therapeutic play or play therapy). Findings indicate that short-term (e.g., one-shot, 30-minute) forms of play in nursing-care contexts generally have been significant in reducing anxiety, although methodology and interpretation of some of the results have been a concern (Phillips, 1988). No studies, however, have determined whether play behaviors or anxiety reduction via play specifically—either in play and activities programs, nursing-care contexts, or occupational therapy—are related to posthospital or treatment behaviors or later adjustment (Thompson, 1985, 1995, 2009).

A few studies have examined play in child life outpatient play and activities programs. Perhaps because outpatient settings are less complex and the children focused on more limited activities for shorter periods of time, serious empirical inquiry is viewed as less complex to conduct. Alternatively, inpatient play and activities programs vary widely in objectives and methods or "curricula." Programs vary from those that are diversionary to those that are therapeutic (Bolig, 1984, 1988; Thompson, 2009), although McCue (2009) argued for additional types, including psycho-therapeutic. Because programs also vary in the extent to which playrooms are the focus for activities, play, preparation, and relationships; the consistency with which staff are available; the educational backgrounds of staff; and the ratio of staff to children, comparative studies are more complex to conduct. Additional factors affecting complexity of description and comparison of programs and play outcomes are (a) age ranges of the children served, (b) variations in the types of illness represented, (c) the equipment and play materials available, and (d) the quality of relationships (Thompson, 2009). All of these variables have been found to be important predictors of variations in programs and of program outcomes in other settings involving children (Frost, Wortham, & Reifel, 2007).

Much research on play in the hospital in the late 1960s through the late 1980s focused on the disruption of play in hospitalized children, aggression in play, and the choice of play materials used by hospitalized children in relation to their anxiety levels. Data on the disruption of play indicate that the hospital environment, at least temporarily, alters the patterns of play of hospitalized youngsters (Cataldo, Bessman, Parker, Pearson & Rogers, 1979; Tisza, Hurwitz, & Angoff, 1970). Findings from a study on aggression in play indicate no increase in aggressive play behaviors with either hospitalization in general or with surgery (Vredevoe, Kim, Dambacher, & Call, 1969). Gilmore (1966) studied the selection of play materials of children suffering from anxiety related to hospitalization. On the whole, research indicates that children who are neither highly anxious nor highly defensive often will select toys that are relevant to their particular situation. Children presented with choices will select hospital play materials if they are not too frightened; the most highly anxious children are least likely to select such toys if they are in a free-play situation. But the presence of an adult can modify this response and help children feel more comfortable with anxiety-producing materials (Bolig, 1992).

A few studies have focused on play interventions and their relationship to children's play behaviors in outpatient settings (Cataldo et al., 1979; Ispa, Barrett, & Kim, 1988; Pearson, Cataldo, Turemen, Bessman, & Rogers, 1980; Williams & Powell, 1980), while others have investigated the effect of play therapy or information and educative play on children's anxiety. More recent inquiry has focused on physiological stress indicators of anxiety and whether the use of virtual reality truly represents play (Li & Lopez, 2008).

Studies focusing on play interventions have found that short supervised play sessions with materials related or unrelated to the medical setting may help children to cope more effectively with hospitalization (e.g., Clatworthy, 1981; Lockwood, 1970; Schwartz, Albino, & Tedesco, 1983). One experimental study, using a control group, examined a nurse's use of medical play with a doll and hospital equipment; results indicated that although the doll play did not reduce children's stress scores, anxiety-defense scores of the experimental group were found to be significantly lower after engaging in the play session (Lockwood, 1970). Clatworthy's (1981) experimental study also investigated the effect of play interventions on anxiety levels. The control group children were found to be more anxious at the final evaluation than were children in the experimental group. However, play intervention did not serve to decrease children's anxiety levels over the course of hospitalization. Instead, the control group children evidenced increased anxiety levels over the course of hospitalization, whereas the experimental group's anxiety levels held constant.

Rae, Worchel, Upchurch, Sanner, and Daniel (1989) found that short sessions of therapeutic play (i.e., nondirective but reflective and interpretative with symbolic objects) were significantly more effective in reducing the self-reported fears of children ages 5 through 12 than diversionary play, verbal support, or no treatment. In a study of latency-age youngsters hospitalized for a minimum of 10 days, Fosson, Martin, and Haley (1990) presented them with a single 30-minute session with medical play or a control of television viewing with the investigator. Findings included a decline in anxiety in both groups, from admission to discharge; although not significant, a greater decline occurred among those children in the medical playgroup.

Schwartz et al. (1983) found in an experimental study that an opportunity to play under the supervision of a supportive adult—whether the play materials were related to the source of stress or not—was somewhat effective in altering children's manifestation of anxiety. Children in a control group received no preoperative preparation from an adult, whereas children in one experimental group were allowed to play with toys unrelated to their upcoming medical procedure in the presence of the child life specialist. Children in a second experimental group were given information by the child life specialist about the upcoming procedure through the use of medical-play techniques. Findings indicated that both groups of children who participated in an adult-supervised play session were consistently more cooperative and less upset than were the control group children. The children in the two playgroups (related to or unrelated to upcoming surgery or procedures) varied significantly in anxiety at only one point—during induction of anesthesia. During this procedure, those children who had been in the playgroup related to the surgical procedure fared better than did those in the unrelated playgroup.

Play and activities (or child life) programs rarely have been studied. In a quasi-experimental study, Clegg (1972) attempted to assess the effectiveness of a comprehensive child life program and reported significant reduction in anxiety levels of children who had participated in child life programs. However, no control groups were used for comparison. Bolig (1980) found that children participating in an activities-based child life program increased in (internal) locus of control, although the level of anxiety was not affected. Wolfer, Gaynard, Goldberger, Laidley, and Thompson (1988), in a quasi-experimental study of a model child life program with a preparation rather than a play focus, found positive effects on a variety of outcome measures, such as coping, adjustment, and recovery variables. Pass and Bolig (1993), in a naturalistic study of children's play in two forms of child life programming foci (i.e., playroom/group versus nonplayroom/individual), found no differences in the frequency and complexity of play, although there was a trend toward significance for therapeutic and educative play occurring more in the playroom-focused setting.

In a field experiment with play type as an outcome variable, Bolig (1992) varied the amount of time a child life–supervised playroom was available and the type of equipment, and found that young children played the majority of the time under any condition. Most of children's play was functional, constructive, and normative, and with a parent, child life specialist, or volunteer. Play type and form was, however, influenced by the addition of symbolic objects and the presence of adults, in interaction with amount of time in the playroom. Both functional and dramatic forms increased with added symbolic material, with significantly more dramatic group play occurring in the 2-hour condition than in the 1-hour condition; and the more time and more adult involvement, the more complex the play. Child life specialists and volunteers were more likely to maintain play at higher levels (i.e., dramatic play and games with rules) than were parents.

Supervised play sessions with materials, whether related or unrelated to the hospital setting, may prove helpful in reducing children's anxiety or distress during hospitalization (Thompson, 1985). Such sessions are the basis of play therapy. A meta-analysis of 800 studies on play therapy (Fisher, 1992) found that this form of play had a significant influence on alleviating children's distress. The type of organized program also appears to affect children differently, although, in the few studies conducted thus far, the outcome variables have differed. Bolig's (1983) typology of child life programs, expanded and amended by McCue (2009) to six types, might provide a characterization useful for further study. The amount of time in the inpatient setting and amount of time in a supervised playroom also influence the amount and types of children's play. Lastly, there is some initial evidence that parents and professionals encourage different levels of play. Whether short periods of no play, maintenance of children's prehospitalization play level, or enhancement of play has any long-term sequalae has yet to be studied.

Variables Affecting Children in Hospitals and Their Play

Many variables have been found to affect the psychosocial and behavioral responses of hospitalized children (Thompson, 1985, 2009) and may have an impact on their play behaviors. These include play environment, parent contact, age, length of hospitalization, type of illness, and gender.

The Play Environment

For many years, researchers and practitioners in child development and early childhood education (e.g., Bruner, Jolly, & Silva, 1976; Frost & Klein, 1979; Piaget, 1962; Shure, 1963; Smith & Connolly, 1981) have recognized that the immediate physical and affective environments affect behavior. Through the presence and permission of adults, young children in particular gain assurance and encouragement to interact with objects and people (see Figure 3.3). Through the stimulation of various concrete, symbolic objects, children first explore and then express uniquely. Knowledge of a particular environment is a more reliable predictor of people's behaviors than knowledge of demographic variables or individual behavior tendencies (Barker, 1968).

However, to date, limited investigation of play environmental factors in hospital settings has taken place. Tisza et al. (1970) found that amount of time in the hospital was related to exhibition of play behaviors. Three days were necessary for the young children studied to begin to play. Harvey and Hales-Tooke (1970) noted that the presence of a play leader was necessary for children to engage in "settled play." Likewise, in outpatient settings, Williams and Powell (1980) found that the presence of a play facilitator was related to more play and less anxious behaviors. Type of play materials was found to be related to children's anxiety and defensiveness. Gilmore (1966) found

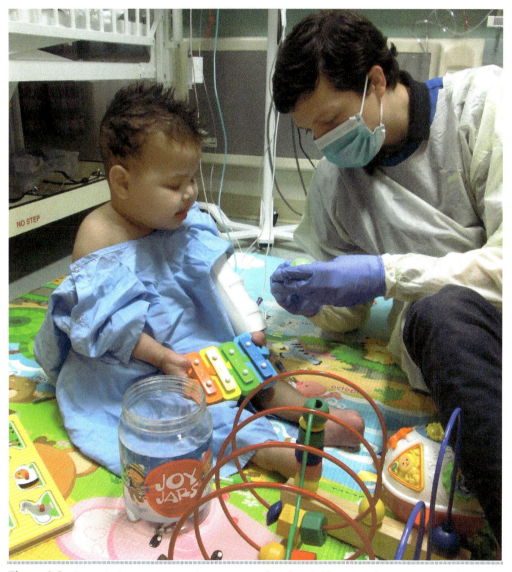

Figure 3.3. Through the presence and permission of adults, children gain the assurance and encouragement to interact with objects and people. *Note.* Photo courtesy of Jessica Uze.

the presence of anxiety to be an important influence on the choice of toys; either a marked increase or decrease in interest was noted. Burstein and Meichenbaum (1979) also found that level of anxiety influenced selection of play materials. Children low in defensiveness prior to hospitalization actively played with relevant materials in the pre-hospital period and displayed minimal anxiety following discharge. Children high in defensiveness avoided one prehospital play with hospital-relevant toys and had higher anxiety following hospitalization.

But the relationships among type of equipment or toys, room arrangement, space, and child behaviors, including play, have not been studied in hospital programs, with one exception: Eisert, Kulka, and Moore (1988) reported that a play structure, developed to facilitate symbolic play of children with disabilities, significantly increased amount of time in partial play, symbolic play, and total play (Eisert et al., 1988). Bolig (1992) found that the longer children were in a (supervised) playroom, the more likely they were to engage in higher levels of play. Also, the presence of symbolic and thematic materials enhanced play, as did the presence of the parent and child life specialist. Contextual factors in one-one hospital room activities or play have yet to be explained (e.g., presence of a roommate, interactions with parents, specific play materials, media).

Parent Contact

Lehman (1975) and Brain and Maclay (1968) reported that "rooming in" (i.e., parents' staying through the hospitalization) has a positive effect on children's responses to hospitalization. The relationship of parent involvement during their child's hospitalization to play behaviors, in either playrooms or other contexts, has been explored only in two field studies (Thompson, 1985). Hall (1977) noted increased parental play with children after the introduction of a supervised playroom; Bolig (1992) found that parental presence was related to increased play, but not as complex forms of play as occurred with a child life specialist. With today's essentially open visiting, future research must account for the quantity and quality of parent (or family) presence as well as parents' degree of involvement with their children in play.

Age

The preschool years are included in the age range most likely to suffer disturbances as a result of hospitalization; the majority of disruption and play intervention studies have been conducted with this age group. As would be anticipated, it is for this developmental stage that play, and especially normative play, may serve the most critical preventive, curative, and equilibration functions. However, for older children, play may also be critical, although different forms may be more effective. Related expressive and efficacy activities, such as music, art and biblio-therapy, drama, and even humor, need investigation (see Chapter 4: The Arts in Children's Health-Care Settings). Computer-assisted preparation, virtual activities, and related interventions with school-age children and adolescents also may be effective (Li & Lopez, 2008).

Length of Hospitalization

Tisza et al. (1970) found evidence that preschool-age children show a disruption in play behavior during the first day of hospitalization. The disruption gradually diminished over the 3-day observation period. Burstein and Meichenbaum (1979) also noted disturbances of play in a study of the relationships among play, anxiety, and defensiveness. They recorded the amount of time each child spent playing with materials for each play session and found that the children spent significantly less time playing with toys during hospitalization than they did either prior to or after release from the hospital. Burstein and Meichenbaum (1979) attributed the disturbance in play behavior to a "disposition not to play" rather than to the distractions of the novel stimuli in the hospital setting. Pass and Bolig (1993) found that the longer children were hospitalized, the more they engaged in educative and rough-and-tumble play and the less they engaged in exploratory behavior. Less time in the hospital—and opportunity to create relationships and become more comfortable in the setting—might relate to even less play.

Type of Illness

Although type of illness (and frequency of admissions) are related to differential psychosocial responses, type of illness has rarely been studied for impact on quantity and quality of play. Pass and Bolig (1993) found that children admitted for surgical procedures engaged in less play, and more unoccupied behavior and reading, than children who were admitted for other medical reasons.

Gender

Pass and Bolig (1987) found that boys engaged in more constructive play than girls in two different child life settings; girls had more onlooker behavior than boys. But the variety of children's play in nonmedical contexts has been found to be influenced by gender, with girls engaging in less rough-and-tumble and aggressive play and showing interest in a wider variety of toys and play materials than boys (Johnson, Christie, & Yawkey, 1999). It is likely that gender differences in play among hospitalized children may be found when other factors are controlled.

Research Questions for Play in Health-Care Settings

Many basic and applied questions about the play of ill or hospitalized children, and in the variety of health-care settings, remain unanswered or have yet to be asked. A survey on the state of play and innovations in North American hospitals (Vilas, 2014) and the 2008 and 2014 reviews of research on therapeutic play in pediatric health care are steps for congruent scientific study. The few other studies that have been conducted have failed to use similar instruments (or definitions of play), populations, methodologies, or comparison groups. Replication is necessary, as is improved methodology, because the methodology or analyses in some early studies may be questionable.

Thus, the major research issues are as follows: (a) whether play (and its different types/forms) occur during health-care encounters and in health-care contexts, and under what conditions play occurs; (b) whether play is a valid measure of children's psychological state during hospitalization or other health-care experiences; (c) what factors contribute to variation in children's play during health-care encounters; and (d) whether children's play during hospitalization, ambulatory care, or even home care contributes to variation in physiological and psychological recovery. Further questions about the types of organized programs (e.g., philosophies, curricula, interactional patterns), variations in facilitative relationships (e.g., professional training, type of relationship, amount of time in relationship), and the physical environment in which play occurs (e.g., where, type of equipment) also need to be addressed. This imperative for a better understanding of the dynamics of play is furthered by today's emphasis on evidence-based practice. The recent (2014) survey of play and innovations in child life has generated additional discipline-specific questions, such as how more opportunities can be provided for child-centered/open-ended play and the level of staff training in play required to optimize various forms of play (Vilas, 2014).

Facilitating Play in Health-Care Settings

The roles of the adult in children's play are especially critical during health-care encounters. Without sensitivity to children's responses, adults can turn "play" into "not play" or fail to help turn "not play" into "play." This adaptation of roles or behaviors of adults in children's play may indeed be one of the most sensitive and nonmedical functions in which health-care practitioners engage. The facilitation of different *types* and *forms* of play may also have various effects on children during hospitalization, and differing posthospital adjustment patterns are likely to be related to these types and forms of play (Rae et al., 1989). The inclusion or exclusion of various types or forms of play may favor one aspect of functioning over another (e.g., cognitive over affective). Typically, adults engaging in play with children favor cognitive functioning, asking questions rather than reflecting children's feelings or intents, for example. Thus, if play provision is to continue to be an integral aspect of health care for children, it must be recognized that not all activities in which children engage are play.

Each theory of play has implications for psychosocial and psychoeducational prevention and intervention strategies. As examples, the psychoanalytic theories support the contention that children need to "express" feelings through play to master events and to avoid repression or fixation, and cognitive theories (e.g., Piaget, 1962) postulate that children acquire knowledge through play. The "expression of feelings" and "acquisition of knowledge" perspectives on play have been the predominant positions on the functions of play, with several subtypes.

There are underlying theoretical principles, particularly related to the environmental aspects required to sustain play, and these may be competing. Unstructured play, for example, congruent with nondirective forms of play therapy and characteristic of psychoanalytic theory, requires different responses from the environment than does guided or co-play, which is characteristic of cognitive theories. Cognitive theories presume a greater transaction between children and their environments—a more or less coequal interaction/impetus by adult and child. However, the psychoanalytic view requires an initial supportive relationship with adults for children to feel secure enough to explore and ultimately play with their environment.

Thus, a cognitive perspective implies a more active adult role in children's play. More active or directive roles have certain dangers; that is, there is a subtle but critical line beyond which adults can turn children's play into "not play," or overstimulate or overwhelm children's regulatory systems. Furthermore, although limited, there is empirical support from studies of children in other settings for the idea that more active play involvement of adults may favor cognitive aspects of development, whereas unstructured and nondirected play might have more social or emotional benefits (Smith,

1995). Alternatively, in health-care settings with little time to develop relationships, the reciprocal play process between adults and children may actually facilitate attachment (Rutter, 1981). This continuum of play to not play is illustrated in Figure 3.4.

Identifying the variety of roles in which adults can engage in children's play and the resultant differences in the quantity and quality of children's play has precipitated another line of research, particularly in school and childcare settings. Enz and Christie (1997) identified six roles that adults engage in with children's play. Roles can be conceptualized on a continuum that ranges from no involvement to complete control (Johnson et al., 1999). Among children in classroom and early childhood education settings, the most productive roles are in the middle range of involvement. These middle-range roles (Johnson et al., 1999, pp. 210–213) are as follows:

- *Stage manager*—While staying on sidelines during play, the adult helps children prepare for play and responds to children's requests for assistance with materials and equipment.
- *Co-player*—The adult becomes a partner in play, taking on less dominant roles than the children, following the children's actions and interactions.
- *Play leader*—The adult extends and expands children's play through suggesting new roles, themes, and elements.

The most effective roles for professionals in health care might be found at the higher end of these middle-range roles, because a greater intensity of interaction might be essential, given limited time and other resources. However, greater sensitivity to individual reactions and issues is required at these higher levels of intensity. Specialized training of staff may be required for engagement in more curative forms of play—similar to play therapy. Using cognitive-behavioral theory, the pending requirement for child life specialists to obtain a master's degree in their specific discipline may provide the depth of knowledge and skills congruent with this level of engagement.

Wolfgang and Bolig (1979) identified specific behaviors congruent with these roles through which adults in play encounters with hospitalized children take on more or

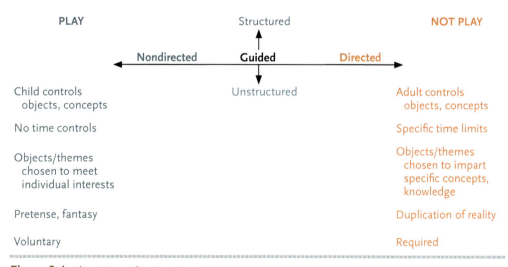

Figure 3.4. Play to Not Play continuum.

less "control," on a continuum from "structured" behaviors, such as physical help or modeling, to verbal directions, to verbal questions, to nondirective statements, and, at the other end, to "open," with visual looking-on behavior. McCue (2009) also described the nature of therapeutic relationships in child life congruent with ethics, standards, and level of training as well as supportive and professional roles.

Similarly, the types of materials selected (and who chooses) may also be viewed as contributing to the degree of structure. Items that are structured, such as puzzles, are most likely to be used in the way the item is intended, whereas "open" or fluid materials, such as sand and water, are more likely to be subject to children's feelings or thoughts (see Figure 3.5). Lastly, symbolic objects, including health-care items, are more likely to elicit unique expressions of feeling and experiencing. In the approach outlined by Wolfgang and Bolig (1979), adults interact and transact with children and their play through modifying their own behaviors and materials as children become more or less expressive. The goal is for children to be in control and fully expressive in symbolic forms of play.

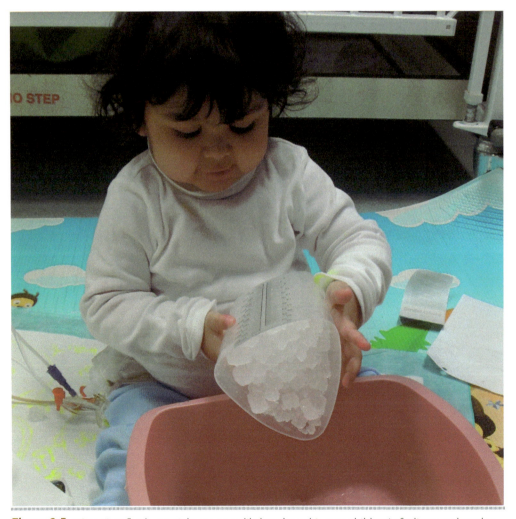

Figure 3.5. "Open" or fluid materials are more likely to be subject to children's feelings or thoughts. *Note.* Photo courtesy of Jessica Uze.

Playing Into the 21st Century

There is a renewed research and advocacy interest in play across disciplines (Johnson, 2015a, 2015b), as the actual time children spend in play is dramatically decreasing. Brain development research has contributed to this heightened concern about play's demise. A 1999 article in *U.S. News & World Report* by Brownlee stated that the study of play has gained a badge of respect as biologists have found increasing evidence that to a variety of species, play is nearly as important as food and sleep. For example, there is increasing evidence that the "locomotion play" of young animals forges connections between neurons in the brain, especially in the cerebellum, the region that controls and coordinates movement. Early evidence suggests that play taps into the brain chemicals involved in pleasure. When rats play, their brains release dopamine, a chemical that in humans induces elation and excitement. There is also an increasing consensus that play experiences help form multiple and hardwired interactions in the brain, and children who do not play may actually have smaller brains (Brown, Sutterby, Therrell, & Thornton, 2002).

And there continues to be an awareness of the importance of research specifically on the changing health services for children:

> The characteristic of childhood as a unique developmental stage of life, the continuity of child health with adult health, and a distinctive child health care system justify a separate focus of health services research on children. Child health services research currently lacks the tools necessary to monitor the impact of the health care system change on children's health and to compare the effectiveness of alternative treatment modalities. (Forrest, Simpson, & Clancy, 1997, p. 1787)

Play continues to be a viable aspect of early childhood education and is still the subject of many books in the field. There are several new journals devoted to play research, conceptualization, and application. Several organizations are concerned with play, as are a number of professional associations (see Appendix 3.1). Moreover, several organizations provide play training.

This renewed interest in play, from its therapeutic functions to its learning functions, is significant, and commitment to its implementation is likely to continue. Brain research, as noted above—especially on critical periods and the effects of trauma—is likely to provide further evidence of the importance of play and its role in relaxation, multiple facets, and internal-control aspects.

Play in Health-Care Settings of the Future

In 1992, Louv talked about each generation of children living a childhood of firsts. Children in today's health-care and early childhood settings, although not different in their basic needs, are different in their experiences. They are the first childcare generation, the first multicultural generation, and the first generation to grow up with the computer. In terms of health care, this is the first generation that is likely to spend only one or two days in the hospital when born, to benefit from gene or immune therapy, or perhaps to undergo laser and robotic surgery. They may be informed about impending experiences online or, someday, by virtual reality in a specially equipped room in which they are guided through an impending experience (Goldstein, 2011). They can seek out websites about their own illness or surgery and perhaps communicate with children all over the world who have a similar disability or disease (Bush, Huchital, & Simonian, 2002). In the future, they may have interactive dolls or plush toys to hold on to that interact with them (Goldstein, 2011). Some children in health-care settings may have a "nurse" robot who attends to their care and responds to their questions. They will spend even less time in acute health-care settings than in ambulatory and home settings. A computer chip implanted into children with diabetes and asthma may monitor their responses and alert their home-health caretakers or parents to an impending crisis. This form of prevention, and more sophisticated knowledge of etiology of illnesses, will lead to fewer diseases affecting children or less acute onset of chronic diseases that are not yet curable.

Less illness and less time in health-care settings may very well enhance quality of life. But as discussed in the beginning of this chapter, children's essential needs for comfort, control, reassurance, information, human support, and play will not change appreciatively, despite all the technological and medical advances. The challenges in providing play and other child-focused ways of learning and expressing will thus continue. Sophisticated and costly virtual experiences may influence certain aspects of children's adjustment and coping but may not be sufficiently different from or better than traditional playroom-based experiences and ensuing relationships to warrant decrease in support for play, including space for congregate and "normative" play (Battles & Wiener, 2002; Goldstein, 2011).

According to Isenberg and Jalongo (1997), adults who facilitate and advocate for play in this increasingly complex and technological future will need to

- develop a wide range of strategies for a wide range of abilities, situational responses, and physical limits to foster play, creativity, and self-expression;
- develop paradigms and approaches to maximize play possibilities in acute-care settings;
- expand and refine communication capacities;
- focus on intrapersonal traits and interpersonal skills for developing and maintaining optimal and therapeutic relationships;
- extend knowledge of child and human development with neurophysiological theory and research;
- document the effect of their professional practices and policies on children's adjustment, recovery, health, and development; and
- assure personal resources and creative energies to face challenges optimistically.

And child life specialists, in particular, will need to provide more evidence of the effectiveness of their practice (and play). In addition to master's degrees requiring more specific therapeutic theory and skills, they may also bring a greater research orientation to practice (Vilas, 2014), thereby facilitating greater professionalism of their discipline. Nurses, occupational therapists, and others in child health care will continue to advance their own psychosocial strategies through increased study.

Play will be revitalized and more clearly understood in health care and other contexts in the years to come, for, as Sutton-Smith (1995, p. 290) stated, "What may be

---

Text Box 3.3
Play for Peace

Play for Peace brings children from different cultures together through cooperative play to promote positive relationships among people who have a history of intercultural tension. The hope is that bringing children with unique backgrounds, values, and beliefs together through the seemingly simple act of play will sow seeds of compassion for a more peaceful today and tomorrow. The objectives of Play for Peace are to promote positive relationships among children from cultures in conflict; to create a nonthreatening environment free from fear, where children can experience the joy of play; and to influence the behavior of adults through the positive example of children at play.

Note. For more information on Play for Peace, visit the website at www.playforpeace.org. Reprinted with permission.

adaptive about play may not be the skills that happen to be a part of it, but the willful belief in one's own capacity for a future." And what may be most important about play is our belief in the uniqueness of children, as well as what we can learn from children's play (see Text Box 3.3).

Conclusion

Life continues to *play* with us all; we are not in full control but use our culture's symbols, relationships, interactions, and resources to *play it (life) back*. Children play to gain not only knowledge but also the culture-bound skills, as well as timeless roles, that enable them to contribute, adapt, heal, and love. In a time of rapidly increasing technology, changing social structures, demands for early achievements, and testing in schools, play may serve a more critical function than in times past, when children and adults had more free time to explore, dream, and experiment with ideas, roles, and relationships. Yet at other times, children were at high physical risk, were viewed as "little adults," or were valued primarily for contributions to the economy of the family; frequently, play might have not been possible. Thus, it is important to understand that play as a behavior and concept is defined by historical, cultural, and economic situations.

Study Guide

1. What is play, and what functions does it serve for the developing child?

2. What are the different types, forms, and themes common to play, and how do age, culture, gender, and environmental factors affect these?

3. What unique functions does play serve for children in health-care settings, and what factors influence children's "playability" in these settings?

4. What evidence do we have, or do we need, to support continued provision of all forms of play in health-care settings, from normative/nondirective to individualized guided play?

5. What are the functions/roles of child life specialists in facilitating various forms of play, and how have these been influenced by societal views of play, health-care policy, and varying theoretical perspectives?

6. What future challenges to play and play provision in health-care settings might there be, and what counteractions/evidence might sustain play as a primary process for children (and adolescents)?

Appendix 3.1

Resources for Play

Play Organizations

The Association for Play Therapy, Inc. (APT)

3198 Willow Avenue #110
Clovis, CA 93612
USA
Phone: 559/294-2128
Fax: 559/294-2129
E-mail: info@a4pt.org
URL: www.a4pt.org
Facebook: 4PlayTherapy
An international organization dedicated to the advancement of play therapy; conducts and makes available play therapy research.

The Association for Study of Play (TASP)

Strong Museum of Play
One Manhattan Square
Rochester, NY 14607
Phone and Fax: 515/263-2700
URL: www.tasplay.org
Facebook: The-Association-for-the-Study-of-Play-TASP
A multidisciplinary group of professionals committed to play research and its application.

Alliance for Childhood

PO Box 20973
Park West PO
New York, NY 10025
USA
Phone: 202/643-8242
E-mail: info@allianceforchildhood.org
URL: www.allianceforchildhood.org
Facebook: Alliance-for-Childhood
A partnership of individuals and organizations committed to fostering and respecting each child's inherent right to a healthy, developmentally appropriate childhood.

National Institute for Play (NIFP)

Stuart Brown, Founder
PO Box 1398
Carmel Valley, CA 93924
USA
Phone: 831/659-1740
E-mail: inquiry/nationalinstituteforplay.org
URL: www.nifplay.org
Facebook: National-Institute-for-Play
Provides a mix of information and resources to give a deeper understanding of the nature and importance of play, and connections to helpful people, organizations, and information.

Children's Play Council

8 Wakley Street
London EC1V 7QE
United Kingdom
Phone: 44 020 7843 6016
Fax: 44 020 7278 9512
E-mail: cpc@ncb.org.uk
URL: www.ncb.org.uk/cpc/
A campaigning and research organization dedicated to raising people's awareness of the importance of play in children's lives and the need for all children to have access to better play opportunities and services.

International Council for Children's Play (ICCP)

Web page: http://www.iccp-play.org/
Promotes research on children's play and toys.

The International Play Advocacy (IPA)

International Membership Secretary
Mr. Gerrit Lekkerkerker, Hoflaan 4
3271 BD Mijnsheerenland
The Netherlands
Phone: 31 10 417 23 58
Fax: 31 10 417 2095
E-mail: scz@bsd.rotterdam.nl
URL: www.ncsu.edu/ipa
Supports dialog on play and advocates for children's right to play throughout the world.

National Lekotek Center

2001 N. Clybourne Avenue
Chicago, IL
USA
Phone: 773-528-5766
TTY: 800/573-4446
Fax: 773-537-2992
E-mail: lekotek@lekotek.org

URL: www.lekotek.org/
Facebook: NationalLekotek
Dedicated to promoting access to developmentally appropriate play and learning for children with special needs and their families.

Play England

c/o Homerton Grove Adventure Playground
Wardle Street
London E9 6BX
Phone: 44 07595271532
E-mail: info@playingengland.net
URL: www.playengland.org.uk
Promotes England as country where all children and young people can fully enjoy their right to play.

Professional Organizations Supporting Play in Practice

American Occupational Therapy Association (AOTA)

4720 Montgomery Lane
PO Box 31220
Bethesda, MD 20824-1220
USA
Phone: 301/652-2682
TDD: 800/377-8555
Fax: 301/652-7711
E-mail: praota@aota.org
URL: http://www.aota.org
A professional association of occupational therapists, occupational therapy assistants, and students of occupational therapy dedicated to helping people regain, develop, and build skills that are essential for independent functioning, health, and well-being.

Association of Child Life Professionals (formerly Child Life Council)

1820 N. Fort Myer Drive, Suite 52
Arlington, VA 22209
USA
Phone: 571/483-4500 or 1/800-252-4515
Fax: 571/483-4482
E-mail: clcstaff@childlife.org
URL: www.childlife.org
Facebook: ChildLifeCouncil
A professional organization composed of child life specialists, educators, students, and others who use play, recreation, education, self-expression, and theories of child development to promote psychological well-being and optimum development of children, adolescents, and their families.

National Association for the Education of Young Children (NAEYC)

1313 L Street, NW, Suite 500
Washington, DC 20005
USA
Phone: 202/232-8777
Toll Free: 866/424-2460
Fax: 202/328-1846
E-mail: naeyc@naeyc.org
URL: www.naeyc.org
An organization of early childhood educators and others dedicated to improving the quality of programs for children from birth through third grade.

National Association for Health Play Specialists (NAHPS)

21 Rosefield Road, Staines
Middlesex, TW18 4NB
United Kingdom
E-mail: hospitalplay@msn.com
URL: www.nahps.org.uk
Facebook: www.facebook.com/pages/Nahps/172764366247991
Twitter: https://twitter.com/nahpsofficial
A charity that provides professional support to hospital play staff to promote the physical and mental well-being of children and young people who are patients in hospital or hospice or receiving medical care at home.

Play Training

The Canadian Association for Child Play Therapy (CACPT)

PO Box 24010
Guelph, Ontario N1E6V8
Canada
Phone: 519-827-1506
E-mail: Elizabeth@cacpt.com
URL: www.cacpt.com
Serves as one of the world's major resources in play therapy, and child psychology. CPTI runs many training programs each year in the field of child psychology and play therapy, with a variety of presenters in many regions of the world.

Chesapeake Beach Professional Seminars (CBPS): Play Therapy Training Institute

3555 Ponds Wood Drive
Chesapeake Beach, MD 20732-3916
USA
Phone: 410/535-4942
Fax: 410/414-9902
E-mail: cbps2006@yahoo.com
URL: www.cbpseminars.org
Provides traditional as well as innovative play therapy/child psychotherapy training for mental health professionals and others providing therapy with children.

The National Institute of Relationship Enhancement (NIRE)

4400 East-West Highway, Suite 28
Bethesda, MD 20814
USA
Phone: 301/680-8977
Fax: 502/226-7088
E-mail: nire@nire.org
URL: www.nire.org
Provides training, supervision, and certification for mental health professionals in the Child-Centered Play Therapy Model, and conducts basic and advanced skills-training workshops in play therapy, as well as offering supervision and certification in this effective intervention with children.

The Play Therapy Training Institute, Inc. (PTTI)

983 Route 33, Building 2
Monroe Township, NJ 08831
USA
Phone: 609/448-2145
Fax: 609/448-1665
E-mail: info@ptti.org
URL: www.ptti.org
Offers a variety of 1- and 2-day Play Therapy Seminars; following a broad-spectrum, eclectic approach to Play Therapy, instruction is available in all the major approaches and techniques.

Play Therapy United Kingdom (PTUK)

The Coach House
Belmont Rd.
Uckfield
East Sussex TN22 IBP
UK
Phone: 44 01825761143
Fax: 44 01825769913
E-mail: ptukorg@aol.com
URL: www.playtherapy.org.uk
Promotes the use of play and creative arts as ways of enabling children to reach their full potential.

The Theraplay Institute (TTI)

1840 Oak Avenue, #320
Evanston, IL 60201
USA
Phone: 847/256-7334
Fax: 847/256-7370
E-mail: theraplay@aol.com
URL: www.theraplay.org
Provides training and research in Theraplay, a dynamic and effective short-term approach to treating children's emotional and behavioral problems. Based on the intimacy and physical interplay that characterize healthy relationships between parent and child, Theraplay techniques use structured play to promote the child's self-esteem, competence, and trust in others.

Play Journals

American Journal of Play: http://www.journalofplay.org/
International Journal of Play: http://www.tandfonline.com/loi/rijp20 - .VkYkxMkynTA
International Journal of Play Therapy: http://www.apa.org/pubs/journals/pla/
Play and Culture Series: www.tasplay.org/studies/

Online Encyclopedias & Open Access Journals

Encyclopedia of Children's Health: www.healthofchildren.com
Encyclopedia of Play Science: http://www.scholarpedia.org/article/Encyclopedia:Play_Science

Online Play Courses/Modules

Future Learn: Exploring Play: The Importance of Play in Everyday Life
https://www.futurelearn.com/courses/play

PowerPoint Presentation

Bolig, R. (2006, May). *Power to the patients.* Presented at the Association for the Study of Play Conference, Ontario, Canada. Retrieved from www.tasplay.org/taspfiles/ppts/bolighospitalplaypaper-1.ppt

Videos

TED TALKS (2014, August 6): *The Decline of Play and Rise of Mental Disorders: NPR (2014): Scientists Say Child's Play Helps Build a Better Brain.* Retrieved from http://www.npr.org/sections/ed/2014/08/06/336361277/scientists-say-childs-play-helps-build-a-better-brain

Recommended Books/ Handbooks

Broadhead, P., Howard, J., Wood, E. A. (Eds.). (2010). *Play and learning in the early years: From research to practice.* Thousand Oaks, CA: Sage.

Hart, R., & Rollins, J. (2011). *Therapeutic activities for children and teens coping with healthcare issues.* Hoboken, NJ: John Wiley & Sons.

Johnson, J. E., Eberle, S. G., Hendricks, T. S., & Kuschner, D. (Eds.). (2015). *The handbook for the study of play.* Lanham, MD: Rowman & Littlefield. (Co-published with the Strong National Museum of Play)

Pellegrini, A. D. (Ed.). (2011). *The Oxford handbook of the development of play.* New York, NY: Oxford University Press.

Thompson, R. H. (Ed.). (2009). *The handbook of child life: A guide for psychosocial care.* Springfield, IL: C. C. Thomas.

Tonkin, A. (Ed.). (2014). *Play in healthcare: Using play to promote child development and well-being.* Oxon, England: Routledge.

Turner, J., & Brown, C. (Eds.). (2014). *The Pips of child life: Early play programs in hospitals.* Dubuque, IA: Kendall Hunt Publishing Company.

References

Alliance for Childhood. (2010). *The loss of children's play: A public health issue.* Policy Brief #1. Retrieved from http://www.habitot.org/museum/pdf/play_research/Health_brief.pdf

Almquist, L., Hellnas, P., Stefansson, M., & Granlund, M. (2006). 'I can play!' Young children's perceptions of health. *Developmental Neurohabitation, 9*(3), 275–284.

American Academy of Pediatrics, Committee on Hospital Care. (2014). Policy statement: Child Life programs. *Pediatrics, 133*(5), e 1471. Retrieved from http://www.pediatrics.aappublications.org/content/5/e1471

Association for Play Therapy, Inc. (2016). *About APT.* Retrieved from http://www.a4pt.org/?page=AboutAPT

Barker, R. G. (1968). *Ecological psychology: Concepts and methods of studying the environment of human behavior.* Stanford, CA: Stanford University Press.

Battles, H. B., & Wiener, L. S. (2002). STARBRIGHT World: Effects of an electronic network on the social environment of children with life-threatening illnesses. *Children's Health Care, 31,* 47–68.

Bergen, D. (1988). Using schema for play and learning. In D. Bergen (Ed.), *Play as a medium for learning and development: A handbook of theory and practice* (pp. 169–180). Portsmouth, NH: Heinemann.

Bodrouz, E., & Leong, D. J. (2015). "A Head Taller than Himself": Vygotskian and post-Vygotskian view on children's play. In J. E. Johnson, S. G. Eberle, T. S. Hendricks, & D. Kuschner, (Eds.). *The handbook of the study of play* (pp. 203–214). New York: Rowman and Littlefield/the Strong.

Bolig, R. (1980). The relationship of personality factors to responses to hospitalization in young children admitted for medical procedures. (Doctoral dissertation: Ohio State University, 1981). *Dissertation Abstracts International, 41,* 3732-B.

Bolig, R. (1984). Play in hospital settings. In T. Yawkey, & A. Pellegrini (Eds.), *Play: Developmental and applied.* Hillsdale, NJ: Erlbaum.

Bolig, R. (1988). Guest editorial: The diversity and complexity of play in health care settings. *Children's Health Care, 16,* 132–133.

Bolig, R. (1990). Play in health care settings: Challenges for the 1990s. *Children's Health Care, 19,* 229–233.

Bolig, R. (1992). *Play in child life contexts: A field experience.* Paper presented at the Association for the Care of Children's Health Conference, Atlanta, GA.

Bolig, R., Yolton, K., & Nissen, H. (1991). Medical play: Issues and questions. *Children's Health Care, 20,* 225–229.

Borrell-Carrio, F. (2004). The biosocial model 25 years later. *Annals of Family Medicine, 2*(6), 576–582.

Brain, D. J., & Maclay, I. (1968). Controlled study of mothers and children in hospital. *British Medical Journal, 1,* 278–280.

Brown, P., Sutterby, J. A., Therrell, J. A., & Thronton, C. D. (2001). *Play is essential to brain development.* Austin, TX: International Play Equipment Manufacturers Association.

Brown, S. L. (2014). Consequences of play deprivation. *Scholarpedia, 9*(5), 30449. Retrieved on from www.scholarpedia/org/article/Consequences_of_ Play_Deprivaton

Brownlee, S. (1997, February 3). The case for frivolity. *U.S. News and World Report,* pp. 45–48.

Bruner, J. S., Jolly, A., & Silva, K. (Eds.). (1976). *Play: Its role in development and evolution.* New York: Basic Books.

Burstein, S., & Meichenbaum, D. (1979). The work of worrying in young children undergoing surgery. *Journal of Abnormal Psychology, 7,* 121–132.

Burghardt, G. M. (2005). *The genesis of animal play: Testing the Limits.* Cambridge, MA: MIT Press.

Bush, J. P., Huchital, J. R., & Simonian, S. (2002). An introduction to program and research initiatives of the STARBRIGHT Foundation. *Children's Health Care, 31,* 1–10.

Camera, L. (2015, December 9). No child left behind has finally been left behind. *U.S News & World Report.* Retrieved from http://www.usnews.com/news/articles/2015/12/09/congress-replaces-no-child-left-behind-shifts-power-to-states

Carlisle, R. (2009). *The encyclopedia of play in today's society.* Thousand Oaks, CA: Sage.

Carlsson-Page, N., McLaughlin, G. B., & Almon, J. W. (2015). *Reading instruction in kindergarten: Little to gain and much to lose.* New York, NY: Alliance for Childhood.

Cataldo, M. F., Bessman, C. A., Parker, L., Pearson, J. E., & Rogers, M. C. (1979). Behavioral assessment for pediatric intensive care units. *Journal of Applied Behavior. Analysis, 12,* 83–97.

Child Life Council. (2015). *Strategic plan.* Retrieved from http://www.childlife.org/About/StrategicPlan

Clark, C. D. (2003). *In sickness and in play: Children coping with chronic illness.* New Brunswick, NJ: Rutgers University Press.

Clatworthy, S. (1981). Therapeutic play: Effects on hospitalized children. *Children's Health Care, 9,* 108–113.

Clegg, R. (1972). Effects of a child life program upon the anxiety levels of children hospitalized for major elective surgery. (Doctoral dissertation, University of Maryland). *Dissertation Abstracts International, 33,* 4882-B.

Copple, C., & Bradekamp, S. (2009). *Developmentally appropriate practice* (3rd ed.). Washington, DC: NAEYC.

Csikszentmihalyi, M. (1990). *Flow: The psychology of optimal experience.* New York: Harper-Collins.

Delpo, E., & Frick, S. (1988). Directed and non-directed play as a therapeutic modality. *Children's Health Care, 16,* 261–267.

Eisert, D., Kulka, L., & Moore, K. (1988). Facilitating play in hospitalized handicapped children: The design of a therapeutic play environment. *Children's Mental Health, 13,* 201–208.

Elkind. D. (2007). *The power of play: Learning what comes naturally.* Boston, MA: DaCapo Press.

Eluvathingal, T., Chugani, H., Behen, M., Juhasz, C., Muzic, O., Maqbool, M., … Makki, M. (2006). Abnormal brain connectivity in children after early severe socioemotional deprivation. *Pediatrics, 117*(6), 20932100.

Encyclopedia of Children's Health. (2015). *Play.* Retrieved from http://www.healthofchildren.com/P/Play.html

Enz, B., & Christie, J. (1997). Teacher play interaction styles: Effects of play behavior and relationships with teacher training and experience. *International Journal of Early Childhood Education, 2,* 55–75.

Erikson, E. (1963). *Childhood and society.* New York, NY: Norton. (Original work published 1950)

Erikson, E. (1972). Play and actuality. In M. W. Piers (Ed.), *Play and development.* New York, NY: Norton.

Fisher, E. P. (1992). The impact of play on development: A meta-analysis. *Play and Culture, 5*(5), 328–331.

Forrest, C. B., Simpson, L., & Clancy, C. (1997). Child health services research: Challenges and opportunities. *Journal of the American Medical Association, 277,* 1787–1792.

Fosson, A., Martin, J., & Haley, J. (1990). Anxiety among hospitalized latency-aged children. *Journal of Developmental and Behavioral Pediatrics, 11,* 324–327.

Freud, S. (1952). *Beyond the pleasure principle.* New York: Norton.

Frost, J. L. (2010). *A history of children's play and play environments.* New York, NY: Routledge.

Frost, J. L., & Klein, B. L. (1979). *Children's play and playgrounds.* Boston, MA: Allyn & Bacon.

Frost, J. L., Wortham, S. C., & Reifel, S. (2007). *Play and development.* Upper Saddle River, NJ: Pearson/Merrill.

Gariepy, N., & Howe, N. (2003). Therapeutic power of play: Examining the play of young children with leukemia. *Child: Care, Health, and Development, 34*(2), 141–144.

Gilmore, J. (1966). The effect of anxiety and cognitive factors in children's play behavior. *Child Development, 37,* 397.

Glickman, C. (1988). Play in public school settings: A philosophic question. In T. D. Yawkey, & A. D. Pellegrini (Eds.), *Child's play: Developmental and applied (pp. 255–271).* Hillsdale, NJ: Erlbaum.

Goldstein, J. (2011). Technology and play. In A. D. Pellegrini (Ed.), *The Oxford handbook of the development of play* (pp. 322–337). New York, NY: Oxford University Press.

Gray, R. (2010). The decline of play and the rise of psychopathology in children and adolescents. *American Journal of Play, 3,* 443–463.

Groos, K. (1901). *The play of man.* New York, NY: Appleton.

Halfon, N., Wise, P. H., Forrest, C. B. (2014). The changing nature of children's health development: New challenges require major policy solutions. *Health Affairs, 33*(12), 2116–2124. Retrieved from http://content.healthaffairs.org/content/33/12/2116 l

Hall, D. J. (1977). *Social relations and innovation: Changing the state of play in hospitals.* London, UK: Routledge & Kegan Paul.

Hall, G. S. (1904). *Adolescence: Its psychology and its relation to physiology, anthropology, sex, crime, religion, and education* (Vol. 1). New York, NY: Appleton.

Harvey, S., & Hales-Tooke, A. (1970). *Play in hospital.* London, UK: Faber & Faber.

Hendricks, T. S. (2015a). Play as self-realization: Toward a general theory of play. In J. E. Johnson, S. G. Eberle, T. S. Hendricks, & D. Kuschner (Eds.), *The handbook of the study of play* (pp. 1–17). New York, NY: Rowman and Littlefield.

Hendricks, T. S. (2015b). Where are we now? Challenges to the study of play. In J. E. Johnson, S. G. Eberle, T. S. Hendricks, & D. Kuschner (Eds.), *The handbook of the study of play* (pp. 381–392). Little Field, NY: Rouman.

Holmes, R. M. (2013). Children's play and culture. *Scholarpedia, 8*(6), 31016.

Hughes, F. P. (2010). *Children, play and development.* Thousand Oaks, CA: Sage.

Isenberg, J. P., & Jalongo, M. R. (1997). *Creative expression and play in early childhood.* Columbus, OH: Merrill.

Ispa, J., Barrett, B., & Kim, Y. (1988). Effects of supervised play in a hospital waiting room. *Children's Health Care, 16,* 195–201.

Johnson, J. E. (2015a). Introduction. In J. E. Johnson, S. G. Eberle, T. S. Hendricks, & D. Kuschner (Eds.), *The handbook of the study of play* (pp. xi-xv) New York: Rowman and Littlefield.

Johnson, J. E. (2015b). What is the state of play? *International Journal of Play, 3*(1), 4-5.

Johnson, J. E., Christie, J. F., & Yawkey, T. D. (1999). *Play and early childhood development.* New York: Longman.

Johnson, J. E., Eberle, S. G., Hendricks, T. S., & Kuschner, D. (2015). *The handbook of the study of play.* New York, NY: Rowman and Littlefield.

King, N. R. (1979). Play: The kindergartner's perspective. *Elementary School Journal, 80,* 81–87.

Koller, D. (2008). *Evidence-based practice statement. Therapeutic play in pediatric health care: The essence of child life practice.* Arlington, VA: Child Life Council. Retrieved from https://www.childlife.org/files/EBPPlayStatement-Complete.pdf

Kossoff, D. (1996). To die with dignity: In sweet memory of a girl named Kasey. *The Advocate, 2,* pp. 29–30. Arlington, VA: Child Life Council

Kuntz, N., Adams, J. A., Zahr, L., Killen, R., Cameron, K., & Wasson, H. (1996). Therapeutic play and bone marrow transplantation. *Journal of Pediatric Nursing, 11,* 359–367.

Lehman, E. J. (1975). The effects of rooming-in on the behavior of preschool children during hospitalization and follow-up. *Dissertation Abstracts International, 36,* 3052-B.

Levin, D. E. (2004, October). Rethinking children's play. *Our Children, 25,* 8–11.

Li, H. C., & Lopez, V. (2008). Effectiveness and appropriateness of therapeutic play intervention in preparing children for surgery. *Journal for Specialists in Pediatric Nursing, 13*(2), 63–73.

Lillard , A. S., Lerner, M. D., Hopkins, E. J., Dove, R. A., Smith, E. D., & Palmquist, G. M. (2013). The impact of pretend play on development: A review of the evidence. *Psychological Bulletin*, *139*(1), 1–34.

Lockwood, N. L. (1970). The effects of situational doll play upon the preoperative stress reactions of hospitalized children. In American Nurses Association *Clinical Sessions* (pp. 133–140). New York, NY: Appleton-Century-Crofts.

Louv, R. (1992). *Childhood's future*. New York, NY: Doubleday.

Marcon, R. (2002). Moving by grade: Relationship of preschool models and later school success. *Early Childhood Research and Practice*, *4*(1), 1–11. Retrieved from http://www.ecrp.unc.edu/u4n17/marcon.html

McCue, K. (1988). Medical play: An expanded perspective. *Children's Health Care, 16*, 157–161.

McCue, K. (2009). Therapeutic relationships in child life. In Thompson. R. (Ed.). *The handbook of child life: A guide to psychosocial care* (pp. 57–77). Springfield, IL: CC Thomas.

Morris, J. (2015). *Position statement: Evidence-based practice*. Retrieved from https://www.childlife.org/files/CLCPositionStatementEBP.pdf

National Association for Health Play Specialists. (2015). *Power of play in health service delivery report*. Retrieved from www.nahps.org.uk

Nicolapoulous, A. (2010). The alarming disappearance of play from early childhood education. *Human Development, 53*, 1–4. Retrieved from http://psychology.cas2.lehigh.edu/sites/psychology.cas2.lehigh.edu/files/disappearance_of_play.pdf

Parten, M. (1932). Social play among preschool children. *Journal of Abnormal and Social Psychology*, *28*, 136–147.

Pass, M., & Bolig, R. (1993). A comparison of play behaviors in two child life program variations. *Child Care, 22*, 5–17.

Patrick, G. T. W. (1916). *The psychology of relaxation*. Boston, MA: Houghton Mifflin.

Pearson, J. E. R., Cataldo, M., Turemen, A., Bessman, C., & Rogers, M. (1980). Pediatric intensive care unit patients: Effects of play intervention on behavior. *Critical Care Medicine, 8*, 64–67.

Pellegrini, A. D. (2009a). Research and policy on children's play. *Child Development Perspectives*, *3*(2), 131-136.

Pellegrini, A. D. (2009b). *The role of play in human development*. New York: Oxford University Press.

Pellegrini, A. D. (2011). *The Oxford handbook of the development of play*. New York: Oxford University Press.

Phillips, R. (1988). Play therapy in health care settings: Promises never kept? *Children's Health Care, 16*, 182–187.

Piaget, J. (1962). *Play, dreams, and imitation in childhood*. New York: Norton.

Pianta, R., Howes, C., Burchinal, M., Bryant, D., Clifford, R., Early, D., & Barbarin, O. (2005). Features of pre-kindergarten programs, classrooms, and teachers. *Applied Developmental Science*, *9*(3), 144–159.

Plank, E. (1962). *Working with children in hospitals*. Cleveland, OH: Western Reserve University.

Po, J. (1992). Nurses, children, play. *Issues in Comparative Pediatric Nursing, 15*, 261–269.

Power, T. G. (2000). *Play and exploration in children and animals*. Mahwah, NJ: Erlbaum.

Quinton, D., & Rutter, M. (1976). Early hospital admissions and later disturbances of behaviour: An attempted replication of Douglas' findings. *Developmental Medicine and Child Neurology, 18*, 447–459.

Rae, W., Worchel, F., Upchurch, J., Sanner, J., & Daniel, C. (1989). The psychosocial impact of play on hospitalized children. *Journal of Pediatric Psychology, 14*, 617–627.

Richards, S. S., & Wolff, E. (1940). The organization and function of play activities in the set-up of a pediatric department. *Mental Hygiene, 24*, 229–237.

Robertson, J. (1958). *Young children in hospitals*. New York, NY: Basic Books.

Roopnarine, J. L. (2011). Cultural variations in beliefs about play, parent–child play, and children's play's meaning for child development. In A. D. Pellegrini (Ed.), *The Oxford handbook of the development of play* (pp. 19–37). New York, NY: Oxford University Press.

Rubin, K. H., Fein, G. G., & Vandenberg, B. (1983). Play. In E. M. Hetherington (Ed.), and P. H. Mussen (Series Ed.), *Handbook of child psychology:* Vol. 4 socialization, personality and social development (pp. 698–774). New York, NY: Wiley.

Rutter, M. (1981). Psychosocial resilience and protective mechanisms. *American Journal of Orthopsychiatry, 57,* 316–331.

Schwartz, B. H., Albino, J. E., & Tedesco, L. A. (1983). Effects of psychological preparation on children hospitalized for dental operations. *Journal of Pediatrics, 102,* 634–638.

Schwartzman, H. (1978). *Transformations: The anthropology of children's play.* New York, NY: Plenum Press.

Shure, M. (1963). Psychological ecology of a nursery school. *Child Development, 34,* 979–992.

Smilansky, S. (1968). *The effects of socio-dramatic play on disadvantaged preschool children.* New York, NY: Wiley.

Smith, P. K. (1995). Play, ethology, and education: A personal account. In A. D. Pellegrini (Ed.), *The future of play theory: A multidisciplinary inquiry into the contributions of Brian Sutton-Smith* (pp. 3–21). Albany, NY: State University of New York Press.

Smith, P. K., & Connolly, K. J. (1981). Social and aggressive behavior in preschool children as a function of crowding. *Social Science Information, 16,* 601–620.

Smith, P., & Vollstedt, R. (1985). On defining play: An empirical study of the relationship between play and various play criteria. *Child Development, 56,* 1042–1050.

Spencer, H. (1870). *Principles of psychology.* New York, NY: Appleton.

Spodek, B., & Saracho, O. N. (1988). The challenge of educational play. In D. Bergen (Ed.), *Play as a medium for learning and development* (pp. 9–22). Portsmouth, NH: Heinemann.

Sutton-Smith, B. (1995). The pervasive rhetorics of play. In A. D. Pellegrini (Ed.), *The future of play theory: A multidisciplinary inquiry into the contributions of Brian Sutton-Smith* (pp. 275-294). Albany: State University of New York Press.

Sutton-Smith, B. (2009). *The ambiguity of play.* Boston, MA: Harvard University Press.

Thompson, R. H. (1985). *Psychological research on pediatric hospitalization and health care: A review of the literature.* Springfield, IL: Thomas.

Thompson, R. H. (1995). Documenting the value of play for hospitalized children: The challenge of playing the game. In E. Klugman (Ed.), *Play, policy, and practice* (pp. 145–158). St. Paul, MN: Redleaf Press.

Thompson, R. (2009). *The handbook of child life: A guide for pediatric psychosocial care.* Springfield, IL: C. C. Thomas.

Tisza, V. B., Hurwitz, I., & Angoff, K. (1970). The use of a play program by hospitalized children. *Journal of the American Academy of Child Psychiatry, 9,* 515–531.

Tonkin, A. (Ed.) (2014). *Play in healthcare: Using play to promote child development and wellbeing.* New York, NY: Routledge.

Trawick-Smith, J. (2009). *Science in support of play: The case for play-based preschool programs.* Willimantic, CT: Eastern Connecticut State University, Center for Early Childhood Education.

Turner, J., & Brown, C. (2014). *The pips of child life: Early play programs in hospitals.* Dubuque, IA: Kendall Hunt Publishing.

Vilas, D. B. (2014). *Report on findings on play practices and innovations survey: The state of play in North American hospitals.* Arlington, VA: Child Life Council.

Vredevoe, D. L., Kim, A. C., Dambacher, B. M., & Call, J. D. (1969). Aggressive post-operative play responses of hospitalized children. *Nursing Research Report, 4,* 4–5.

Vygotsky, L. (1978). *Mind in society.* Cambridge, MA: Harvard University Press.

White, R. E. (2012). *The power of play.* Minnesota Children's Museum. Retrieved from http://www.mcm.org/uploads/MCMResearchSummary.pdf

Williams, Y. B., & Powell, M. (1980). Documenting the value of supervised play in a pediatric ambulatory care clinic. *Journal of the Association for the Care of Children's Health, 9,* 15.

Wilson, J. M. (2014). A new era: From play activities to child life at Johns Hopkins Hospital. In J. Turner & C. Brown. (Eds.), *The pips of child life: Early play programs in hospitals* (Chapter 8). Dubuque, IA: Kendall/Hunt.

Wilson, J. M., & Chambers, E. (1996). Child life can (and must) adapt to the new healthcare environment. *The Advocate, 2,* 36–37.

Wing, L. A. (1995). Play is not the work of the child: Young children's perceptions of work and play. *Early Childhood Research Quarterly, 10*(2), 223–247.

Wolfer, J., Gaynard, L., Goldberger, J., Laidley, L., & Thompson, R. (1988). An experimental evaluation of a model child life program. *Children's Health Care, 16,* 244–254.

Wolfgang, C. H., & Bolig, R. (1979). Play techniques for preschool age children under stress. *Journal of the Association for Care of Children in Hospitals, 7,* 3–10.

4 The Arts in Children's Health-Care Settings

Judy A. Rollins

Objectives

At the conclusion of this chapter, the reader will be able to:

1. Discuss the theoretical and cultural explanations for using the arts for emotional, social, and cognitive adaptation and coping.
2. Review historical and current thinking about the use of the arts in the healing process with children and youth.
3. Define various forms and relevant functions of creative arts therapy.
4. Summarize the current body of research on the use of the arts with children in health-care settings and during health-care encounters.
5. Outline resources and supports for the use of the expressive arts in health-care settings.

Health-care experts agree that hospitalization and other health-care experiences can have serious emotional consequences for children. However, with appropriate support, children can weather, and even grow from, these experiences. The arts can play a significant role in this support.

Although the arts may lack the power to cure, they can promote healing. To more fully understand the use of the arts in health-care settings, it is important to understand the distinction between "curing" and "healing." Curing is to bring about recovery from a disease (i.e., to eliminate the disease). Healing is a process of becoming physically and psychologically whole; healing can take place even as the body weakens (Graham, 1993). Some of the most powerful experiences with the arts can occur when cure is no longer an option and impending death is a reality.

The concept of using the arts in health-care settings is not new. Music greeted the ancient Greeks when they entered their temples of healing. But even before then, art was a healing force. Human beings have always used pictures, stories, dances, and chants as healing rituals (Graham-Pole, 2000). As Western medicine developed with an emphasis on disease processes and cure, the arts were cast aside. Today, however, there is renewed interest in complementary, alternative, or integrative medicine practices, of which the arts often are considered a part. Recognizing the need to investigate and evaluate such practices, the U.S. Congress mandated the establishment of the Office of Alternative Medicine at the National Institutes of Health (NIH) in 1991, which in 2014 became the National Center for Complementary and Integrative Health (NCCIH) (National Institutes of Health, 2016).

Children use the arts in health-care settings much in the same way they use play (see Chapter 3: Play in Children's Health-Care Settings); however, a distinction can be made. According to Greaves (personal communication, February 1996), "Of course art is play. . . . It all starts off that way, playing around with ideas. Creativity is play. And children use play as a creative tool. After the play though, the production of the artwork then becomes hard work." Offering a combination of creativity and discipline, the arts start from where children are, but make them raise their sights (Rogers, 1995).

This chapter addresses the *therapeutic use of the arts* with children in health-care settings. "Art itself is in many ways therapeutic, for it permits the discharge of tension and the representation of forbidden thoughts and feelings in socially acceptable forms" (Rubin, 1982, p. 57). It is important to distinguish between the therapeutic use of the arts and *creative* (art, music, dance, poetry, drama) *therapy*. In the first instance, artists and other caring adults facilitate children's engagement in expressive activities that may be therapeutic. For example, children may communicate verbally or nonverbally their thoughts, feelings, and concerns through or while engaging in these expressive activities, or use such activities as a distraction to cope with pain. However, *creative arts therapists*, who receive special training that prepares them to prescribe and interpret specific expressive activities, conduct *creative arts therapies*. These highly trained professionals use the wide range of arts modalities and creative processes to enhance self-awareness; foster health communication and expression; promote the integration of physical, emotional, cognitive, and social functioning; and facilitate behavioral and personal change (National Coalition of Creative Arts Therapies Associations, n.d.). Called creative arts therapies because of their roots in the arts and theories of creativity, these therapies are a unique domain of psychotherapy and counseling and are defined as

> the use of art, music drama, dance/movement, poetry/creative writing bibliotherapy, play, and sandplay within the context of psychotherapy, counseling, rehabilitation, or medicine. Additionally, the expressive therapies are sometimes referred to as "integrative" when various arts are purposively used in combination in treatment. (Malchiodi, 2014)

A certification and/or licensing process is involved. Professional artists without these credentials can do meaningful work with children, but they must be aware of their limitations and not cross the boundary into territory for which they are unprepared. Bucciarelli (2016) points out that, increasingly, artists in residence or artists in healthcare (University of Florida Center for Arts in Medicine, 2017) and creative arts therapists are working together in health care settings.

The term *arts* often first brings to mind the visual arts, yet all forms of the arts (e.g., music, dance, storytelling, poetry, drama, photography) can be used and even mixed when working with children who are ill, disabled, or dying. This chapter begins with a discussion of ways children use the arts as tools for coping with illness and health-care experiences and describes related research findings and applications. Recommendations for using the arts with children and for establishing arts programming in children's health-care settings follow.

The Arts as Tools for Coping With Illness and Health-Care Experiences

Health-care experiences have long been recognized as stressful for everyone, but research indicates that these experiences can have serious emotional consequences for the developing child (Rollins & Mahan, 2010). These consequences often are the result of the many stresses inherent in children's health-care experiences. For example, children rarely are permitted to refuse treatments, medications, and procedures. They are constant recipients of "things" being done to them. They may have to "hold still" for a painful procedure, one that they may not understand, and be left feeling powerless and confused. Placed in a passive role with limited opportunities to make meaningful choices, they often experience emotions that are intense and confusing.

Creative outlets give children an opportunity to express the many emotions associated with illness and health-care experiences. These emotions can include troublesome ones, such as fear, confusion, anger, or guilt, as well as happier ones that reflect joy, satisfaction, and personal growth. The creative process is used to transform pain and conflict and foster self-awareness and growth. In the art experience, the person, process, and product are equal.

Participating in the arts can help children deal with several realities of illness and health-care experiences (see Table 4.1). For example, engaging in art experiences can distract children from pain and discomfort. By being positioned in active roles, children are empowered and in control of their world as "doers" instead of "receivers." The arts can provide children opportunities to explore safe methods of emotional expression; help them make the most of their present abilities; engage them in something familiar and enjoyable; and help them learn, grow, and develop in many significant ways (Rollins, 2016).

Pain and Discomfort

Most children who are ill experience some pain or discomfort. Some children engage in play and other expressive activities in an effort to distract themselves from these and other health-care stressors, such as nausea. Although not a substitute for appropriate pharmacological support, the arts can be integrated into a child's pain-management routine. Children often use drawing as a valuable tool to communicate the location and degree of pain, and reports indicate that the arts have been effective to some degree for relief of even severe pain. According to Gerik (2005), children particularly respond to pain-control strategies that involve their imaginations and senses of play.

Gate control theory can serve as a conceptual framework for using the arts to help children cope with pain (Wall, 1973). This theory proposes that pain impulses are moderated by a gating mechanism that opens to allow nerve impulses to reach the brain or closes to decrease or prevent impulse transmission, depending on the extent to which the gate is open. There is central control, which is the influence that cognitive or higher central nervous system processes have on pain perception via descending fibers to the gating system. Anxiety, anticipation, and excitement may open the gate and thus increase the perception of pain. However, cognitive activities such as distraction, suggestion, relaxation, and imagery tend to close the gate and prevent sensory transmission of pain.

Table 4.1

Key Concepts: Meeting Psychosocial/Developmental Needs of Children in Health-Care Settings Through the Arts	
In health-care settings, children	The arts provide opportunities for children to
1. May experience pain and discomfort	Develop new coping strategies Distance and distract themselves
2. Have limited opportunities to make decisions	Make choices Be independent
3. Are in passive roles, where they are led, dressed, doctored, and are the constant recipients of things being done to them	Be the active ones Be the ones in charge
4. Experience many emotions, such as fear, confusion, anger, guilt, happiness, joy, and pride	Communicate feelings, both pleasant and unpleasant Safely let go Relive and master traumatic experiences
5. May be physically limited	Draw on their remaining abilities Imagine what they may be unable to do physically
6. Are in a health-care atmosphere with confusing sights, sounds, smells, and strangers	Do something "normal" and familiar Share experiences with others Experience the pleasure and joy of childhood
7. Are in a situation that provides opportunities for learning and growth	Demonstrate understanding of their condition and treatment Experience closure Develop potential for a lifelong interest in the arts and creative expression

Note. Adapted from *Art is the HeART: An Arts-in-Healthcare Program for Children and Families in Home and Hospice Care* (p. 53), by J. Rollins and L. Riccio, 2001, Washington, DC: WVSA Arts Connection. Copyright 2001 by WVSA Arts Connection. Adapted with permission.

Reduced Opportunities to Make Decisions

Children are rarely permitted to refuse or reschedule treatments, medications, and procedures. The ability to make choices gives children a much-needed sense of control over something in their lives and therefore helps relieve stress. Engaging in the arts, children have endless opportunities to make choices. They can choose colors, what to paint, which musical instrument to play, which dance move to make, the ending to a story, poem, or song, and so on (see Figure 4.1). They can even choose not to participate in an activity. This decision, too, has great value; it may be the only real choice the child has had honored that day.

Passive Role

Many of the things that are done to children when they are ill—being poked, prodded, led, doctored, nursed, or dressed—are unpleasant or even painful. Again, children

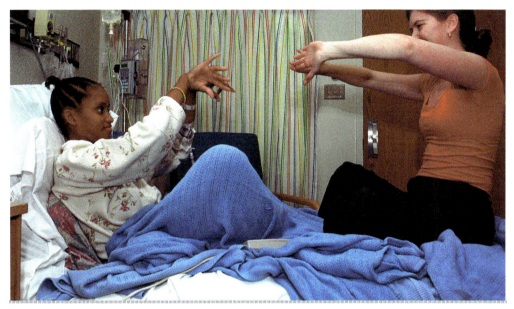

Figure 4.1. The arts provide many opportunities for children to make choices.

usually have no choice. When children are creating, they are the ones in charge. They can squish lumps of clay and form animals or whatever they wish, pound nails into wood and build airplanes, sing as loudly or softly as they like. For that moment, *they* are in control, the captains of their ship, the masters of their universe.

Emotions

Children can experience unpleasant emotions when ill. It is difficult to have to "hold still" for a painful procedure, to be nauseated all the time, to get shots, or to miss school graduation. Health-care experiences are especially confusing for young children. They may wonder why their parents are letting these terrible things happen to them and be bewildered by their feelings of anger toward people as well as events. They often express anger in misbehavior or refusal to cooperate.

Children often find it easier to express these feelings and concerns through the arts. Something as simple as the health-care professional or artist saying to a child after a difficult procedure, "Children sometimes tell me that having their blood drawn can be kind of hard. I wonder if you could draw a picture of what it was like for you and we can talk about it," can provide an opportunity for the child to process the experience and the emotions that surround it.

In many social settings, such as family or school, children receive the message that expression of strong emotion—anger, fear, grief—will exacerbate interpersonal tensions and hasten rejection. Research indicates, however, that habitual repression of strong emotions can lead to immune deficits that reduce resistance to infection and neoplastic disease (Pert, Dreher, & Ruff, 1998) and poor mental health (Hu et al., 2014).

The creative process facilitates a more honest reflection of what children are thinking and feeling—their hopes, dreams, and fears (see Figure 4.2). Looking at the sequence of cognitive development, children think first in images; as they grow older they learn to translate these images into words. Then they learn to play it safe with words, guarding what they reveal about their thoughts, ideas, or feelings.

Not all the emotions children experience while ill, hospitalized, or dying are unpleasant. Engaging in the arts can take children, sometimes only for a moment, to a different place—a place of joy and contentment. Children can use the arts to express these good feelings, too.

Physical Limitations

Children may be physically limited, some temporarily (an arm immobilized for an intravenous line), some permanently. Also, certain conditions, such as cystic fibrosis or cancer, can sap a child's energy and therefore limit activity.

Methods for engaging in an art activity can usually be adapted to meet special needs. For example, children without the use of their arms can learn to hold a paintbrush with their mouths or feet. In other cases, tools can be adapted. For example, foam rubber can be wrapped around crayons or pencils and secured with a rubber band. This shapes the child's hand around the implement, making it harder to drop. Often the children themselves suggest adaptations, recognizing that methods or equipment they use for other activities, for instance, holding a spoon for feeding, can be transferred to arts experiences, such as holding a paintbrush.

Redefining the arts experience is another method of adapting. For example, what exactly is "dancing"? We typically think of moving across space on our feet. However, children can dance using only their arms or even simply their eyes. Much of what children take away from an arts experience is the good feeling that comes from self-expression, which is acting at whatever level possible in whatever way they decide. Even if a child is unable to physically participate in a particular activity, often he or she can still decide the important factors, such as choice of colors for a painting, where a line goes in a drawing, what song to sing, and so on, while directing someone else in the actual execution (see Text Box 4.1 and Figure 4.3).

Some children (e.g., children undergoing bone marrow transplants), although physically able to move about, may be physically confined and isolated in their hospital room for infection control or protection. Art experiences can be designed to help them feel less isolated and part of a "community." For example, an artist can go from room to room asking every child for a line to a poem or a move for a dance routine and afterwards return to each room to share the completed project.

Physical limitations may take on added dimensions for children with special health-care needs. Throughout the course of childhood, most children will miss at least one party or other anticipated event because of illness. For the child with a

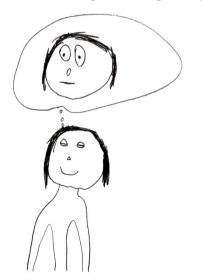

Figure 4.2. Drawing provided an excellent communication tool for this 7-year-old boy to express a common presurgery fear: waking up in the middle of the operation.

Text Box 4.1
Artist by Proxy

The practice of drawing by proxy goes back at least to the 17th century. It has been said that Peter Paul Rubens had others do preliminary drawings for him when his hands became crippled with arthritis. Because of the complex directions he provided, the resultant painting was truly his; the drawer simply acted as a tool. Artist and children's book author and illustrator Joan Drescher applies this technique with interactive sessions using her book, *The Moon Balloon*. Research confirmed the benefits of these sessions with hospitalized children. Rollins, Drescher, and Kelleher (2011) conducted a study with 50 hospitalized children (ages 6 to 19 years) who participated in 45- to 60-minute artist-by-proxy sessions based on *The Moon Balloon*. During the individual sessions in the children's hospital room, children chose balloons that represented different feelings, and Drescher drew the balloons with the child's requested images inside. She continually asked the child to describe details to generate richness and enhance interaction (e.g., "What color is your dog?"), and after drawing, asked for verification. Findings revealed that the sessions improved children's perceptions of their present quality of life as measured by PedsQL Present Functioning Visual Analogue Scales (Sherman, Eisen, Burwinkle, & Varni, 2006), and provided an effective method for children to express their thoughts about the hospital, illness, and unrelated issues.

Note. Adapted from "Exploring the Ability of a Drawing by Proxy Intervention to Improve Quality of Life for Hospitalized Children" by J. Rollins, J. Dresher, and M. Kelleher, 2011, *Arts & Health, 4*(1), 55–69.

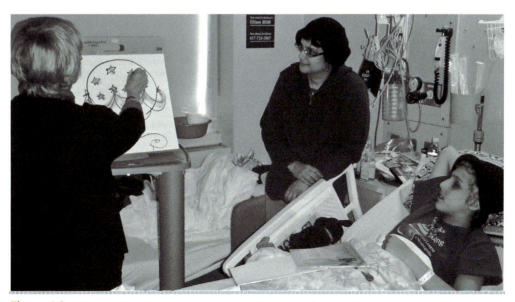

Figure 4.3. Children tell artist Joan Drescher exactly what to draw and how to draw it in Moon Balloon drawing-by-proxy sessions.

chronic illness or disability, this may not be a once-in-a-childhood occurrence but something that happens all the time—something the child comes to expect. These factors all contribute to the enormous sense of isolation many children with special needs and their families experience.

Health-Care Atmosphere

The health-care atmosphere may mean confusing sights, sounds, and smells, and strangers entering the hospital room, treatment room, or even the sanctity of the child's home. This atmosphere does little to foster the normal experiences of childhood. Like play, creating art or engaging in other expressive activities is normal, the essential "work" of childhood. The creative process allows children to escape from their situation and return to the world they know. Children often can share these expressive experiences alongside family members and friends. Parents frequently report that watching their children engaged in normal childhood activities gives them a real sense of hope. As opposed to particularized hope, which relates to a specific outcome such as recovery from a condition, this sense of generalized hope can be seen as a state that gives life meaning and protects against despair (Wiles, Cott, & Gibson, 2008).

Learning and Growing

Children in health-care settings have the opportunity to learn about physical concerns and about themselves. They can communicate their understanding of their condition and treatment in expressive activities, which gives parents and health-care professionals opportunities to discuss a child's understanding and concerns and correct misconceptions. For example, a 10-year-old girl with heart disease was scheduled to have some teeth extracted in preparation for future orthodontic work. Because of her heart condition, the dental surgery was taking place in a hospital to enable appropriate monitoring. She was asked to draw a picture of why she had come to the hospital, which she depicted accurately and somewhat humorously, in Figure 4.4. Next, she was asked to draw a picture of how she thought the operating room would look. Although she had been hospitalized in the past, she had never been in an operating room. She produced the drawing in Figure 4.5. When she was asked about the obvious hole in the patient's chest, she expressed her concern that because previous hospitalizations were always for her heart condition, the doctor might mistakenly operate on her heart instead of her teeth. This information was passed on to the dental surgeon and the anesthesiologist, both of whom assured her of which parts of her body would be involved and which parts would not. Drawing allowed her to communicate what she had been unable to express in words. Perhaps Bernie Warren, a professor of Dramatic Art at the University of Windsor, Canada, said it best: "Things that are scary are often beyond words" (B. Warren, personal communication, November 2000).

The arts have a unique role for children with chronic conditions who face a lifetime of health-care experiences. Having the opportunity to complete an art activity, with a final product, allows such children to experience a much-needed sense of closure, plus the personal satisfaction that comes from a job well done. A lifelong interest in the arts might begin in the hospital, clinic, home, or hospice care setting. For children with chronic or disabling conditions whose occupational choices may be limited, this may be the most important benefit of all.

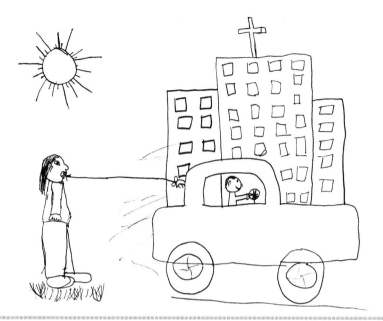

Figure 4.4. Through her drawing, a 10-year-old girl communicates her knowledge of the reason for her coming to the hospital.

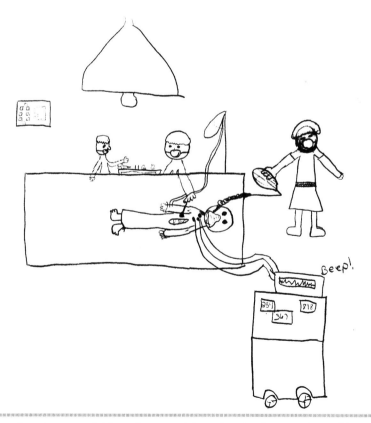

Figure 4.5. In their drawings children often reveal fears that they have not been able to put into words.

Although having special meaning for children in health-care settings, creative expression plays a critical role in growth and development for *all* children. Evidence indicates that the arts, particularly music, dance, and the visual arts, develop neural connections and body/brain connections, which further learning in many areas, including math, reading, writing, and general language development (Hanna, Patterson, Rollins, & Sherman, 2011). The very nature of creative activities—there is no one right way to express something—promotes success and all the good feelings that go along with it. Certain experiences also can help children develop large and small muscle skills. The creative process itself promotes mental or cognitive development, for creating is a series of problem solving and decision-making. Creative expression also fosters emotional and social development. Art is a universal language, and children express themselves more naturally and spontaneously through art than through words.

Research Findings and Applications

Limited research, particularly quantitative research, has been conducted regarding the impact of the arts with children in health care. With exceptions, much of the evidence available to date is anecdotal, but with the rapid development of the arts and health/arts in the health-care field, that situation is changing. In recent years, because of increasing interest in complementary, integrative, and mind–body medicine, and greater acceptance of alternative practices, more funding has become available for research in these areas. The development of new quantitative tools and greater acceptance of more sophisticated qualitative measures hold great promise for answers to many of our questions in the near future.

There is, however, much research activity in the use of some creative arts therapies, particularly music therapy. Please note that creative arts therapists conducted some of the research cited here (as noted), and thus some findings may not be applicable when such arts experiences are facilitated by individuals who do not have the specific knowledge and skills that professional creative arts therapists have.

A small but growing body of research indicates that a physiological process may actually take place through contact with certain images and other forms of the arts. Goldstein (1980) described "thrills"—tingling sensations individuals may experience when exposed to emotionally arousing stimuli. His findings show a relationship between these experiences and the release of endorphins—which serve as the body's own pain reliever, relaxer, and mood enhancer. An emerging science that is part of this physiological research is psychoneuroimmunology (PNI), which is concerned with the correlation between stress and health. Specifically, PNI refers to the study of the relationship between the mind and the brain, nervous system, endocrine system, and immune system (Linton, 1995). Research findings in this field clearly demonstrate that the mind, brain, and nervous system can be directly influenced, either positively or negatively, by sensual elements in the environment (Crawford, Lee, Bingham, & Active Self-Care Therapies for Pain, 2014).

Schoeller (2015) discusses occurrences that sound similar to Goldstein's thrills. He defines chills: "a muscular phenomenon best described as the sensation of coldness created by a rhythmic oscillating tremor of skeletal muscles" (p. 1). Such events are referred to as *aesthetic chills* when they are associated with a positive, pleasant process and are often associated with goose bumps and shivers down the spine. Although mainly studied in the field of musicology, aesthetic chills also may be elicited by visual arts, literature, scientific research, and religious practices. It is hypothesized that aesthetic chills correspond to a satisfaction of humans' internal drive to acquire knowledge about the external world and perceive objects and situations as meaningful. This need to explore and understand environmental conditions is a biological prerequisite for survival.

Although there is much to learn, the literature on stress provides some rationales for the efficacy of the use of the arts in children's health-care settings. Ryan-Wenger (1992) described 15 categories of strategies children use to cope with stress. Of these, the use of at least five strategies—"behavioral distraction," "cognitive distraction," "emotional expression," "self-controlling activities," and "social support"—can be fostered by engaging in the arts. For example, painting, listening to music, or laughing at a funny story can help children set aside the need to deal with stressors for a time.

Much overlap exists between the arts, and often more than one modality is used concurrently in practice and research (e.g., singing and drama as a part of storytelling, dancing to music). For example, Madden, Mowry, Gao, Cullen, and Foreman (2010) found that a combination of art therapy, music therapy, and dance/movement therapy improved response to such factors as pain and nausea and improved children's mood. However, for organizational purposes, what follows is a selection of research findings categorized loosely by art modality.

Music

Music-based interventions hold promise for overriding emotional and behavioral reactions to stress for the following reasons: (1) an extensive body of research has established music as an effective medium for altering mood states and diminishing state anxiety; (2) music-based interventions have been shown to be effective in directing and sustaining children's attention during stressful medical procedures; and (3) music's social qualities have been used in clinical situations to foster family communication and interaction (Robb et al., 2008). Below are examples of research in these areas as well as others related to health-care conditions and circumstances.

Music therapy research supports inclusion of the evidence-based neonatal intensive care unit (NICU) music therapy protocols in best-practice standards for treating preterm infants (Standley, 2012). Music therapy with live sound and parent-preferred lullabies improved infants' cardiac and respiratory function (Loewy, Stewart, Dassler, Telsey, & Homel, 2013) and enhanced parent–child bonding, thus decreasing parental stress (Loewy, 2015; Loewy et al., 2013). Live harp music led to increased weight gain in stable premature infants (Kemper & Hamilton, 2008), and, when combined with kangaroo care (KC) (see Chapter 1: Children's Hospitalization and Other Health-Care Encounters), reduced mothers' anxiety more than KC alone (Schlez et al., 2011). Schwilling and colleagues (2015) reported significantly lower salivary cortisol level, reduced apneas and oxygen desaturations, and improved pain scores for premature infants exposed to 15 minutes of live harp music on 3 consecutive days. A pacifier-activated lullaby system (PAL)—a pacifier fitted with a pressure transducer that activated 10 seconds of recorded music—increased feeding rates of premature infants (Standley, 2003) and significantly shortened the length of gavage feeding for 34-week-old babies

(Standley et al., 2010). The music of Mozart limited infants' pain increase during heel-lance procedures for blood collection (Bergomi et al., 2014).

Several studies have dealt with children's use of music for coping with disease-related stressors. Regarding asthma, school-age children with asthma say that listening to music is one of the most effective and frequently used strategies for coping with their disease (Fley & Beier, 2006). In one study, playing a brass or wind instrument or singing decreased asthma symptoms, depression, and anxiety (Sliwka, Wloch, Tynor, & Nowobilski, 2014). For pediatric oncology patients, music can alleviate adverse cancer experiences and promote resilience and normal development, and the positive effect may carry over to the home environment and vicariously support families (O'Callaghan, Baron, Barry, & Dun, 2011). In an outpatient pediatric oncology clinic, 20 minutes of music improved relaxation significantly more than 20 minutes of rest (Kemper, Hamilton, McLean, & Lovato, 2008).

O'Callaghan, Barry, and Thompson (2012) remind us that adolescents and young adults (AYAs) with cancer require special care "because of intensified challenges related to developmental vulnerability, treatment toxicity effects, and slower improvements in survival rates compared to other age groups" (p. 687). When asked for their perspectives about music's role in their lives, most AYAs mentioned music's calming, supportive, and relaxing effects, which alleviated hardships associated with their diagnosis. Music offered supportive messages, enabled personal and shared understandings about cancer's effects, and elicited helpful physical, emotional, and imaginary states. Music therapy helped promote normalization and supportive connections with others.

Robb et al. (2014) examined the efficacy of a therapeutic music video (TMV) intervention delivered to AYAs during the acute phase of hematopoietic stem cell transplant. The multisite randomized controlled trial assigned 113 AYAs ages 11–24 years to either a six-session intervention with a music therapist to create a music video or the control group, which allowed participants to choose from 15 audiobooks selected by a librarian with expertise in AYAs, listen to and discuss the books, and exchange books as desired. The TMV group reported significantly better courageous coping, social integration, and family environment.

Kemper and McLean (2008) investigated parents' attitudes and expectations regarding music's effect on their children with cancer. Of those responding to their survey ($N = 45$), 82% reported playing music for their child at home within the previous week. Reasons cited for playing music included (1) to entertain, (2) to help the patient feel better, (3) to keep the patient comfortable, (4) to provide comfort, (5) to distract the patient from pain, and (6) to distract the patient from nausea.

Music also has proved beneficial in establishing treatment routines as positive experiences for children and their families (Grasso, Button, Allison, & Sawyer, 2000). Routine chest physiotherapy (CPT, an important component of prophylactic therapy for children with cystic fibrosis) requires a significant commitment of time and energy. Grasso and colleagues evaluated the effect of using recorded music as an adjunct to CPT and compared effects of the use of music specifically composed and compiled by a music therapist, familiar music, and no audiotape on children's and parents' enjoyment of CPT. Findings indicate that enjoyment of CPT significantly increased after the use of specifically composed and recorded music as an adjunct.

Marley (1984) found that music reduced stress-related behaviors in infants and toddlers who were hospitalized. (See Text Box 4.2.) Music also has produced relaxation for children during cardiac catheterization (Micci, 1984) and decreased preoperative anxiety (Kain et al., 2004) and preprocedure anxiety (Liu et al., 2007). Music can provide channels through which children can express the fear, anger, sadness, and loneliness of hospitalization. Peter Alsop and Bill Harley's album *In the Hospital*, which features children talking and singing about their feelings and hospital experiences, helps hospitalized children communicate their own thoughts and feelings (Grimm & Pefley, 1990). Hearing about others through story or song helps children realize that they are not alone in a particular situation.

Music can be used before, during, and after procedures. Procedural-support music therapy achieved a 100% success rate in eliminating the need for sedation for children receiving echocardiograms (ECGs) (Walworth, 2005). In a study of 108 unpremedicated children ages 4–13 years who underwent venipuncture, those who interacted with a musician had significantly lower distress and pain intensity than those in the control group (Caprilli, Anastasi, Grotto, Abeti, & Messeri, 2007). Balan, Bavdekar, and Jadhav (2009) reported similar findings using recorded classical instrumental music. The use of postoperative music medicine (see Text Box 4.3) was found to reduce morphine consumption for school-age children who had undergone day surgery (Nilsson, Kokinsky, Nilsson, Sidenvall, & Enskar, 2009).

The type of music used is an important consideration. McCraty, Barrios-Choplin, Atkinson, and Tomasino (1998) investigated the effects of different types of music on tension, mood, and mental clarity. Participants completed psychological profiles before and after listening to 15 minutes of four types of music: grunge rock, classical, New Age, and designer (music designed to have specific effects on the listener). Feeling shifts among participants were observed with all types of music. Of the four types, designer music was most effective in increasing positive feelings and decreasing negative feelings. The findings are summarized in Table 4.2 and suggest that designer music may be useful in the treatment of tension, mental distraction, and negative moods.

Table 4.2

Effects of Four Different Types of Music on Tension, Mood, and Mental Clarity	
Type of Music	**Impact**
Grunge rock	Significant increases in hostility, sadness, tension, and fatigue Significant reductions in caring, relaxation, mental clarity, and vigor
Classical	Mixed
New Age	Mixed
Designer	Significant increases in caring, relaxation, mental clarity, and vigor Significant decreases in hostility, fatigue, sadness, and tension

Note. Adapted from "The Effects of Different Types of Music on Mood, Tension, and Mental Clarity," by R. McCraty, B. Barrios-Choplin, M. Atkinson, and D. Tomasino, 1998, *Alternative Therapies in Health and Medicine, 4*(1), pp. 75–84.

Text Box 4.2
Heartbeat Lullabies: Heartbeat Music Therapy

Heartbeat Lullabies—arrangements of songs that incorporate actual human heartbeat with music and singing—have been used in a variety of ways with children:

- to help decrease the amount of sedative medications,
- to help relax claustrophobic children undergoing magnetic resonance imaging,
- to calm babies who are born dependent on cocaine,
- to calm fussy, irritable babies,
- to help ease premature infants' transition to the home, and
- to help normal, healthy children who have trouble sleeping.

Research findings indicate positive results from the use of Heartbeat Music Therapy recordings (Research, n.d.). Nurses in a newborn nursery used the tape with 59 infants over a 6-week period in 1985. They found that 94% of the infants stopped crying or went to sleep within 2 minutes when the Heartbeat Music Therapy recording was played.

Researchers in the NICU at Children's Hospital Medical Center of Akron, in Akron, Ohio, used the Heartbeat Music Therapy recordings in their study of the effects of music enhancement and sound reduction on the growth and development of premature babies.

Previous studies on music enhancement and on sound reduction showed that noise increases a newborn's heart rate and blood pressure and decreases oxygen saturation levels. Noise also causes babies to spend more time awake or crying. They miss the important sleep time in which they conserve the energy and calories they need for healthy growth.

The Akron study included NICU babies who were born at 25 to 30 weeks' gestation, weighed less than 2 lb. 12 oz. at birth, and were medically stable. Babies were divided into three groups. Group 1 babies heard the Heartbeat Music Therapy recordings, Group 2 babies wore foam-plastic earmuffs, and babies in Group 3 received standard NICU care. Participation in the study began by the time an infant was 7 days old and continued until discharge. The results of the 3-year study showed that babies who received the music treatment had better sleeping patterns, had steadier heart rates and respiration, and were released from the hospital 2 weeks earlier than babies who did not receive musical stimulation.

In a randomized, double-blind study of 23 neonates undergoing circumcision at a large university hospital, Joyce, Keck, and Gerkensmeyer (2001) found that pain intensity rates were less for the babies listening to Heartbeat Music Therapy recordings than for babies hearing no music. Further, the heart rates for babies who had the music intervention remained stable, resulting in higher oxygen saturation rates throughout the procedure.

The results of this and other studies can have important implications for use of music therapy in a variety of health-care settings. For more information on Heartbeat Music Therapy and a sample of the intervention, see the website http://babygotosleep.com/ or contact Terry Woodford at terry@audiotherapy.com or 1-800-537-7748.

Note. Used with permission of Audiotherapy Innovations, 2519 W. Pikes Peak Avenue, Colorado Springs, CO 80904.

‖‖‖

Text Box 4.3
MusiCure

MusiCure is music created by composer and oboist Nils Eje. MusiCure consists of genre-less soundscapes intended to appeal to all listeners, regardless of musical tastes and everyday listening habits. The compositions combine acoustic instrumental solos and ensemble work with recordings of nature sounds that have been carefully selected and integrated into the music. The entire MusiCure series is evidence based and has two primary goals: (1) to have a physically soothing, calming, and relaxing effect and (2) to simulate the mind in a positive way, providing mental inspiration and optimistic inner journeys in nature.

‖‖

Note. Retrieved from http://musicure.com/category/about-musicure-6/

Certain types of music are used in palliative care. Therese Schroeder-Sheker (1993), a pioneer in the field of music thanatology, explained that music for the living is meant to engage the listener, while music for the dying is meant to free the listener. Although music is individualized for each patient, chants frequently are used because of their freeing tendency:

> The plainchant or Gregorian chant is sung without being attached to rhythm; one cannot count a pulse. There is no rhythmic accent. The body of sung prayer is in neither 4/4 nor 3/4 (3 or 4 beats per measure); therefore, the chants are not stimulating, they are calming. Almost always, symmetrical music in 4/4, regardless of tempo, helps sustain metabolic activity and support the general binding tendency to deepen incarnation and relationship to physical body. (p. 45)

Parents have claimed that palliative music therapy provided comfort and stimulation for their child as well as a positive experience for the family (Lindenfelser, Hense, & McFerran, 2012). Palliative care music therapy interventions can also assist in pain management and encourage bonding and legacy building (Duda, 2013).

Visual Arts

Archibald, Scott, and Hartling (2014) reported on the use of visual art as a mechanism to facilitate or reduce specific child attributes (e.g., self-efficacy, anxiety) and to facilitate understanding through communication or assessment. For children with asthma, for example, 7 weeks of 1-hour art therapy group sessions decreased anxiety and increased quality of life (Beebe, Gelfand, & Bender, 2010).

Art therapists, play therapists, child life specialists, psychologists, medical social workers, clinical counselors, psychiatric nurses, and other mental health-care professionals have widely used art expression in therapy with children in medical environments, yet until recently very little has been written specifically about "medical art therapy." Medical art therapy is the use of art expression and imagery with individuals who are physically ill, experiencing trauma to the body, or undergoing aggressive medical treatment such as surgery or chemotherapy (Malchiodi, 1993). In the first book devoted to medical art therapy with children (Malchiodi, 1999), contributing authors discussed the use of medical art therapy using mandalas (Delue), with children with eating disorders (Cleveland), cancer (Councill), asthma (Gabriels), HIV/AIDS (Piccirillo), burns (Russell), and arthritis (Barton). In a final chapter, Malchiodi discussed the somatic and spiritual aspects of children's art expressions.

Drawing, painting, sculpture, and other visual art modalities offer a means of nonverbal communication. The visual arts can bring out mixed, poorly understood feelings, in an attempt to bring them to order and clarity. Visual art activities provide a vehicle for children to express their anxiety and other feelings related to health-care experiences and illness. Rubin (1999, p. 10) pointed out that not only art therapists could make the healing capacity of art available to children: "Many people can—and should—offer children art material in situations of medical stress." Although the use of projective artwork and other art therapy techniques are often best left to certified art therapists, other caring adults can use other techniques, such as the illuminative artwork technique. In this method, the facilitator does not impose analysis of the child's work, but instead encourages the child to use the artwork as a communication tool (Spouse, 2000). The child renders a drawing based on a certain topic or theme and is then asked to explain its significance.

Rollins (2003) found that children used this type of drawing as a means of direct expression, and/or as a focal point from which conversation would flow. She calls this second way the "campfire effect," the result of an activity or experience that provides a focal point shared by the individuals involved and serves to increase conversation in both quality and quantity (see Case Study 4.1 and Figure 4.6).

A similar method, "draw-and-write," involves inviting children to draw pictures and then write about what is happening in their pictures. Data for this method are richer and more insightful than those obtained through writing alone. This method has proven effective in exploring young children's perceptions about health and illness; it helps the less verbally able to communicate their own health perceptions because

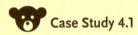 Case Study 4.1

"I was a scared girl."

A 12-year-old girl with a brain tumor created the drawing in Figure 4.6. She used her drawing both as a means of direct expression and as a conversation starter. She said she was the girl in her drawing and this is what she looked like when she was told she had cancer: "I was a scared girl." She said that she had been afraid of dying and then looked up, saying, "And I am again right now." She sensed she was dying and, with no treatment options left, in fact was, but had not been told. Her parents were reluctant to give her the news and asked the physician to hold back as well. After seeing her drawing, the physician convinced the family that now was the appropriate time to have that conversation.

Figure 4.6. A 12-year-old girl used her drawing as both direct expression of her fears and a tool for communication, the "campfire effect."

the method allows them to draw and then seek adult help to express their thoughts in writing (Pridmore & Lansdown, 1997).

For example, to explore school-age children's early understanding of basic genetic/genomic concepts, Driessnack and Gallo (2013) used "Draw-and-Tell Conversation" interviews. Children were asked to draw the inside of their bodies using a provided body outline and then to talk about their drawings, followed by specific questions and probes. Using this technique, children shared their emerging awareness of basic genetic concepts through drawing and conversation without hesitation. The researchers concluded that this approach can be used to support parents as they approach and discuss genetic concepts with their children.

While the process of visual expression creates an opportunity for catharsis, at the same time the artwork itself offers a tool to monitor the child's emotional and developmental state and progress. Children who are stressed tend to show more emotional indicators in their drawings than do children who are not stressed. Rae (1991) used the *ipsative method* for analyzing children's drawings for the purpose of assessment. The ipsative method is a procedure whereby psychosocial adjustment and coping are assessed by using the child's own drawings as a standard for comparison. Rather than looking solely at traits, content, or themes in a single drawing, the health-care professional evaluates children's psychosocial and emotional progress as a function of the changes in the drawings over time. Because children's emotional status can change quickly, repeated drawings can offer a more realistic, multidimensional assessment of functioning at a particular time or over a length of time.

Children with cancer have reported engaging in drawing and painting as a means of effectively distracting themselves from even severe pain (Rollins, 1995). In addition to the mechanism in gate control theory, described earlier, brain research over the past four decades may offer another explanation for this occurrence. We now know that

Table 4.3

A Comparison of Left-Mode and Right-Mode Characteristics	
Left Mode	**Right Mode**
Verbal—Using words to name, describe, define	*Nonverbal*—Awareness of things, but minimal connection with words
Analytic—Figuring things out step-by-step and part-by-part	*Synthetic*—Putting things together to form wholes
Symbolic—Using a symbol to stand for something (e.g., the sign "1" stands for the process of addition)	*Concrete*—Relating to things as they are, at the present moment
Abstract—Taking out a small bit of information and using it to represent the whole thing	*Analogic*—Seeing likenesses between things; understanding metaphoric relationships
Temporal—Keeping track of time, sequencing one thing after another; doing first things first, second things second, and so on	*Nontemporal*—Without a sense of time
Rational—Drawing conclusions based on reason and facts	*Nonrational*—Not requiring a basis of reason or facts; willingness to suspend judgment
Digital—Using numbers as in counting	*Spatial*—Seeing where things are in relation to other things and how parts go together to form a whole
Logical—Drawing conclusions based on logic: one thing following another in logical order (e.g., a mathematical theorem or a well-stated argument)	*Intuitive*—Making leaps of insight, often based on incomplete patterns, hunches, feelings, or visual images
Linear—Thinking in terms of linked ideas, one thought directly following another, often leading to a convergent conclusion.	*Holistic*—Seeing whole things all at once; perceiving the overall patterns and structures, often leading to divergent conclusions.

Note. From *Drawing on the Right Side of the Brain* (p. 40), by B. Edwards, 2012, Los Angeles: J. P. Tarcher, Inc. Copyright 1979 by J. P. Tarcher, Inc. Reprinted with permission.

each hemisphere (left and right) of the brain has its own way of knowing and perceiving external reality (see Table 4.3; Edwards, 2012).

Drawing is largely a right-brain function. The ability to draw may depend on whether one has access to the capabilities of the right hemisphere (i.e., whether one can "turn off" the dominant verbal left hemisphere and "turn on" the right). And so, while operating in the right hemisphere, the child who is drawing may be aware of pain but with the left side turned off, he or she does not focus on the words to name, describe, or define it; the focus is on the drawing. The process of creating makes it difficult to think or worry about other things at the same time. Furthermore, with the right hemisphere's sense of timelessness, individuals often emerge from a drawing session surprised at the passage of time and how comfortable they were during that period.

Although children who are ill often communicate thoughts, feelings, fears, or concerns about their illness through their drawings, just as often the content of their drawings may be unrelated to disease. In some cases children's drawings refer to non-disease-related stressors that are common in the lives of many of today's children: parental divorce and remarriage, geographic mobility, maternal employment and alternative sources of child care, competitive pressures, and various forms of parental insufficiency (Rollins, 1990). Coping with stressors of this nature may be as difficult as, or even more difficult for the child than, coping with disease-related stressors.

The use of the arts in health-care settings typically focuses on process over product. But at times the product itself can take on importance. While the process can create relaxation, distraction, or excitement, the finished products of painting, printmaking, sculpting, and other visual arts experiences can bring the child great satisfaction. There is much joy and pride in successfully creating what one set out to create, or even pleasant surprise when something turns out better than expected. Finally, product is important for legacy activities (see Chapter 6: The Child Who Is Dying and Chapter 9: Spiritual Issues in Children's Health-Care Settings), and every effort should be made to provide quality materials and expert facilitation to create these precious memories.

Storytelling

Many children find storytelling or reading helpful in coping with stress. Stories can offer a means of dealing with unfaceable fears and untenable realities by doing so indirectly (Freeman, 1991). When a child's unique knowledge and imagination is coupled with an adult's knowledge of child development, fantasy skills can be used as tools for coping, even when the situation is grave. A well-chosen story permits children to discuss their issues and situations if they wish. Other children simply enjoy stories as a fantasy escape that need not be analyzed and as an opportunity to set things aside for a time (see Case Study 4.2). In other words, children take from a story only what they are ready to find. They may find meaning in their experiences and renewed hope (Heiney, 1995).

 Case Study 4.2

Setting Things Aside

When I think about a child setting things aside for a time, 4-year-old Jamal comes to mind. Off and on, Jamal had spent most of the winter in the hospital. An aggressive course of chemotherapy meant that frequently he felt pretty lousy and just stayed in his room. On one good day that had followed a string of very bad ones, Jamal joined us for a story. For a brief time Jamal was not the sickly little boy dealing with nausea and fatigue from the powerful drugs intended to kill the cancer inside him. His single focus was to be the best frog he could possibly be. He puffed out his chest and strutted about the "swamp" with a "gribbitt" that surely would have convinced most any frog that he was kin. Jamal's visit with us was short, but he returned to his room with a sense of pride and renewed vigor, which perhaps empowered him to believe that he could handle more of whatever was required so that he could have that chance of getting well.

Storytelling has been used to help children deal with both mental and physical pain (Heiney, 1995). For example, Kuttner (1988) found that a hypnotic method using the child's favorite story was more effective statistically than behavioral distraction and standard medical practice in alleviating distress, pain, and anxiety during painful bone marrow aspirations.

Indeed, the power of story to distract should not be taken lightly. In 1794, before the use of anesthetics, a young boy had surgery to remove a tumor. He was told such an interesting story during his operation that it absorbed his attention and removed pain from conscious awareness. Eighteen years later, this true believer in the power of story, Jacob Grimm, wrote *Snow White* (Hilgard & LeBaron, 1984).

Storytelling can offer catharsis, which may occur vicariously as feelings of despair, anger, and anxiety are released through the characters in the story (Heiney, 1995). Further, the tone of stories children tell can provide clues to their emotional state. Research indicates that children with higher anxiety levels and poorer adjustment to hospitalization, as measured through observation, tend to tell more negative stories (Hudson, Leeper, Strickland, & Jesse, 1987).

The very structure of an individual story—with a beginning, a middle, and an end taking place in a definite time frame—as well as the structure of a storytelling session itself, can provide a much-needed sense of predictability and closure for children who are ill. This can be especially important for children with chronic conditions who must deal with the ongoing saga of health-care experiences. This same sense of predictability can be enhanced through the telling of familiar stories, old favorites such as *Goldilocks and the Three Bears*, *The Three Little Pigs*, and *The Three Billy Goats Gruff*. Hearing something familiar, especially when attempting to cope with an unpredictable illness or the strange surroundings of a hospital, can provide children with a sense of comfort and safety.

Digital storytelling is becoming a popular intervention with children who are ill, and research findings indicate positive benefits. In a randomized intervention with 28 children with cancer (ages 7–17 years), Akard et al. (2015) reported that children in the digital storytelling group showed slightly better emotional and school functioning compared with those in the control group. Parents saw benefits as well: Their child's digital story provided emotional comfort to them, facilitated communication, and helped their children express their feelings, cope, and feel better emotionally. Digital storytelling has also been used to promote health outcomes for children. Wyatt and Hauenstein (2008) described "Okay with Asthma," a digital story to help children learn about asthma, which includes the feelings and emotions that may be associated with having the disease. Children watch the animated story and then build their own digital story by inserting texts into scenes presented in comic-strip style. For more information, see Appendix 4.1.

Dance and Movement

Dance, described simply, is a statement of emotion expressed through movement. All living organisms, including human beings, at least once in their lives exhibit behaviors that could be referred to as dancing (Warren & Coaten, 1993, p. 58):

Within all of us there is a dancer. Washing our faces, digging the garden or baking bread can all be viewed as our own personal pieces of choreography, our own special dances.

According to Warren and Coaten (1993), the body is an instrument of expression; in childhood it is through the movement of our bodies that we start to build a picture of our world. We grow and develop and discover what our bodies can do, which ultimately leads to a growing awareness of our body's structure and to the growth of body image. Perhaps of greatest importance is the link between dance/movement and emotion. Our movements—the way we move, the way we stand, our gestures—reflect our inner emotional state. This emotional link is what differentiates dance/movement from the purely mechanical level of physical exercise. At times, intense emotions erupt spontaneously out of a free imaginative movement process; at other times, a particular emotion may be deliberately evoked through the music and physical action (Chodorow, 1992).

Dance and movement help the individual (a) gain greater control of isolated body parts, (b) improve body image, (c) achieve controlled emotional release, and (d) become more socially adept (Warren & Coaten, 1993). Hanna (1995) believes that dance may help the healing process as a person gains a sense of control through (a) possession by the spiritual in dance; (b) mastery of movement; (c) escape or diversion from stress and pain through a change in emotion, states of consciousness, and physical capability; and (d) confronting stressors to work through ways of handling their effects.

Although research findings supporting the proposition that dance movement improves a person's body image have been contradictory, previous work focused on styles such as ballet, jazz, and modern dance. Lewis and Scannell (1995) argued that creative dance movement, with its less structured approach and absence of predetermined performance standards, has a positive effect on body image. Given the potential for widespread clinical use of creative dance movement with children having body-image disturbances, empirical research on the relationship between creative dance movement and body image is warranted.

Koshland and Curry (1996) described the following four general goals dance/movement therapy can address that can be applied universally to children who are hospitalized:

- *Establishing trust*—Movement, voice tone, sound, gestures, and kinesthetic empathy may be used to tune into the child's nonverbal messages. A peekaboo game is a simple way to accomplish this goal with young children.

- *Enhancing body awareness*—Dialogue with the body, dialogue between the child and dance/movement therapist, and movement props, such as a feather duster, yarn ball, colorful wand, stretch band, or sounds of bells and music, are used.

- *Identifying body sensations*—Although the child has become aware in a general way with what is going on in his or her body, the next step is to learn to identify sensations that may have resulted from the child's illness or injury. A child may learn to regulate breath, physical sensation, or circulation. The facilitator can join in with the child's movement, or exaggerate the child's movement to intensify and clarify emerging themes and issues.

- *Enabling the expression of feelings*—After a relationship has developed and the child is more aware of and able to identify bodily sensations, he or she is ready to learn how to express feelings. The use of colorful props, stories, and music provides a focus, especially for a child who is frightened, angry, or tired.

Dance/movement therapy has been used successfully with children and adolescents with a variety of acute and chronic diagnoses. For example, Goodill and Morningstar (1993) discussed its use with a 2-year-old boy with cellulitis of the legs to help him express anger and other feelings about his illness; with a 4-year-old who was isolated as a result of exposure to chicken pox and was demonstrating boundary and body-image issues; and with two school age girls—one with cystic fibrosis and the other with epilepsy—to help them express hope and experience exchanging a positive caregiving activity. Dance/movement has proven effective when used with children and adolescents with autism (Koch, Mehl, Sobanski, Sieber, & Fuchs, 2015), cancer (Madden et al., 2010; see Case Study 4.3), adolescents with eating disorders (Carraro, Cognolato, & Bernardis, 1998), and children with muscular dystrophy (Biricocchi, Drake, & Svien, 2014).

Creative Writing

Although a great deal has been said about children's use of nonverbal art forms, many children use creative writing to cope with the stresses of health-care experiences. Children diagnosed with life-threatening diseases often are encouraged to keep a journal to record what is going on in their lives and how they feel about it. Unlined paper also invites drawing to accompany children's words, if they choose. When children review their journals at a later date, they receive encouraging evidence from their entries that they are not "in the same place," but have indeed been successful at adapting to some degree to their disease and treatment.

The link between reading literature and writing is storytelling. Children too young or otherwise unable to write can dictate a story for an adult to record. Individual books

 Case Study 4.3

Learning to Focus Free-Floating Anxiety Through Meaningful Action

Madden et al. (2010) presented a case study of a 13-year-old boy with cancer who was just beginning chemotherapy. His subcutaneous infusion port had been surgically placed the day before. "He was pale, spoke in a shaky voice, and claimed to be nauseous. He moved in a rigid, guarded manner and isolated his port side as if he were paralyzed" (pp. 139–140). The boy was quite sad and tearful, explaining that he would be unable to play baseball this year. The dance/movement therapist began by throwing balls to him, encouraging him to use both hands to catch the balls, which were various sizes, colors, and textures. Over the next 10 minutes he began to relax. When the therapist asked about his physical symptoms, he was surprised and relieved to say the nausea and pain were gone. He then expressed hope that he might be able to play ball sooner than he had expected.

for children featuring their likes and dislikes have become popular over the years in pediatric settings. In a hospital, a group of children can participate in writers' workshops. The goal is to immerse children in a richly literate environment and encourage them to write as real-life authors do.

Writing and reading poetry helps children give voice to situations that touch their hearts (see Case Study 4.4). Children may be particularly responsive to writing poetry because its nature allows them to express themselves more readily in metaphor. Children's poems can be displayed through "sky writing" that is placed on the ceiling over their beds (see Figure 4.7). Poetry can be used to address many health issues and is appropriate for all content areas.

Bibliotherapy promotes the deliberate use of a preselected poem that puts the reader in the shoes of the poet, who, having revealed him or herself, makes it safe for the reader to do likewise. Goldstein (2011) proposed that school guidance counselors can use poetry therapy as a tool to increase empathy and promote awareness in both staff and students to combat bullying.

Another avenue for creative writing is writing music and lyrics, which may hold special appeal for teenagers. The research findings of North, Hargreaves, and O'Neill (2000) have indicated that music is important to adolescents because it allows them to (a) portray an "image" to the outside world and (b) satisfy their emotional needs.

Writing is a wonderful way for children to make sense of their world. Children often are surprised by the insights that emerge as they write. Writing is about discovery. Writing is thinking. Writing is life discovery (Froehlich, 1996).

Drama

Drama, from the Greek word that means "to do" or "act" (Graham-Pole, 2000), has been used successfully with children to address a variety of concerns. For example,

---

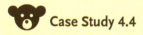 **Case Study 4.4**

Heartsongs

Mattie Stepanek, who had a rare genetic disease that took his life at the age of 13, began writing poetry at the age of 3 to cope with the death of his brother, who had the same disorder. Many of his poems speak of "heartsongs," which he described as "your inner beauty, the song in your heart that wants you to help make yourself a better person and to help other people do the same. Everybody has one" (*Wisdom Beyond His Years*, 2004, p. 2). During one of his many hospitalizations at Children's National Medical Center in Washington, DC, Mattie's wish to have his poetry published was fulfilled. Within weeks, the book was on the *New York Times* best-seller list. He wrote four additional books of poetry. A peacemaker as well as a poet, Mattie established a close friendship with former president Jimmy Carter, who described Mattie as "the most extraordinary person I ever met" (Wood, 2004, p. 1). Although Mattie used a wheelchair and relied on a feeding tube, a ventilator, and frequent blood transfusions to stay alive, his poetry provided the voice for him to fulfill his life mission to spread peace through the world.

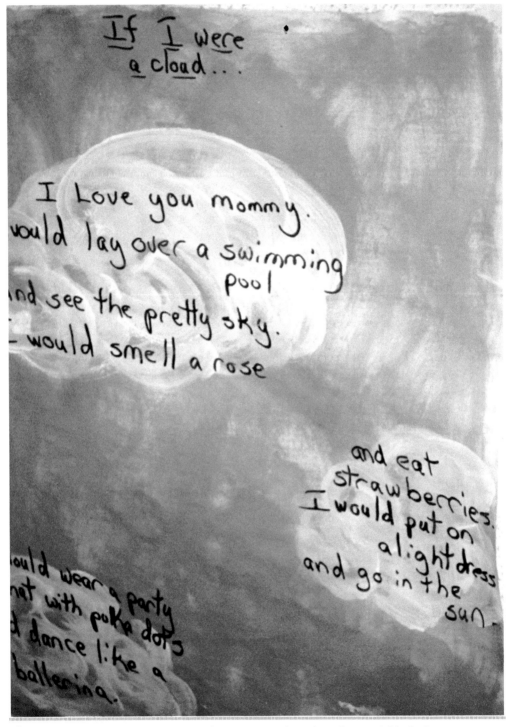

Figure 4.7. Poetry can be displayed as "sky writing" on the ceiling above a child's bed.

drama programs have been designed to increase AIDS awareness (Harvey, Stuart, & Swan, 2000), to reduce epilepsy-related stigma among school-age children (Brabcova, Lovasova, Kohout, Zarubova, & Komarek, 2013), to promote social and personal well-being in children with communication difficulties (Barnes, 2014), to increase preschoolers' knowledge of sun protection (Seidel et al., 2013), and to promote healthy relationships for teenagers (Fredland, 2010).

Drama also has been used successfully to address the issue of bullying at school. A matched design study was conducted with 190 children (mean age 10.4 years) from two schools (Joronen, Konu, Rankin, & Astedt-Kurki, 2012). One school received the drama-program intervention, which included classroom drama sessions, follow-up activities at home, and three parents' evening sessions concerning issues of social well-being during the school year. The control school carried out a common school curriculum. Bullying victimization decreased 20.7% from pretest to posttest in the intervention group, but increased 1.6% in the control group.

Drama therapy may be an excellent fit for children with autism spectrum disorder. Chasen (2011) pointed out the benefits a child with ASD brings to the theater. Children classified as higher functioning already speak with a unique expressive intonation. Some children are able to reproduce specific vocal intonations and qualities, perfectly capturing the essence of a character. Others have unique skills, such as the ability to memorize dialogue (echoic abilities), to adhere to rules, and to adapt to routines required for rehearsal and plot performance. O'Leary (2013) reported that all seven children with ASD in a 6-week theater program made positive advances in certain social and behavioral skills. In a more recent study, Corbett et al. (2016) randomly assigned 30 children with ASD (8- to 14-year-olds) to a 10-week, 40-hour theater intervention group or a wait-list control group. Children in the theater group showed significant differences in social ability compared with children in the control group.

Drama also is an effective intervention for individuals with chronic illness or disability. Graham-Pole (2000) described a professor of theater and literature's drama session with depressed teenagers with diabetes who refused to take their injections. The teens were asked to play parts: "We're going to act—like we're having fun. Fake it till you make it." The professor was after their self-consciousness:

> This is self-awareness of a productive kind. It's getting them to really see themselves right here and now, perhaps for the first time. It's getting them to start taking some real pride in their appearance and their performance. (p. 130)

In time, the previously reluctant and self-pitying teens were trying to outdo each other, expressing themselves, and enjoying the release from their real-life selves.

A discussion of drama and children would be incomplete without a mention of puppetry. Puppets are used in a variety of pediatric health-care settings because they provide safe, vicarious outlets for impulses and fantasies. In working with children and puppetry, it has been observed that the puppet becomes the actual personality of the child. Brounley (1996) explained the significance:

> Since the puppet exhibits no personality conflicts with the child, there is no reason for the child to feel threatened when speaking for the puppet. People speaking through puppets tend to assert themselves more than if they were speaking for themselves. Individuals listening to puppets also tend to accept more from a puppet than they would from another human being, even though they realize that the

other human being is speaking. The responses to puppets are possible because they do not threaten. (p. 178)

Puppets are used to educate, entertain, and provide opportunities for expression of emotions, fears, and fantasies. Puppetry is frequently used in preparing children for health-care encounters.

Humor

Because many forms of the arts are fun and produce laughter, humor has become a popular topic of research in health care. Lambert and Lambert (1995) reported increases in immunoglobulin A (IgA) levels when school-age children participated in a humor program. Having a sense of humor was included in the list of themes adolescents identified as important for health professionals in caring for adolescents with chronic illness (Woodgate, 1998). Researchers have even devised a scale to measure sense of humor. Thorson, Powell, Sarmany-Schuller, and Hampes (1997) found that scores on the *Multidimensional Sense of Humor Scale* (MSHS) are related positively to a number of factors associated with psychological health, such as optimism and self-esteem, and related negatively with signs of psychological distress, such as depression. They conclude that humor is a multidimensional construct that seems to be intimately related to quality of life.

Dowling (2002) provided an extensive account of children's use of humor as a coping strategy, which included the developmental aspects of humor. Piaget's (1962) cognitive stages of development are compared with McGhee's (1979) proposed stages of humor development. For example, children in the concrete operations stage (7 to 11 years) can (a) understand more abstract and implied incongruities, (b) search for multiple meanings, and (c) explain the reason for their amusement. On the other hand, children in the formal operations stage (11 to 15 years) have the cognitive ability to appreciate the complex structure of humor and the motivations behind its use.

Humor can be incorporated into everyday interactions with children. Hart and Rollins (2011) devoted an entire chapter to methods and activities for implementing humor in a hospital setting. Many hospitals offer special programs that involve humor. Two such programs, clown-doctors and magicians, are described below.

Clown-Doctors

Picture a clown at the bedside of a sick child, and one imagines the smiling face of a delighted child. However, in past years some child development specialists expressed concern about the practice, citing the fact that some children are afraid of clowns or that some typical clown antics are inappropriate for sick or hospitalized children. These fears, for the most part, can be put to rest if specially trained clowns are used, such as those in New York's Big Apple Circus Clown Care Unit (CCU), who have been prepared to work with children in hospitals. Founded in 1986, the CCU provides clowns with special training in the needs of children who are ill and hospitalized. This model clown program has been replicated in a dozen countries, including Canada, the United States, France, and Brazil (Oppenheim, Simonds, & Hartmann, 1997).

The clown programs work in close partnership with medical staff at each host hospital, tailoring the program to meet the needs of the facility. Clowns visit each hospital 3 to 5 days each week, 50 weeks per year. Clown "doctors," like their medical colleagues, are highly skilled practitioners of their profession. Each member of the clown program is a professional artist—not a volunteer—selected via intensive auditions for high-quality artistry and sensitivity. The clowns work in teams of two or three, with a supervising clown on each team.

Inspired by the Big Apple Circus Clown Care Unit, Caroline Simonds founded Le Rire Médecin (The Laughter Doctor) in Paris, France, in 1991. A few years after its founding, Le Rire Médecin decided that it was important to define the basic principles of the group's work and to create some rules—a code of ethics—for clowns performing in hospitals. To professionalize its mission, the group made formal distinctions between the standards required for a "walk-around" clown job, family entertainment, and in-depth work interacting with a medical team. The final document consists of 11 basic articles that delineates standards of professionalism, boundaries of artistic expression, limits of the creative role, responsibility of each artistic act, respect for patients as well as health-care workers, privacy, emotional parameters and distance from patients, basic safety, and even hygiene (Simonds, 1999). To view the code of ethics, see http://www.hospitalclown.com/archives/vol-09/vol-9-1and2/vol9-1_code%20of%20ethics.pdf.

Randomized controlled studies confirm that clown-doctors can reduce children's anxiety prior to surgery (Fernandes & Arriaga, 2010; Golan, Tighe, Dobija, Perel, & Keidan, 2009; Vagnoli, Caprilli, & Messeri, 2010). One study found that a clown and parent accompanying the child to the operating room were more effective in reducing anxiety than oral sedation (midazolam) and parent accompaniment (Vagnoli et al., 2010). Fernandes and Arriaga reported reduction of preoperative worries and emotional responses not only in children but also in their parents. Through interviews with hospitalized children and observations, Mansson, Elfving, Peterson, Wahl, and Tunell (2013) concluded that the clowns brought play and humor into the hospital and that this gave children the opportunity to focus on something other than their illness, aiding their well-being and recovery.

Magic

At Rush University Medical Center in Chicago, a child life specialist and a magician developed an innovative hospital-based program to address the psychosocial issues children and adolescents often experience as a result of illness and hospitalization (Hart & Walton, 2010). The program features (1) magicians using interactive close-up magic and humor as a technique to promote socialization, enhance self-esteem, and increase opportunities for choice and control, and (2) magicians providing the personal instruction and materials that enable chronically ill and long-term patients to learn and perform magic in order to promote a sense of empowerment and feelings of mastery. Magicians use tricks that incorporate two of the fundamental principles of comedy: surprise and humorous self-deprecation on the part of the comedian. The program's success led to the creation of the nonprofit children's foundation Open Heart Magic, which now maintains and staffs bedside interactive therapeutic-magic programs in five hospitals in the Chicago area.

Magic has many benefits for children, particularly children challenged in behavior, social cognition, linguistics, motor coordination, and sensory abilities (Spencer, 2013). Learning magic tricks

- Encourages children to be sociable, flexible, and cooperative with other children;

- Helps children recognize and implement the codes of social conduct;
- Encourages children to have meaningful conversation, recognize and respond to facial expressions, and improve the understanding and expression of emotion;
- Encourages children to understand different perspectives and the thoughts and feelings of others;
- Provides positive social experiences;
- Educates children on the value of listening, giving and receiving compliments, giving appropriate criticism, and acknowledging when they are wrong and learning from mistakes; and
- Improves gross and fine motor skills.

Relationship-Centered Care

Intense moments in our lives cry out for human contact. Simply offering a storybook or art supplies to a child who is hospitalized may be helpful and appreciated, but research tells us that people-directed activities are more effective (Banks, Davis, Howard, & McLaughlin, 1993). This makes sense, because the term *relationship-centered care* stresses the concept that interactions among people are the foundation of any therapeutic or healing activity (The Pew-Fetzer Task Force, 1995). In other words, the presence of an artist, musician, storyteller, parent, teacher, child life specialist, nurse, volunteer, or other concerned and caring adult is likely to enhance the child's ability to use the arts in a therapeutic way.

As mentioned earlier, a child's artwork can serve as a communication tool between the child and the caring adult. Through conversation with the adult in an atmosphere of empathy and honest consideration, the child can become more aware of his or her reactions, behavior, intentions, and ambitions. According to Pinchover (1998), the child derives new abilities from these contacts, which moderate anxieties and strengthen healthy energies. Better collaboration and sounder ways of coping with intrusive medical treatment, as well as more trust and hope, seem to emerge from the relationships.

For some activities, such as storytelling, the storyteller's presence is critical. There is a close, caring communication implicit in the storytelling relationship (Freeman, 1991). An analysis of music research in medical treatment determined that the provision of live music was more effective than recorded music when selected and performed by trained music therapists (Bailey, 1983). It is reasonable to assume that a live musician and recorded music would produce different experiences for children. If the interactions among people are the foundation for a therapeutic or healing activity, then perhaps this difference, too, may be attributed to the interaction between the musician or other artist and the individual.

Olson (1998) wrote that bringing live music to the bedside can be a way of extending the caring tradition of nursing practice, pointing out that bedside musical care is consistent with a holistic nursing philosophy and can be used during pregnancy, childbirth, and in neonatal care. Live music at the bedside can become a part of a treatment plan to foster integrity, well-being, and health.

Schiller and colleagues (2003) found that drawing could provide an additional dimension of depth and enrichment in the relationship between school-age children with cancer and their nurses. Twenty children, ages 7 to 14 years, were asked to draw self-portraits representing both how they looked before they became ill and their current appearance. The children used the process to share their feelings with their nurses and, through their drawings, contributed greatly to understanding how the children viewed themselves throughout the various stages of the disease and treatment.

Greaves (1996) offered an additional benefit of personal interaction between the artist and child. In the health-care environment, children can receive more individual attention in art instruction than would be possible from a teacher in the classroom. Interacting with an artist provides an opportunity for children to develop a potential for artistic interest and expression that can be explored throughout a lifetime (Rollins, 2016).

Professional Artwork

Children, especially, may respond to artwork created by professional artists as tools for coping. Prescott and David (1976) reported that children, who live according to the information provided by their senses, remember places and sensations more than they remember people. Thus, they are likely to be more sensitive to their surroundings than are adults, and may be affected deeply and for a long time by details of which adults are unaware.

Little research has been undertaken to date regarding children and young people's opinions about artwork in hospitals. We do know that adolescents want age-appropriate artwork that avoids childhood emblems such as cartoon characters, clowns, balloons, and teddy bears, and prefer less permanently fixed art and more opportunity to add their own posters and artwork (Blumberg & Devlin, 2006). In a study seeking the opinions of 31 hospitalized children ages 9 to 17 years, Bishop (2012, p. 83) reported that participants found art to be a key environmental attribute with a number of functions in the children's hospital experience, including providing a rich source of aesthetic variation, entertainment, distraction, engagement, and identity that supported their capacity to maintain a positive frame of mind and remain positively engaged in their experience. (For more about the health-care environment, see Chapter 8: The Health-Care Environment.)

Most guidance for the selection of art for hospitals has suggested the use of realistic art. Research to date is slim and primarily anecdotal, but findings indicate that patients use abstract, non-nature, and ambiguous artwork in very specific ways and find such artwork helpful in coping with health-care settings and experiences (Rollins, 2011). We know that images can be powerful tools for healing. Simonton, Matthews-Simonton, and Creighton (1981) recommended a program of relaxation, attitude change, and mental imaging as an adjunct to standard cancer therapies. They suggested that patients form a mental picture of their cancer and of the immune system's victory over the disease. The basis for this technique is an ancient notion that a picture or image held in the mind can effect bodily change (Buttler, 1993):

> Psychologists have long recognized that images are preverbal, deeply linked to our emotions and unconscious mind. . . . Artists also have recognized that images can communicate feelings in ways our thinking minds cannot understand. Whenever we say that a painting, a photograph, a piece of music, or the smell of a flower

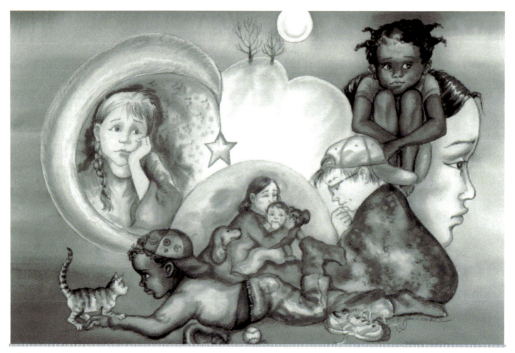

Figure 4.8. *Symbols of Courage,* murals at the Floating Hospital for Children at New England Medical Center in Boston, Massachusetts, empower children with cancer to tell their stories. *Note.* Photograph by Joan Drescher. Used with permission.

moves us in a way we cannot express, we are acknowledging the power of images. (p. 117)

Artist and author Joan Drescher, a specialist in murals for healing environments, uses positive images in paintings she creates for children's health-care settings. Her objective is to use these positive images to support the healing process: kites as symbols of courage and hope, air balloons as symbols of freedom and transcendence, and community-based images and nature images as regenerative symbols (Drescher, 1993).

She created the Symbols of Courage Project—a series of seven murals for the Children's Hematology/Oncology Clinic at the Floating Hospital for Children at New England Medical Center in Boston, Massachusetts. In the process of developing the murals, she spent many hours in the clinic talking with the children and their families and sketching her impressions of the experience. The murals illustrate the journey that children with cancer and their families go through, from the first diagnosis through the complete treatment protocol (see Figure 4.8).

Through the use of symbols within the murals, children are empowered to tell their story. In addition to helping children and their families through this difficult journey, the Symbols of Courage Project demonstrates to caregivers and the world what patients and their families go through. According to the clinic's medical director, the murals magnify the ability of all caregivers to understand and even experience the healing process with families, which brings new insight and power to the doctor–patient relationship (L. Wolfe, personal communication, May 1997).

Vara Kamin specializes in creating works of art that unlock the body's natural healing, soothing, and self-nurturing capabilities. Rich in color, movement, and texture,

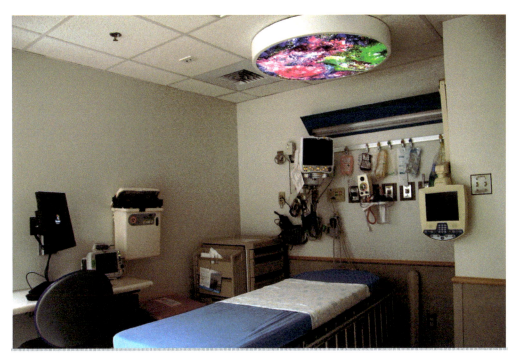

Figure 4.9. *Touching Petals,* in the Sedation Unit of the Children's Hospital of Philadelphia.

Kamin's paintings provide a positive point of focus while stimulating active imagination and inviting the viewer to a place of self-reflection. Replicated images of Kamin's paintings have been placed in hospitals and healing centers throughout the United States and abroad. The Children's Hospital of Philadelphia (CHOP) has installed Kamin's images in interventional radiology, magnetic resonance imaging (MRI), fluoroscopy, and sedation rooms (see Figure 4.9). Pre-sedation, children gaze at the images, focusing on favorite colors, finding images, naming them, and sometimes narrating stories about them; child life specialists lead them in guided imagery or relaxation exercises such as breathing in the calm colors and breathing out the pain (Rollins, 2011). The images also are used during procedures such as IV starts, injections, and catheter placements (M. Hoynoski, personal communication, March 16, 2016).

Interactive art can empower children, offering a sense of control in a place where so much is out of their control. With advances in technology, artists are able to create sophisticated interactive art for children's health-care settings. Art dans la Cité in Paris installs contemporary visual art in hospitals. The organization commissioned the artist Santiago Torres to create interactive digital paintings for the waiting room of the pediatric surgical department in Nantes University Hospital in Nantes, France. By touching the digital screen, children can transform the colors, shapes, and design of the work, themselves becoming creators (see Figure 4.10).

Facilitating the Creative Process

Children in health-care settings are, first and above all else, children. Therefore, techniques used to facilitate the creative process in such settings are similar to those used

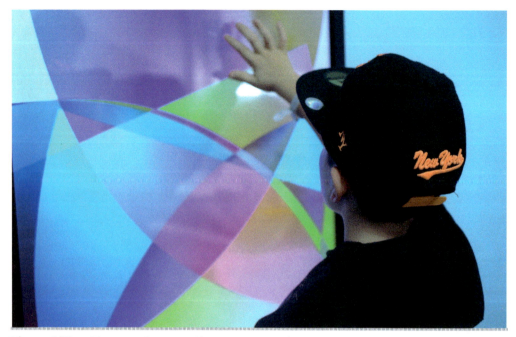

Figure 4.10. *Tableaux tactiles interactifs* (interactive tactile paintings), Santiago Torres, 2013. Digital installation in the waiting room of the pediatric surgical department, Nantes University Hospital, Nantes, France.

Table 4.4

Development of Drawing	
Approximate Age (years)	**Characteristics of Drawing**
0–1	The infant has reflex responses to visual stimuli. The infant brings a crayon to the mouth but does not draw.
1–2	At approximately 13 months, the infant makes a first scribble: a zigzag. The infant watches the movement of the crayon leaving its marks on a surface.
2–4	Circles appear and gradually predominate. The circles then become discrete. In a casually drawn circle, the child envisages an object. The child makes a first graphic symbol, usually between 3 and 4 years.
4–7	In this stage of intellectual realism, the child draws an internal model, not what is actually seen. The child draws what is known to be there. Transparencies that show people through walls and the hulls of ships are commonly produced. Drawings are expressionistic and subjective.
7–12	During this stage of visual realism, subjectivity diminishes. The child draws what is actually visible. Human figures are more realistic and proportionate. Colors are more conventional. The child distinguishes between the right and left sides of the figure drawn.
12+	With the development of the critical faculty, most children lose interest in drawing. The gifted tend to persevere.

Note. Adapted from *Interpreting Children's Drawings* (p. 38), by J. DiLeo, 1983, New York, NY: Brunner/Mazel. Copyright 1983 by Brunner/Mazel. Adapted with permission.

with children everywhere. However, children's conditions and the setting itself often require special consideration. For example, as noted in Chapter 1, children often regress when ill or hospitalized. This may be evident in the type of arts experience they are willing to engage in, and often in an art product itself (see Table 4.4 for developmental characteristics of children's drawings).

Children who are ill usually have lower energy levels than their healthy counterparts and therefore may not appear very enthusiastic about participating in an arts experience. Their responses or affect—the nonverbal expression of their inner state—may be swift, subtle, and therefore difficult to see. Because children's responses usually help artists set the pace for, or even decide to abandon, a particular project, it is important to become familiar with these subtle and fleeting responses. Also, because we often gauge the success of our work by a child's response, knowing that the child may be having a wonderful time and yet be unable to show it can help us to continue doing this meaningful work without the satisfying feedback that is commonplace with healthy children.

Psychosocial Assessment

Even for artists operating in the role of facilitator and not "therapist," familiarity with various elements of psychosocial assessment can be helpful in planning activities for individual children, monitoring children's responses and progress, and making adaptations and recommendations. The basics of psychosocial assessment include (a) affect; (b) temperament; (c) the ability to communicate and interact with peers, adults, and family; (d) personal or family stressors; (e) coping style; (f) the amount and types of defense mechanisms used; and (g) self-concept and level of self-esteem (Rollins & Riccio, 2001).

After considering the child's temperament, for example, a visual artist may want to suggest a weaving project for a child who is highly persistent. A child with a low level of persistence might do better with a quick printmaking project that allows him or her to see results almost instantly. Considering temperament can help the artist break out of the habit of using the child's age as the sole consideration. For instance, some 6-year-olds have temperaments that welcome very sophisticated, lengthy art projects, while some teenagers would quickly lose interest and prefer creating something that can be completed in one session.

Knowledge of Preceding Events

Children live very much in the here and now. Knowledge of what the child has experienced that day can be an important piece when planning an appropriate arts experience. For example, a child who has just received an injection may be agitated and angry. An activity that allows the child an opportunity to express some of his or her anger, such as pounding on a drum or a lump of clay, may be more appropriate at that moment than attempting to paint with watercolors and a tiny brush.

Basic Concepts

There are several basic guidelines to encourage children's creativity and enjoyment of an arts experience (Rollins & Mahan, 2010, p. 82).

1. *Offer children a wide range of media to explore.* They may never arrive at a finished product, but it's the process that is important.

2. *Erase the line between modalities.* Use music during a visual art activity; sing while dancing; combine singing and chanting with storytelling and drama.

3. *Encourage children to consider as many details as possible.* Ask questions about their work, such as "Who lives in that tree?"

4. *Provide suggestions for activities.* Provide a list of things the child might wish to draw. Offer ideas for songs or poetry, such as writing a poem about "Where I'm From."

5. *Respect the importance and uniqueness of a child's emotional life.* Engaging in an expressive activity can bring out all sorts of thoughts, concerns, and feelings, which the child may be reluctant to share, at least at that moment. For example,
   - When giving children sketchbooks, give them a supply of paper clips as well. They can express their thoughts and feeling through writing and drawing and then clip together the pages they do not want others to see. They still will experience the benefits of expressing their thoughts.
   - When encouraging children to talk about their artwork, ask, "Would you like to tell me about your drawing?" rather than saying, "Tell me about your drawing."

6. *Accept the feelings, honest responses, or fantasies that children express symbolically or verbally.* At times, a child's response is unexpected, bizarre, regressive, or messy, but as long as there is no actual harm, the child will get the most benefit from the experience if these responses can be accepted and respected.

7. *Be an extension of and for the child who is physically unable to do all or parts of an activity or project.* The child will still have a sense of empowerment from having the opportunity to problem solve and engage in decision-making.

8. *Encourage any special interest or talent in the arts.* Suggest or provide books or tools, or refer the child to a particular artist or artist's work. The curious moment should be captured, for interest is the best motivation for learning.

9. *Help children celebrate their art.* Display their art informally and formally; encourage performances such as mini-plays, concerts, or puppet shows; help them create beautiful books for their stories.

Children with special needs may need extra help getting started on a project. Once started, they may not work as quickly as other children. It is important to resist interfering with the child's creative process but also to keep alert for signs that the child is struggling and may want help. In such cases it may be best to acknowledge the difficulty of the task and say, for example, "That's a really tough part. Would you like me to help hold the pieces together while you glue them?" Often a simple strategy, such as taping a piece of paper to the table to anchor it for drawing or painting, is all that is needed to adapt an activity for a child's special needs.

Safety Issues

Safety considerations when using the arts with children typically fall under one or more of the following categories: (a) the art materials, (b) the techniques or activities,

(c) the child's age and developmental level, and (d) the child's condition (see Table 4.5). Before beginning an activity with a child,

1. *Read the label on art supplies.* Remember that *nontoxic* refers to acute, short-term health effects.

2. *Use your senses.* Paint, for example, can get moldy, and moldy paint should not be used. When in doubt, throw it out.

3. *Remember that smell is not a good indicator of toxicity.* Some materials, such as markers, can have a strong odor but be nontoxic. Others may have no odor or smell sweet but may be toxic.

4. *Think through each step of an activity.* Consider all equipment needed and techniques to be used.

5. *Consider the child's condition.* Certain odors may bother children who are nauseated. Often, children whose immune systems are depressed should not be exposed to certain fresh fruits and vegetables commonly used in children's printmaking activities.

6. *Assess the surroundings.* Some activities require more space than others. Excessively noisy activities may disturb others close by.

7. *Consider supervision requirements.* Some activities require greater supervision than others. When working with a group of children or conducting an activity that requires close supervision, extra help may be needed.

See Appendix 4.1 for resources on safety and the arts.

Table 4.5

Safety Considerations When Planning Arts Experiences for Children	
Variable	**Considerations**
Materials	Toxic substances can be inhaled, ingested, or absorbed through the skin.
	Exposure to toxins can cause acute or chronic illness, an allergic reaction, or skin damage.
Techniques/Activities	Physical agents such as noise, vibration, repetitive motion, heat, and electrical equipment can cause injury and illness (e.g., loud music might adversely affect hearing).
Child's age and developmental level	Children under the age of 12 may not understand the need for precautions or carry them out consistently and effectively.
	Preschool-age children will sometimes deliberately put things into their mouths and swallow them.
	Habits such as nail-biting or thumb-sucking increase the risk.
Child's condition	Exposure to art materials or processes or participation in art activities that exceed an individual child's physical limitations may place the child, especially a child with disabilities, at high risk for further illness or injury.
	Many of the hazards can be eliminated or reduced with one-to-one supervision or other appropriate measures.

Note. Adapted from *Artist Beware*, by M. McCann, 1992, Guilford, CT: The Lyons Press.

Home Care Considerations

Artists experienced in working with children in hospitals will find that many of their skills transfer quite easily to the home health or home hospice care setting. Although similar to working with children in hospitals, working with children in the home is different in several ways (Rollins & Riccio, 2001, 2002):

- *Artists cannot assume that simple supplies will be available, and even if they are, that these supplies are available for the artist's use.* For example, the artist who needs an oven to bake polymer clay beads should bring along a toaster oven. Although most homes have ovens, it could be in use or not available for the artist's use.
- *Artists need to ask permission before using anything.* This includes something as simple as filling a container of water to rinse a paintbrush.
- *Paint spills and other accidents may be more consequential in the home.* In the hospital, paint spilling on the bed linen is not a major issue; a quick trip to the linen cart or closet for replacements usually is all that is required. In the home, bed linens may be cherished heirlooms, so bringing along a vinyl tablecloth or other covering is helpful.
- *To make best use of their time, artists need to be totally prepared for the activity, including being ready to offer alternatives.* Carefully thinking through each step of the planned activity and bringing along whatever may be needed, including something as basic as a container to hold water, will help ensure a good experience for the child, family, and artist.

Perhaps the biggest difference when visiting a child in the home is immediately seeing so many more sides to the child and the family—what they like, how they live, what is important to them—than is seen in the hospital room. In some cases this seems to help establish a bond more quickly, which can contribute significantly in the development of meaningful arts experiences (Rollins & Riccio, 2001).

Starting an Arts Program

Arts programs in pediatric settings come in all shapes and sizes. Learning about existing programs, what they do, and how they got started can be a helpful exercise. There is no one best way to start a program, and, although there often are many similarities, no two programs are ever exactly alike. Some programs pay their artists; others use volunteers. Some programs are hospital-based; others are community-based, with artists serving children in health-care settings—including the home—through arts organizations or museum schools.

The logical entry point for hospital arts programs is in, or in coordination with, child life, which all children's hospitals in the United States and many general hospitals with sizable pediatric units have. In fact, several child life departments today also include "arts" or "creative arts" in their department titles. In children's rehabilitation or long-term care facilities, recreation therapy may be the point of contact. In smaller health-care facilities, the department of nursing is an appropriate place to start the conversation. See Appendix 4.2 for helpful resources on starting arts programming.

Selecting Artists

Spending adequate time to select appropriate artists is critical. Without certain basic characteristics, no amount of preparation and supervision will make a difference. Rollins and Mahan (2010) believe that the following are essential characteristics:

1. A genuine interest in children, a caring attitude, and sensitivity to cultural differences. Without an appreciation for the uniqueness of each child, the trust needed to establish a helpful and enjoyable relationship with children will be absent.

2. Knowledge and experience in a chosen art form. If the artists are confident in their ability to do what they do best, they can communicate that to children and help them be successful in what they are trying to accomplish. Although it is desirable for the artist to have experience in more than one art form or medium, sometimes it is fun for children and the artist to explore new possibilities together.

3. A respect for the child's creative process and products. Respect for the uniqueness of the individual includes respect for each individual's creative process and products of that process. Artists must want to facilitate rather than interfere with that process. In the absence of this quality, disastrous consequences can result.

4. An appreciation and respect for the power of the arts and an understanding of personal limitations. Art is a powerful communicator, one that carries both a tremendous potential and an equally great responsibility. (See the earlier section on differences in roles of artists and creative arts therapists.)

5. Flexibility. Artists need to be able to adapt to a variety of children and situations that may change during the course of an activity with an individual child or group of children.

6. A sense of humor. Artists who can laugh at themselves and humorous situations convey a sense of warmth that facilitates trusting relationships with children.

7. The ability to collaborate with others. Helping children through health-care experiences, illness, dying, and death is a team effort. If artists are to be considered members of the health-care team, they need to be able to work effectively with hospital or health-care agency staff, volunteers, and family members for the most successful outcome.

8. No health condition that could result in harm to the children or to the artist. Hospitals and health-care agencies require persons who will have regular contact with children to undergo a limited health screening, which typically includes a PPD test for tuberculosis and proof of either having been immunized against or having had certain childhood diseases, such as measles, mumps, rubella, and chicken pox. On the other hand, artists with certain chronic health conditions need to be aware of the possibility that their health may be compromised by exposure to children with particular diseases or conditions.

Most artists who are interested in working in pediatric health-care settings will bring some experience working with children. However, the desire to work with children is probably more important than experience. And because working with children often means working with family members, it is a plus if the artist seems to be comfortable with people of all ages.

Preparing Artists

Professionals who work with children generally agree that the special circumstances and needs of children in health-care settings require some sort of preparation beyond a general hospital orientation for the following reasons (Rollins & Mahan, 2010):

- Children are not simply smaller versions of adults, but are growing and changing constantly.
- Children experience illness and health-care experiences very differently than adults do.
- Health-care staff members, parents, and even the artists themselves worry that, lacking preparation, artists with even the very best intentions run the risk of hurting children emotionally and perhaps even physically.
- Preparation brings a level of comfort to the artists and therefore helps them derive more satisfaction from their work.

What kind of and how much preparation is needed? This depends on several factors:

- *What is the population?* Will artists be working with children in hospitals, in hospice care, in the home, in a community agency? Will artists be working with parents and other family members as well?
- *What role will the artists assume?* Will they be there primarily to entertain and someone will always be with them for supervision? If this is the case, a review of Text Box 4.4, A Checklist for Hospital Entertainment Activities, may be all that is needed. Will artists be conducting groups, working with individual patients, or both? Will they be working with families, groups of families, staff, or all of the above?
- *Is it clear what role the artists will assume?* Often roles evolve or expand once a program is in place. For example, the original intent of a Washington, DC– area program was to have artists work with children who were ill or dying in home and hospice care and their siblings. Within weeks after the program was implemented, it became clear that another group served by the referral agency—children who had parents or other family members in hospice care—could also benefit from artists' visits. Very quickly the artists' role was expanded, and additional training was supplied.
- *What are some ways to find out what role the artists might assume?* There are informal and formal ways to assess what is needed. The population (including children, families, and staff) can be asked informally or through focus groups and surveys. Having an ongoing advisory group that includes all of these stakeholders also can be helpful.

Conclusion

A growing number of health-care professionals share the vision that storytelling, music, painting, poetry, dance, and other forms of the arts will one day be considered

|||||||||||||||||||||||||||||||||||||||||||||||||||||||||||||||||||||||||||||||||||||||||||||||||||||||||||||||

Text Box 4.4
A Checklist for Hospital Entertainment Activities

This checklist can be used to ensure that entertainment activities for children in the hospital and their families are developmentally appropriate.

1. Does the hospital (and each pediatric unit) have established policies for entertainment and visits from celebrities?

2. Is a team that includes child development or child life specialists, direct care providers, and parents available to monitor visiting groups?

3. Is each visiting group given a copy of the departmental policies concerning such events?

4. Are visiting individuals and groups asked the following questions about their proposed entertainment?

   • Is it appropriate for the developmental ages of the children?

   • Could it cause confusion or misconceptions about anything that might happen in the hospital?

   • Might it engender fears or fantasies about being harmed in any way?

   • Does it contain religious themes or content that might trouble some families?

   • Does it avoid any suggestion of violence (including the use of weapons) or death?

   • Does it avoid the use of masks or costumes that might frighten young children?

   • Does it invite children's participation in appropriate and noncompetitive ways?

5. Are visiting groups or celebrities oriented to the needs of children who are hospitalized and their families and how to approach and talk to them?

|||||||||||||||||||||||||||||||||||||||||||||||||||||||||||||||||||||||||||||||||||||||||||||||||||||||||||||||

essential elements of quality health care. The current health-care climate requires that all services show just cause for every dollar spent. Because pediatric care costs more to provide than adult care, most pediatric services, including arts programs, are faced with justifying their very existence.

Hospitals put a strong emphasis not only on quality and cost but also on patient satisfaction. We know the arts can play a significant role in improving patients' satisfaction with their care (Karnik, Printz, & Finkel, 2014). Hospitals are beginning to see that patient satisfaction is an area where arts programming can make a major contribution. When documented research verifies the true benefits of arts programming, such programs will become commonplace in children's health-care settings and funding for these services will cease to be such a struggle.

Study Guide

1. What functions do expressive arts experiences serve for children, and in particular, children who are ill or hospitalized?

2. Compare and contrast creative arts and play of children, discussing when one or the other might be most beneficial for children in health-care settings.

3. Define creative arts therapies and outline their various forms and functions.

4. Explain the processes by which the arts can be tools for (a) coping, (b) reducing stress or pain, (c) adapting, (d) feeling empowered, and (e) learning.

5. Discuss the current status of research on the arts in health care and the healing of children.

6. What factors influence selection of type of expressive arts for children?

7. What characteristics of artists or arts facilitators prove most effective for working with children in health-care settings?

8. What are the barriers and resources for arts facilitation and arts programs in child health-care settings?

Appendix 4.1

Resources for Safety and the Arts

Organizations

Arts, Crafts, & Theater Safety
181 Thompson Street, #23
New York, NY 10012-2586
Phone: 212/777-0062
E-mail: ACTSNYC@cs.com
http://artscraftstheatersafety.org/

The Art and Creative Materials Institute
99 Derby Street, Suite 200
Hingham, MA 02043
Phone: 781/556-1044
Fax: 781/207-5550
E-mail: debbieg@acminet.org
www.acminet.org/safety.htm

Publications

McCann, M. (2005). *Artist beware, Updated and revised: The hazards in working with all art and craft materials and the precautions every artist and craftsperson should take* (4th ed.). New York, NY: The Lyons Press.

Rossol, M. (2001). *The artist's complete health and safety guide* (3rd ed.). New York: Allworth Press.

Rossol, M. (2000). *The health & safety guide for film, TV & theater* (2nd ed.). New York, NY: Allworth Press.

Shaw, S., & Rossol, M. (1991). *Overexposure: Health hazards in photography*. New York, NY: Allworth Press.

Appendix 4.2

Resources for Pediatric Arts-in-Health-Care Programs

General

Clift, S., & Camic, P. (2015). *Oxford textbook of creative arts, health, and wellbeing*. Oxford, UK: Oxford Press.

Lambert, P. (Ed.). (2016). *Managing arts programs in healthcare*. London, UK: Routledge.

Malchiodi, C. (Ed.). (2012). *Art therapy and health care*. New York, NY: Guilford Press.

Ridenour, A. (2001). Art for health's sake. A step-by-step approach to developing a facility arts program. *Health Facilities Management, 14*(9), 21–24.

Rollins, J. (2004). *Arts activities for children at bedside*. Washington, DC: WVSA Arts Connection.

Rollins, J., & Mahan, C. (2010). *From artist to artist-in-residence: Preparing artists to work in pediatric healthcare settings*. Washington, DC: Rollins & Associates.

Sadler, B., & Ridenour, A. (2009). *Transforming the healthcare experience through the arts*. San Diego, CA: Aesthetics, Inc.

Digital Storytelling

Lambert, J. (2013). *Digital storytelling: Capturing lives, creating community* (4th ed.). New York, NY: Routledge.

Holyoake, D. (2013). Once upon a time there was an angry lion: Using stories to aid therapeutic care with children. *Nursing Children and Young People, 25*(7), 24–27.

Okay with Asthma
URL: http://okay-with-asthma.org/

Organizations

MusiCure–Gefion Records
ApS 2830 Virum
Copenhagen Denmark
Telephone: 45 45854948
E-mail: contact@musicure.com
URL: http://musicure.com/
Go to website to hear music.

References

Akard, T., Dietrich, M., Friedman, D., Hinds, P., Given, B., Wray, S, & Gilmer, M. (2015). Digital storytelling: An innovative legacy-making intervention for children with cancer. *Pediatric Blood & Cancer, 62*(4), 658–665.

Archibald, M., Scott, S., & Hartling, L. (2014). Mapping the waters: A scoping review of the use of visual arts in pediatric populations with health conditions. *Arts & Health, 6*(1), 5–23.

Bailey, L. (1983). The effects of live music versus tape-recorded music on hospitalized cancer patients. *Music Therapy, 3*, 17–28.

Balan, R., Bavdekar, S., & Jadhav, S. (2009). Can Indian classical instrumental music reduce pain felt during venipuncture? *Indian Journal of Pediatrics, 76*, 469–473.

Banks, S., Davis, P., Howard, V., & McLaughlin, T. (1993). The effects of directed art activities on the behavior of young children with disabilities: A multi-element baseline analysis. *Art Therapy: Journal of the American Art Therapy Association, 10*(4), 235–240.

Barnes, J. (2014). Drama to promote social and personal well-being in six- and seven-year-olds with communication difficulties: The Speech Bubbles project. *Perspectives in Public Health, 134*(2), 101–109.

Beebe, A., Gelfand, E., & Bender, B. (2010). A randomized trial to test the effectiveness of art therapy for children with asthma. *Journal of Allergy and Clinical Immunology, 126*(2), 263–266.

Bergomi, P., Chieppi, M., Maini, A., Mugnos, T., Spotti, D., Tzialla, C., & Scudeller, L. (2014). Nonpharmacological techniques to reduce pain in preterm infants who receive heel-lance procedure: A randomized controlled trial. *Research & Theory for Nursing Practice, 28*(4), 335–348.

Biricocchi, C., Drake, J., & Svien, L. (2014). Balance outcomes following a tap dance program for a child with congenital myotonic muscular dystrophy. *Pediatric Physical Therapy, 26*(3), 360–365.

Bishop, K. (2012). The role of art in a paediatric healthcare environment from children's and young people's perspectives. *Procedia-Social and Behavioral Sciences, 38*, 81–88.

Blumberg, R., & Devlin, A. (2006). Design issues in hospitals: The adolescent client. *Environment and Behavior, 38*(3), 293–317.

Brabcova, D., Lovasova, V., Kohout, J., Zarubova, J., & Komarek, V. (2013). Improving the knowledge of epilepsy and reducing epilepsy-related stigma among children using educational video and educational drama—a comparison of effectiveness of both interventions. *Seizure, 22*(3), 179–184.

Brounley, N. (1996). Puppet and drama therapy with hospitalized and abused children. In M. Froehlich (Ed.), *Music therapy with hospitalized children* (pp. 177–193). Cherry Hill, NJ: Jeffrey Books.

Bucciarelli, A. (2016). The arts therapies: Approaches, goals, and integration in arts and health. In S. Clift, & P. Camic (Eds.), *Oxford textbook of creative arts, health, and wellbeing: International perspectives on practice, policy, and research* (pp. 271–279). Oxford, UK: Oxford Press.

Buttler, K. (Ed.). (1993). *The heart of healing*. Atlanta, GA: Turner.

Caprilli, S., Anastasi, F., Grotto, R., Abeti, M., & Messeri, A. (2007). Interactive music as a treatment for pain and stress in children during venipuncture: A randomized prospective study. *Journal of Developmental and Behavioral Pediatrics, 28*, 399–403.

Carraro, A., Cognolato, S., & Bernardis, A. (1998). Evaluation of a programme of adapted physical activity for ED patients. *Eat Weight Disorders, 3*(3), 110–114.

Chasen, L. R. (2011). *Social skills, emotional growth and drama therapy*. Philadelphia, PA: Jessica Kingsley.

Chodorow, J. (1992). Sophia's dance. *American Journal of Dance Therapy, 14*(2), 111–123.

Corbett, B., Key, A., Qualls, L., Fecteau, S., Newson, C., Code, C., & Yoder, P. (2016). Improvement in social competence using a randomized trial of a theatre intervention for children with autism spectrum disorder. *Journal of Autism and Developmental Disorders, 46*(2), 658–672.

Crawford, C., Lee, C., Bingham, J., & Active Self-Care Therapies for Pain (PACT) Working Group. (2014). Sensory art therapies for the self-management of chronic pain symptoms. *Pain Medicine, 15,* s66–s75.

Dowling, J. (2002). Humor: A coping strategy for pediatric patients. *Pediatric Nursing, 28*(2), 123–131.

Drescher, J. (1993). Murals for healing. *Child Health Design, 7,* 9–10.

Driessnack, M., & Gallo, A. (2013). Children 'draw-and-tell' their knowledge of genetics. *Pediatric Nursing, 39*(4), 173–180.

Duda, L. J. (2013). Integrating music therapy into pediatric palliative care. *Progress In Palliative Care, 21*(2), 65–77 13p. doi:10.1179/1743291X13Y.0000000049

Edwards, B. (2012). *Drawing on the right side of the brain* (4th ed.). Los Angeles, CA: Tarcher.

Fernandes, S., & Arriaga, P. (2010). The effects of clown intervention on worries and emotional responses in children undergoing surgery. *Journal of Health Psychology, 15*(3), 405–415.

Fredland, N. (2010). Nurturing healthy relationships through a community-based interactive theater program. *Journal of Community Health Nursing, 27,* 107–118.

Freeman, M. (1991). Therapeutic use of storytelling for older children who are critically ill. *Children's Health Care, 20*(4), 208–215.

Froehlich, M. (1996). Bibliotherapy and creative writing as expressive arts with hospitalized children. *Music therapy with hospitalized children: A creative arts child life approach* (pp. 195–206). Cherry Hill, NJ: Jeffrey Books.

Gerik, S. (2005). Pain management in children: Developmental considerations and mind-body therapies. *Southern Medical Journal, 98*(3), 295–305.

Golan, G., Tighe, P., Dobija, N., Perel, A., & Keidan, I. (2009). Clowns for the preventions of preoperative anxiety in children: A randomized controlled trial. *Pediatric Anesthesia, 19*(3), 262–266.

Goldstein, A. (1980). Thrills in response to music and other stimuli. *Physiological Psychology, 8*(1), 126–129.

Goldstein, M. (2011). Social implications of bullying. *The Arts in Psychotherapy, 39,* 206–208.

Goodill, S., & Morningstar, D. (1993). The role of dance/movement therapy with medically involved children. *International Journal of Arts Medicine, 2*(2), 24–27.

Graham, B. (1993). Wounded healers. In N. Vahle (Ed.), *Healing and the mind with Bill Moyers: A resource guide for the field of mind/body health.* Sausalito, CA: Institute for Noetic Sciences.

Graham-Pole, J. (2000). *Illness and the art of creative self-expression.* Oakland, CA: New Harbinger.

Grasso, M., Button, B., Allison, D., & Sawyer, S. (2000). Benefits of music therapy as an adjunct to chest physiotherapy in infants and toddlers with cystic fibrosis. *Pediatric Pulmonology, 29*(5), 371–381.

Greaves, B. (1996). Visual expression for the child in hospital. *Children in Hospital, 22*(1), 9–11.

Grimm, D., & Pefley, P. (1990). Opening doors for the child "inside." *Pediatric Nursing, 16*(4), 368–369.

Hanna, G., Patterson, M., Rollins, J., & Sherman, A. (2011). *The arts and human development: Framing a national research agenda for the arts, lifelong learning, and individual well-being.* Washington, DC: National Endowment for the Arts.

Hanna, J. (1995). The power of dance: Health and healing. *Journal of Alternative and Complementary Medicine, 1*(4), 323–331.

Hart, R., & Rollins, J. (2011). *Therapeutic activities for children and teens coping with health issues.* Hoboken, NJ: John Wiley & Sons.

Hart, R., & Walton, M. (2010). Magic as a therapeutic intervention to promote coping in hospitalized pediatric patients. *Pediatric Nursing 36*(1), 11–16.

Harvey, B., Stuart, J., & Swan, T. (2000). Evaluation of a drama-in-education programme to increase AIDS awareness in South African high schools: A randomized community intervention trial. *International Journal of Sexually Transmitted Disease and AIDS, 11*(2), 105–111.

Heiney, S. (1995). The healing power of story. *Oncology Nursing Forum, 22*(6), 899–904.

Hilgard, J., & LeBaron, S. (1984). *Hypnotherapy of pain in children with cancer.* Los Altos, CA: William Kaufman.

Hu, T., Zhang, D., Want, J., Mistry, R., Ran, G., & Wang, X. (2014). Relation between emotion regulation and mental health: A meta-analyis review. *Psychologial Reports, 114*(2), 341–362.

Hudson, C., Leeper, J., Strickland, M., & Jesse, P. (1987). Storytelling: A measure of anxiety in hospitalized children. *Children's Health Care, 16*(2), 118–122.

Johnson, B., Jeppson, E., & Redburn, L. (1992). *Caring for children and families: Guidelines for hospitals.* Bethesda, MD: Association for the Care of Children's Health.

Joronen, K., Konu, A., Rankin, H., & Astedt-Kurki, P. (2012). An evaluation of a drama program to enhance social relationships and anti-bullying at elementary school: A controlled study. *Health Promotion International, 27*(1), 5–14.

Joyce, B., Keck, J., & Gerkensmeyer, J. (2001). Evaluation of pain management interventions for neonatal circumcision pain. *Journal of Pediatric Health Care, 15*(3), 105–114.

Kain, Z., Caldwell-Andrews, A., Krivutza, D., Weinberg, M., Gaal, D., Wang, S., & Mayes, L. (2004). Interactive music therapy as a treatment for preoperative anxiety in children: A randomized controlled trial. *Anesthesia & Analgesia, 98*, 1260–1266.

Karnik, M., Printz, B., & Finkel, J. (2014). A hospital's contemporary art collection: Effects on patient mood, stress, comfort, and expectations. *HERD, 7*(3), 60–77.

Kemper, K. J., & Hamilton, C. (2008). Live harp music reduces activity and increases weight gain in stable premature infants. *Journal of Alternative and Complementary Medicine, 14*, 1185–1186.

Kemper, K., Hamilton, C., McLean, T., & Lovato, J. (2008). Impact of music on pediatric oncology outpatients. *Pediatric Research, 64*(1), 105–109.

Kemper, K., & McLean, T. (2008). Parents' attitudes and expectations about music's impact on pediatric oncology patients. *Journal of the Society for Integrative Oncology, 6*(4), 146–149.

Koch, S., Mehl, L., Sobanski, E., Sieber, M., & Fuchs, T. (2015) Fixing the mirrors: A feasibility study of the effects of dance movement therapy on young adults with autism spectruem disorder. *Autism, 19*(3), 338–350.

Koshland, L., & Curry, L. (1996). Dance/movement therapy with hospitalized children. In M. Froehlich (Ed.), *Music therapy with hospitalized children* (pp. 161–175). Cherry Hill, NJ: Jeffrey Books.

Kuttner, L. (1988). Favorite stories: A hypnotic pain-reduction technique for children in acute pain. *American Journal of Clinical Hypnosis, 30*(4), 289–295.

Lambert, R., & Lambert, N. (1995). The effects of humor on secretory immunoglobulin A levels in school-aged children. *Pediatric Nursing, 21*(1), 16–19.

Lewis, R., & Scannell, E. (1995). Relationship of body image and creative dance movement. *Perceptive Motor Skills, 81*(1), 155–160.

Lindenfelser, Hense, C., McFerran, K. (2012). Music therapy in pediatric palliative care: Family-centered care to enhance quality of life. *American Journal of Hospice and Palliative Care, 29*(3), 219–226.

Linton, P. (1995). Creating a total healing environment. In S. Marberry (Ed.), *Innovations in healthcare design* (pp. 121–132). New York, NY: Van Nostrand Reinhold.

Liu, R., Mehta, P., Fortuna, S., Armstrong, D., Cooperman, D., Thompson, G., & Gilmore, A. (2007). A randomized prospective study of music therapy for reducing anxiety during cast room procedures. *Journal of Pediatric Orthopaedics, 27*, 831–833.

Loewy, J. (2015). NICU music therapy: Song of kin as critical lullaby in research and practice. *Annals of the New York Academy of Sciences, 1337*, 178–185.

Loewy, J., Stewart, K., Dassler, A., Telsey, A., & Homel, P. (2013). The effects of music therapy on vital signs, feeding, and sleep in premature infants. *Pediatrics, 131*, 902–918.

Madden, J., Mowry, P., Gao, D., Cullen, P., & Foreman, N. (2010). Creative arts therapy improves quality of life for pediatric brain tumor patients receiving outpatient chemotherapy. *Journal of Pediatric Oncology Nursing, 27*(3), 133–145.

Malchiodi, C. (1993). Introduction to special issue: Art and medicine. *Art Therapy Journal of the American Art Therapy Association, 10*(2), 66–69.

Malchiodi, C. (Ed.). (1999). *Medical art therapy with children.* Philadelphia: Jessica Kingsley.

Malchiodi, C. (2014, June 30). Creative arts therapy and expressive arts therapy. *Psychology Today.* Retrieved from https://www.psychologytoday.com/blog/arts-and-health/201406/creative-arts-therapy-and-expressive-arts-therapy

Mansson, M., Elfving, R., Peterson, C., Wahl, J., & Tunell, S. (2013). Use of clowns to aid recovery in hospitalized children. *Nursing Children and Young People, 25*(10), 26–30.

Marley, L. (1984). The use of music with hospitalized infants and toddlers: A descriptive study. *Journal of Music Therapy, 21,* 126–132.

McCann, M. (2005). *Artist beware* (4th ed.). Guilford, CT: The Lyons Press.

McCraty, R., Barrios-Choplin, B., Atkinson, M., & Tomasino, D. (1998). The effects of different types of music on mood, tension, and mental clarity. *Alternative Therapies in Health and Medicine, 4*(1), 75–84.

McGhee, P. (1979). *Humor: Its origin and development.* San Francisco, CA: Freeman.

Micci, N. (1984). The use of music therapy with pediatric patients undergoing cardiac catheterization. *Art Psychotherapy, 11,* 261–266.

National Coalition of Creative Arts Therapies Associations. (n.d.). *About NCCATA.* Retrieved from http://www.nccata.org/#!aboutnccata/czsv

National Institutes of Health. (2016). *National Center for Complementary and Integrative Health (NCCIH).* Retrieved from http://www.nih.gov/about-nih/what-we-do/nih-almanac/national-center-complementary-integrative-health-nccih

Nilsson, S., Kokinsky, E., Nilsson, U., Sidenvall, B., & Enskar, K. (2009). School-aged children's expereinces of postoperative music medicine on pain, distress and anxiety. *Paediatric Anaesthesia, 19*(12), 1184–1190.

North, A., Hargreaves, D., & O'Neill, S. (2000). The importance of music to adolescents. *British Journal of Educational Psychology, 70* (Pt. 2), 255–272.

O'Callaghan, C., Baron, A., Barry, P., & Dun, B. (2011). Music's relebane for pediatric cancer patients: A constuctivist and mosaic research. *Supportive Care in Cancer, 19*(6), 779–788.

O'Callaghan, C., Barry, P., & Thompson, K. (2012). Music's relevance for adolescents and young adults with cancer: A constructivist research approach. *Supportive Care Cancer, 20*(4), 687-697. DOI: 10.1007/s00520-011-1104-1

Olson, S. (1998). Bedside musical care: Applications in pregnancy, childbirth, and neonatal care. *Journal of Obstetric Gynecology and Neonatal Nursing, 27*(5), 569–575.

Oppenheim, D., Simonds, C., & Hartmann, O. (1997). Clowning on children's wards. *The Lancet, 350,* 1838–1840.

Pert, C., Dreher, H., & Ruff, M. (1998). The psychosomatic network: Foundations of mind–body medicine. *Alternative Therapies, 4*(4), 30–41.

Piaget, J. (1962). *Play, dreams, and imitation in childhood.* New York, NY: Norton.

Pinchover, E. (1998). Art therapy for hospitalized children inspired by Elizabeth Kuebler-Ross' approach. *Harefuah, 135*(7–8), 257–262, 336.

Prescott, E., & David, T. (1976). *The effects of the physical environment on day care.* Pasadena, CA: Pacific Oaks College.

Pridmore, P. J., & Lansdown, R. G. (1997). Exploring children's perceptions of health: Does drawing really break down barriers? *Health Education Journal, 56,* 219–230.

Rae, W. (1991). Analyzing drawings of children who are physically ill and hospitalized using the ipsative method. *Children's Health Care, 20*(4), 198–207.

Research. (n.d.). *Baby-go-to-sleep.* Retrieved January 1, 2004, from www.babygotosleep.co.uk/research.html

Robb, S., Clair, A., Watanabe, M., Monahan, P., Azzouz, F., Stouffer, J., … Hannan, A. (2008). Randomized controlled trial of the active music engagement (AME) intervention on children with cancer. *Psycho-Oncology, 17,* 699–708.

Robb, S., Rurns, D., Stegenga, K., Haut P., Monahan, P. Meza, J., … Haase, J. (2014). Randomized clinical trial of therapeutic music video intervention for resilience outcomes in adolescents /young adults undergoing hematopoietic stem cell transplant. *Cancer, 120*(6), 909–917.

Rogers, R. (1995). In need of a guarantee. *Children & Society, 9*(4), 32–51.

Rollins, J. (1990). Childhood cancer: Siblings draw and tell. *Pediatric Nursing, 16*(1), 21–27.

Rollins, J. (1995). Art: Helping children meet the challenges of hospitalization. *Interacta, 15*(3), 36–41.

Rollins, J. (2003). *A comparison of the nature of stress and coping for children with cancer in the United States and the United Kingdom.* Unpublished doctoral dissertation, DeMontfort University, Leicester, England.

Rollins, J. (2011). Arousing curiosity: When hospital art transcends. *Health Environments Research & Design Journal, 4*(3), 72–94.

Rollins, J. (2016). The arts in pediatric healthcare settings. In P. Lambert (Ed.), *Managing arts programs in healthcare* (pp. 172–188). London, UK: Routledge.

Rollins, J., Drescher, J., & Kelleher, M. (2011). Exploring the ability of a drawing by proxy intervention to improve quality of life for hospitalized children. *Arts & Health: An International Journal for Research, Policy and Practice, 4*(1), 55–69.

Rollins, J., & Mahan, C. (2010). *From artist to artist-in-residence: Preparing artists to work in pediatric healthcare settings* (2nd ed.). Washington, DC: Rollins & Associates.

Rollins, J., & Riccio, L. (2001). *ART is the heART: An arts-in-healthcare program for children and families in home and hospice care.* Washington, DC: WVSA Arts Connection.

Rollins, J., & Riccio, L. (2002). ART is the heART: A palette of possibilities for hospice care. *Pediatric Nursing, 28*(4), 355–362.

Rubin, J. (1982). Art therapy: What it is and what it is not. *American Journal of Art Therapy, 21*, 57–58.

Rubin, J. (1999). Foreword. In C. Malchiodi (Ed.), *Medical art therapy with children*. Philadelphia, PA: Jessica Kingsley.

Ryan-Wenger, N. (1992). A taxonomy of children's coping strategies: A step toward theory development. *American Journal of Orthopsychiatry, 62*(2), 256–263.

Schiller, T., Bachval, I., Dana, Z., Hadad, S., Gross, J., & Shalev, J. (2003). 2002 APON conference proceedings: Draw me a picture: Children with cancer draw for the nurses. *Journal of the Association of Pediatric Oncology Nurses, 20*(2), 101.

Schlez, A., Litmanovitz, I., Bauer, S., Dolfin, T., Regev, R., & Arnon, S. (2011). Combining kangaroo care and live harp music therapy in the neonatal intensive care unit setting. *Israel Medical Association Journal, 13*(6), 354-358.

Schoeller, F. (2015, October 20). Knowledge, curiosity, and aesthetic chills. *Frontiers in Psychology.* Retrieved from http://dx.doi.org/10.3389/fpsyg.2015.01546

Schroeder-Sheker, T. (1993). Music for the dying: A personal account of the new field of music thanatology—History, theories, and clinical narratives. *Advances, The Journal of Mind–Body Health, 9*(1), 36–48.

Schwilling, D., Vogeser, M., Kirchhoff, F, Schwaiblmair, F. Boulesteix, A., Schulze, A., & Flemmer, A. (2015). Live music reduces stress levels in very low-birthweight infants. *Acta Paediatrica, 104*(3), 360–367.

Seidel, N., Stoelzel, F., Garzarolli, M., Herrmann, S., Breitbart, E., Berth, H., … Ehninger G. (2013). Sun protection training based on a theater play for preschoolers: An effective method for imparting knowledge on sun protection? *Journal of Cancer Education, 28*(3), 435–438.

Simonds, C. (1999). Clowning in hospitals is no joke. *British Medical Journal, 319*, 792.

Simonton, O. C., Matthews-Simonton, S., & Creighton, J. (1981). *Getting well again.* New York: Bantam Books.

Sliwka, A., Wloch, T., Tynor, D., Nowobilski, R. (2014). Do asthmatics benefit from music therapy: A systematic review. *Complementary Therapies in Medicine, 22*, 756–766.

Spencer, K. (2013). Magic tricks benefit children with autism? *KidzEdge Magazine*. Retrieved from http://kidzedge.com/recent-issues/magic-tricks-benefit-children-with-autism/

Spouse, J. (2000). Talking pictures: Investigating personal knowledge through illuminative artwork. *NT Research, 5*(4), 253–261.

Standley, J. (2003). The effect of music-reinforced nonnutritive sucking on feeding rate of premature infants. *Journal of Pediatric Nursing, 18*(3), 169–173.

Standley, J. (2012). Music therapy research in the NICU: An updated meta-analysis. *Neonatal Network, 31*, 311–316.

Standley, J., Cassidy, J., Grant, R., Cevasco, A., Szuch, C., Nguyen, J., … Adams, K. (2010). The effect of music reinforcement for non-nutritive sucking on nipple feeding of premature infants. *Pediatric Nursing, 36*(3), 138–145.

The Pew-Fetzer Task Force. (1995). *Health professions and relationship-centered care*. San Francisco: The Pew Health Professions Commission.

Thorson, J., Powell, F., Sarmany-Schuller, I., & Hampes, W. (1997). Psychological health and sense of humor. *Journal of Clinical Psychology, 53*(6), 605–619.

University of Florida Center for Arts in Medicine. (2017). *Talking about arts in health: A white paper addressing the language used to describe the discipline from a higher education perspective*. Gainesville, FL: Author.

Vagnoli, L., Caprilli, S., & Messeri, A. (2010). Parental presence, clowns or sedative premedication to treat preoperative anxiety in children: What could be the most promising option? *Pediatric Anesthesia, 20*(10), 937–943.

Wall, P. (1973). The gate control theory of pain mechanism. A re-examination and restatement. *Brain, 101*, 1–18.

Walworth, D. (2005). Procedural-support music therapy in the healthcare setting: A cost-effectiveness analysis. *Journal of Pediatric Nursing, 20*(4), 276–284.

Warren, B., & Coaten, R. (1993). Dance: Developing self-image and self-expression through movement. In B. Warren (Ed.), *Using the creative arts in therapy* (2nd ed., pp. 58–83). London: Routledge.

Wiles, R., Cott, C. & Gibson, B. (2008). Hope, expectations and recovery from illness: A narrative synthesis of qualitative research. *Journal of Advanced Nursing, 6*(6), 564–573.

Wisdom Beyond His Years. (2004). Retrieved June 23, 2004, from www.oprah.com/tows/pastshows/tow_past_20011019_b.jhtml

Wood, T. (2004). *Memories, jokes and respect mark Mattie's services*. Retrieved June 28, 2004, from www.mdausa.org/mattie/remember.cfm

Woodgate, R. (1998). Health professionals caring for chronically ill adolescents: Adolescents' perspectives. *Journal of the Society of Pediatric Nurses, 3*(2), 57–68.

Wyatt, T., & Hauenstein, E. (2008). Enhancing children's health through digital story. *CIN: Computers, Informatics, Nursing, 26*(3), 142–148.

5 Children and Youth With Special Health-Care Needs

Elizabeth Ahmann and Judy A. Rollins

Objectives

At the conclusion of this chapter, the reader will be able to:
1. Define "children and youth with special health-care needs."
2. Discuss factors contributing to the numbers of children and youth with special health-care needs.
3. Identify and describe theoretical frameworks typically used in the care of children and youth with special health-care needs and their families.
4. List and discuss key principles in the care of children and youth with special health-care needs.
5. Draw implications for partnering with children and youth with special health-care needs and their families to optimize positive outcomes.

Medical and technological advances have resulted in increased life expectancy for children with chronic and disabling conditions. For example, polio survivors, the first generation of children with technology dependency, have entered the ranks of senior citizens. Advances made during the poliomyelitis era have led to today's progress in neonatology, critical care, and rehabilitation medicine, resulting in the second generation of children with technology dependency. Children with acute or chronic life-threatening illnesses and premature and low-birth-weight infants never expected to survive in the not-so-distant past now survive to grow into adulthood and, as did many polio survivors, have children of their own.

In many instances, survival has come at a high physical and emotional cost for children and their families. For children and youth with special health-care needs, health-care encounters are not a one-time event but a series of ongoing events. The experiences themselves are not only more numerous but also often more invasive, uncomfortable, or painful than those encountered by other children. Additionally, transition to adult care, when it occurs, can be fraught with challenges.

The nature of children's conditions and ongoing treatments translates into often challenging and complex psychosocial and family considerations. The effect may be found in several aspects of life, including psychological well-being and emotional and behavioral development. This chapter will address psychosocial issues for children and youth with special health-care needs in hospitals, the home, and the community.

Overview of Children and Youth With Special Health-Care Needs

Several conceptual approaches have been used to classify children with chronic health problems: condition lists, functional status assessments, an elevated need for health-related services, and limitations in social roles, such as school or play. Numerous definitions of the term *chronic illness* have been used, and specific terms such as *disability*, *impairment*, and *technology dependence* have also been applied to children with special needs. These varied conceptual approaches and definitions have contributed to challenges both in gathering data to describe the population of children with special needs and in planning and advocating for services.

In 1998, in part because eligibility for health and educational services is determined by whether a child is considered to have "special health-care needs," the federal Maternal and Child Health Bureau's Division of Services for Children with Special Health Care Needs developed the following definition:

> Children with special health care needs are those who have or who are at an increased risk for a chronic physical, developmental, behavioral, or emotional condition and who also require health and related services of a type or amount beyond that required by children generally. (McPherson et al., 1998, p. 138)

Approximately 27% of children and youth ages 0 to 19 have a chronic condition requiring services that typically extend beyond those needed by healthy children (Robert Wood Johnson, 2010). One in 15 (6.7%) of children have two or more chronic conditions, with an associated higher rate of activity limitations, including more school absences and more days spent in bed, as well as higher costs of care. Respiratory diseases and asthma are the most common chronic conditions in children (Robert Wood Johnson Foundation, 2010). Approximately 13% of those ages 8 to 15 years and 20% of youth ages 13 to 18 experience severe mental disorders in a given year, and additional numbers have less severe mental illness that still has a significant impact on their lives (National Alliance on Mental Illness [NAMI], 2013).

Many factors contribute to a continuing increase in the prevalence of chronic conditions in young people: increased survival rates for prematurely born infants; improved life-prolonging treatments for previously fatal childhood illnesses (e.g., cystic fibrosis); environmental changes affecting rates of respiratory conditions and obesity; the development of "late effects" of treatments such as chemotherapy; an increase in diagnosis of behavior and learning conditions, such as attention-deficit/hyperactivity disorder; and improved case-finding for both medical and mental health conditions (Van Cleave, Gortmaker, & Perrin, 2010).

The impact of chronic illness and disability in children and youth is far-reaching. Some may experience effects in developmental, social, emotional, and physical realms, frequently with long-lasting consequences (Rezaee & Pollock, 2015). Family members—parents, siblings, and even grandparents—often make accommodations and adjustments when a young person has special health-care needs. The larger social fabric is also affected. This group of children and youth has an increased use of health-care services and associated higher health-care costs; makes use of special federal programs; and may require specialized local health, developmental, and educational services. Care coordination is an important, and sometimes neglected, service.

Theoretical Frameworks

Theoretical frameworks, including normalization, stress and coping theory, a more recent emphasis on hope and resilience, and various applications of systems theory all have relevance in the care of children and youth with special health-care needs and their families.

Normalization

Normalization strategies have long been emphasized in the care of children and youth with special needs. Based on a review of the literature, Knafl and Deatrick (1986) outlined four defining characteristics of normalization:

- acknowledging the existence of the illness,
- defining family life as normal,
- defining the social consequences of the illness as minimal, and
- engaging in behaviors consistent with a view of family life as "normal."

Normalization has been considered important for a child's optimal development and for encouragement of family stability. Protudjer, Kozyrskyj, Becker, and Marchessault (2009) found that children with asthma use the following strategies to normalize their lives: minimizing the health impact, stressing normality, emphasizing abilities, making adaptations in daily living, and managing symptoms with medications. Parents can promote normalization by encouraging self-care and age-appropriate choices and decision-making; promoting normal development, with modifications as needed, including participation in out-of-home/extracurricular activities; and supporting age and development-appropriate participation in family rules, chores, and social activities. Additional strategies to normalize family life include maintaining family routines, planning parental "dates," and going on family vacations.

Research by Knafl and colleagues (1996) examined how families manage a young person's chronic condition. Those families considered to be "thriving" were characterized by a focus on normalcy and a feeling of confidence in their ability to meet illness-related demands. At the same time, this model may not always be applicable. Normalizing life for a child and family with special needs can pose challenges and require a balance of competing demands on time and energy. For some families, the required treatment regimen is a significant burden and entails behaviors that make their family feel quite different from other families. For example, in a study of families with children dependent on ventilators, Toly, Musil, and Carl (2014) found that functional status and amount of home health-care nursing were two factors predicting normalization efforts; others were maternal depressive symptoms (related to the child's functional status), race/ethnicity, and the child's age.

Additionally, it may be unreasonable to expect all families to try to maintain life as "normal" in all phases and circumstances of caring for a child or youth with chronic illness. A "new normal," or a "variable normal" may be a more reasonable expectation. Rehm and Bradley (2005) studied families with children who were both medically fragile and developmentally disabled, finding that "parents recognized normal and positive aspects of their lives while acknowledging the profound challenges that their families faced. Parents concluded that it was possible to have a good life that was not necessarily normal by usual standards" (p. 807). In particular, during times of upheaval—such as when obtaining a diagnosis, during exacerbations of symptoms, or during a phase of terminal care—deviations from a practice of "normalizing" family life may be quite understandable and appropriate (see Case Study 5.1). These may, in fact, be times during which children and families need extra support.

Stress and Coping Theory

Lazarus and Folkman's (1984) stress and coping framework has been widely used in research on children with special needs and their families. In fact, for years, research on this population focused on stressors. As a result, many potential stressors for families of children with special needs have been identified. In broad categories, these include the following (Walker, 1999):

- aspects of the illness trajectory,
- role strain,
- role confusion,
- financial stressors,
- time constraints,
- energy demands,
- psychosocial stressors, and
- sustained uncertainty.

Research indicates that parents' response to these stressors can range from mild to severe. For example, in one study of mothers of adolescents and young adults with disabilities, Seltzer and colleagues (2009) found that the mothers experience chronic strain comparable to that of combat soldiers. Measurements of their daily cortisol patterns showed higher-than-normal chronic stress on days when they spent more time with their children. The researchers concluded that the mothers might be at risk for the long-range health consequences of cortisol dysregulation and would benefit from stress-reduction strategies.

In an attempt to determine why some families do well when others, exposed to similar stressors, struggle to keep family life running, McConnell, Savage, and Breitkreuz (2014) surveyed a random sample of 538 families raising children with disabilities and behavior problems. Results indicate that families do well under conditions of high social support and low financial hardship, while families with low levels of social support and high levels of financial hardship typically struggle, even when the number or intensity of child behavior problems is low. The researchers concluded that strengthening social relationships and ameliorating financial hardships might be more important than other types of interventions.

Researchers have also used stress and coping theory to explain the stressors and responses of children and youth with special needs. In addition to physiological stressors related to their condition and treatment, young people may face psychosocial stressors such as stigma, bullying, and being pitied, patronized, undervalued, or left out. Raghavendra, Newman, Grace, and Wood (2013) pointed out that youth with

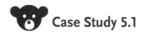 **Case Study 5.1**

One Family's Experience

A family presented Sam, their 14-month-old son, to a hospital emergency department with an accidental strangulation injury. Sam's first admission to the pediatric intensive care unit (PICU) focused on lifesaving measures and preserving brain and respiratory function. He was discharged after 2 weeks and the family was advised to continue care with the ear, nose, and throat (ENT) surgeon to follow the healing injury to Sam's trachea. The family planned to resume life as usual with their son and his 3-year-old sister, Alice. The child's mother expressed immense feelings of gratitude that her child suffered no brain injury as a result of the accident, and was quite relieved to be able to go on with life as usual.

However, 2 weeks after discharge, the family again presented to the emergency department with their son, who was experiencing increasing breathing difficulties. He was again admitted to the PICU, where the decision was made to urgently perform a tracheostomy. This admission lasted 2 weeks, during which time the family had to learn to care for their child and his new tracheostomy. Sam's mother was very anxious—afraid she would not be able to care for him at home.

During these 2 weeks, Sam's mother learned to care for the tracheostomy, identified other caregivers who needed to be trained, and set up the home to accommodate the new equipment that would be needed to care for Sam. In addition, she identified and sought assistance with a number of developmental issues for both of her children. The child life specialist worked with her to prepare Alice for having a brother with a tracheostomy. Medical, social work, nursing, and case management staff taught the family to provide Sam's care, and helped to arrange the home care he would need. Child life and speech pathology staff worked with Sam and his family to begin using sign language as an alternative means of communicating while this child, at a sensitive age for language acquisition, had a tracheostomy and was prevented from speaking.

As the magnitude of the life changes required for this family became clearer, the mother began to identify areas of her life that could be simplified, and changes she would need to make in her daily routines. Again, the transdisciplinary team helped her work with these issues and become more comfortable with this major life transition. It is anticipated that Sam will have a successful tracheal reconstruction and be decannulated within 18 to 24 months. If that happens, the family will be able to resume life as it was before the accident. If not, they seem to have the skills and the desire to make life as normal as possible for everyone in the family.

This family's experience illustrates the shift from life with healthy children, to life with a child who has special needs. The family appears to be adapting very quickly, but each family will approach this differently, according to their own preferred coping styles. Health-care professionals can help family members identify effective coping strategies and encourage them to use these strategies to manage caring for the family in these new circumstances.

certain disabilities worry about having friends, have reduced social networks and fewer reciprocated friendships, and are more isolated than their peers without disabilities. Increasingly, children and youth with disabilities are coping with these challenges through online social networking. As a result, increased self-esteem and overall mental health often follow (Steinfield, Ellison, & Lampe, 2008).

Much of the same literature that identifies parental and child stress also suggests that most parents and children appear to cope well and remain relatively resilient. Perceived control, the ability to use social support, and other psychosocial resources seem to be important in helping parents support healthy development for their children (Barnett, Clements, Kaplan-Estrin, & Fialka, 2003).

Hope and Resilience

Because individuals and families perceive their own situations differently, what is stressful to one family may not be stressful to another. Additionally, individuals and families bring a variety of coping abilities to a situation, and, despite the stressors they face, most families cope effectively with the demands of raising a child with special needs. As a result, the recent trend in research on children and youth with special health-care needs and their families involves a focus on resilience. As an example, a recent study of parents of children with cancer found low rates of post-traumatic stress—rates similar to those of parents of healthy children in the comparison group (Phipps et al., 2015). Additionally, higher measures of psychological growth were found among the parents of children with cancer, a sign of resilience.

Rosenberg, Starks, and Jones (2014) suggested that an understanding of multiple factors is needed to promote resilience, including person-level perspectives, individual resources, processes of adaptation, and emotional well-being. Some approaches Rosenberg, Baker, Syrjala, Back, and Wolfe (2013) suggested for supporting resilience include the following:

- assuring effective communication with health-care providers,
- helping families find sources of hope,
- supporting spirituality,
- promoting social support,
- assisting family members in setting realistic goals,
- adapting and learning new skills as needed, and
- aiding parents in developing coping strategies over time.

Parent training may be particularly efficacious in promoting coping and resilience when young people have behavior-related conditions (Pourmohamadreza-Tajrishi, Azadfallahs, Hemmati Garakani, & Bakhshi, 2015; Zwi, Jones, Thorgaard, York, & Dennis, 2011). Other strategies, such as participating in a group intervention led jointly by a mental health professional and trained parent of an older child, have been shown to help parents of infants and toddlers with disabilities navigate the adaptation process (Barnett et al., 2003). Because the primary focus is on the parent or family's psychosocial adaptation and not the child's condition, parents of children with a variety of conditions can attend together.

Encouraging efforts at meaning-making is another resilience-promoting strategy. Meaning-making can take any variety of form(s) that express a parent's or family's talents, needs, and values. For example, making meaning might consist of any of the following (Ahmann, 2013b; Dokken, 2013; Rosenberg et al., 2013):

- living in a purposeful way as a legacy to one's child,
- writing—whether poetry or stories about one's child or one's own journey,
- becoming a parent advocate or support-group leader,
- educating others,
- starting an organization or a foundation, and
- engaging in public or inspirational speaking related to one's journey.

Additionally, an ethnographic study of families of children with special needs identified the theme of hope as critical to families: "Coping with a seriously ill child is enormously difficult for parents, and having hope that they can meet their child's needs and that their child's health and well-being will improve is vital to managing day to day" (Lucile Packard Foundation for Children's Health, 2012, p. 16). Sometimes hope will simply take the form of knowledge that the family is providing the best care possible, whatever the outcome. Sensitivity to the important role of hope is critical. Health-care providers can promote hope by offering informed guidance, helping family members draw on resources such as supportive cultural and spiritual traditions, and offering realistic support regarding the child's health and comfort (Lucile Packard, 2012).

Systems Theory

Systems theory suggests that all human systems consist of interdependent, interacting parts characterized by a dynamic steady-state balance between the parts and their environment (Bronfenbrenner, 1979; VonBertalanffy, 1968). Early on, Olson, Sprenkle, and Russell's (1979) circumplex model of family systems suggested that in family life, the dynamic balance occurring between cohesion and adaptability determines adjustment.

Other applications of systems theory to the care of children and youth with special needs allow researchers to examine multiple dimensions of child and family life and help clinicians recognize the interconnections between the young person, the family, the health-care system, and the social environment, and to conduct comprehensive assessments. Using systems theory as a framework to examine the interconnections between families and the health-care system, Rolland (2015, p. 104) identified an ongoing need for progress: "In my view, the ability of the health-care consumer (patient and his or her family members) and professional worlds to collaborate in a more egalitarian and less hierarchical and wary manner remains a significant constraint to progress."

Friction with the health-care system increases as children shift from acute to chronic care. The Lucile Packard Foundation (2012) described four different styles families tend to use when interacting with the health-care system (see Table 5.1). Families sometimes move back and forth between the styles, depending on their changing circumstances and the support they receive.

For more on the application of family systems theory within the family itself, see Chapter 7: Families in Children's Health-Care Settings.

Table 5.1

Family–System Interaction Styles		
Style	Definition	Characteristics
Vulnerable	Limited or incapacitated by cultural and/or psychological conditions	May be fearful of and/or unfamiliar with health-care system May be overwhelmed by anxiety about child's condition May become almost incapacitated
Compliant	Follows instructions, is accepting, doesn't ask for more	Exhibits strong dependence on health-care professionals Tends to do as told, neither more nor less Accepts instruction and does best to comply Asks few questions Unassertive in seeking additional help
Advocate	Purposefully makes and uses relationships to obtain resources	Actively engages in child's care Participates in decision-making Advocates effectively for child Tends to seek out other families that have similar experiences and the need to increase knowledge of their child's condition, the health-care delivery system, and community resources
Activist	Sees self as an active part of health-care team; may eventually use expertise to help others	Becomes part of the health-care team Uses expertise to advocate on behalf of others Teaches others to advocate for themselves May find opportunities to work professionally within the system May find opportunities to educate local, state, and federal policy makers

Note. Adapted from *Six Models for Understanding How Families Experience the System of Care for Children With Special Health Care Needs: An Ethnographic Approach,* by Lucile Packard Foundation for Children's Health, 2012, Palo Alto, CA: Author.

Principles of Care

First and foremost, the care of children and youth with special needs must be sensitive to their normal and unique/special needs. Listed below are the six Maternal and Child Health Bureau principles of care for children and youth with special health-care needs (CYSHCN) plus a seventh principle, cultural competence, which was added by experts in the field (National Consensus Framework, 2014, p. 7):

- *Family-professional partnerships*—Families of CYSHCN will partner in decision-making at all levels and will be satisfied with the services they receive;
- *Medical home*—CYSHCN will receive family-centered, coordinated, ongoing comprehensive care within a medical home;

- *Insurance and financing*—Families of CYSHCN have adequate private and/or public insurance and financing to pay for the services they need;
- *Early and continuous screening and referral*—Children are screened early and continuously for special health-care needs;
- *Easy-to-use services and supports*—Services for CYSHCN and their families will be organized in ways that families can use them easily and include access to patient and family–centered care coordination;
- *Transition to adulthood*—Youth with special health-care needs receive the services necessary to make transitions to all aspects of adult life, including adult health care, work, and independence;
- *Cultural competence*—All CYSHCN and their families will receive care that is culturally and linguistically appropriate (attends to racial, ethnic, religious, and language domains).

A key principle in the care of children with special health-care needs is recognizing that these children have the same developmental needs as all children and are more like their unaffected peers than different from them. Seeing each child as a whole child, rather than as a "diabetic" or "asthmatic" is important in providing meaningful, relevant care. In a book titled *Building the Healing Partnership*, one mother explained,

> Many professionals seem to forget sometimes that Laura is not only a little girl with Turner Syndrome or congenital heart disease or malformed kidneys or complications of surgery or multiple orthopedic problems. . . . She is also a Girl Scout, a student of the viola, a reader of great books, a sister who comforts a crying brother, a daughter who sweeps the kitchen, a granddaughter who crafts homemade Valentines, a niece who tickles a cousin—all of the things that are more important about her than the string of diagnoses that we can choose from. (Leff & Walizer, 1992, pp. 209–210)

Promoting Normal Development

Children with chronic illnesses or disabilities have been described as "normal children in abnormal situations" (Patterson & Geber, 1991, p. 150). Although they have the same developmental needs as all children, an extra set of demands and hardships associated with the chronic condition makes accomplishing their developmental tasks more difficult. This is true at all stages, from infancy through the young adult years.

To promote normal development in a child with special needs, parents first benefit from a thorough understanding of the child's condition. Providing parents with complete and accurate information about their child's condition will support optimal understanding, confidence, and a sense of competence.

Parents also benefit from understanding what normal development is like for children of different ages. This will help each family in normalizing opportunities for their own child, including (a) emphasizing the child's abilities and de-emphasizing limitations; (b) structuring the environment to provide developmentally appropriate opportunities and activities; and (c) providing appropriate expectations, guidance, and discipline.

A related area of family education addresses how the young person's condition may affect activities of daily living, including eating, dressing, toileting, and sleeping.

Depending on the complexity of care requirements, families may need help in arranging to meet the therapeutic needs of their child or teen within the context of family life. For example, whenever possible, medication schedules should be arranged to allow parents to sleep through the night. Families can be helped to learn how to accommodate special dietary needs in family menu preferences. Special feeding requirements (e.g., tube feeding) can be scheduled to coincide with family mealtimes when appropriate. Physical therapy exercises can be incorporated into dressing and other daily routines rather than be scheduled at other times.

Table 5.2 lists some developmental aspects of chronic conditions, by developmental stage, along with potential supportive interventions. An example of one family's journey in promoting normal development is included below (see Case Study 5.2). More on promoting normal development is discussed later in this chapter.

Noncategorical Approach

Another key principle in care for children and youth with special needs, called a "noncategorical approach," was first suggested by Stein and Jessop (1982) and then re-emphasized by Vessey and Maguire (1999). A noncategorical approach means that, in many ways, the concerns and problems faced by young people with various chronic conditions are similar regardless of the condition. Although specific chronic conditions may pose unique challenges and require particular solutions (for example, a child who is deaf may need instruction in sign language, a young person who has asthma may need daily medication, a child or teen with depression may need weekly therapy), all young people with or without chronic conditions face the same general challenges: (a) functioning in developmentally appropriate ways, (b) maintaining self-esteem, and (c) participating in family and community life.

When a young person has special needs—whether medical, developmental, or behavioral/emotional—the journey to independent functioning can sometimes be challenging for both parent and child. Yet, increasing independence is crucial for developing self-efficacy and self-esteem and for full participation in family and community life. Models such as the Leadership Model, the "consultant" parent model, and the "coaching" model can provide guidance to families on how to sequence steps toward independence.

Leadership Model

Kieckhefer and Trahms (2000) developed a Leadership Model, which illustrates the path of parent and child/youth through a planned and systematic transition of responsibility. Figure 5.1 shows the directions of systematic planned shifting of responsibility for the care of the chronic condition from the parent to the young person. The bold arrows depict the need for the parent to guide this movement and the important idea that both parent and child or teen has an active role to play.

1.　Initially, the parent provides all the necessary care to the child, regardless of the child's age.
2.　As the child grows in cognitive and physical skill development, experience with the condition, and management competence, the parent transfers

(text continues on p. 182)

Table 5.2

Developmental Aspects of Chronic Illness or Disability in Children

Developmental Tasks	Potential Effects of Chronic Illness or Disability	Supportive Interventions
Infancy		
Develop a sense of trust	Multiple caregivers and frequent separations, especially if hospitalized	Encourage consistent caregivers in hospital or other care settings
	Deprived of consistent nurturing	Encourage parents to visit frequently or "room-in" during hospitalization and to participate in care
Attach to parent	Delayed because of separation, parental grief for loss of "dream" child, parental inability to accept the condition, especially a visible defect	Emphasize healthy, perfect qualities of infant
		Help parents learn special care needs of infant to enable them to feel competent
		Expose infant to pleasurable experiences through all senses (touch, hearing, sight, taste, movement)
Learn through sensorimotor experiences	Increased exposure to more painful experiences than pleasurable ones	Encourage age-appropriate developmental skills (e.g., holding bottle, finger feeding, crawling)
	Limited contact with environment from restricted movement or confinement	Encourage all family members to participate in care to prevent overinvolvement of one member
Begin to develop a sense of separateness from parent	Increased dependency on parent for care	Encourage periodic respite from demands of care responsibilities
	Overinvolvement of parent in care	
Toddlerhood		
Develop autonomy	Increased dependency on parent	Encourage independence in as many areas as possible (e.g., toileting, dressing, feeding)
Master locomotor and language skills	Limited opportunity to test own abilities and limits	Provide gross-motor-skill activity and modification of toys or equipment, such as a modified swing or rocking horse
Learn through sensorimotor experience, beginning preoperational thought	Increased exposure to painful experiences	Institute age-appropriate discipline and limit-setting
		Recognize that negative and ritualistic behaviors are normal
		Provide sensory experiences (e.g., water play, sandbox, finger paint)

(continues)

Table 5.2 (*continued*)

Preschool	
Develop initiative and purpose	Encourage mastery of self-help skills
Master self-care skills	Provide devices that make tasks easier (e.g., self-dressing)
Begin to develop peer relationships	Encourage socialization, such as inviting friends to play, day-care experiences, trips to park
Develop sense of body image and sexual identification	Provide age-appropriate play, especially associative play opportunities
Learn through preoperational thought (magical thinking)	Emphasize child's abilities; dress appropriately to enhance desirable appearance
Limited opportunities for success in accomplishing simple tasks or mastering self-care skills	Encourage relationships with same-sex and opposite-sex peers and adults
Limited opportunities for socialization with peers; may appear "like a baby" to age-mates	Help child deal with criticisms; realize that too much protection prevents child from learning realities of world
Protection within tolerant and secure family may cause child to fear criticism and withdraw	Clarify that cause of child's illness or disability is not his or her fault or a punishment
Awareness of body may center on pain, anxiety, and failure	
Sex-role identification focused primarily on mothering skills	
Guilt (thinking he or she caused the illness or disability, or is being punished for wrongdoing)	

School Age	
Develop a sense of accomplishment	Encourage school attendance; schedule medical visits at times other than school; encourage child to make up missed work
Form peer relationships	Educate teachers and classmates about child's condition, abilities, and special needs
Learn through concrete operations	Encourage sports activities (e.g., Special Olympics)
Limited opportunities to achieve and compete (e.g., many school absences or inability to join regular athletic activities)	Encourage socialization (e.g., Girl Scouts, Campfire, Boy Scouts, 4-H Clubs, having a best friend or a club)
Limited opportunities for socialization	Provide child with knowledge about his or her condition
Incomplete comprehension of the imposed physical limitations or treatment of the disorder	Encourage creative activities (e.g., VSA arts)

Table 5.2 (*continued*)

Adolescence

Develop personal and sexual identity	Increased sense of feeling different from peers and less able to compete with peers in appearance, abilities, special skills	Realize that many of the difficulties the teenager is experiencing are part of normal adolescence (rebelliousness, risk taking, lack of cooperation, hostility toward authority)
		Provide instruction on interpersonal and coping skills
Achieve independence from family	Increased dependency on family; limited job or career opportunities	Encourage socialization with peers, including peers with special needs and those without special needs
Form sexual relationships	Limited opportunities for sexual friendships; fewer opportunities to discuss sexual concerns with peers	Provide instruction on decision making, assertiveness, and other skills necessary to manage personal plans
Learn through abstract thinking	Increased concern with issues such as why he or she got the disorder, whether he or she can marry and have a family	Encourage increased responsibility for care and management of the disease or condition, such as assuming responsibility for making and keeping appointments (ideally alone), sharing assessment and planning stages of health-care delivery, and contacting resources
	Decreased opportunity for earlier stages of cognition may impede achieving level of abstract thinking	Encourage age-appropriate activities, such as attending mixed-gender parties, sports activities, driving a car
		Be alert to cues that signal readiness for information regarding implications of condition on sexuality and reproduction
		Emphasize good appearance and wearing stylish clothes, use of makeup
		Understand that adolescent has same sexual needs and concerns as any other teenager
		Discuss planning for future and how condition can affect choices

Note. From *Whaley and Wong's Nursing Care of Infants and Children–Sixth Edition* (pp. 1006–1007), by D. Wong, M. Hockenberry-Eaton, D. Wilson, M. Winkelstein, and E. Ahmann, 1999, St. Louis, MO: Mosby. Adapted with permission.

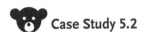 **Case Study 5.2**

Promoting Normal Development

Naomi's daughter Hailey not only was born at 28 weeks' gestation but also was diagnosed with moderate asthma and severe food allergies by the time she was 3 years old. Managing her conditions at home was challenging enough but, when Hailey started school, Naomi strategized about how to normalize her daughter's life while still protecting her against asthma flare-ups and life-threatening allergic reactions. Key strategies included:

• Continuity of specialist

Soon after Hailey's diagnosis, Naomi selected a pediatric allergist/immunologist who has followed Hailey for almost 20 years. The specialist has come to know Hailey well and, therefore, has been helpful in averting serious crises. For example, Hailey's asthma is exacerbated by sinus infections. Early on, the specialist identified the antibiotic that would treat the infection quickly, and used it consistently for Hailey over the years.

• Providing information and tools to key individuals

From the time that Hailey started school, Naomi met with teachers and the school nurse at the beginning of each academic year. She provided them with treatment plans for asthma flare-ups and allergic reactions and a Ziploc bag containing needed medications (e.g., inhaler, spacer, EpiPen, Benadryl). As Hailey got older and was involved in sports, the coach became another key individual included in the loop.

• Promoting normal development

Naomi followed the same strategy she used at school in normalizing Hailey's social life (play dates, birthday parties, sleepovers). She provided treatment plans and medications to the parents hosting the events. Eventually, the parents of Hailey's best friends "knew the drill" and would even call Naomi to review menus ahead of time!

• Making choices with consideration of health conditions

From the time Hailey was 5 years old until her freshman year in high school, she swam competitively. When Hailey began to have more sinus infections, the specialist ascertained that the flip turns required in competitive swimming were causing sinus infections. Hailey and Naomi, together with the specialist, decided that swimming was not the best sport for Hailey, and she switched to cross-country.

As Hailey grew older and could manage more aspects of her own asthma and allergies, the key care strategies remained the same but Hailey herself took over increasing responsibility for implementing them, for example:

• Transition of responsibility

Beginning in high school, Naomi still provided the school and the track coach with the treatment plans and a supply of medications, but Hailey also carried her own supply and knew what to tell people to do in an emergency.

(continues)

Case Study 5.2 (*continued*)

• Self-management

Near the end of high school, Naomi shifted responsibility to Hailey for contacting the specialist's office when she needed a prescription refilled or routine appointments scheduled.

• Self-advocacy

Hailey began interacting more independently with her specialist, discussing her treatment plan and any proposed changes. Because Hailey had been doing so well, at the time she entered college, the specialist suggested reducing the dose of her asthma medication. Hailey said no, because she intended to continue running!

• Independent management

When Hailey entered college, *she* informed her roommates and close friends about her asthma and food allergies and was very much the one in charge. As an example, during her sophomore year in college, Hailey was out running and realized she was having an allergic reaction. She quickly went to a Starbucks, told the staff to call 911, and was able to tell the EMTs exactly what she needed!

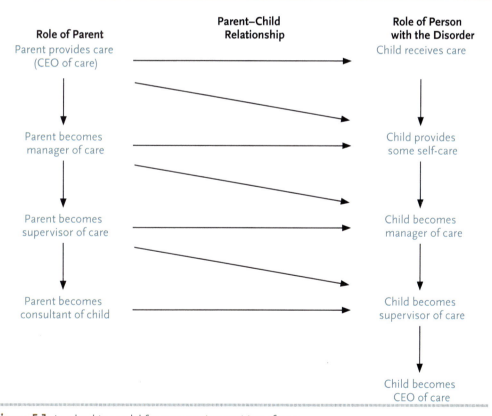

Figure 5.1. Leadership model for systematic transition of care.

Note. From "Supporting Development of Children with Chronic Conditions: From Compliance Toward Shared Management," by G. Kieckhefer and C. Trahms, 2000, *Pediatric Nursing, 26*(4), p. 358. Copyright 2000 by Janetti Publications. Granted with permission.

some of the responsibility for self-care to the child. The parent becomes the "manager" and the child the "provider" for these carefully articulated, skill-appropriate responsibilities. The parent is available to support the child's provider skills and stands ready to reassume some of these tasks for a short time if necessary because the child is ill or other life complications require additional parent support.

3.   As the child becomes more confident and competent in self-management, the parent and child negotiate the next step. The parent becomes the "supervisor" and the child becomes the manager of specific tasks. The parent is, again, poised to resume the managerial role or specific tasks for a short time, if necessary. However, the parent and child must both understand and agree that the child does not regress to a previous stage; the parent provides additional support during times of stress, and the child continues to progress in self-management skills and self-management responsibility development.

4.   Eventually, the parent assumes a "consultant" role in the child's management of the disorder, and the child becomes the "supervisor," manager, and provider of care. The parent supplies information, support, decision-making guidance, and resources, but the child assumes ultimate responsibility for his or her health care as the "CEO." (Kieckhefer & Trahms, 2000, pp. 356–357)

Although the child as CEO of his or her own care is often a step that happens in conjunction with emancipation from the family, there is no specific age ascribed to the leadership stages because young people progress at an individual cognitive and emotional pace concurrent with their experiences (Kieckhefer & Trahms, 2000). Young people may be in a particular stage for a relatively long time as they develop cognitively and emotionally. A premature shift in leadership responsibilities can be just as detrimental as delayed progress. Consequently, the parent–child relationship during effective management of a chronic disorder is dynamic in nature.

The Leadership Model can be integrated with a developmental model. Table 5.3 illustrates a developmental model by listing activities one could expect children of various ages to be able to do and the actions parents could take to support the child's growing capabilities, moving the family forward to increasing child leadership.

"Consultant" Parent Model

Cline and Greene (2007)—a psychologist–parent team—encourage use of a similar model, the "consultant" parent model, urging the development of parent effectiveness through strategies such as "setting loving limits; avoiding power struggles and overprotection; managing a child's resistance to cooperation with health-care routines; easing communication about difficult health issues such as quality and length of life; and navigating both sibling concerns and relationship issues" (Ahmann, 2013a, p. 44). The "consultant" model assists a child in achieving gradual independence through example, experience, empathy, expectations, and encouragement, as illustrated in Table 5.4.

Coaching Model

A "coaching" model for promoting independence in a young person incorporates assessment of current skill levels; both child/youth and parental strengths and weaknesses;

(text continues on p. 188)

Table 5.3

Pragmatic Actions That Support Leadership Skills

Stage/Age	Child Capabilities and Actions That Form the Basis for Leadership Skills	Parent's Leadership Actions to Support the Child's Growing Capabilities
Infant (0–12 months)	Though dependent on parents for care, the child can help by giving clear cues of distress so parents can grow in the recognition of emergent needs and appropriate responses.	Learn ramifications of the condition and how or what resources can help.
		Learn how to ask questions that can assist in managing the condition in the context of an overall healthy living pattern.
	For example, clear cues of hunger and satiety help the parent understand when to offer formula and when to withdraw it. Similarly, clear cues of increasing respiratory effort (e.g., grunting, use of accessory muscles) provide parents with a sign of respiratory distress in asthma.	Participate in support activities to increase knowledge of the disorder and its management.
		Develop daily treatment routine that fits with family life patterns.
		Recognize signs of immediate distress and seek emergency care.
		Recognize signs of early distress and seek evaluation.
	Clear cues of optimal health (e.g., adequate growth, development, social interaction) also enable parents to identify the positive impact of their actions to promote good management.	Learn to acknowledge those challenges that are developmentally typical for most children versus challenges specific to the child's condition.
		Learn how to share information with extended family and day-care providers.
		See and acknowledge evidence that the child is thriving under attentive management.
		Assume the role of repository for condition-specific information regarding the child's reaction to the treatment.
Toddler (1–3 years) If condition initially diagnosed at this age (e.g., asthma), the earlier child capabilities and parental support actions need to be addressed before attempting to accomplish or master those listed in this section.	Cooperate with routine treatments.	Develop rituals regarding treatment so that child knows what to expect and can begin to learn through repetition.
	Help hold equipment and work with parent to make equipment function as needed (e.g., use of blender to prepare formula for PKU or the nebulizer for asthma medication delivery).	Begin to recognize the child needs to have roles in the management of the condition.
	Develop a sense that parents are a source of help and comfort.	Identify possible roles the parents are willing to begin to share with the child.
	Accept constraints of condition and treatment with limited behavioral acting out (e.g., "yes foods" and "no foods" for PKU or trigger avoidance with asthma).	Change the established management routine based on the child's growing capabilities and areas of cooperation.
	Understand firm limits of parents (e.g., "No").	Continue to build clinical and community support network.

(continues)

Table 5.3 (continued)

Stage/Age	Child Capabilities and Actions That Form the Basis for Leadership Skills	Parent's Leadership Actions to Support the Child's Growing Capabilities
Preschool (4–5 years)	Identify body parts important to early identification of a problem or treatment.	Acknowledge regressions, allow very brief period of reorganization, and then resume and praise prior skill performance.
	Test limits of cooperation.	Set fair and appropriate limits.
	Use magical thinking, which may lead to fears.	Model acceptance of the management routines and limits.
	Imitate adult's behaviors.	Encourage some flexibility in rituals of treatment so child begins to experience multiple ways to accomplish same goal.
	Learn labels for condition-specific "problems" to enable communication about treatment needs.	Develop relationships with school personnel regarding specific needs.
	Learn labels for feelings associated with condition and its treatment to enable communication about feelings.	
Early school age (6–9 years)	Recognize and act on 1 or 2 major internal body cues of a problem.	Continue to label cues and give positive reward for child's recognition.
	Participate actively in concrete monitoring of condition.	Start negotiating with child for what each party will do regarding management and set criteria for forward movement that fit with family life.
	Increase understanding of condition, cause and effect, concrete level of what's going on inside the body to necessitate management.	Be prepared to renegotiate for cause.
		Establish logical consequences for actions.
		Negotiate the "rules" for working together to get all necessary treatments completed.
		Be positive and reinforcing about what needs to get done.
		Avoid overemphasis on condition.
		Support normative activities and integrate treatment needs.
		Model telling others about the disorder for the child.
		Discuss the approach to telling teachers, friends, coaches, and others about the disorder and the amount of detail necessary to share.

Table 5.3 (continued)

Stage/Age	Child Capabilities and Actions That Form the Basis for Leadership Skills	Parent's Leadership Actions to Support the Child's Growing Capabilities
Late school age (10–12 years)	Increase level of understanding of condition; begin to understand long-term needs. Develop new labels that are medically articulate to enable effective discussion with providers. Learn how and when to respond to peer pressure yet still take care of self. Enact most psychomotor skills associated with treatment with parental support. Learn more sophisticated system for reporting symptoms, management steps, and outcomes. Develop specific set of self-management tasks that are completed independently.	Remain present for the child; that is, be involved in care and monitoring decision-making. Accept the manager versus CEO role in much of treatment. Ensure that child has told important others (e.g., friends, parents, coaches) of the condition and what assistance they could provide if needed. Be there in case of emergencies or new presentation, out-of-the-routine needs, changes and maybe even the doing of some aspects. Provide the tools so the child can self-manage (e.g., get the formula, get the prescriptions). Support the child in actively communicating with his or her provider, encouraging discussion of the child's monitoring system to help the child grow in understanding.
Early adolescent (13–15 years)	Become main manager of daily, routine care. Develop strategies to ensure completion of all necessary routine management tasks. Know how to effectively ask for assistance in complex situations. Know when to be flexible versus not flexible, and be able to enact the flexibility when appropriate.	Shadow, or observe the performance closely to offer immediate corrective feedback. Negotiate and renegotiate who does what. Become the consultant versus remaining the manager. Discuss new issues (e.g., sex, drugs, alcohol) for their normative and any special condition effects.
Late adolescent (16–18 years)	Make a commitment to lifetime treatment. Increase understanding of the disorder and its long-term as well as short-term consequences on other aspects of life (e.g., vocations, intellectual achievement, well-being). Achieve sense of self as capable manager of disorder. Integrate the realities of the condition with the invincible nature of their years. Appreciate that the constraints of the management allow. Continue to develop more independent clinic and community-support network as transition to adult-based care services.	Develop a flexible way of communicating with the child to stay informed while not seen as interfering. Remain "present" for support and problem-solving with the youth. Provide support and guidance as the youth transitions from pediatric to adult-care services.

Note. From "Supporting Development of Children with Chronic Conditions: From Compliance Toward Shared Management," by G. Kieckhefer and C. Trahms, 2000, *Pediatric Nursing, 26*(4), pp. 354–363. Copyright 2000 by Jannetti Publications. Reprinted with permission.

Table 5.4

Strategies Used in Cline and Greene's "Consultant" Parent Model

Goal	Try	Avoid
1) Help a child learn to value self-care by providing an *example* of optimistic and responsible behavior.	Verbalizing one's own self-care: "I have a cold, so I am going to take care of my body by drinking extra water and juice and going to bed early."	Being preachy: "You really need to take better care of yourself."
2) Build a child's self-concept by having high enough *expectations* and by asking the child's opinion.	Setting expectations: "I know it is frustrating to miss school again, but if anyone can handle it, you can." Evoking ideas and opinions: "How do you think you might handle your bedtime meds at the sleepover?"	Placing demands: "You need to take your medicine right now so that we can leave." Babying: "Don't worry, I know it's hard. I'll pack a healthy lunch for you."
3) Share control—especially important for children with medical challenges – through offering choices and using *enforceable* statements rather than threats.	Offering choices: "Would you like your treatment before or after you get your pajamas on?" Using enforceable statements: "I will take you to the party after you have checked your blood sugar."	Making threats: "You can't go to the game if you don't take your medicine." Nagging: "I have to tell you every night: Wear that retainer!"
4) Provide *empathy* before following through with consequences, whether natural or imposed.	Offering empathy: "I am sorry that didn't work out for you." Giving empathy and consequences: "I know it is disappointing to miss the class trip because your symptoms are flaring up, but it might be better than getting hospitalized away from home where you'd be all alone because we couldn't visit you."	Showing anger: "I can't believe you went out for recess when I said not to!" Laying blame: "I told you you'd be sorry you didn't plan ahead for your meds." Giving unreasonable consequences: "You are grounded for a month for . . ."

Table 5.4 (*continued*)

Goal	Try	Avoid
5) Provide *experience* in thinking and problem solving through the use of curiosity, offering guidance, exploring consequences, and allowing the child to make a final decision and then experience the consequence of that decision.	Showing curiosity: "How concerned are you about skipping your nebulizer treatment before soccer practice?" Offering guidance: "One way some kids handle this is . . ." Exploring consequences: "I wonder what some options are for helping with the science fair project if you have to miss school today?" Allowing the child to decide: "So how did you decide to handle that?"	Giving endless reminders: "Don't forget your afternoon Adderal!" Fixing the problem: "You need to keep your inhaler in your backpack."
6) Promote competence and confidence by offering *encouragement* as often as possible for a job well done.	Offering encouragement: "You must be proud of yourself for the choice you made. That's what I'd call very responsible behavior."	Doing for an older child: "Here, let me check your blood sugar now." Belittling: "You never write down your peak flows! You know you are supposed to do that every day."

Note. From Cline and Green's "Parenting Children with Health Issues: Essential Guidance," by E. Ahmann. In Ahmann, E. (2013). *Pediatric Nursing, 39*(1) pp. 44—45. Reprinted with permission.

joint goal-setting between parent and the young person, as appropriate; and development of plans for teaching gradual step-wise skill attainment. The model was developed in an educational context for use with children with ADHD and executive-skills deficits (Dawson & Guare, 2009; Guare, Dawson & Guare, 2013). Maitland and Quinn (2013) applied the model to preparing teens with ADHD and learning disabilities for college. The model has relevance for children with other special needs as well.

Related principles in planning care and support of the child with special needs include encouraging the development of self-efficacy and resilience and focusing on strengths rather than weaknesses. When children have challenging emotional or behavioral issues, several specialized resources may be particularly useful to parents navigating their children's care and increasing independence (see Appendix 5.1: Resources).

Family–Professional Partnerships

The principles of patient- and family-centered care provide an overarching framework for the care of children with or without special needs (see Text Box 5.1). The federal Maternal and Child Health Bureau Division of Services for Children with Special Health Needs (2005, p. 2) defined family-centered care as follows:

> Family-Centered Care assures the health and well-being of children and their families through a respectful family-professional partnership. It honors the strengths, cultures, traditions and expertise that everyone brings to this relationship. Family-Centered Care is the standard of practice that results in high quality services.

The Institute for Patient- and Family-Centered Care outlines four core concepts in this model (Institute, n.d.):

- Patient- and family-centered care is an approach to the planning, delivery, and evaluation of health care that is grounded in mutually beneficial partnerships among health-care providers, patients, and families. It redefines the relationships in health care.
- Patient- and family-centered practitioners recognize the vital role that families play in ensuring the health and well-being of infants, children, adolescents, and family members of all ages. They acknowledge that emotional, social, and developmental support are integral components of health care. They promote the health and well-being of individuals and families and restore dignity and control to them.
- Patient- and family-centered care is an approach to health care that shapes policies, programs, facility design, and staff day-to-day interactions. It leads to better health outcomes and wiser allocation of resources, and greater patient and family satisfaction.

Core concepts include:

- *Respect and dignity.* Health-care practitioners listen to and honor patient and family perspectives and choices. Patient and family knowledge, values, beliefs and cultural backgrounds are incorporated into the planning and delivery of care.

Text Box 5.1
Commonly Accepted Family-Centered Care Principles

- Information Sharing: The exchange of information is open, objective, and unbiased.
- Respect and Honoring Differences: The working relationship is marked by respect for diversity, cultural and linguistic traditions, and care preferences.
- Partnership and Collaboration: Medically appropriate decisions that best fit the needs, strengths, values, and abilities of all involved are made together by involved parties, including families at the level they choose.
- Negotiation: The desired outcomes of medical care plans are flexible and not necessarily absolute.
- Care in Context of Family and Community: Direct medical care and decision-making reflect the child within the context of his/her family, home, school, daily activities, and quality of life within the community.

NOTE: Groups such as Family Voices, the Maternal and Child Health Bureau, the American Academy of Pediatrics, and the Institute for Patient- and Family-Centered Care have developed principles of family-centered care. Despite some variation, the general principles above are shared by these organizations.

Note. From "Family-Centered Care: Current Applications and Future Directions in Pediatric Health Care," by D. Z. Kuo, A. J. Houtrow, P. Arango, K. A. Kuhlthau, J. M. Simmons, & J. N. Neff, 2012, *Maternal and Child Health Journal, 16*, pp. 297–305. Reprinted with permission of Springer.

- *Information sharing.* Health-care practitioners communicate and share complete and unbiased information with patients and families in ways that are affirming and useful. Patients and families receive timely, complete, and accurate information in order to effectively participate in care and decision-making.
- *Participation.* Patients and families are encouraged and supported in participating in care and decision-making at the level they choose.
- *Collaboration.* Patients and families are also included on an institution-wide basis. Health-care leaders collaborate with patients and families in policy and program development, implementation, and evaluation; in health-care facility design; and in professional education, as well as in the delivery of care.

The goal of patient- and family-centered care is to provide for optimal care of young people by encouraging partnerships between health-care providers, the child, and family. In fact, the American Academy of Pediatrics policy statement on family-centered care states that "the perspectives and information provided by families, children, and young adults are essential components of high-quality clinical decision-making, and that patients and family are integral partners with the health-care team" (AAP, 2012, p. 394).

Patient- and family-centered care is often "insufficiently implemented in clinical practice" (Kuo et al., 2012, p. 297). Nonetheless, the American Academy of Pediatrics

(2012, p. 395) concludes that "[p]atient- and family-centered approaches lead to better health outcomes and wiser allocation of resources as well as to greater patient and family satisfaction." For these reasons, family-centered care is considered the gold standard in inpatient as well as in outpatient primary care, specialty care, emergency care, and chronic care (Kuo et al., 2012).

Further, many health-care systems and state and federal legislative bodies, as well as both the Institute of Medicine and Healthy People 2020, have recognized the benefits and importance of patient- and family-centered care (Kuo, et al., 2012). In fact, patients and families are increasingly being involved not only in relation to the care of themselves or their family members but also in advisory roles regarding practice and policy more broadly:

> Some hospital systems . . . incorporate families at different levels of clinical care and education on a formal, systematic basis. Specific examples include family advisory boards and family/peer support groups, family presentations on care experiences at Grand Rounds, and hiring family members as consulting staff to specific programs. [Some hospitals] . . . incorporate experienced family leaders as peer consultants or staff. (Kuo et al., 2012, p. 300)

Similarly,

> in a federally funded medical home project using a quality-improvement model, families served by 13 community-based pediatric practices are collaborating with pediatricians and office staff to enhance the practices' capacity to provide care to children with special health-care needs and to be more responsive to the priorities and needs of these children and their families. These practices have permanently integrated family input into decisions about their processes of care. (AAP, 2012, p. 397)

In clinical practice, patient- and family-centered care recognizes that family members know their child best. Family members care for their children's health, developmental, social, and emotional needs across settings and over a period of many years. Although it is common for health-care providers to focus on an immediate crisis and see the young person and family primarily in that limited context, families must balance their child's health-care needs with both the child's other needs and interests and other family members' needs and interests, in the short and long term. Because of this, family members should be active participants in assessing needs, in planning, and in implementing care. Health-care providers should ensure opportunities for families to participate as fully as they wish in decision-making and care provision.

Insurance and Financing

The American Academy of Pediatrics supports the concept that all children, including children and youth with special needs, should have access to medically necessary services to (1) promote optimal growth and development; (2) maintain and avert deterioration in functioning; and (3) prevent, detect, diagnose, treat, ameliorate, or palliate the effects of physical, genetic, congenital, developmental, behavioral, or mental conditions, injuries, or disabilities (AAP, 2013). Yet, financial concerns do pose a challenge for many families that have children or youth with special needs and do, at times, interfere with access to timely and appropriate care. Porterfield and DeRigne (2011) cite data suggesting that out-of-pocket medical expenses for children with special health-care needs are estimated to be twice the amount required for children without chronic conditions. These expenses can include the costs of evaluations, nonstandard therapies, mental health co-pays, special supplies and equipment, medications, special formulas or foods, transportation, home modifications, insurance costs, and unreimbursed bills. Not surprisingly, more severe conditions are associated with higher out-of-pocket expenditures.

On average, families of children and youth with special needs spend approximately 2% of their household income on unreimbursed medical costs; for 3% to 4% of families, these costs exceeded 10% of household income, and more than 20% of families receiving public insurance reported that their child's medical expenses led to family financial problems (Porterfield & DeRigne, 2011). An additional concern is that burdensome costs of care can lead to delayed care and unmet needs.

Families with private insurance may need help to understand and advocate for the maximum benefits from their insurance company or managed-care organization. Additionally, receiving care-coordination for medical or behavioral conditions, often from a medical home, appears to be a factor in reducing the economic burden of care for families (Porterfield & DeRigne, 2011; Ronis, Baldwin, Blumkin, Kuhlthau, & Szilagyi, 2015).

Additional considerations loom as a young person with special health-care needs reaches adolescence. Insurance coverage may change in young adulthood, so financial issues should be considered in late adolescence. Some individuals with disabilities will qualify for Supplemental Security Income (SSI) or Medicaid; otherwise, options under the Affordable Care Act should be investigated. As another financial consideration, some families may need to investigate independent living arrangements and in-home support services for the transition to adulthood. Financial implications of educational, vocational, and employment training options should also be considered as part of transition planning. In other circumstances, residential placement options and advance financial planning should be considered for the time when aging parents may no longer be able to care for their child.

Early and Continuous Screening and Referral

Federal guidelines require early and continuous screening of children for health-care conditions through several programs: Early and Periodic Diagnosis and Treatment (EPSDT), Medicaid managed care for CYSHCN, and the Patient Protection and Affordable Care Act.

For children enrolled in Medicaid, EPSDT provides comprehensive and preventive health-care services for children under age 21 who are enrolled in Medicaid, with the following screening requirements at periodic, age-appropriate levels (Early and Periodic, n.d; National Consensus Framework, 2014, p. 8):

- comprehensive health and developmental history
- comprehensive unclothed physical exam

- vision and hearing screening
- referral to a dental provider
- appropriate immunizations
- lead screening
- lab tests
- developmental and behavioral screening
- anticipatory guidance

An increasing number of states are moving children and youth with special health-care needs into their Medicaid managed-care programs. As of 2010, 32 states required that at least one Medicaid managed-care program or geographic area enroll CYSHCN (Lee, 2014). The Federal Medicaid managed-care regulations mandate screening for these children (National Consensus Framework, 2014).

Additionally, since 2010, the Patient Protection and Affordable Care Act requires that Bright Futures Guidelines for Health Supervision of Infants, Children, and Adolescents be followed in all pediatric settings, with no family cost-sharing, as the standard that provides the basis for eligible preventive services (National Consensus Framework, 2014). Developed by the American Academy of Pediatrics, Bright Futures is a set of theory-based, evidence-driven guidelines that address the key issues in child health and development. (For more information, about Bright Futures, see Appendix 5.1: Resources.)

Easy-to-Use Services and Supports

For most families, community-based services are easier to use than services located at a distance, such as at a tertiary-care center. Ideally, CYSHCN and their families could access to comprehensive home and community based support services, through their health plan or medical home, perhaps in partnership with other community agencies. These agencies might include family organizations, public health, education, early intervention, special education, child welfare, mental health, and home health-care organizations (National Consensus Framework, 2014).

Antonelli (2012, cited in National Consensus Framework (2014, p. 18) suggested that agreements between health systems and relevant community agencies and programs—including respite care, home care, and palliative and hospice care—should ideally be structured to

- promote family support through linking families to family organizations and other services and supports,
- promote shared financing,
- establish systems for timely communications and appropriate data sharing,
- ensure access and coordination of services for individual children and their families,
- promote collaboration between community-based organizations and agencies, providers, health-care systems, and families, and
- specify responsibilities across the various providers and community-based agencies serving children and their families.

As these principles suggest, care coordination is a critical support for families of children and youth with special needs. The next section on the medical home addresses this issue in more detail.

Medical Home

It is generally understood that comprehensive, coordinated, multidisciplinary management facilitates optimal care, especially for the child with multiple, complex problems. Care of children and youth with special needs should be comprehensive and multidisciplinary in that it addresses not only medical concerns and needs but also emotional, developmental, educational, social, financial, and familial concerns and priorities.

Care coordination is important for families of children and youth with multiple and/or complex needs and serves several purposes: (a) ensuring continuity for the child and family across care settings (i.e., inpatient, outpatient, educational, and therapeutic); (b) improving interdisciplinary communication and, thus, reducing fragmentation of care when multiple providers are involved; and (c) both prioritizing and consolidating care requirements, thus reducing the burden of care for the family. Goals should focus not only on short-term management but also on long-term plans. For the young person with multiple and complex needs, care coordination is also important to ensure that health maintenance needs, such as primary care and developmental and emotional support, are not overlooked. Care coordination is a typical service provided by a medical home.

The American Academy of Pediatrics Council on Pediatric Practice first introduced the concept of the medical home in 1967 to promote optimal care for children and youth with special health-care needs. The medical home concept became a priority when the federal government included it as a goal in Healthy People 2020, encouraging that all young people with special health-care needs receive regular ongoing comprehensive care within a medical home. The medical home has come to mean promoting comprehensive for children and youth with special needs through care coordination centered on active participation of the child and family (Thrall et al., 2012). A medical home has three key components (Improving, n.d., p. 1):

- an approach to providing comprehensive primary care,
- a partnership between the pediatric care team, the child/youth, and the family to ensure that all medical and nonmedical needs are met, and
- a way to help the child/youth and the family access, coordinate, and understand specialty care, educational services, out-of-home care, family support, and other public and private community services.

See Text Box 5.2 for a more detailed outline of the medical home concept.

Data suggest that approximately 50% of children and youth with special health-care needs have a medical home (Porterfield & DeRigne, 2011). Research findings document that quality of care, patient and family experiences of care, access to care, timeliness of care, and costs of care improve with the use of a medical home (Grumbach, Bodenheimer, & Grundy, 2009; Mosquera et al., 2015; Overview, 2014; Ronis et al., 2015). Outcomes of care, including improved health status and overall quality of life for the young person and family, also improve for medical and certain behavioral conditions (Adams & Tapia, 2013; Mosquera et al., 2015; Overview, 2014).

||||||||||||||||||||||||||||||||||||||||||||||||||||||||||||||||||||||||||||||||||||||||||||||||||||||||||||||||||||||||||||||||||||||||||||||

Text Box 5.2
Medical Home Standards

The medical home is ready and willing to provide well, acute, and chronic care for all children and youth, including those affected by special health-care needs or those who hold other risks for compromised health and wellness.

The medical home comprises a primary care provider and/or pediatric subspecialist and, as part of an integrated care team, does the following:

1. Provides access to health-care services 24 hours a day, 7 days a week

2. Provides health-care services that encourage the family to share in decision-making, and provides feedback on services provided

3. Performs comprehensive health assessments

4. Promotes an integrated team-based model of care coordination

5. Maintains and updates a comprehensive, integrated plan of care that has been developed with the family and other members of a team; addresses family care clinical goals; encompasses strategies and actions needed across all settings; and is shared effectively with families and among providers

6. Conducts activities to support CYSHCN and their families in self-management of the child's health and health care

7. Promotes quality of life, healthy development, and healthy behaviors across all life stages

8. Integrates care with other providers and ensures that information is shared effectively with families and among providers

9. Performs care tracking, including sending of proactive reminders to families and clinicians of services needed, via a registry or other mechanism

10. Provides care that is effective and based on evidence, where applicable

||||||||||||||||||||||||||||||||||||||||||||||||||||||||||||||||||||||||||||||||||||||||||||||||||||||||||||||||||||||||||||||||||||||||||||||

Transition to Adulthood

Between 50% and 90% of children with special health-care needs reach adolescence and live into adulthood (Tysbina, Kingnoth, Maxwell, Bayley, & Lindsey, 2012). Yet, the majority of these young people (some 60%) do not receive adequate support to transition from pediatric to adult medical care (Harris, Freeman, & Duke, 2011; McManus et al., 2013). Summarizing several studies, Hopper, Dokken, and Ahmann (2014, p. 250) report that inadequate transition planning has been shown to result in "poor treatment adherence, lack of adequate care, in some cases no care at all, an increased risk of secondary complications, an increase in emergency department use and hospitalization, and even diminishment of productive participation in society . . . [placing] a significant burden on both young people and families."

Transition preparation is often best addressed in a medical home but is important in any setting. Family-centered transition strategies include the following (Hopper, Dokken, & Ahmann, 2014, pp. 251–252):

- Provide advance, perhaps gradual, preparation for all aspects of the transition process well before it happens.
- Determine the timing and length of the transition process according to the patient's needs [including health status] as opposed to a set age or time frame.
- Offer transition planning that addresses not only medical but also psychosocial and educational [and vocational] needs of young adult patients, [staggering these transitions if possible].
- Teach patients and their families about case management as part of transition planning.
- Develop opportunities for information sharing among families [such as] transition "forums" and peer support groups.
- Prepare portable transition summaries for patients and families with information about condition(s), medications, treatments, hospitalizations, and surgeries.
- Educate adult-care providers about the important and evolving role of young adult patients in their own health care [as well as] the role parents continue to play in the health care of young adults with special medical needs.
- Allow for a period of overlap in services.

See Appendix 5.2: Transition Resources for a number of useful materials to aid the transition from pediatric to adult care for youth with special health-care needs.

Cultural Competence

It is well understood that culture and ethnicity affect access to care, use of services, the perceived meaning of illness, health-care practices, and communication. Cultural traditions and spiritual beliefs are often the foundation of a family's life and provide guidance, support, comfort, and meaning (Weiner, McConnell, Latella, & Ludi, 2013). These traditions can become even more important in stressful or challenging circumstances. Yet, providing appropriate care for individuals with different life experiences, beliefs, value systems, religions, languages, and notions of health care it can be a challenge (Weiner et al., 2013). Weiner and colleagues (2013, p. 48) described cultural competence as follows:

> Research shows that cultural competence is more than accumulated knowledge of cultural practices; it encompasses a need for medical practitioners to consider their own constructs of bias and belief. . . . Cultural competence must be considered in context of the diverse personal, medical, and practitioner cultures that abound in clinical settings. . . . Moreover, cultural practices cannot be taken out of patient context. It is easy to oversimplify cultural or religious practices. Social factors, such as class and literacy, differentiate individuals within cultural norms. . . . Likewise, practitioners must be aware of the contrary effect of perpetuating rigid stereotypes about what members of a particular "culture" believe, do, or want, and how that translates to provision of care. The modern view of cultural competence emphasizes its fluidity: a process that bridges care and patient need as a vital link in communication with patients and families during tragic circumstances.

A focus on family-centered care can encourage partnership with family members in gaining knowledge of a family's value systems, beliefs, structure, decision-making approaches, religion, ethnic roots and cultural norms, group cultural practices and, of course, language translation needs, as a basis for demonstrating respect and providing culturally competent care (Weiner et al., 2013)

While language is only one piece of culture, communication in health care is critical and is a cornerstone of family-centered care. For this reason, all health-care settings should ensure timely access to professional interpreting services whenever a language or communication barrier exists. Using family members or friends as interpreters risks faulty communication and patient safety and potentially compromises privacy (Dudley, Ackerman, Brown, & Snow, 2015).

Family Adaptive Tasks

Most families with children or youth with special needs have a number of challenges to manage. *Adapting* is defined as an ongoing process whereby parents are able to sensitively read and respond to their child's signals in a manner conducive to healthy development (Barnett et al., 2003). Drawing from theoretical research and clinical literature, Clawson (1996) identified eight adaptive tasks of families having a child with a chronic illness or disability, each of which will be addressed below.

Accepting the Condition

Depending on a young person's condition, families may face a period of uncertainty prior to obtaining a final or definitive diagnosis. Even if it relieves uncertainty, the diagnosis itself can be challenging to face for parents and professionals alike. Once a diagnosis is made, family members face an often challenging period of learning to understand and manage the condition and to adapt family life to incorporate care needs (Smith, Cheater, & Bekker, 2013).

For some family members, *accepting* the condition may carry implications of going beyond adaptation, to being able to say to oneself, for example, "My child has a disability, and this is OK." This may be particularly difficult for parents of children and youth with developmental disabilities and mental illness. It may take years before parents are comfortable fully accepting the reality, and there will also be times when it does not feel OK. It may be more helpful to think in terms of *acknowledgement*, perhaps a more accurate term for this mental task than *acceptance*. Health-care providers can support families by recognizing the difficulty of this task and preparing them for possible periods of chronic—recurrent—sorrow. In an article addressing research on the issue, several family stories illustrated the challenges involved in living with chronic sorrow; one parent described life with her daughter, who has a neuromuscular disorder and requires a gastrostomy tube, a tracheostomy, and a ventilator (Gordon, 2009, p. 118):

> Any dream of a happy "white picket fence" existence is definitely gone. At some level, you are mourning the loss of a typically developing child all the time. You also get up every day not knowing what will happen. I had a friend who was pregnant at the same time as I was. For a long time, I couldn't be around her and see her daughter going through typical developmental milestones—and so directly face

the reality of what Felicia could not do. Birthdays and holidays are not good times. What can I buy my daughter as a gift? She can't play with dolls or other toys! On more than one occasion, I've bawled my eyes out in an aisle in Toys"R"Us.

The father of a child with medulloblastoma and a severe head injury that occurred as a result of a fall during treatment also shared his experience (Gordon, 2009, p. 118):

[As a parent] you have a broken heart. Sometimes you're jealous when you see other kids Chris's age who are in school or getting married. Chris didn't get to go to the prom or play sports; it does get to you sometimes. When you get tired, you might get aggravated with the situation. "Chronic sorrow" really sums it up.

See also Appendix 5.1: Resources for videos related to families' experiences.

Providing Daily Management of the Condition

Parents ultimately are responsible for the day-to-day management of a child's special needs. Daily management of these needs will vary greatly depending on the diagnosis, severity of the condition, and therapeutic treatments. Some conditions, such as diabetes, epilepsy, or asthma, require "controlling" as well as managing, and certain nonprogressive conditions, such as cerebral palsy, require more vigilance to prevent associated complications. To varying degrees, parents may need education about the child or young person's condition, education and training in the child's special care requirements, help organizing their time and incorporating specific care requirements into the family's daily plan, and assistance in developing collaborative working relationships with health-care providers. Nightingale, Friedl, and Swallow (2015) recommend asking individual parents directly about their learning needs and preferences as the most reliable way of addressing needs related to managing their child's long-term condition.

A continuum of five family management styles has been identified that includes *thriving, accommodating, enduring, struggling,* and *floundering* (Knafl et al., 1996). Thriving families experience normalcy and feel confident about being able to handle the demands posed by the illness. Families in between thriving and floundering are characterized by conflict and uncertainty about how to manage the illness. Enduring families have a negative view of the situation and feel burdened even if they are capable. Education and support, including parent-to-parent support, can benefit families managing complex care.

Meeting Normal Developmental Needs of the Child/Youth

To promote normal development, young people should be provided age-appropriate activities. Even those with serious medical problems can be helped to engage in appropriate developmental experiences. In the 1990s, when children began to go home from the hospital with complex conditions requiring the use of medical technology in the home, several principles were articulated to optimize their developmental planning; these principles apply, as well, to any young person with special needs (Ahmann & Klockenbrink, 1996; Ahmann & Lierman, 1992; Glass & Blinkoff, 1996). The first principle involves using a full understanding of the medical condition to plan developmental opportunities both at a time when the young person has the most energy and endurance and during activities, to observe for signals of stress. Second, flexibly tailor plans to individual abilities, interests, and needs. Finally, creatively adapt any required medical equipment to meet developmental needs.

The following examples of interventions for a child who is ventilator-dependent demonstrate developmental support at various stages. Among their various developmental needs, infants need a range of motor experiences and have a strong need to suck. To respond to these needs, health-care providers and parents can vary the ventilated infant's positioning to encourage freedom of movement and, if oral feeding is not tolerated, to encourage non-nutritive sucking as long as the infant shows no signs of distress. As the toddler years approach, freedom and mobility to explore become paramount. A safe environment, including covers on medical supplies and equipment, should be provided, and equipment modifications, such as lengthy oxygen or ventilator tubing, should be made to encourage mobility. Mounting the ventilator on a wheelchair or wheeled wagon or cart will also allow the toddler maximum freedom of movement.

Later, as the preschool-age child begins to master many new skills, providing ways for the young person to help with medical treatments (e.g., opening packages, arranging supplies, holding tubing) can be developmentally supportive. The school-age child should increasingly be taught self-care skills, such as suctioning and medication administration, under supervision. In addition, the school-age child should carry identification, a medical bracelet, and emergency supplies and equipment, such as saline, portable suction, and a replacement tracheostomy tube, so that attending school, visiting friends, and participating in other social activities is safely facilitated. Meeting same-age peers with similar medical conditions, through a camp or support group, may also be beneficial at this age.

Adolescents can begin to master self-care, though some monitoring from afar may still be needed. Teens should also begin to participate in decision-making regarding their medical care. Additionally, information about any sexual limitations of the condition (e.g., a spinal cord injury) should be addressed openly; options regarding education, vocation, and employment should be considered; and plans should be made for gradual transition to adult health-care providers.

As is true for all young people, promoting coping and self-efficacy can buffer stress and contribute to mental health and self-esteem in the presence of special needs. No matter what the age, health-care providers and parents can help young people understand their medical conditions and can instruct and encourage their participation in self-care. Although the Piagetian framework has been used for over three decades to outline children's illness concepts in a stage-based approach (Bibace & Walsh, 1980), somewhat more recent research (Yoos, 1994) suggests that the illness experience influences one's ability to acquire specific knowledge and reasoning capabilities about the disease and its treatments, no matter what the developmental stage. Further, Vygotsky's theory of social development points out that with the help of a more knowledgeable person, young people can be brought to a deeper level of understanding of concepts, exceeding what they would be able to attain on their own (Vygotsky, 1962, 1978).

In a study related to spina bifida, the severity of a child's condition was a factor in expected age of self-care skill development (Greenley, 2010). Thus, individual assessments of a child's knowledge base and knowledge needs are important. Effective teaching for self-care must be informed by developmental stage but also directed to the young person's individual level of understanding and account for complexity of care.

Meeting the Developmental Needs of Other Family Members

Over the years, research related to families of children and youth with special needs has identified numerous stressors related to family coping. Many of these fall into the realm of meeting the developmental needs of other family members. Simply making efforts to maintain family rituals and activities that foster cohesiveness and closeness (e.g., celebrating birthdays, sharing meals together) can decrease some of the strains of day-to-day care.

Parents may face emotional stress because of the diagnosis, changes in the young person's condition, unmet developmental milestones, and the impact of managing the condition on a daily basis. Role strain is common as parents learn care procedures, medical terminology, and case management tasks, and continue to manage other family and employment responsibilities. Parents may face time constraints in juggling their child's care needs with employment demands and the needs of other family members. Financial stressors can include inadequate insurance coverage, unreimbursed medical expenses, and employment constraints resulting from the need to maintain insurance coverage. Parental health can also be affected by the demands of caring for children and youth with certain conditions. Any of these stressors may interfere with parents meeting their own normal developmental needs.

In two-parent families, mothers and fathers may react differently to a diagnosis and prognosis, to the demands of daily care, to long-term concerns, and to financial burdens of care (see Appendix 5.1: Resources for videos of parents' reactions). Parents may also have different, and sometimes gender-based, coping mechanisms. Recognizing each other's strengths and contributions to the family and accepting each other's coping mechanisms as valid can help parents in keeping these various coping differences from becoming a source of conflict. Additionally, the marriage or partnership relationship needs nurturing. Single-parent families may face particular financial, physical, and emotional burdens when providing care for a child with special needs.

Research findings about the effects on siblings of a young person with special needs have been inconsistent and even contradictory. While earlier studies suggested greater adjustment problems, many of those studies did not use control groups; more recent and better-designed studies tend to suggest fewer problems. For example, in a study of over 300 children with a brother or sister with a disability, Neely-Barnes and Graff (2011) found no statistically significant group differences in sibling psychological problems. However, most published research studies are based on parent reports, which may lead to incomplete conclusions about the experiences of siblings themselves (Hastings & Petalas, 2014). Some differences in sibling coping are associated with age, birth order, and gender. See Text Box 5.3: Potential Stressors and Coping Strategies for Siblings. Aware health-care providers and parents can promote coping and positive outcomes. The national Sibling Support Project, founded in 1990, provides a variety of resources to support siblings, including its "SibShop" workshops that are offered in many states (www.siblingsupport.org). For more about issues for family members, see Chapter 7: Families in Children's Health-Care Settings.

Text Box 5.3
Potential Stressors and Coping Strategies for Siblings

Stressors

- Less attention from parents
- Emotional realignments within the family
- Physical and emotional separation from parents and the sibling with special needs
- Lack of information or information that is understandable at their developmental level
- Disrupted family communication
- Perceived sense of guilt over causing the illness or disability
- Negativity between how the ill child and siblings are disciplined
- Assumption of more household responsibilities and chores, often including caregiving functions for the child with special needs
- Fear of the unknown (e.g., fear of what the treatments and hospitalizations are like, fear of death, fear of self or other family members becoming ill)
- Changes in family routines
- Changes in recreation activities

Coping Strategies

- Seeking out information
- Using social support resources
- Having an outlet separate from the ill child and family as a means of distraction and source of self-esteem (e.g., school, recreation activities, clubs, friends)
- Expressing emotions
- Engaging in thought stopping: the forced substitution of positive thoughts for negative ones
- Developing empathy: the ability to assume the perspective of another
- Having other well siblings with whom to share feelings, concerns, and household tasks
- Using available social support network to provide physical and emotional care when needed
- Having open communication within family that promotes expression of feelings

Note. From "Chronic Conditions: Effects on the Child's Family," by C. Walker, 1999, in M. E. Broome and J. A. Rollins (Eds.), *Core Curriculum for the Nursing Care of Children and Their Families.* Pitman, NJ: Jannetti Publications, pp. 262–263. Copyright 1999 by Jannetti Publications. Reprinted with permission.

Coping With Ongoing Stressors and Periodic Crises

Anticipatory guidance for children and youth with special needs and their families can promote coping with ongoing stressors and periodic crises. Some conditions will pose new challenges at different developmental stages, and families can be helped to feel prepared to manage the changes.

Developmental disabilities, for example, may have a greater effect on functioning as the child ages and normal developmental expectations change. Anticipatory guidance can help families prepare for potentially difficult or disappointing transitions, such as school entry. Some conditions will have periods requiring crisis management (e.g., acute asthma) and other periods of less intense management. Families can be alerted to signs and symptoms of acute exacerbations and be given protocols to assist decision-making in these difficult situations. Still other conditions will have periods of remission and recurrence (e.g., cancer), and families should be prepared in advance for these possibilities as well as for a potential terminal phase. Children with severe disabilities or behavioral problems may at some point require residential treatment or placement, and these options should be discussed with the family as warranted

Periodic ongoing assessment with the young person and the family is important to ensure optimal outcomes. All planning should be undertaken as a collaborative, patient- and family-centered process. Family members should be provided with information and support for decision-making as necessary on an ongoing or crisis basis. Information should be shared fully and openly and in terms that all family members can understand. Family members can be helped to identify and evaluate their options and to gain the information and skills they need to sustain their decisions. Finally, all support offered in decision-making should promote the family's own goals, values, and interests.

Managing Feelings

Both the professional literature and family reports indicate a wide range of feelings common to families of children and youth with special needs. Some previous research has suggested stages of adaptation, but it is now understood that there is wide variability in how families adjust to a diagnosis.

At the time of diagnosis, shock and denial are common. Denial may last for some time and is not always maladaptive. In fact, it can be a useful protective mechanism for some families who continue to provide appropriate care for their children, allowing the family to adjust over time to a diagnosis while they mobilize their energies and coping resources.

Adjustment to the diagnosis may involve feelings of guilt, bitterness, and anger as the family acknowledges the presence of the diagnosed condition. Understanding family, friends, and professionals can provide the support needed for family members to process these strong feelings as they acclimate to the new family circumstances. Parent-to-parent support is particularly valuable.

As families adjust and gather information, realistic expectations for the young person can be formed, and family life can be reintegrated with the new perspective imposed by the illness or disability. A focus on family strengths, the promotion of normalization, encouragement and promotion of family cohesion, and involvement of the family members as collaborators in assessment and planning related to care of their child can support family empowerment.

Cognitive, behavioral, and emotional tasks all comprise the adaptive coping process. Cognitive tasks include learning about the condition, the prognosis, and the care requirements. Behavioral tasks include providing for the child or youth's therapeutic needs, monitoring the condition, and supplying day-to-day management. Emotional tasks include grieving the loss of the "perfect child," managing anger, and addressing the limitations the condition places on the parents and the family as a whole.

Family members also have to navigate often complex and contradictory feelings in relation to health-care providers and the health-care system. Parent-to-parent support often introduces families to others who have advocate or activist styles and can encourage parents to develop these more assertive approaches.

Educating Others About the Chronic Illness or Condition

Parents may want help knowing how to explain a disability or illness to the child/youth or to siblings of various ages. They may want guidance on how much to tell and how to tell friends and neighbors about a condition so that the young person can be understood but not teased or stigmatized. The child or teen may need similar guidance. Parents also may need to train home-care nurses and respite workers in how to meet special needs. They may need to be prepared to explain an uncommon condition to either physicians providing emergency care or other physicians who may not be knowledgeable about their child's diagnosis and care requirements. All of this should be considered when educating families and providing anticipatory guidance.

Establishing a Support System

Social support has repeatedly been shown to positively influence coping and health-care outcomes. Families can benefit from professional support, support from family and friends, and the unique support of peers.

Support provided by peers, such as family-to-family or parent-to-parent support, can provide families with information, emotional support, a sense of being understood, friendship, mentoring, role modeling, assistance with problem solving, and a base for advocacy efforts. Professionals can facilitate family-to-family support by (a) making referrals to local and national support groups; (b) facilitating meetings by providing space, transportation, and child care; (c) developing peer support networks; and (d) linking interested parents one-on-one when no formal support group is available. See Appendix 5.1: Resources for information about locating a "support parent" for parents of children with special needs.

Additional Issues in the Care of Children and Youth With Special Health-Care Needs

Children and youth with special needs are not only part of their families but also part of their communities. Comprehensive coordinated care, based in their communities, is essential for promoting optimal outcomes. Two additional issues of importance when a young person has special health-care needs are educational issues and, in cases of complex chronic illness, home care services.

Educational and Developmental Issues

One important aspect of normal activity is formal education. The Education for All Handicapped Children Act (PL 94-142), passed in 1975, emphasizes the right of all young people, ages 5 to 21 years, to a free, public education in the "least restrictive environment," and provides for related services, such as physical and occupational therapy, as necessary, to maximize benefit from the educational program. In 1986, PL 99-457, the Education of the Handicapped Amendment, extended PL 94-142 to children with disabilities between the ages of 3 and 5 years. The title of the act was later changed to the Individuals with Disabilities Education Act (known as IDEA). In 1993, Part H of PL 103-382, amendments to IDEA, strengthened the federal commitment to provision of early intervention services by extending services to infants and toddlers from birth to 3 years of age.

As part of IDEA, children ages 0 to 3 years old with or at risk of disabilities are entitled to a comprehensive evaluation and, if the child is eligible for early intervention services, the development of an individualized family service plan (IFSP). When a child approaches 3 years of age, he or she can be referred to community programs, or, if intervention services are still needed, can be transitioned to Part B of IDEA, which serves young people ages 3 to 21 years with special needs, and an individualized education plan (IEP) will be developed. Note that some children with ADHD or other less involved learning disabilities may qualify for educational accommodations under a 504 plan, which falls under different legislation: Section 504 of the Rehabilitation Act of 1973. Section 504 defines disability more broadly than IDEA.

Over the years, states have interpreted the provisions of IDEA differently, in particular the meaning of "related" services. In the Supreme Court case *Cedar Rapids v. Garret F.* (1999), the family of a child dependent on a ventilator wanted the school district to pay for a registered nurse to care for the child at school, but the school district did not think that such a provision was required by IDEA. The Supreme Court ruled that IDEA requires schools to provide health supports for students who need them as long as the care is not medical and not performed by doctors (Questions and Answers, 1999).

In many cases, students with special educational or developmental needs can easily be incorporated into the general education classroom. Some may be "pulled out" of the classroom to be provided special services, such as occupational, physical, or speech therapy. In certain situations, preparation of the young person for the school experience or for school reentry after a hospitalization may be helpful. Preparation of classmates and teachers can also be helpful when a child or teen has noticeable physical changes or differences (e.g., loss of hair due to chemotherapy, use of a wheelchair). Other planning and preparations to ensure safety and appropriate care may be necessary when a young person requires complex health-care services. Students with severe cognitive or behavioral problems may require placement in specialized educational settings. Additionally, parents may need assistance to develop the skills required to effectively advocate for their child or teen in the educational setting.

Home-Care Services

Some young people with special health-care needs will require home-care nursing and therapeutic services. In fact, pediatric home care has been among the fastest growing components of the home-care industry. Plans to transition a young person from hospital to home should begin early during a hospitalization to allow family members to learn and demonstrate all aspects of care.

Principles of patient- and family-centered care must also apply in the home setting. The home is the family's domain and home care providers must respect family choices and values, and work in collaboration with the family in efforts to care for their child. The family should be seen as a partner in care. An effective family/professional collaborative relationship will feature the following characteristics: (a) a shared purpose, (b) mutual respect and trust, (c) communication, (d) dialogue, (e) active listening, (f) awareness and acceptance of difference, and (g) negotiation. These characteristics are important considerations for nurses or other health-care providers in the home-care setting.

Part of the collaborative process should involve establishing "house rules" that allow the family to maintain a feeling of control over their environment when health-care providers are present (Klug, 1993). House rules, or guidelines with which families and professionals are comfortable, also serve to frame, from the beginning, the working relationship between the family, home health agency, nurses, and other professionals who come into the home (Wegener, 1996). Establishing these guidelines helps ease the potential tension between parents and professionals around boundary and authority issues.

Respecting parental expertise is also an essential principle in the home-care setting. Parents are not always supported in their role as manager for their child's long-term condition, nor is their expertise and contribution to care always valued (Smith et al., 2013). Yet, parents often will have more specific training in care for their particular child's needs than will a home-care nurse. Additionally, parents are most familiar with their child's personality, communication, and symptom patterns. Partnership in the home-care setting is essential not only for respect of the family members but also for optimal care of the young person.

Conclusion

Steadily since the 1970s or so, the survival of youth with special health-care needs has markedly improved, and most of these children now live into early adulthood or beyond. With a commitment to family-centered care and, increasingly, the medical home, with its emphasis on care coordination—a seamless system that offers continuity of care from birth through childhood into the teen and young adult years, and bridges medical, educational, and social services—quality of life, rather than merely survival, can be the goal for young people and their families.

Study Guide

1. Discuss factors that have contributed to an increased prevalence of children and youth with major chronic illnesses or special health-care needs.

2. Describe the impact of chronic illness or disability on the young person, the family, and the health-care system.

3. Identify and discuss major principles in care of children and youth with special health-care needs.

4. Describe several theoretical frameworks for providing care for children and youth with special health-care needs.

5. Define medical home and discuss its advantages for children and youth with special health-care needs and their families.

6. List and discuss key adaptive tasks for families who have a young person with special health-care needs.

7. There are several legal or policy requirements in the care and schooling of students with special health-care needs. Cite these acts and explain the implications for health-care providers.

8. Does the research support any one approach to assisting families of children and youth with special health-care needs?

9. What quality-of-life issues for children and youth with special needs and their families are underaddressed either in the research or in support systems?

10. Hypothesize future health-care advances that might create an increase in the number of young people with special needs or change the course of the lives of children and youth who today have those conditions.

Appendix 5.1

Resources

Publications

DeGangi, G. & Kendall, A. (2008) *Effective parenting for the hard-to-manage child*. New York, NY: Routledge.

A skills-based book for parents who need practical advice from experts, without all the jargon and generalizations. The book provides specific strategies and techniques for children who are intense, highly reactive, and unable to self-calm. Focused on the younger child.

Donvan, J., & Zucker, C. (2015). *In a different key: The story of autism*. New York, NY: Random House.

The story of the discovery of autism and the first child diagnosed with the disorder draws on extensive research to trace how understandings about the condition have evolved through eight decades and how it has affected families in different historical periods.

Harvey, P., & Penzo, J. (2009). *Parenting a child who has intense emotions: Dialectical behavior therapy skills to help your child regulate emotional outbursts and aggressive behaviors*. Oakland, CA: New Harbinger Publications, Inc.

Harvey. P., & Rathbone, B. (2015). *Parenting a teen who has intense emotions: DBT skills to help your teen navigate emotional and behavioral challenges*. Oakland, CA: New Harbinger Publications, Inc.

Effective guides to de-escalating young peoples' emotions and helping them express feelings in productive ways. Strategies are drawn from dialectical behavior therapy (DBT), including mindfulness and validation skills.

Organizations

Parent to Parent USA
http://www.p2pusa.org/p2pusa/sitepages/p2p -home.aspx
Provides emotional and informational support to families of children who have special needs, most notably by matching parents seeking support with an experienced, trained "Support Parent."

Videos

Bright Futures
https://brightfutures.aap.org/about/Pages /About.aspx

Me and My Disabled Child
https://www.youtube.com/watch?v=bl_ZxlXo ZxYPart 1: Before the News

Father's Days: A cartoonist's journey into first-time fatherhood by Bob Moran
http://s.telegraph.co.uk/graphics/projects/ fathers-days/index.html

Welcome to Holland by Emily Perl Kingsley
https://www.youtube.com/watch?v=r15Pu YoID94

Appendix 5.2
Transition Resources

Adolescent Health Transition Project (AHTP)
A website with a variety of resources, including a video, Transition Planning Guide, Health History Summary, and Health Care Skills Checklist developed by the Adolescent Health Transition Project of the University of Washington, funded by the Washington State Department of Health, Children with Special Health Care Needs Program.

http://depts.washington.edu/healthtr
/resources/tools.html

Got Transition/Center for Health Care Transition
A website developed through a cooperative arrangement between the Maternal and Child Health Bureau, The National Alliance to Advance Adolescent Health, and other partners. Offers a variety of tools (in English and Spanish) organized by six core elements of health-care transition.
http://www.gottransition.org/resources/index
.cfm

Healthy Transitions NY
A website developed for youth with developmental disabilities 14 to 25 years of age, family caregivers, service coordinators, and health-care providers. Provides tools for coordinating care, keeping a health summary, and setting priorities during the transition process.
http://www.healthytransitionsny.org

National Diabetes Education Program (NDEP)
A website to help teens with diabetes make a smooth transition to adult health care through a variety of materials, including a transition planning checklist, health status summary, and links to other resources.
http://ndep.nih.gov/transitions/index.aspx

Supporting the Health Care Transition from Adolescence to Adulthood in the Medical Home
A clinical report from the American Academy of Pediatrics, American Academy of Family Physicians, and American College of Physicians, Transitions Clinical Report Authoring Group representing expert opinion and consensus on the practice-based implementation of transition for all youth beginning in early adolescence. Provides a structure (including a decision-making algorithm, age-specific guidelines, and attention to provider, family, and youth readiness, including youth with special health-care needs) for training and continuing education to further understanding of the nature of adolescent transition and how best to support it. Encourages health-care providers to adopt these materials and make this process specific to their settings and populations.

American Academy of Pediatrics, American Academy of Family Physicians, and American College of Physicians, Transitions Clinical Report Authoring Group. (2011). Supporting the health care transition from adolescence to adulthood in the medical home. *Pediatrics, 128*(1), 182–200. doi:10.1542/peds.2011-0969. Retrieved from http://pediatrics.aappublications.org/content/128/1/182.full

Note. From Schlucter, J. Dokken, D., & Ahmann, E. (2015). Transitions from pediatric to adult care: Programs and resources. *Pediatric Nursing, 41*(2), p. 87.

References

Adams, R. C., Tapia, C., & the Council on Children with Disabilities (2013). Early intervention, IDEA Part C services and the medical home: Collaboration for best practice and best outcomes. *Pediatrics, 132*(4), e1073–e1088. doi:10.1542/peds.2013-2305

Ahmann, E. (2013a). Cline and Green's Parenting Children with Health Issues: Essential guidance. *Pediatric Nursing, 39*(1), 43–46, 49.

Ahmann, E. (2013b). Making meaning when a child has mental illness: Four mothers share their experiences. *Pediatric Nursing, 39*(4), 202–205.

Ahmann, E., & Klockenbrink, K. L. (1996). Developmental assessment and intervention in the home. In E. Ahmann (Ed.), *Home care for the high risk infant: A family-centered approach* (pp. 293–304). Gaithersburg, MD: Aspen.

Ahmann, E., & Lierman, C. (1992). Promoting normal development in technology dependent children: An introduction to the issues. *Pediatric Nursing, 18*(2), 143–148.

American Academy of Pediatrics (AAP) Committee on Child Health Financing. (2013). Policy statement: Essential contractual language for medical necessity in children. *Pediatrics, 132*(2), 398–401. doi:10.1542/peds.2013-1637

American Academy of Pediatrics (AAP) Committee on Hospital Care and the Institute for Patient- and Family-Centered Care. (2012). Patient- and family-centered care and the pediatrician's role. *Pediatrics, 129*(2), 394–404. doi:10.1542/peds.2011-3084

Antonelli, R. C. (2012). Integration for children with special health needs: Improving outcomes and managing costs. Presentation for the National Governors Association, July 12, 2012. Unpublished. Cited in Association of Maternal & Child Health Programs. (2014). *Standards for systems of care for children and youth with special health care needs.* Washington, DC: Author, p. 18. Retrieved from http://www.amchp.org/AboutAMCHP/Newsletters/member-briefs/Documents/Standards%20Charts%20FINAL.pdf

Barnett, D., Clements, M., Kaplan-Estrin, M., & Fialka, J. (2003). Building new dreams: Supporting parents' adaptation to their child with special needs. *Infants and Young Children, 16*(3), 184–200.

Bibace, R., & Walsh, M. (1980). Development of children's concept of illness, *Pediatrics, 66,* 912–917.

Bronfenbrenner, U. (1979). *The ecology of human development.* Cambridge, MA: Harvard University Press.

Clawson, J. (1996). A child with chronic illness and the process of family adaptation. *Journal of Pediatric Nursing, 11*(1), 52–61.

Cline, F. W., & Greene, L. (2007). *Parenting children with health issues.* Golden, CO: Love and Logic Institute.

Dawson, P., & Guare, R. (2009). *Smart but scattered.* New York, NY: The Guilford Press.

DeGangi, G. and Kendall, A. (2008). *Effective parenting for the hard-to-manage child: A skills-based book.* New York, NY: Routledge.

Dokken, D. (2013). Making meaning after the death of a child: Bereaved parents share their experiences. *Pediatric Nursing, 39*(3), 147–150.

Dudley, N., Ackerman, A., Brown, K. M., & Snow, S. K. (2015). Patient- and family-centered care of children in the emergency department: Technical report. *Pediatrics, 135*(1), e255–e272. doi:10.1542/peds.2014-3424.

Early and Periodic Screening, Diagnostic, and Treatment. (n.d.). *Medicaid.gov.* Retrieved from http://www.medicaid.gov/Medicaid-CHIP-Program-Information/By-Topics/Benefits/Early-and-Periodic-Screening-Diagnostic-and-Treatment.html

Glass, P., & Blinkoff, R. (1996). Overview of developmental issues. In E. Ahmann (Ed.), *Home care for the high risk infant: A family-centered approach* (pp. 285–292). Gaithersburg, MD: Aspen.

Gordon, J. (2009). An evidence-based approach for supporting parents with chronic sorrow. *Pediatric Nursing, 35*(2), 115–119.

Greenley, R. N. (2010). Health professional expectations for self-care skill development in youth with spina bifida. *Pediatric Nursing, 36*(2), 98-102.

Grumbach, K., Bodenheimer, T., & Grundy, P. (2009). *The outcomes of implementing patient-centered medical interventions.* [Information sheet]. Washington, DC: Patient-Centered Primary Care Collaborative. Retrieved from https://pcmh.ahrq.gov/sites/default/files/attachments/The%20 Outcomes%20of%20Implementing%20Patient-Centered%20Medical%20Home%20Interven tions.pdf

Guare, R., Dawson, P., & Guare, C. (2013). *Smart but scattered teens.* New York, NY: The Guilford Press.

Harris, M. A., Freeman, K. A., & Duke, D. C. (2011). Transitioning from pediatric to adult health care. *American Journal of Lifestyle Medicine, 5*(1), 85–91.

Hastings, R., & Petalas, M. (2014). Self-reported behavior problems and sibling relationship quality by sibling of children with autism spectrum disorder. *Child: Care, Health and Development, 40*(6), 833–839.

Hopper, A., Dokken, D., & Ahmann, E. (2014). Transitioning from pediatric to adult health care: The experiences of patients and families. *Pediatric Nursing, 40*(5), 249–252.

Improving the medical home through the use of technology. (n.d.). [Fact sheet]. Retrieved from http:// www.medicalhomeinfo.org/downloads/pdfs/HITMedicalHomeFactSheet.pdf

Institute for Patient- and Family-Centered Care. (n.d.). *Frequently asked questions.* Accessed at http://www.ipfcc.org/faq.html

Kieckhefer, G., & Trahms, C. (2000). Supporting development of children with chronic conditions: From compliance toward shared management. *Pediatric Nursing, 26*(4), 354–363.

Klug, R. M. (1993). Clarifying roles and expectations in home care. *Pediatric Nursing, 19*, 374–376.

Knafl, K., Breitmayer, B., Gallo, A., & Zoeller, A. (1996). Family response to childhood chronic illness: Description of management styles. *Journal of Pediatric Nursing, 11*(5), 315–326.

Knafl, K., & Deatrick, J. (1986). How families manage chronic conditions: An analysis of the concepts of normalization. *Research in Nursing and Health, 9*, 215–222.

Kuo, D. Z., Houtrow, A. J., Arango, P., Kuhlthau, K. A., Simmons, J. M., & Neff, J. N. (2012). Family-centered care: Current applications and future directions in pediatric health care. *Maternal and Child Health Journal, 16*, 297–305. doi:10.1007/s10995-011-0751-7

Lazarus, R. S., & Folkman, S. (1984). *Stress, appraisal and coping.* New York, NY: Springer.

Lee, J. (2014, February). Medicaid managed care for children and youth with special health care needs. *State Health Policy Blog.* National Academy for State Health Policy. http://www.nashp .org/medicaid-managed-care-children-and-youth-special-health-care-needs/

Leff, P., & Walizer, E. (1992). *Building the healing partnership: Parents, professionals, and children with chronic illnesses and disabilities.* Cambridge, MA: Brookline Books.

Lucile Packard Foundation for Children's Health. (2012). *Six models for understanding how families experience the system of care for children with special health care needs: An ethnographic approach* [Report]. Retrieved from http://cshcn.wpengine.netdna-cdn.com/wp-content/uploads/2012/12 /enthographic_03-01-13.pdf

Maitland, T. E. L., & Quinn, P. O. (2011). *Ready for take-off: Preparing your teen with ADHD or LD for college.* Washington, DC: Magination Press.

Maternal and Child Health Bureau Division of Services for Children with Special Health Needs (2005). *Definition of family-centered care.* Retrieved from http://fndusa.org/wp-content /uploads/2015/05/What_is_Family_Centered_Care.pdf

McConnell, D., Savage, A., & Breitkreuz, R. (2014). Resilience in families raising children with disabilities and behavior problems. Research in *Developmental Disabilities, 35*, 833–848.

McManus, M. A., Pollack, L. R., Cooley, W. C., McAllister, J. W., Lotstein, D., Strickland, B., & Mann, M. Y. (2013). Current status of transition preparation among youth with special needs in the United States. *Pediatrics, 131*(6), 1090–1097.

McPherson, M., Arango, P., Fox, H., Lauver, C., McManus, M., Newacheck, P. W., . . . Strickland, B. (1998). A new definition of children with special health care needs. *Pediatrics, 102*(1), 137–140.

Mosquera, R. A., Avritscher, E. B. C., Samuels, C. L., Harris, T. S., Pedroza, C., Evans, P., Tyson, J. E. (2015). Effect of an enhanced medical home on serious illness and cost of care among high-risk children with chronic illness: A randomized clinical trial. *Journal of the American Medical Association, 312*(24), 2640–2648.

National Alliance on Mental Illness (NAMI). (2013). *Mental illness: Facts and numbers.* (Factsheet). Retrieved from https://www.nami.org/getattachment/Learn-More/Mental-Health-by-the-Numbers/childrenmhfacts.pdf

National Consensus Framework for Systems of Care for Children and Youth with Special Health Care Needs Project. (2014, March). *Standards for systems of care for children and youth with special health care needs.* Retrieved from http://www.amchp.org/AboutAMCHP/Newsletters/member-briefs/Documents/Standards%20Charts%20FINAL.pdf

Neely-Barnes, S. L., & Graff, J. C. (2011) Are there adverse consequences to being a sibling of a person with a disability? A propensity score analysis. *Family Relations, 60,* 331–341.

Nightingale, R., Friedl, S., & Swallow, V. (2015, May 27). Parents' learning needs and preferences when sharing management of their child's long-term/chronic condition: A systematic review. *Patient Education and Counseling, 98*(11), 1329–1338. doi:10.1016/j.pec.2015.05.002

Olson, D. H., Sprenkle, D., & Russell, C. S. (1979). Circumplex model of marital and family systems: I. Cohesion and adaptability dimensions, family types, and clinical applications. *Family Process, 18,* 3–28.

Overview of data related to the pediatric medical home. (2014, February 18). [Fact sheet, American Academy of Pediatrics]. Retrieved from https://www.aap.org/en-us/Documents/practicesupport_data_pedatric_medical_home.pdf

Patterson, J. M., & Geber, G. (1991). Preventing mental health problems in children with chronic illness or disability. *Children's Health Care, 20*(3), 150–161.

Phipps, S., Long, A., Willard, V.W, Okado, Y., Hudson M., Huang, Q., ... Noll, R. (2015, May 20). Parents of children with cancer: At-risk or resilient? *Journal of Pediatric Psychology, 40*(9), 914–925. doi:10.1093/jpepsy/jsv047

Porterfield, S. L., & DeRigne, L. (2011). Medical home and out of pocket medical costs for children with special health care needs. *Pediatrics, 128,* 892–900.

Pourmohamadreza-Tajrishi, M., Azadfallah, P., Hemmati Garakani, S., & Bakhshi, E. (2015). The effect of problem-focused coping strategy training on psychological symptoms of mothers of children with Down Syndrome. *Iranian Journal of Public Health, 44*(2), 254–62.

Protudjer, J. L. P., Kozyrskyj, A. L., Becker, A. B., & Marchessault, G. (2009). Normalization strategies of children with asthma. *Qualitative Health Research, 19*(1), 94–104.

Questions and Answers about the Garret F. Supreme Court Case. (1999, March–April). *Family Voices* (newsletter). Algodones, NM: Family Voices.

Raghavendra, P., Newman, L., Grace, E., & Wood, D. (2013). 'I could never do that before': Effectiveness of a tailored Internet support intervention to increase the social participation of youth with disabilities. *Child: Care, Health and Development, 39*(4), 552–561.

Rehm, R. S., & Bradley, J. F. (2005). Normalization in families raising a child who is medically fragile/technology dependent and developmentally delayed. *Qualitative Health Research, 15*(6), 807–820.

Rezaee, M., & Pollock, M. (2015). Multiple chronic conditions among outpatient pediatric patients, Southeastern Michigan, 2008–2013. *Preventing Chronic Disease, 12,* 140397. doi:http://dx.doi.org/10.5888/pcd12.140397.

Robert Wood Johnson Foundation. (2010). *Chronic care: Making the case for ongoing care.* [Report]. Retrieved from www.rwjf.org/pr/product.jsp?id=50968

Rolland, J. S. (2015). Advancing family involvement in collaborative health care: Next steps. *Family Systems & Health, 33*(2), 104–107.

Ronis, S. D., Baldwin, C. D., Blumkin, A., Kuhlthau, K., & Szilagyi, P. G. (2015, May 29). Patient-centered medical home and family burden in Attention-Deficit Hyperactivity Disorder. *Journal of Developmental and Behavioral Pediatrics* [Abstract]. Retrieved from http://www.ncbi.nlm.nih.gov/pubmed/26035140

Rosenberg, A. R., Baker, K. S., Syrjala, K. L., Back, A. L., & Wolfe, J. (2013). Promoting resilience among parents and caregivers of children with cancer. *Journal of Palliative Medicine, 16*(6), 645–652.

Rosenberg, A. R., Starks, H., & Jones B. (2014). "I know it when I see it." The complexities of measuring resilience among parents of children with cancer. *Support Care Cancer, 22*(10), 2661–2668.

Seltzer, M., Almedida, D., Greenberg, J., Savla, J., Stawski, R., Hong, J., & Taylor, J. (2009). Psychosocial and biological markers of daily lives of midlife parents of children with disabilities. *Journal of Health and Social Behavior, 50*, 1–15.

Smith, J., Cheater, F., & Bekker, H. (2013, January 14). Parents' experiences of living with a child with a long-term condition: A rapid structured review of the literature. *Health Expectations.* Advance online publication. doi:10.1111/hex.12040

Stein, R. E. K., & Jessop, D. J. (1982). A noncategorical approach to chronic childhood illness. *Public Health Reports, 97*, 354–362.

Steinfield, C., Ellison, N., & Lampe, C. (2008). Social capital, self-esteem, and use of online social network sites: A longitudinal analysis. *Journal of Applied Developmental Psychology, 29*, 434–445.

Thrall, R. S., Blumberg, J. H., Beck, S., Borgoin, M. D., Votto, J. J., & Barton, R.W. (2012). Beyond the medical home: Special Care Family Academy for children and youth. *Pediatric Nursing, 38*(6), 331–335.

Toly, V. B., Musil, C. M., & Carl, J. C. (2012). Families with children who are technology dependent: Normalization and family functioning. *Western Journal of Nursing Research, 34*(1), 52–71.

Tysbina, I., Kingnoth, S., Maxwell, J., Bayley, M., & Lindsey, S. (2012). Longitudinal Evaluation Transition Services ("LETS Study"): Protocol for outcome evaluation. *BMC Pediatrics, 12*, 51. doi:10.1186/1471-2431-12-51

U.S. Department of Health and Human Services. (2010). *Healthy People 2020.* Washington, DC: U.S. Government Printing Office. Retrieved from http://www.healthypeople.gov/2020/topics-objectives2020/pdfs/HP2020objectives.pdf

Van Cleave, J., Gortmaker, S. L., & Perrin, J. M. (2010). Dynamics of obesity and chronic health conditions among children and youth. *Journal of the American Medical Association, 301*(7), 623–630.

Vessey, J., & Maguire, M. (1999). In M. Broome, & J. A. Rollins (Eds.), *Core curriculum for the nursing care of children and their families* (pp. 243–256). Pitman, NJ: Jannetti.

VonBertalanffy, L. (1968). *General systems theory.* New York, NY: Braziller.

Vygotsky, L. (1962). *Thought and language.* Cambridge, MA: MIT Press.

Vygotsky, L. (1978). *Mind in society.* Cambridge, MA: Harvard University Press.

Walker, C. L. (1999). Chronic conditions: Effects on the child's family. In M. E. Broome & J. A. Rollins (Eds.), *Core curriculum for the nursing care of children and their families* (pp. 257–266). Pitman, NJ: Jannetti.

Wegener, D. (1996). A social work perspective. In K. Gunter, & R. Manago (Eds.), *Beyond discharge: Interdisciplinary perspectives for transitioning children with complex medical needs from hospital to home* (pp. 19–24). Bethesda, MD: Association for the Care of Children's Health.

Weiner, L., McConnell, D. G., Latella, L., & Ludi, E. (2013). Cultural and religious considerations in pediatric palliative care. *Palliative and Supportive Care, 11*(1), 47–67.

Yoos, H. L. (1994). Children's illness concepts: Old and new paradigms. *Pediatric Nursing, 20*(2), 131–140.

Zwi, M., Jones, H., Thorgaard, C., York, A., & Dennis, J. A. (2011, Dec. 7). Parent training interventions for Attention Deficit Hyperactivity Disorder (ADHD) in children aged 5 to 18 years. *Cochrane Database of Systematic Reviews, 12*, CD003018. doi:10.1002/14651858.CD003018.pub3

6

The Child Who Is Dying

Lois J. Pearson

Objectives

At the conclusion of this chapter, the reader will be able to:

1. Discuss the theories and research on grief and the implications for understanding and supporting children and families.
2. Delineate children's understanding of death at various stages of development and the typical responses at each stage.
3. Relate the historical and current views of health-care professionals on supports for children who are dying and their families, citing social, economic, medical, cultural, and religious factors that have contributed to changing ideas.
4. Summarize preparation and support strategies for children and their families.

The birth of a child represents fulfillment in the creation of a family, not only for the present but also for the future. The attachment between a parent and child is stronger than any other relationship (Doka, 1995). The connecting bond formed at conception is intensely developed before the child is born, not only in the life of each parent but also in the life of the child who will soon become a big brother or big sister. Grandparents also anticipate new life as the fulfillment of hope into a new generation. The family is forever changed with each addition of a new member and relationship. It is for all of these reasons that the event of critical illness or injury and death of an infant, child, or adolescent can be a devastating experience.

Health-care professionals are in a critical position to support families in a time of such great stress. This may be either at the time of diagnosis with a serious and potentially terminal illness or at the time of catastrophic injury or sudden illness with little hope for survival. Being familiar with the characteristics of grief for each member of the family and interventions that may promote positive coping is essential for the provision of family-centered care. This sensitive caring should be a component of health care intended to cure, but also care that is provided when no cure is possible. A growing number of health-care facilities are providing death and bereavement seminars to prepare clinicians and increase their confidence in caring for seriously ill and dying children and their families.

This chapter will look at the unique characteristics of grief for parents, siblings, grandparents, and others. The impact of death at home or in the hospital will be explored within the context of palliative care. The dying child's particular needs and issues will also be considered. (Note: Spiritual care is discussed in Chapter 9: Spiritual Issues in Children's Health-Care Settings.) In each circumstance, special attention will focus on interventions by health-care professionals that may have lasting effects for families facing the loss of a child.

The Grief of Parents

For parents, the agony of losing a child is unparalleled. When their child dies, a vital part of time has been severed. Parents grieve the lost child for the rest of their lives, never to be whole again. A parent's grief is forever. Only memories remain.

—Rando, 1986, p. 11

It does not matter at what age a child dies, for the loss of a child is always unnatural. For a parent, the loss of a child reflects the loss of part of the parent and the parent's hopes and dreams for the future. It is an assault on the parent's role as protector and provider and results in a diminished sense of self. The loss of a child even has an impact on the promise that children will be the caregivers for the parent in his or her old age. In the instance of genetic factors responsible for a child's death, a parent may experience guilt about not being able to produce a child that could survive to old age (Rando, 1986).

"Grief is the internal meaning given to the experience of bereavement" (Wolfelt, 1996, p. 322). Mourning is "grief gone public," and involves taking the internal experience of grief and expressing it outside oneself (Wolfelt, 1996, p. 322).

The grief of a parent is described as "the most difficult, painful, and time-consuming loss anyone can survive" (Doka, 1995, p. 73). Grief comes in overlapping phases, the first of which is shock. It includes devastating disbelief, helplessness, and bewilderment, which cause a state of physiological and emotional alarm. The second phase begins when the state of shock wears off and the actuality of the child's absence is realized. Rando (1986) described the emotion of this phase as "angry sadness." This may include feelings of panic and extreme fear, guilt, and anger directed at God, medical personnel, or even the dead child for leaving. During this phase of increased awareness of the loss, there are often acute physical feelings of emptiness and longing with vivid visual and auditory recall or dreams. The third phase, conservation and withdrawal, is often the longest phase of the grieving process. It is a time characterized by despair when grieving parents finally realize the loss and that life will be forever changed. Parents may withdraw from external activities to regain strength and energy. Strengthened by this renewed energy, bereaved parents enter the phase of "searching for meaning" characterized by attempts to put the loss of a child into some natural order, which begins the process of healing. Rando (1986) described a similar "reestablishment phase," when parents are finally able to reengage in everyday activities and begin "growing up" with the loss. Parental loss affects the marital relationship as severe grieving takes emotional energy away from the relationship. Grief responses may be very dissimilar between spouses, and reactions to the loss will have different effects based on specific marital roles.

Parental loss of a child also has tremendous societal impact, as the devastating grief of parents is out of all proportion to the expectations of society based on responses to other losses. Rando (1986) highlighted the fact that while a grieving spouse is referred to as "widow" or "widower" and a child who has lost parents as an "orphan," there is no accepted specific term in reference to a grieving parent. Perhaps this omission reflects the challenge experienced in trying to be supportive of grieving parents. And finally, the ability to be supportive of grieving parents often is difficult when society members fear even contemplating the loss of their own child.

Children's Understanding of Death

For the past half-century, researchers have attempted to study the child's understanding of death. Certainly the concept of death is complex and acquired over a lifetime (see Figure 6.1). To be able to support a child facing his or her own death or the death of a sibling requires knowledge of the degree to which a child's understanding of death differs from that of adults. The provision of family-centered care requires not only the ability to answer children's questions, but also, and more important, an understanding of what questions a child may ask and why (see Table 6.1. Children's Understanding of Death, by Age).

Age-appropriate attention to a child's understanding of death is found in Piaget's work detailing cognitive development (Piaget, 1960). His classic study of the way children acquire and process information helps adults realize what children are capable of understanding about death at each developmental level.

The first stage, sensorimotor, describes an infant's ability to respond to feelings associated with separation from those who love him or her, rather than understanding

(text continues on p. 219)

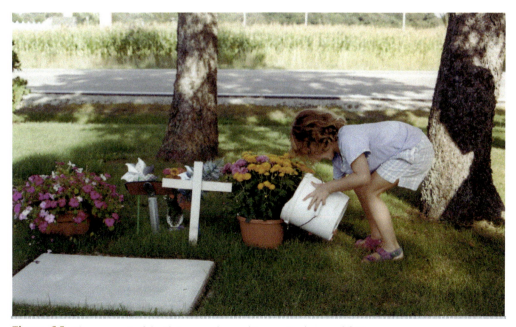

Figure 6.1. The concept of death is complex and is acquired over a lifetime.

Table 6.1

Children's Understanding of Death, by Age

Age	Understanding of Death	Characteristic Behaviors	Language/Approach	Interventions
Newborn to 3 Years				
A 2-year-old has begun having temper tantrums each morning 2 weeks after the death of her 1-week-old sister. Her mother admits that she cries each morning upon awakening to another day of grieving. When the 2-year-old is questioned about why she is acting that way, she replies that she "wants Mommy not to be sad anymore!"	• Does not comprehend death • Aware of a constant buzz of activity in the house • Aware of Mom and Dad looking sad and teary-eyed • Aware that someone in the home is missing	• Has altered eating and sleeping patterns • Is irritable • Clings	• Use the D words: *dying, death, dead.* • Avoid euphemisms such as "lost, passed away, gone to sleep," which confuse young children. • Explain in physiological terms (i.e., a person who is dead does not eat or drink or have feelings, like being cold after burial in the ground). • Expect questions to change. • Expect repeated questioning and testing to confirm information.	• Maintain routines but allow for flexibility. • Choose familiar and supportive caregivers. • Assign a support person for each child during funeral, burial, and other rituals. • Acknowledge all feelings of the child and adults by naming feelings and giving permission to express anger and sadness in developmentally appropriate ways. • Give extra hugs when needed to help the child feel secure.
3 to 5 Years				
A 4-year-old was thought to not know anything about the anticipated death of her soon-to-be-born baby brother until she was observed playing "dead baby" with her dolls. It was only then that the family realized how perceptive this 4-year-old was to the surrounding grief.	• Sees death as temporary and reversible; child continually asks if person will return • May feel ambivalent • Through magical thinking, may assume responsibility for the death	• Is concerned about own well-being • Feels confused and guilty • May use imaginative play, reenacting scene of CPR, etc. • Withdraws • Is irritable • Regresses	• Explain cause of death factually; that which is mentionable is manageable. • Answer questions honestly (e.g., clarify wellness of sibling, unlike that of dying child). • Avoid abstracts. • Diffuse magical thinking. • Be consistent and persistent.	• Reinforce that when people are sad, they cry; crying is natural. • Read stories (see bibliography of children's books). • Provide materials so that the child can draw pictures. • Encourage dialogue and family meetings. • Expect misbehavior as the child struggles with confusing feelings and issues. • Offer play with themes of death while providing supportive guidance.

Table 6.1 (*continued*)

Age	Understanding of Death	Characteristic Behaviors	Language/Approach	Interventions
6 to 9 Years				
A 6-year-old boy who has just returned from the bedside of his dying newborn sister explains in a matter-of-fact style to his 5-year-old sister, "We cannot go to heaven after Mindy goes there, because you would have to have a spaceship. Heaven is way farther away. You have to go past Mars."	• Begins to understand concept of death • Feels it happens to others • May be superstitious about death • May be uncomfortable in expressing feelings • Worries that other important people will die	• May seem outwardly uncaring, but is inwardly upset • May use denial to cope • May attempt to "parent" parent • May act out in school or at home • May play death games	• Look for questions within questions. • Expect a more global view. • Encourage the child to answer his or her own questions. • Explore feelings by asking questions such as "What do you think?"	• Listen to determine what kind of information the child is seeking. • Increase physical activity while role-modeling stress-reducing behaviors. • Work on identifying feelings, which are becoming more sophisticated (i.e., frustration, confusion). • Encourage creative outlets for feelings (i.e., drawing, painting, clay, blank books).
9 to 12 Years				
A 10-year-old girl describing her feelings following the unexpected death of her father: "Sure I thought he would die before me. He was older than I am. But I certainly didn't expect him to die when I was only 10 years old!" A 9-year-old boy, in explaining why his baby sister did not look like herself at the open casket visitation, stated, "Her soul is gone, and that's what gives people their light."	• Accepts death as final • Has personal fear of death • May be morbidly interested in skeletons, gruesome details of violent deaths • Concerned with practical matters about child's lifestyle	• May appear tough or funny • May express and demonstrate anger or sadness • May act like adult but regress to earlier stage of emotional response	• Provide more detail as needed, especially to explain the cause of death in a physiological context. • Probe for thoughts and feelings. • Allow for spiritual development. • May answer questions about an afterlife by stating, "We don't really know, but we believe that . . ."	• Encourage creative expressions of feelings. • Explore support group and peer-to-peer connection. • Establish family traditions and memorials. • Incorporate children into rituals not just at time of death, but at important anniversaries (e.g., taking balloons to the cemetery; creating a special ornament for the Christmas tree, which is always hung first; having birthday dinners and memory nights).

(continues)

Table 6.1 (*continued*)

Age	Understanding of Death	Characteristic Behaviors	Language/Approach	Interventions
Adolescents				
An adolescent girl wrote these words after her father died and her mother was diagnosed with cancer: "While I was tending to my mom, all I felt was anguish and despair. I tried to kill myself in an adverse way by driving my Firebird at 100 mph on a winding road. It was stupid, but it was the only way to rid myself of my anger. I had bad feelings that my mom was going to leave me alone and I would be without the two people I loved the most, my mom and dad." (Snoddy, 1992, p. 13)	• Has an adult concept of death, but the ability to deal with loss is based on experience and developmental factors • Experiences the thrill of recklessness • Focuses on present • Is developing strong philosophical views • Questions the existence of an afterlife	• Increased reliance on peers instead of family • Moody and irritable • May engage in risk-taking behaviors • Appears rebellious and tests limits • May act impulsively or without common sense	• Treat the young person as an adult, with information, respect, and responsibility. • Role-model adult behaviors. • Allow the adolescent to make informed choices.	• Allow for informed participation. • Encourage peer support. • Suggest individualized and group expressions of grief (i.e., school memorials). • Support group advocacy for causes (e.g., Students Against Drunk Driving [SADD]). • Recommend creative outlets (e.g., writing, art, music).

Note. From "Separation, Loss, and Bereavement," by L. Pearson, 1999, in *Core Curriculum for the Nursing Care of Children and Their Families* (pp. 77–92), by M. Broome and J. Rollins (Eds.), 1999, Pittman, NJ: Jannetti. Copyright 1999 by Jannetti. Reprinted with permission.

death itself. Attention to comfort and care routines is important in this stage. Piaget described the next period in two stages: preoperational and concrete operational. In the preoperational stage, children 2 to 6 years of age do not process thought logically, but instead function within an egocentric world. Children in this stage perceive death as temporary and reversible, somewhat like the concept of sleep. Questions in this stage often center on issues of the dead person's ability to eat, sleep, stay warm under the ground, and so on. In the second stage, concrete operational, children 7 to 12 years of age begin to think more logically. They are increasingly able to process events less egocentrically and learn by observation. Their understanding of death also is affected by their experience. Questions may relate to physiological processes of dying as their knowledge of the body and its function increases. In this developmental stage, children begin to role-model adult behaviors related to grief while also gaining support from religious beliefs and practices shared within the family (Piaget, 1960).

Finally, in Piaget's formal operational stage, children over the age of 12 years begin to integrate adult concepts of death. They can differentiate causes with increased intellectual capacity and also are able to acknowledge feelings and beliefs about death, and life after death, based on their ability to handle abstract concepts (Davies, 1999).

Components of the Concept of Death

A child's concept of death does not consist of a single complex concept, but rather may be broken down into three components or subconcepts (Davies, 1999). The first component, the understanding that once something is dead it will not come alive again, is termed *irreversibility*. Before grasping the concept of irreversibility, a child thinks that a sibling who dies today will be back tomorrow, similar to the idea of waking from sleep. The 4-year-old at the bedside of her dead newborn brother, shaking a stuffed animal energetically as if attempting to wake him from his sleep, has not yet developed the concept of irreversibility.

Nonfunctionality refers to a child's understanding that all external and internal functions have stopped (i.e., breathing, thinking, moving) (Speece & Brent, 1996). The child who is capable of understanding nonfunctionality will be supported by attention to the physiological explanations of dying (i.e., the heart stops beating, the lungs stop breathing, and the brain stops thinking). The child no longer questions what the body will feel or do when buried under the ground.

The third component is *universality*, the understanding that all living things eventually die. At this level children will understand that they, too, will one day die. Magical thinking or the belief that one may avoid dying by being smart or lucky no longer protects children in this stage. Death is universal.

Two other components are not as clear. One component is *causality*, the ability to understand both internal and external events that may bring about a death. The last component is the belief in some form of life after death, which can characterize a child's or adult's concept of death. However, this belief in an *afterlife* is still the subject of discussion among researchers (Davies, 1999).

Speece and Brent (1996) concluded that the "model age" for acquiring all three concepts is at about 7 years. They report that 60% of children achieve a mature understanding of all three concepts between 5 and 7 years of age. Perhaps the most helpful aspect of this research for health-care professionals is the knowledge that what is happening when a child is dying must be explained in terms of death as universal, and more important, must focus on the differences between being alive and being dead.

Talking to Children About Death

Like all grief work with families, the responsibility of explaining death to children carries great significance for a child and family's future grief work. Role-modeling appropriate language and behavior may make the critical difference when a child is dying. When the medical environment describes a critical illness or injury as "incompatible with life," it is up to child life professionals, nurses, social workers, and pastoral care staff to provide age-appropriate explanations for children. It may be necessary to begin a conversation with parents by acknowledging their grief, while identifying the need to be honest and accurate in talking to children. The reality of the *D* words, *dying, dead, death*, may seem insensitive to grieving parents without preparatory explanations.

The most important consideration is that children hear the words from people they trust or in the presence of people they trust. Parents may be too distraught or exhausted to actually say the words telling of a child's death but may be able to provide their physical presence and supportive touch while a health-care professional, extended family member, or friend actually says the words. It is doubtful that children will remember who said the words, but they will remember in whose lap they were sitting at the time. Words will need to be repeated, and a child's questions may be repeated to many people as the child continually seeks to integrate what is happening and being communicated.

Communication should be focused on physiological happenings. Explaining present medical conditions age-appropriately will help children understand impending death in terms of what is happening to a person's body. Explaining the inability of a person's heart to work or that an injury to someone's brain cannot be fixed with medicines helps a child understand the impossibility of continuing to live.

Communication often may be enhanced by first asking a child what is happening. A child's explanation of the present situation will help health-care professionals begin preparation at the level of the child's understanding. This approach also helps identify the information that has already been conveyed to the child directly by other family members, or indirectly, by overhearing telephone conversations or observing family members' behaviors. Many families truly believe that they have protected a child from the tragic events that are happening to the family, only to witness the child's explanation of all that they know in response to a staff member's assessment and initial intervention.

The next step in communicating an impending death includes reframing explanations so that they are developmentally appropriate, while clarifying misconceptions. A young school-age child who has been told that his or her sibling is going to heaven so great-grandma can take care of him may have difficulty. It is not necessary to deny concepts that bring comfort to a family in the acceptance of the loss, but these concepts should be augmented by more age-appropriate explanations. "Because baby brother's heart did not grow right inside Mom's tummy and the doctors and nurses are not able to fix it, his body may stop working, and he will die. Mommy and Daddy believe he will be in heaven with Great-grandma." The ability to process the abstract concept of heaven is one that the child may need to "grow into" as he or she matures in developmental understanding of death, but that does not take away the comfort of family beliefs.

It is important to avoid euphemisms in communicating with children of all ages. Using words that relate to sleep, journeys, or being lost often confuse young children and may cause difficulties after the death. Children's drawings illustrate how easily children confuse death with sleep, drawing coffins that look like beds under the ground. Even the concept of an open casket at a funeral visitation may confuse a child unless statements are clear (e.g., "She may look like she is sleeping, but she is dead. Her head and body are cold because no parts of her body are working"). Using appropriate words helps children clarify these misconceptions. For example, a child life specialist relates the confusion over terminology at the death of her uncle when she was 4 or 5 years old. Her parents told her that Uncle Bob had been killed in a car crash, but during the long trip to her grandparents' home she recalls asking over and over again, "Was Uncle Bob killed?" While her parents' frustration level continued to escalate, what she really needed to know was whether the term "killed" meant the same as "died."

The ability to identify a cause for the death, again using age-appropriate language, is another important aid to children's understanding of death. If the death is a result of an illness, it is important to address the child's basic and often unspoken questions:

- Did I cause it to happen?
- Can it happen to me?
- Who will take care of me now?

The tendency toward magical thinking in young children involves children believing that their thoughts, wishes, or actions may have caused the illness, injury, or accident. Clarification of the cause of illness or injury often helps. If it is not entirely possible to give an explanation, for example, if the cause of the death is not known, reassuring children by presenting the known factors should help (e.g., "Usually children get special medicine to make them better and go home from the hospital, but the medicine that doctors have didn't work for the kind of illness your brother had"). Death from an unexplainable illness complicates grieving for adults; it is even more complex for children with less developmental understanding. Providing reassurance that the dying child's illness is much different than the kind of illness that a child brings home from day care or school involves talking about how sick the child is and how medicine that the doctors have does not work for this kind of illness. Even with this reassurance, children may be expected to react differently the first time that they are ill or a parent is ill after the death of a family member. Finally, it is most important while communicating with children about any death, to provide a caring presence for reassurance, extra love and support, trusted adults to answer questions, and time to integrate information.

The Grief of Siblings

Approximately 73,000 children in the United States die each year, and an estimated 83% leave a sibling survivor (Machajewski & Kronk, 2013). The unique bond of siblings lasts a lifetime, longer than any other relationship. The bond between siblings begins before birth, as the family eagerly anticipates the new baby and a child prepares to become a big brother or sister; it strengthens as the siblings spend time together. Siblings may spend 80%–100% of their lifetimes with each other and use each other to determine their own personal identity and understand the world around them (Packman, Horsley, Davies, & Kramer, 2006). No life experience prepares a child for a sibling's death. A young girl sitting with a child life specialist in the ICU where her teenage brother had just died remarked, "Ah, Buddy (her pet name for him), we had such great times together, but he never died before!"

Situational, individual, and environmental factors all affect sibling bereavement (Davies, 1999). Situational factors include the cause of death, sudden death versus long-term illness, and whether the death was accidental or a homicide. Individual factors include age, gender, past experiences, and coping styles. The involvement of an extended support network of family and friends, and communication among family members of both factual and emotional responses, constitute environmental factors. A study in Sweden of 174 young adults who had lost a sibling 2 to 9 years earlier found that the majority (54%) of siblings had not worked through their grief (Sveen, Eilegard, Steineck, & Kreicbergs, 2014).

Even after a long-term illness, the actual death still may be perceived as a surprise. While parents continue to hope that their child will be the one to survive, the timing of the death may be unexpected (e.g., "We expected him at least to live through Christmas"). Siblings tend to revise their appraisal of the sick child's state of health in a positive direction unless they continue to be exposed to negative reminders. For example, a 9-year-old girl visited the bedside of her dying newborn baby brother in the ICU. The child life specialist often asks siblings whether they would like to create memory books (see Figure 6.2). After several sad visits to the bedside in the presence of her grieving family, the girl remarked to the child life specialist that she was going to leave a few blank pages in the memory book she was creating for her brother, stating that her brother could then "tell his own story when he grows up." Whether this reflected wishful thinking or her inability to process the events that indicated that the infant's death was imminent is unknown, but her comment identified the need to gently clarify this expectation: "Everybody wishes that your baby brother would grow up to write his own book, but we do not think that he will be alive much longer. When his heart stops working, he will die. That is why everyone is very sad."

Helpful Interventions for Siblings When a Child Has a Life-Threatening Illness

The responsibility of parenting both healthy and ill children can be an overwhelming task. Siblings whose brother or sister is being treated for cancer report feelings of loneliness, guilt, jealousy, sadness, anger, and anxiety. These feelings may be present independent of whether the sibling survives or dies. Most siblings will ultimately recover from these feelings of emotional distress, while only a small percentage will experience post-traumatic stress symptoms of anxiety, depression and/or poor quality of life (Rosenberg et al. 2015). Parents struggle to be present for both the sick child and well siblings. Sharing information is challenging for parents during this time, and withholding information as a way to protect siblings may actually make bereavement more difficult for siblings. Preparing siblings for their brother or sister's death and offering an opportunity to say good-bye are also factors associated with fewer inferior outcomes.

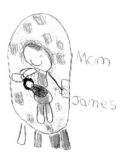

My mom had a baby in her tummy. We didn't know the baby was very sick.

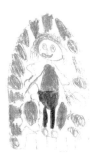

My mom had to go to get her pictures checked for her tummy once in a while. The baby got bigger and bigger.

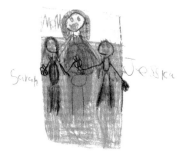

We felt him kicking and then we made up his name. His name was James. He was very sick.

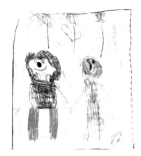

When mama had the baby, he felt even sicker. Somebody said if he goes up to heaven he would feel much better. We only got to stay with him for two days. The next day he died at 1:00.

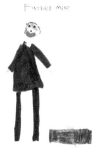

Then Father Mike, who is always our priest in the church. He had a box where James was in and somebody buried him up.

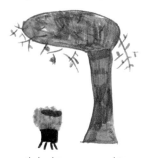

We put a wreath by his grave and it was very pretty. We still have the wreath on. We put snow on it to make it look very pretty. We always go and see James Louis.

Figure 6.2. "My Brother," by Sarah, age 6 years.

Health-care professionals can help parents by encouraging the inclusion of siblings during the stages of illness. Interventions that health-care professionals can use to help parents and siblings include the following (Davies, 1999):

- Encourage siblings to participate in family meetings with health-care professionals.
- Inquire about siblings' coping and provide positive reinforcement for coping behaviors.

- Allocate time to be spent alone with siblings. (In one hospital, physicians in the ICU have been known to sit alone with a sibling in the playroom to answer questions and provide information and support for the sibling without the presence of other adult family members.)
- Encourage siblings to participate in bedside cares.
- If siblings cannot be at the hospital, include them in indirect participation (e.g., phone calls, letters, e-mails, video calls via Skype or FaceTime).
- Offer age-appropriate teaching sessions to help them understand the illness process.
- Develop sibling groups and special sibling events to provide peer-to-peer support.
- Encourage open discussion between parents and their well children.
- Facilitate children's healthy relationships with their peers.
- Encourage hospital visiting and school involvement.

Sibling Responses at the Time of Death

Nearly all children, regardless of the circumstances of a sibling's death, experience certain characteristic responses. Davies's studies (1999) indicated that the greatest incidence of behavioral problems after the death of a sibling was noted in preschool and young school-age children. Attention-seeking behavior and irritability were common. One fourth of siblings in the study reported "crying a lot." Generally, crying or not crying was attributed to individual coping styles and the attitude of a family toward tears as emotionally and physiologically healing. Forty-four percent of siblings reported an inability to concentrate in school, and that the longer they stayed away from school, the harder it was to re-enter the school routine. Siblings reported that a week was the right amount of time before returning to school.

Sleeping difficulties are frequent, especially the ability to fall asleep, although insomnia is uncommon in children (Eilegard, Steineck, Nyberg, & Kreicbergs, 2013). Davies (1999) reported that guilt also was universal, in terms of siblings' perceptions of the cause of death. Some siblings feel survivor guilt that perhaps they should have died instead of the one who did. These feelings may be difficult to resolve if the surviving child feels as though he or she is competing with the dead child's memory within the family (Grollman, 1995). Siblings may also feel a double loss as they experience the death of a brother or sister and a loss of parental protection and attention when parents are overwhelmed by grief (Eilegard et al., 2013). Health complaints are often reported and, like other responses, may be observed up to 3 years after the death. Aches and pains are common in siblings and may be similar to the symptoms or medical condition of the ill sibling (Grollman, 1995). Finally, surviving siblings may be confused about their role in the changed family. Becoming the oldest child or only child often challenges the sibling's perception of his or her own identity.

The majority of studies of bereaved siblings have looked at deaths caused by cancer. An unusual U.S. study compared parents' reports of the reactions of children who experienced a sibling's death in the pediatric intensive care unit (PICU) or the neonatal intensive care unit (NICU) (Youngblut & Brooten, 2013). Data were collected at 7 months after the death. Parent comments were clustered around six themes:

1. Changed behaviors (38%)
2. Not understanding what was going on (23%)
3. Maintaining a connectedness with the sibling (14%)
4. Not enough time to be with the sibling and/or to say good-bye (9%)
5. Believing the sibling was in a good place (9%)
6. Not believing that the sibling would die (6%).

Changed behaviors included the expected emotional and physical responses of crying, not talking, and avoiding activities that had been shared with the sibling. Parents reported that comments on the theme of not understanding what was going on were exhibited by preschool and young children, as would be developmentally appropriate. The theme of not believing that the sibling would die was observed mostly in adolescents. This may be another developmental factor reflecting the typical adolescent's feelings of invincibility (Youngblut & Brooten, 2013). The study concluded that the majority of parental responses about siblings' reactions to a death were about losses experienced in the PICU, presumably because most of those children had spent time at home with their siblings, while those infants who died in the NICU probably had spent limited time with their older surviving siblings. Bereaved siblings who have offered advice to health-care professionals emphasize the importance of being able to be present at the bedside with adult family members (Steele et al., 2013).

Helpful Interventions for Siblings at the Time of Death

Despite the research examining the difficulty of reconciling children's grief, there have been factors identified in the literature that may prove beneficial. As health-care professionals, it is important to support these behaviors at the time of death and help families access known resources and supports. Siblings who are included at the time of death and in the rituals following the death are better able to reconcile the loss. Providing stable caregivers and supportive extended family during the first days of a parent's acute grief also helps. Often, at the bedside of a dying child in the ICU, the child life specialist or other staff members may gently enlist the strong arms of an uncle, aunt, or other family member to hold a younger sibling who may be lost in the group of mourners at the bedside. Being the recipient of a child's trust at such a time will certainly help the adult in whose care a sibling might be placed, as well as help the child.

Role-modeling feelings is another area where caregivers begin the process of helping children and adults. "Daddy is having a hard time talking right now because he is feeling very sad. People express sadness in many ways, and they are all OK ways to help get feelings out." Suggesting appropriate ways to express anger is also important at the start of grief work. Being able to identify particular behaviors that help reduce stress is important for staff and families. For example, an ICU staff member obtained a pass to a nearby athletic club so that an adolescent boy and his cousin could go over to shoot baskets while the rest of the family sat at the bedside of his dying younger brother.

For younger children, the ability to retreat to a playroom and draw, write, play with toy emergency vehicles, or simply feel comfortable is a significant factor in helping family members meet children's needs. The theoretical base of all psychosocial care is that child's play is the mode of expression and communication. Acknowledging the importance of play within the critical care setting begins the long process of helping children heal though play opportunities.

Siblings who are included in caretaking during illness, are prepared and present at the time of death, participate in family rituals, and are supported by family in their grief work demonstrate higher self-concepts (see Figure 6.3). They also demonstrate psychological growth and move on in life with the ability to reach out to others with greater sensitivity while valuing life and people (Davies, 1999). Sensitive and age-appropriate preparation is required before a child visits his or her sibling who is dying. For guidance, see Text Box 6.1, Preparing Children for the Death of a Sibling in the ICU, and Case Study 6.1.

The Grief of Adolescents

On a cognitive level, adolescents may be able to integrate the death of a loved one like an adult, but their response will be influenced by additional developmental tasks of adolescence. Adolescents feel invincible and may react to a death by increasing risk-

(text continues on p. 230)

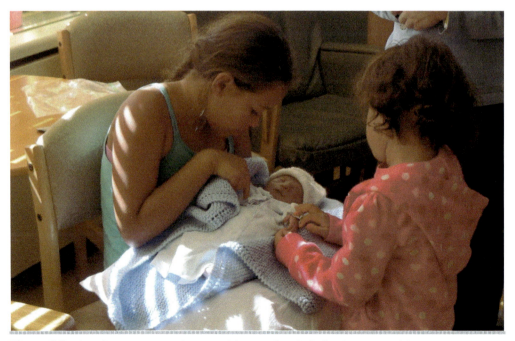

Figure 6.3. Alex's big sisters spend time with him as the whole family says good-bye.

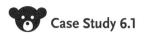 **Case Study 6.1**

Fulfilling a Family's Wishes

The anticipated birth of a new baby into the family was filled with happy preparation because an early ultrasound documented that this new infant would not be born with the same congenital kidney disease that had caused the death of a baby girl 7 years earlier. That baby had lived only 4 hours, and her mother's grief had been complicated by the fact that the mother did not reach the tertiary care hospital where the baby died until after her death. Their 9-year-old son, though only 2 years old at the time of his sister's birth and death, grew up in the midst of the family's grief. Their daughter, who had been born 5 years ago, understood less of the circumstances of the earlier loss experience but was able to state that she "had a sister in heaven."

When this fourth infant was born in severe respiratory distress, he was immediately transported by helicopter to a metropolitan hospital and placed on a ventilator. The two older children were able to see and touch him before he was flown again to a children's hospital in a city about 2 hours from home. Efforts at this third hospital focused on diagnosing his medical condition and placing him on ECMO, a high-tech system that allows the heart and lungs to be supported mechanically, not unlike cardiac bypass used during surgery.

The family was devastated to hear that their newborn did indeed have the same disease as his sibling and his survival was unlikely. Yet this time the family knew what they wanted—to be with the baby and hold him as much as possible while photographing every moment of his short but significant life. The siblings were prepared by the child life specialist and were able to spend much valuable sibling time at the bedside, reading books, singing lullabies, and making dolls.

The fourth grader was able to understand what was wrong with the baby when given age-appropriate information about the infant's kidneys and lungs. He amazed the physicians by appearing to understand the reason why the mechanical support needed to be discontinued after the baby suffered bleeding in his head. The 5-year-old daughter was less able to process so much information but took her cues from the tears and coping of her mother.

For many hours, each family member held the precious baby. Although only his parents were at the bedside when the baby died, the siblings and extended family returned to the bedside for more holding and picture taking. While staff people were somewhat uncomfortable with this extended time at the bedside, especially for the children, every family member expressed gratitude that "this time" at least they had been allowed the experience of holding their baby. And they were certain that their grief work would be helped by the collection of photographs. The older son took one of the baby's pictures to school so his classmates might see "how his baby brother should have looked without all those tubes."

Ultimately, this family, whose members supported one another and did what felt right for them, told the hospital staff that the infant's father, grandfather, uncle, and big brother actually dug the grave together in a final expression of their love.

Note. Courtesy of James and Catherine Hackbarth.

||||||||||||||||||||||||||||||||||||||||||||||||||||||||||||||||||||||||||||||||||||||||||||||||||||||||||||||||||||||||||||||||||||

Text Box 6.1

Preparing Children for the Death of a Sibling in the ICU

Choices related to the ICU experience:
- To visit or not to visit
- With whom and for how long
- What type of preparation is required
- Availability of support persons other than parents

Information to be gathered from parents, if possible:
- Desire to have siblings visit
- Ages and stages of siblings
- Present understanding of situation
- Previous experience with hospitalization or loss
- Person(s) to bring children to hospital and relationship to child
- Availability of person(s) for follow-up
- Members of hospital staff parents want present
- Role of hospital staff at visit

Before the visit:
- Identify cause of accident, nature of illness, and other important factors for siblings.
- Determine present medical condition.
- Know immediate medical and family plans, expected outcomes.
- Find a private, quiet place with easy access to unit.
- Identify and assemble all who will be present.
- If possible, have one staff person for children, another for adults.
- Have children's resources available:
  – Preparation photographs
  – Paper and markers
  – Cloth dolls
  – Blank books
- Look at the patient from visiting child's perspective.
- Arrange to reduce scary details, if possible.

During the visit before going to ICU:
- Arrange seating of children to be close to supportive person.
- Introduce self and meet children.
- Begin by acknowledging frightening nature of situation.
- Acknowledge tears and grief behaviors of surrounding adults.
- Explain present situation by first asking if children understand what has happened so far.
- Respond to child's comments, remembering the three biggest fears of children:
  – Did I do anything to cause this to happen?
  – Could it happen to me?
  – What will happen to me now?
- Clarify cause of injury or illness.
- Explain where sibling is and what is being done.

Text Box 6.1 (*continued*)

- Be honest but do not take away family's hope.
- Explain medical details in simple physiological terms.
- Describe ICU's physical environment: size, windows, number of doctors and nurses, presence of other children and families, some very sick.
- Briefly and simply describe medical equipment—function, look, and sound.
  - Ventilator, IVACs, catheter bag, chest tubes. Reassure that although scary-looking, they are helping sibling.
  - Monitors and alarms—describe place where attached to body, as well as sounds and meanings.
- Describe neurological condition of patient. Describe that coma unlike sleeping; patient cannot walk or talk but can hear.
- Identify what child can do at bedside (i.e., talk, touch).
- Incorporate decorating cloth doll, drawing, or journaling in blank book.

At the bedside:
- Encourage child's entrance into room.
- Facilitate child's easy viewing (e.g., step stool, chair, parent lifting).
- Review equipment that is present. Point out important pieces, especially the ventilator.
- Identify familiar or comforting objects (e.g., photographs, stuffed animal).
- Be sure that child is physically supported by adult family member or yourself.
- Allow family time alone in rooms if members are handling situation well.
- Observe family members, especially children, for cues that the visit has been long enough. Intervene if necessary.

After visit to the room:
- Sit with the children while they process the visit.
- Listen for questions within questions.
- Turn questions back if needed to clarify concerns.
- Acknowledge feelings of all.
- Continue to build trust by being honest and caring.
- Attend to physical needs of children. Offer juice, crackers.
- Be prepared, and help adults understand that children grieve in different ways.

If patient dies:
- Continue interventions in same style that has allowed children to place their trust in you.
- Be honest and explain using physiological terms.
- Clarify cause of death according to original explanation.
- Ask if children want to see sibling again.
- Acknowledge spiritual beliefs if proffered by family and clergy. Avoid abstract images if not age appropriate.
- Encourage drawing and writing in blank books to help children express feelings.
- Offer children a chance to leave the bedside if adults are not ready. Maintain a presence with the children.
- If you knew the child, recall characteristics you liked.
- Reinforce what a great brother or sister the survivor has always been.
- Encourage child to leave something with the patient if desired (e.g., cloth doll, book, drawing).

(*continues*)

Text Box 6.1 (*continued*)

- Provide for sibling a comfort object that was with the patient (e.g., stuffed animal, quilt—one for each surviving sibling).
- Always accompany the family when they leave the hospital after a death.
- If possible, follow up with the surviving siblings by attending the visitation or funeral, writing a note, or calling the children.

Note. From "Separation, Loss, and Bereavement," by L. Pearson, in *Core Curriculum for the Nursing Care of Children and Their Families* (pp. 77–92), by M. Broome and J. Rollins (Eds.), 1999, Pittman, NJ: Jannetti Publications. Copyright 1999 by Jannetti. Reprinted with permission.

taking behaviors. Anger at life's unfairness may encourage acting-out behaviors. Other teens may withdraw, using art, writing, or music to express complex feelings.

Teens frequently struggle in finding support systems. At a time when adolescents are pulling away from the family structure and relying on the support of peers, the experience of loss and its associated emotions may frighten friends away. Family members also may be unavailable because of their personal grief. Wolfelt (1996) has described both "normal" behaviors of grieving adolescents and "red flag" behaviors that indicate when a teen needs help (see Table 6.2, Behaviors of Grieving Adolescents).

In a study conducted through the Compassionate Friends Organization, Hogan and DeSantis (1994) asked adolescents what helped them and what made their grief work harder. Each had experienced the death of a sibling within the last five years. Things that helped adolescents cope were related to themes of self, specific individuals, and a social network. Having a personal belief system and being able to engage in activities that were known to reduce stress were helpful. Parental support, sharing memories, and the support of friends were identified as important. In the previously mentioned study of deaths in the PICU or NICU, comments focused on adolescents' need to continue connectedness with the sibling (e.g., wearing a guardian angel pin, wearing a sibling's favored article of clothing) (Youngblut & Brooten, 2013). Things that hindered their efforts to cope included intrusive thoughts, feelings of guilt, loneliness, insensitivity in the actions or words of others, and parental discord. Researchers noted that these resilient teens were able to identify both family and friends who helped them cope, but also noted the lack of school personnel or community resources in providing support for these grieving adolescents.

Rosenberg et al. (2015) surveyed teens and adults, ages 16 and older (mean age was 26 years), who had experienced the loss of a sibling from cancer. The mean age of the sibling at the time of the loss was 12 years. Of those surveyed, 88% reported that the loss of their sibling continues to affect their lives. The majority listed positive effects: approximately 36% of the sibling survivors felt that they became better communicators, 43% acted more maturely, 45% were more kindhearted, and 17% felt more confident. Almost half indicated that the loss had an impact on their choice of work or career. The researchers summarized that siblings generally recover and find meaning for the loss in their lives, while also concluding that younger siblings are more likely to be seen as vulnerable in the early bereavement period but older siblings are more likely to suffer long-term effects.

Table 6.2

Behaviors of Grieving Adolescents	
Type	Behaviors
Normal	Some limit-testing and rebellion
	Increased reliance on peers for problem-solving
	Egocentrism
	Increased sexual awareness
	Increased moodiness
	Impulsiveness, lack of common sense
Red flag	Suicidal thoughts or actions
	Chronic depression, sleep problems, low self-esteem
	Isolation from family and friends
	Academic failure or overachievement
	Dramatic changes in attitude
	Eating disorders
	Drug or alcohol abuse
	Fighting or legal problems
	Inappropriate sexual behaviors

Note. Adapted from *Healing the Bereaved Child* (pp. 281–282), by A. D. Wolfelt, 1996, Fort Collins, CO: Companion Press. Copyright 1996 by Companion Press. Adapted with permission.

The Grief of Grandparents

The loss of a grandchild presents particular concerns. It is a grief that is unique and complex, as a grandparent mourns the loss of the grandchild but also feels helplessness in witnessing the grief of their adult child (Roose & Blanford, 2011). Grandparents grieve as do parents over the loss of future experiences of the child and the natural order of life, which assumes that young children do not die. Survivor guilt is common, wherein grandparents question why they should go on living in old age, and why a young child should die.

Grandparents feel intense sadness for the loss felt by their adult children. Often they do not know how to support the child's parents in the face of such overwhelming sadness (O'Leary, Warland, & Parker, 2011). They may feel as though they have failed by not protecting the family or recognizing symptoms or hazards leading to the death. Communication between parents and grandparents may be strained as the strong feelings of acute grief are expressed. Feelings of helplessness may be exaggerated if grandparents are excluded from the grieving family. If grandparents are physically or emotionally unhealthy, bereavement may be more complex.

Including grandparents in the support of families is an important consideration. Assessing grandparents' role and availability within the family structure helps identify particular strengths that may be used to support parents. Sharing information with grandparents as well as parents helps the family to process events together, relying on mutual support. Encouraging families to use the wisdom and solid presence of extended family, including grandparents, aids in coping while reducing feelings of helplessness. The comforting care of grandparents is often critical to the coping of siblings who are unable to maintain a continuous presence at the bedside. Finally, bereavement programs need to address the particular grief of grandparents. Resources and support services, such as support groups for grandparents, make an important contribution to a family's reconciliation of loss.

One midwestern hospital has developed a highly successful intergenerational perinatal bereavement program that includes not only parents but also grandparents and siblings. The Still Missed Program offers a monthly support group for parents and a separate support group for grandparents, an annual memorial service and memorial walk, and various rituals and keepsakes. A multidisciplinary staff provides the services and resources, and includes a section for Spanish-speaking families. Program evaluation revealed that grandparents participated in 62% of programs and reported participation to be almost 100% helpful. Similar results were reported for siblings. An important aspect of the program, including grandparents, encouraged their participation to resolve their own grief, learn helpful ways to support their grieving adult children, and especially to recognize and accept that bereavement practices today are very different from those of their generation (Roose & Blanford, 2011).

Anticipatory Mourning

Anticipatory mourning, formerly termed *anticipatory grief*, is "the phenomenon encompassing the process of mourning, coping, interaction, planning, and psychological reorganization that are stimulated and begun in part in response to the impending loss of a loved one and the recognition of associated losses in the past, present and future" (Rando, 2000, p. 29). Offering a critical distinction between grief and mourning, Rando explains that grief refers to a reaction, but anticipatory mourning reveals the complexities of the intra/interpersonal struggles through loss. During this period of anticipating death, the person begins the task of mourning and experiences various grief responses, the most common psychological expressions being feelings of despair, hopelessness, and worthlessness (Al-Gamal & Long, 2010).

Rini and Loriz (2007) explored anticipatory mourning with 11 parents of children who had died while hospitalized. Analysis of the interview data revealed that six factors emerged as facilitating or impeding anticipatory mourning: (1) giving of information to parents, (2) the effect of the attitudes and actions of health-care professionals, (3) physical presence with the dying child, (4) the location of the child's death, (5) issues of hospital policy, and (6) the existence of anticipatory mourning and its relationship with bereavement. Findings suggest that providing a system in which the family, not just the dying child, becomes the focal point of the dying process may facilitate anticipatory mourning.

Sudden Grief

A child's sudden and unexpected death as the result of an accident or injury throws the entire family into chaos. For parents, sudden accidental death usually carries with it some implication of fault or preventability that may or may not be resolved within the family. Violent and traumatic deaths raise anxiety levels and may negatively affect the grief process (Davies, 1999). Siblings involved in a traumatic death often feel much more vulnerable and require additional support before achieving a sense of being safe in similar circumstances. The inability to provide factual information regarding accidental deaths (e.g., the drowning death of a strong swimmer) may cause greater confusion for children.

The response of grieving siblings may be different if the death has been sudden and unexpected. According to Wolfelt (1996), the more sudden the death, the more likely the child is to mourn in doses and to push away the pain at first. Caring adults may be concerned by the siblings' apparent lack of feeling and fewer outward expressions of grief.

Therapeutic interventions should be aimed at assessing the patient and family situation, mobilizing coping resources, and discovering coping strategies. The presence of a trauma response team to provide a total psychosocial assessment should include social work, pastoral care, and child life to help meet the needs of all family members. Team members can identify feelings, restate and clarify responses of family members, listen quietly, and validate a family's loss.

Major Areas of Intervention

Jones (1978) helped identify four major areas of intervention at the time of sudden death. The first intervention occurs at the time of the family's arrival at the hospital. Family members should be met immediately and escorted to a private area where a staff member stays with the family. All known information is shared, especially the extent of the child's injuries. Additional updates on medical conditions should be provided at prearranged intervals of time.

Notification of the death by an honest and compassionate physician is the next crisis intervention point. Nonverbal communication is also significant, with physical touch important, if a family will accept it. Clarification of misconceptions and feelings of guilt should be included in the interaction, with adequate time for questions by parents and other family members. It is crucial to give reassurance that everything was done that could be done (Jones, 1978).

The next area of critical intervention is viewing of the body (Jones, 1978). Generally, it is accepted that long-term outcomes are better for those who are able to see the body of a loved one because it helps them come to terms with the death (Haas, 2003). Family members need to be prepared for changes in the body. A single staff member should provide a supportive presence during viewing of the body while allowing some private time. No time limits need apply. Each family determines its own schedule. Studies indicate that, for most families, the opportunity to see and touch the body helps actualize the death and is reported by grieving families as a choice they were glad to have made (Back, 1991).

Finally, Jones (1978) identified the concluding process as the last important intervention following death in the emergency department. A formalized sequence of signing papers, including the body release form, helps bring closure to this initial portion of grief. Families should be directed in the process of funeral home notification, if appropriate, and told what needs to happen in the following hours or days. It is also beneficial to provide informational resources about initial grief responses and available support services.

Policies for Best Practice

Because the deaths of children and young people under 18 have continued to decrease significantly in recent years as a result of improved health care and safety measures, a child's death in the emergency department (ED) is relatively rare and staff may be less well prepared to provide compassionate family-centered care. In 2014 the American Academy of Pediatrics (AAP), the American College of Emergency Physicians (ACEP), and the Emergency Nurses Association (ENA) issued a Joint Technical Report entitled "Death of a Child in the Emergency Department" (O'Malley et al., 2014). The report outlines principles of family-centered care and policies for best practice.

The report cites a lack of training of health professionals for critical health-care communication and stresses that parent surveys indicate that the way in which news of their child's death is delivered is most important to the long-term coping of family members (O'Malley et al., 2014). The value of family presence at the time of resuscitation of a child has been proved in research and appears to be well supported in hospital policies and procedures in the setting of effective staff preparation, appropriate policy development and implementation, and provision of designated personnel to support the family (Meeks, 2009; O'Malley et al., 2014).

Although family presence at time of resuscitation is accepted, a new debate is focused on family presence at the time of death pronunciation. This issue is complicated by questions of whether a death is pronounced at the scene versus in the hospital, whether resuscitation efforts would be extensive while awaiting family presence, and other policies regarding initiation or termination of resuscitation, all factors for which more research is indicated. The report summarizes that what may be defined as a "good death" in the ED for families would be "caring for the survivors of a child's death in a way that affirms their trust, allowing them to understand the events leading up to the death, to exert some control in the situation, and to say good-bye to their child in whatever way is meaningful to them" (O'Malley et al., 2014, p. e8). These principles are identified as most significant in family bereavement, and can be supported by other members of the ED team with assistance, compassion, and information. (See the Joint Technical Report for helpful appendices, including guidelines for professional staff development and resources for families.) The report concludes with a final example of a closing ritual for staff, noting that there may be healing potential in a communal rather than private ritual following the death of a child in the ED.

Supportive Interventions at the Time of Death in the Hospital

Most inpatient deaths occur in the PICU. Parents report that when their child is dying in the PICU, it is most challenging for them to reclaim their parental role and be allowed to share in the care of their child. Being a parent in the PICU means forging a parental role, keeping informed, preserving the child's personhood, and creating a family environment (Butler, Hall, Willetts, & Copnell, 2015). Having a sense of privacy and control of lighting, noise, and visitors, helped parents feel less disempowered. Price, Jordan, Prior, and Parkes (2011) identified bereaved parents' coping themes of having to keep "doing" throughout their child's illness and dying:

1. *Piloting*—parents navigate their way through the journey of a child's critical illness, and subsequent death while trying to retain some measure of control.

2. *Providing*—parents try to give physically and emotionally to all the needs of their ill child and the family.

3. *Protecting*—parents keep their child, their family, and others from real or potential harm or hurt.

4. *Preserving*—parents seek to maintain roles and cohesiveness of family functioning in the face of extreme emotional and practical chaos.

Supportive interventions at the time of a child's death in any unit within the hospital should be detailed in policies that reflect the philosophy of family-centered care. The parents' ability to make as many choices as possible is of ultimate importance because it restores parenting roles in a situation where everything may appear to be out of control. The word *choices*, rather than *decisions*, may be helpful to indicate that the parent did not have to "decide" about ending treatment, only the manner and timing. This may help reduce grieving parents' guilt about giving up too soon, which is a common concern in later grief work.

Health-care professionals may help parents identify significant support persons and encourage their presence at the bedside when a child is dying. Providing a private place close to the unit but away from the bedside allows family members opportunities to talk, support one another, and make necessary phone calls. A staff person should check frequently to answer questions and respond to needs, while giving the family time to grieve together. The ability to voice empathy by acknowledging feelings of family members is important while listening a lot and talking less (Pearson, 1999).

Providing access to available resources is also important: (a) social work for crisis intervention and support; (b) pastoral care to offer spiritual support; (c) child life to address issues of surviving siblings and other children involved in the death; (d) bereavement counselors for the complex needs of particular family members; and (e) hospice or palliative-care staff, if appropriate. The process at the time of death should be described, as well as choices the family may have about saying good-bye, either at the bedside or in another suitable place. Parents should be encouraged to participate in cares at the time of the death (e.g., holding, bathing, dressing). Staff and parents should also discuss including siblings and extended family, especially grandparents. Some families may need reassurance that all requests, rituals, or plans at the time of the death are acceptable and based only on the parents' needs and wishes.

The concept of memory making is a critical part of supportive caring at the time of the death. In a survey of 77 teaching children's hospitals across the United States, nearly all providers reported offering legacy-making activities to ill children and their families, with patients and families usually completing the activity together (Foster, Dietrich, Friedman, Gordon, & Gilmer, 2012). Although most activities were offered before a patient died and when cure was no longer being sought, the researchers reported a need for additional research to examine activities across different age groups and conditions, the best time to offer such activities, and associations with the positive and negative outcomes of ill children, their family members, and the bereaved.

Legacy-making activities may include a Memory Box containing

- a lock of hair,
- an ink or plaster hand- or footprint (see Figure 6.4),
- photographs of the family and child before and/or after the death,
- comfort objects used at the time of the death (e.g., stuffed animals, quilt), and
- the gown worn at time of the death. (Butler et al., 2015).

One child life specialist is careful to place an extra stuffed animal at the bedside for each surviving sibling so that they have their own comfort objects to cherish after the death. Clergy members sometimes use a seashell for baptisms and blessings, thus providing another memento for the family to keep.

As mentioned earlier, private time at the bedside following a child's death may vary greatly, depending on the family's needs. Providing this time may seem troublesome for staff of busy critical care units, but accommodations need to be made for this critical time. Sometimes a family also may need staff help to actually conclude this final visit. One mother described her feelings of knowing that it was time to leave her child, but of not being able to actually lay the child back in bed. She recalls, years after the death, the precious memory of the ICU physician holding her child and rocking quietly as the family left the unit. Similarly, it may help the family a great deal if they are reassured that a favorite staff member will accompany the child to the morgue after the family has left.

Finally, parents need to be accompanied out of the hospital when leaving after their child's death. After all personal belongings, photos, and so on have been gathered

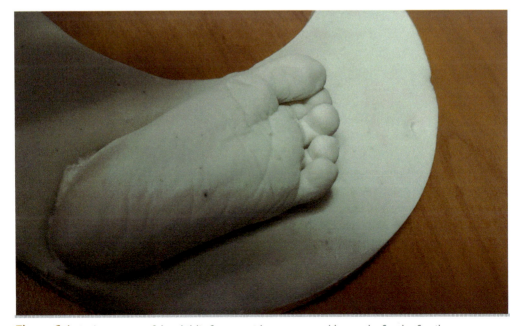

Figure 6.4. A plaster cast of the child's foot provides a treasured keepsake for the family.

and packed, and good-byes said to unit staff, the actual process of leaving might be extremely difficult for family members. Walking the family to the car offers physical and emotional support. Pastoral care staff members in one hospital provide a new teddy bear for mothers to clutch when leaving the hospital after her infant has died. This object of physical touching may help fill the void of empty arms and is reported to be especially comforting for some parents.

In keeping with evidence-based practice, an accurate measure of the dying and death experience in the pediatric intensive care setting is needed to illuminate how nurses, physicians, and psychosocial staff can better manage end-of-life care for the benefit of children, their families, and caregivers. In a retrospective cohort study with 159 clinicians representing five disciplines, the Pediatric Intensive Care Unit-Quality of Dying and Death 20 showed promise as a valid and reliable measure (Sellers, Dawson, Cohen-Bearak, Solomond, & Truog, 2015).

The Dying Child

For many years, child development experts believed that children younger than 10 years of age did not have the cognitive ability to express feelings or experiences related to their own death. Research into the fatally ill child's awareness of death began with Waechter's classic study in 1971. Results of her study indicated that children who are terminally ill are most often protected by adult silence, but, if given both the encouragement and the opportunity, they will talk about their understanding of their illness and fears (Waechter, 1971).

In 1978, Bluebond-Langner studied the interactions of children who were patients on an oncology unit. Her observations and interviews, published in her book, *The Private Worlds of Dying Children*, provide great insight into how children learn about their illness, treatment, and prognosis in stages, each marked by the acquisition of important information. The stages are as follows:

1. Realization that "it" is a serious illness
2. Understanding of the names of the drugs, uses, and side effects
3. Knowledge of the procedures and treatments, relationships between symptoms and procedures, each viewed as unique and isolated events
4. Realization that the disease is a series of remissions and relapses
5. Understanding that the disease will cause death when drugs are no longer effective

As a child passed through each of the above stages, Bluebond-Langner observed that the child went through similar stages related to differing self-concepts:

1. Well at diagnosis
2. Seriously ill and will get better (evidenced by responses of family and friends, and physical changes in themselves)
3. Always ill and will get better

4. Always ill and will never get better (relapses and drug complications threatened child's sense of well-being)

5. Dying (only realized when child heard of the death of a peer)

The stages of acquisition of information and stages of changes in self-concept correspond and may be charted on a continuum (see Figure 6.5). Points on the continuum depict catalytic experiences and events in the child's illness journey.

Despite the parents' refusal to acknowledge the impending death and engage the child in preparation, the children's behaviors provided clues that they did actually realize their imminent death. The children Bluebond-Langner observed exhibited nine types of behavior (Bluebond-Langner, 1978, p. 234):

1. Avoidance of deceased children's names and belongings

2. Lack of interest in nondisease-related conversations or play

3. Preoccupation with death and disease imagery in play, art, and literature

4. Engagement of selected individuals in either disclosures, conversations, or disclosure speeches

5. Anxiety about increased debilitation and about going home, but for different reasons than earlier on in the disease process

6. Avoidance of talk about the future

7. Concern that things be done immediately

8. Refusal to cooperate with relatively simple, painless procedures

9. Establishment of distance from others through displays of anger or silence

The children in her study exhibited a complex form of mutual pretense between themselves and their parents, and between themselves and medical personnel. The author challenges health-care professionals to develop a policy that allows children to talk openly about their illness or prognosis with those whom they choose while still protecting those people, such as their parents, whom they may wish to protect in order to keep them close. Additionally, the child who is terminally ill may not directly disobey societal restrictions to talk openly about the death, but rather will approach the process of gaining information through highly symbolic questions and interactions (Bluebond-Langner, 1978; Sourkes, 1995).

The spiral of grief and anticipatory grief often begins when another child patient dies. Previously unexpressed fears and thoughts of separation begin to be more openly evident or observed. Children may become increasingly sensitive to the effects of separation as though in preparation for the separation caused by death. Play themes may focus on disappearance and return, or elaborate games of hide-and-seek, which test whether the child's absence would be noticed or missed (Sourkes, 1995).

The terminal phase is described as the point when the child's illness no longer responds to conventional treatment. The child becomes aware that there are few remaining options, and attention turns from cure to palliative care. This phase may last for days or weeks or months, with experimental treatment or no treatment. During this phase, the most important choices may be related to pain management and the exploration of palliative-care options (Sourkes, 1995). (See section on palliative care.)

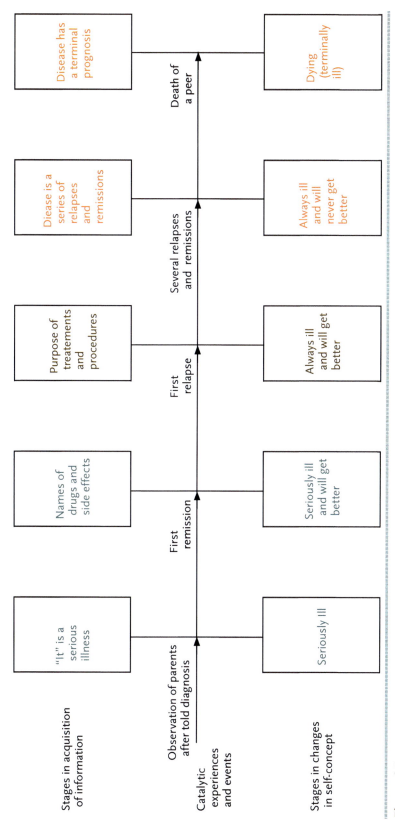

Figure 6.5. Children acquire knowledge of their disease's process, treatment, and prognosis in stages. *Note.* From *Children Mourning: Mourning Children,* by K. J. Doka, 1995, Bristol, PA: Hospice Foundation of America. Copyright 1995 by Hospice Foundation of America. Reprinted with permission.

The child gradually turning inward marks the end of the terminal phase. His or her physical energy is directed toward physical survival and there may be few opportunities for talking. The child may retreat from physical contact and pull into him- or herself and away from others. Preparing parents for these new behaviors as normal and expected as the child nears death will help avoid feelings of rejection often felt by the parents. Rephrasing this concept as the child pulling "into" him- or herself rather than "away" from others may also lessen a parent's reaction to this experience (Sourkes, 1995). For other guidelines on intervening with a child who is dying, see Text Box 6.2.

Bluebond-Langner's more recent work looks at the emerging focus on the child's role in decisions about care and treatment. Whereas originally the most important approach was focused almost exclusively on physical care, there has been a shift in overall aspects of care to look at the impact of illness on the whole person, including social, emotional, and spiritual factors affecting care and treatment plans (Bluebond-Langner, Belasco, & Wander, 2010). In their study, Bluebond-Langner and colleagues addressed the challenges of involving children within the ethical context of parental and physician roles and responsibilities. The following factors are identified as critical for including children in decision-making: (1) children's knowledge and understanding, (2) age and stage of development, (3) experiences, (4) views of illness, and (5) options for care and treatment. The researchers suggest that using age or developmental stage may not accurately predict what children know. Children's experiences and length of illness, as indicated in Figure 6.5, are important indicators of their understanding, even if treatment may have caused cognitive deficits. Also noted, children, like their parents, may remain hopeful despite all indications that no further options for cure are available. The concept of mutual pretense, described in Bluebond-Langner's previous work, also has an impact on a child's willingness to interact with parents, including the child's making choices about treatment based on recognition of a parent's hopefulness about a cure, a new clinical trial, etc., at a time when there is little hope remaining for a meaningful recovery (Bluebond-Langner et al., 2010). For parents, the role of protector usually means engaging in exhaustive research, tests, and clinical trials in an effort to find a cure.

Ultimately the decision-making process respects the value of considering the child/patient, parent, and physician and the inherent relationships. The process requires both talking and listening to one another at a time when such conversation is extremely difficult. Although legally it is the parent who makes the final decisions for the child, giving the child a voice may affect grieving after the loss (Bluebond-Langner et al., 2010).

A study conducted in the Netherlands analyzed why parents did or did not discuss the impending death with their child. Sixty-four percent of parents chose not to talk to their child based on their desire to protect the child, views on talking with children, views of their child's characteristics, the child's refusal to have that conversation, the child's disability, and lack of opportunities to talk with the child (Van der Geest et al., 2015). Some parents reported that they lacked confidence in their ability to talk about death with their child and often waited until it was too late to have the conversation. In addition, parents were frightened about how the child might react. Would he or she be angry or frightened, and would it prevent the child from enjoying his or her final days? Some parents noted that they felt that their child was aware of his or her impending death based on their actions or comments and thus did not feel that it was necessary

||||||||||||||||||||||||||||||||||||||||||||||||||||||||||||||||||||||||||||||||||||||||||||||||||||||||||||||||||||||||||||||||

Text Box 6.2
Guidelines for Intervention With a Child Who Is Dying

1. Do not underestimate the child's capacity to understand.
2. Create open communication but do not force it.
   - Listen first, then offer support.
   - Provide honest information.
   - Remember that it is OK to say "I don't know."
   - Answer only what the child wants to know.
3. Provide creative outlets for anger, such as art.
4. Follow the child's lead.
5. Be honest with the child about impending death.
6. Allow the child time to say good-byes.
7. Permit the child to decide when he or she wants to share the pain of grief.
8. Remember that the child may choose to protect the parent (mutual pretense).
9. Help the dying child to live.
   - Make the child comfortable
     - Arrange physical setting for the child to be with family.
     - Create space for the child in the family living area.
     - Plan family activities for the child to participate in or observe.
     - Arrange for medical equipment only as needed.
   - Create special memorable moments.
   - Continue some routine.
   - Surround the child with people who mean the most to the child.
   - Help the child maintain peer friendships.

||||||||||||||||||||||||||||||||||||||||||||||||||||||||||||||||||||||||||||||||||||||||||||||||||||||||||||||||||||||||||||||||

Note. From "Separation, Loss, and Bereavement," by L. Pearson, in *Core Curriculum for the Nursing Care of Children and Their Families* (p. 87), by M. Broome and J. Rollins (Eds.), 1999, Pittman, NJ: Jannetti. Copyright 1999 by Jannetti. Reprinted with permission.

to talk about it. Of those who did talk with their child about death, some used a spiritual context or symbolic story or book to introduce the concept. These parents felt as though talking with their child allowed them to reassure the child, answer questions, and permit the child to participate in funeral planning. Parents felt that talking about impending death in an open and honest way brought their family closer together. Interestingly, parents reported positive feelings about their decision, whether they decided to talk with their child or chose not to talk (Van der Geest et al., 2015).

It is not unusual for children who are dying to continue to fight death long beyond their expected endurance. This process can be exhausting for the child and for the family and staff at their side. One explanation for this struggle is that the child is trying to stay alive for some particular reason. See Case Study 6.2: Permission to Say Good-Bye.

The Dying Adolescent

Doka defines distinct phases as an adolescent navigates the challenges of illness—the prediagnostic, diagnostic, chronic, recovery, and terminal phases (Doka, 2014). How the adolescent and family manage the early stages may provide insight into behaviors and reactions of the terminal phase. Once the adolescent understands that the goals of care are no longer focused on treatment and are shifting to comfort care, the following tasks need to be addressed:

- Dealing with symptoms, discomfort, pain, and incapacities
- Managing health procedures and institutional procedures
- Managing stress and examining coping
- Dealing effectively with caregivers
- Preserving self- concept
- Preserving relationships with family and friends
- Ventilating feelings and fears
- Finding meaning in life and death
- Preparing for death and saying good-bye

For an adolescent, the experience of living with a life-threatening illness requires the development of ongoing coping skills. One intervention that is often effective is involvement in peer support groups. Opportunities to share common experiences and explore coping strategies may help boost an adolescent's self-esteem and facilitate adjustment to treatment. Giving permission to express fears and concerns as well as difficulties in daily living related to diagnosis and prognosis is found in peer support within the group setting. Providing a social structure within which adolescents are able to develop coping skills and respond proactively to illness-related causes also helps teens feel empowered and in control of their lives and futures.

When an adolescent realizes that a cure is no longer possible and begins the process of saying good-bye, health-care professionals may make a difference by using techniques of empathetic listening. To be the person that the adolescent chooses to help prepare others for his or her upcoming death is indeed a privileged role.

Decision-making for adolescents at end of life is complex. In one study, very few adolescents or parents wanted adolescents to make treatment decisions independently (Knopf, Hornung, & Slab, 2008). While the adolescents clearly stated that they wished to receive technical information as "straight talk when delivering bad news," the teens did not wish to make the final decisions about their care. Some studies have suggested that this trend to have parents and physicians lead the decision-making process may be based in the adolescents' advanced understanding of all of the issues involved (Knopf, Hornung, & Slab, 2008).

Hospice and Palliative Care

The task of understanding the complexity of the child and family as they live through the experience of a child's dying is enormous. The need to give care and

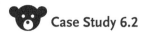 **Case Study 6.2**

Permission to Say Good-Bye

John, a 12-year-old boy, had been in the intensive care unit for the past 4 weeks. Admitted to the hospital for seizures following a brief viral illness, his medical course had been incredibly complex. Each test, treatment, and surgery resulted in a further decline in his condition, leaving him with multisystem failure. His parents and adolescent brother sat by his bedside almost continuously and had come to realize that he would not survive. The choice to provide supportive care until his death is one that this family approached with the same control and information-based approach that they had used since his very first hospital day.

After discussing the details of supportive care, especially concerns about pain control, his mother turned her attention to meeting the needs of extended family and friends. She invited four of John's best friends to gather at the bedside to say good-bye to John. Staff and John's parents prepared these sixth-graders in the supportive presence of their parents for this difficult bedside visit. The boys undertook their task with age-appropriate style, talking and laughing about shared experiences while looking at the many photographs surrounding John's bedside. Following the modeling of John's parents, the friends gained strength and comfort from the belief that John was able to hear their expressions of friendship and love, despite his unresponsiveness. As is often the case, this touching scene was extremely emotional for gathered adults and staff, while the boys managed the visit in an easy style.

Supportive care without aggressive treatments began on Thursday, and John died 2 days later. In the words of John's mother, "We had been telling John that he would be going home soon. Our interpretation of 'home' was heaven. It wasn't until we talked to Dr. P., one of John's physicians, in the ICU on Saturday morning that we realized what we were telling John was probably being interpreted differently by John. Our son was an incredible fighter, as he had demonstrated over the weeks of his hospitalization. We realized that John was fighting to stay alive so that he could go home from the hospital. Dr. P. asked us if we would feel comfortable talking to John and giving him permission to stop fighting. We went back to John's room and told him that it was OK to stop fighting. We told him that he would be going to heaven to be with God, and we would be with him again one day. Within minutes after we had this conversation with John, his breathing pattern changed, and he became diaphoretic. Family was called back to his bedside, and within a few hours John died. That moment when his respirations changed and he broke out in a sweat will be forever engrained in my memory. It was a powerful moment for his father and me. We were sure he heard us, and he was relieved to have Mom and Dad's permission to say good-bye."

Note. Courtesy of Kris and Bob Koebele.

attempt the relief of suffering is just as great as the need to cure and should be no less an ultimate goal of medicine.

—Liben, 1996, p. 28.

The concept of hospice dates back to ancient times. The U.S. hospice movement began in the 1960s. Martinson established one of the earliest hospice-like programs in the United States in 1972 for children with cancer (Buckingham, 1983). It was developed as an alternative to hospital care and its associated costs at a time when the overwhelming effects of hospitalization on children were being extensively examined. The program helped focus on the importance of patients' rights and the ability of parents to maintain control with the continuous availability of medical and nursing resources. Procedures were fully explained to parents, who then provided cares as much as possible. Parents were given information as to potential complications and possible scenarios. Parents also were able to employ those comfort measures that seemed most helpful to their child and appeared to reduce the child's perception of pain.

Martinson's program proved to be cost-effective while demonstrating psychosocial benefits for families as well. Children with cancer reported feeling more secure in the comfortable setting of home and more involved in the activities of all members of the family. Of the children with cancer in her study who were old enough to express an opinion, all preferred being at home to being in the hospital. Parents reported that they felt more in control and less stressed in meeting the needs of all family members when not forced to spend time at the hospital and at home (Grollman, 1995).

Ann Armstrong-Daily founded Children's Hospice International in 1983 because there were only three hospices in the United States that accepted children (O'Quinn & Giambra, 2014). There are now more than 3,000 residential sites that care for children. The goal of Children's Hospice International is to provide education, support, and training to hospices that care for children with life-threatening illnesses and their families. Programming and philosophies focus on the needs of the child, siblings, and parents.

Trend Toward Palliative Care

In recent years, the term *palliative care* has been gradually replacing the term *hospice care*. Up until the 1980s the two terms were interchangeable, but hospice care remained firmly linked with cancer services immediately before a death (Stayer, 2012). Changes in health care and improved technologies meant a longer trajectory of illness and led to a distinction between hospice and palliative care. In the 1990s palliative care become a specialty as programs began to develop. The term *palliative* is derived from the word *palliate*, which means "to lessen the severity of [a disease] without curing or removing it." Palliative care is a broad philosophy of total, compassionate care that meets the physical, social, psychological, and spiritual needs of the patient and family that emerge when a child is diagnosed with a life-threatening illness. It should be instituted at diagnosis and continue through treatment, even when cure is a possibility. The American Academy of Pediatrics statement on palliative care defines the concept as "seeking to enhance quality of life in the face of an ultimately terminal condition" (AAP, 2000, p. 351). It includes the control of pain and other symptoms while addressing a broad spectrum of family and patient needs, also defined as achievement of the best quality of life consistent with a family's values, regardless of the location of the patient (AAP, 2000). The foundation of palliative care rests on the following principles:

1. Respect for the dignity of patients and families
2. Access to competent and compassionate palliative care
3. Support for the caregivers
4. Improved professional and social support for pediatric palliative care
5. Continued improvement of pediatric palliative care through education and research

Ideally, palliative care principles provide support for the child and family through treatment, end of life, and after death. Minimum standards for palliative care require a multidisciplinary team that includes a physician, nurse, social worker, spiritual advisor, and a child life specialist (AAP, 2000). Mature teams would be expected to also include a case manager and bereavement specialist (AAP, 2013). Himmelstein, Hilden, Boldt, and Weissman (2004, p. 1753) noted that the "complex of life-threatening illness occurs within the context of growth and development" because of the nature of the child. Therefore, expressive therapies, such as drawing, writing, journaling, playing, and expressing his or her dreams, wishes, and fears, are of critical importance to the developing child.

Palliative care broadens the scope to apply to other illnesses that are life-limiting (e.g., neurodegenerative and metabolic disorders, severe congenital abnormalities, muscular dystrophy, organ failures, HIV/AIDS). In a multicenter cohort study of more than 500 pediatric palliative-care patients, 40% of the primary medical conditions were genetic/congenital. Of these 500 children, almost 40% had neurological conditions, 20% had cancer, 13% had respiratory conditions, and 8% had gastrointestinal conditions. Five per cent of the patients were less than 1 month of age, and 15.5% were 19 years and older. The median time from consult to death was 107 days, and most palliative-care patients were still alive after 1 year. These statistics contrast greatly with similar studies of adult palliative care (Feudtner et al., 2011).

Using the term *palliative care* (as opposed to *hospice*) helps reduce the assumption that death will occur soon, and for children this is especially important, as it is more difficult to predict length of life. Palliative care may be provided in the hospital or at home and serves as a complement to primary-care medicine. See Text Box 6.3, World Health Organization Definition of Palliative Care for Children.

In the hospital setting, palliative care may not involve stopping all technological support, but rather, changing the focus to less active and technologically intense forms of medical care. Even in the neonatal intensive care unit, families may be provided privacy, a comfortable environment that is physically removed from the sounds of high-tech equipment alarms and the demands of intensive care. It is important to shift the focus from the needs of the patient to the needs of the grieving family. A less restrictive visiting policy, especially for siblings, should be encouraged. Attention to the requested wishes of parents is part of family-centered care and may require some accommodations on the part of staff to support family choices. For example, after making the difficult decision to withdraw ventilator support from their infant born with a devastating genetic abnormality, a family was moved from the private room in the neonatal

Text Box 6.3
World Health Organization
Definition of Palliative Care for Children

World Health Organization Definition of Palliative Care for Children

- Palliative care for children is the active total care of the child's body, mind, and spirit, and it also involves giving support to the family.
- It begins when illness is diagnosed and continues regardless of whether a child receives treatment directed at the disease.
- Health providers must evaluate and alleviate a child's physical, psychological, and social distress.
- Effective palliative care requires a broad multidisciplinary approach that includes the family and makes use of available community resources; it can be successfully implemented even if resources are limited.
- It can be provided in tertiary care facilities, in community health centers, and even in children's homes.

Note. Adapted from "Cancer Pain Relief and Palliative Care in Children," by the World Health Organization & International Association for the Study of Pain, 1998. Geneva, Switzerland: World Health Organization.

intensive care unit to a larger room on another unit. This move accommodated the family's wish to videotape the final hours of the infant's life with the surrounding presence of extended family.

Although at times staff may struggle with family wishes for supportive end-of-life care, at other times sensitive and caring staff may make critical decisions that provide great support for families. A mother and father whose newborn son was dying in the intermediate intensive care unit of a hospital recall "the one good night" they shared as a couple with their newborn son. An insightful nurse rearranged the room to accommodate two daybeds pushed together to form a double bed and allowed both parents to sleep there with the baby between them (Pearson, 1997).

Preferred Place of Death

Much research conducted in the 1960s to 1980s tended to focus on the comparison of death in the hospital to death at home, with a certain presumption that death at home was perceived as more favorable and produced a better outcome for grieving families. Most of the studies focused on children with cancer, and more children with cancer do die at home than do children dying of other diseases. Questions have been raised about whether the care required for cancer patients is more compatible with care and death at home. Also, community services and home outreach are most highly developed in oncology (Bluebond-Langner, Beecham, Candy, Langner, & Jones, 2013).

Bluebond-Langer and colleagues conducted a systematic literature review of preferred place of death for children and young people with life-limiting and life-threatening conditions in England, Australia, Germany, France, Canada, and the

United States. The review yields interesting questions about place of death identified by families at various points along the trajectory of illness as well as detailing actual places of death, mostly based on retrospective parental interviews (Bluebond-Langner et al., 2013). All the families cited the choice they made as the best to meet their needs, and they expressed no regret. Yet the conclusion of the review indicated that none of the studies provided specific evidence that home, a hospital, or a hospice is the best place of death. The researchers suggested that the opportunity to choose place of death may be better aligned with palliative-care principles than the actual place of death. Lowton, who studied parents of adults with cystic fibrosis, wrote that "focusing on place of death per se appeared to be of far less importance to parents than focusing on factors that influenced positively experiences of care at end-of-life" (Lowton, 2009, p. 1061).

Although no one individual or group can provide all the necessary services—whether end-of-life care is planned for home, hospice, or hospital—institutions and agencies that provide palliative-care services should develop a comprehensive palliative care package to ensure that the certain components of "good death" are available, and that the child, family, and health professionals have access to them. The following services can be achieved by combining available resources and sharing established expertise through partnerships among various individuals and agencies (Frager, 1996):

- Ongoing supportive care linked to the child and family at the time of diagnosis
- Early and continuing intervention for psychosocial and spiritual support
- Management of pain and other symptoms
- Liaison between tertiary care center and local health community
- A sibling support program
- Support for staff in dealing with critically ill children
- A school reintegration program
- A humanistic approach within high-tech arenas of care
- A school visitation program for schoolmates and teachers of terminally ill children
- An ethics committee approachable by any concerned member of the caregiving team
- Anticipatory grief counseling and bereavement follow-up
- A speakers bureau to share information about palliative care with the medical and lay communities

Perinatal Palliative Care

One emerging area of palliative care is that of perinatal care for families carrying a fetus with a life-limiting diagnosis. In 2013, the infant mortality rate was 5.96 per 1,000 live births, and the neonatal mortality rate was 4.4 per 1,000 live births (Mathews, MacDorman, & Thoma, 2015). Twenty percent of infant deaths are caused by congenital malformations, deformities, and chromosomal abnormalities. Many of these diagnoses may be made prenatally. For the family whose pregnancy is suddenly and forever changed with the diagnosis of a lethal anomaly, the choices are exceedingly difficult. Perinatal hospice has been proposed as an alternative to termination of a pregnancy. Palliative care has been supported for infants with congenital anomalies incompatible with life, newborns born at the limits of viability, and infants with an overwhelming illness that does not respond to life-sustaining interventions (Munson & Leuthner, 2007). Because a family will have very limited time for bonding with a baby who will not live for long, continuing a pregnancy will provide time for the family to create memories with their as-yet unborn baby and set the stage for normal grieving. After much discussion of all the possibilities, a family might choose a palliative birth plan, knowing that perinatal death is the likely outcome but making time to determine their wishes for the birth experience, family involvement, memory activities, and rituals at time of death (Munson & Leuthner, 2007).

Culturally Sensitive Grief Work

Culturally sensitive grief work requires particular attention to the needs of every family and its unique cultural heritage. There is a great deal of diversity even within a single ethnic group. In immigrant families, children may represent a new generation that is partially assimilated into the dominant culture.

For many families, the practices associated with medical care and decision-making in critical care settings may be difficult. Family culture may not encourage assertiveness in relation to medical authority. Family and extended family support for a child may require leniency in terms of restricted visitation and hospital policies. Treatment decisions may have both medical and moral consequences and tremendous impact on a family's subsequent grief or family members' ability to come to terms with the death. Translators must be provided to help families understand not just the present medical treatment but also the family's options to say no to medical treatments that are not consistent with religious or cultural beliefs.

To provide culturally supportive care requires the realization that normal indicators of previous experience with death may not apply. People from different cultural backgrounds may be grieving significant losses on a chronic basis (e.g., loss of homeland, loss of possessions, loss of native language, tradition).

A series of questions has been developed for health-care professionals to address in making plans for supporting parents and families facing the death of a child (National Cancer Institute, 2013):

- What are the prescribed rituals for handling dying, the dead body, the disposal of the body, and rituals to commemorate the loss?
- What are the group's beliefs about what happens after death?
- What do people believe about appropriate emotional expression and integration of a loss experience?
- What does the family consider to be the roles of each family member in handling the death?
- Are certain deaths particularly stigmatized (e.g., suicide) or traumatic for the group?

An experience in one setting illustrates the changing awareness and respect for culturally diverse grief practices. A Native American adolescent died in the intensive care unit of a pediatric hospital. A large group of family and friends were gathered at the bedside. The family's religious beliefs required that a shaman perform a ceremony using eagle feathers to fan smoke from a fire to ensure the passage of the teen's soul beyond death. Arrangements were made to allow this ceremony to occur in an undeveloped building space close to the ICU but with safety factors also considered.

In a far more unsettling acquiescence to cultural demands and differences, a child life specialist in the same unit spent several hours working with two school-age siblings whose younger brother had become suddenly and seriously ill and was not expected to survive. The children in the playroom were interactive and quite knowledgeable about the beliefs of their Middle Eastern heritage in terms of a life after death for their brother who had chronic health concerns and special needs. They engaged in creating a memory book about their brother and were allowed to visit at the bedside in the presence of both parents and many young uncles and male family friends. After a period of time, the children returned to tell the child life specialist that they would be leaving the hospital soon. Conversations between the child life specialist and the uncle who had emerged as the spokesperson for the family failed to convince him that the children might better handle the sad nature of the sibling's death if allowed to stay with the family at the hospital. The children left a short time later. When the mother and all the female relatives were also sent home before the anticipated death of the young son, it became clear to the child life professional that the decisions to send both the children and the mother home were made not out of failure to understand the grief needs of children but rather in accordance with strict cultural beliefs about the death of a child.

Ethical Issues and End-of-Life Decisions

No issue is more difficult in the scope of meeting the psychosocial needs of children and families than the decisions related to end-of-life care. To recognize that a child is dying requires consummate energy and emotional investment on the part of families and caregivers. The realization that the intensity of high-tech medical care might be more appropriately replaced by supportive care signifies the abandonment of hope for a cure. It is at this most stressful time that decisions must be made, and it is a time that is filled with ethical and moral conflicts. The goals of decision-making require that any decision be made with the child's best interests in mind and that decisions must be shared—a philosophy that has evolved with the focus of family-centered care.

According to Rushton and Glover (1990),

> To respect a child is to acknowledge the importance of his or her world and the relationships that are central to it. Unilateral decision-making by health-care professionals based solely on "medical indications" would deny the fullness of a child's life and the value of the relationships that also benefit to sustain the child. (p. 207)

Thus, it is most important to create a partnership between the family, nursing staff, and physicians. Parents need professional guidance to face the issues of quality of life, knowing that the results of these decisions will have lifelong effects on the family. The ability to participate actively in decision-making is often complicated by feelings of shock and disbelief when a child suddenly becomes critically ill or severely injured. Parents struggle with the transition from parenting a well child to parenting a critically ill child. Other factors that can affect decision-making include inadequate information, emotional upheaval, uncertainty of diagnosis or prognosis, and distrust of medical professionals.

One of the most difficult decisions health-care providers and parents may face involves life-support withdrawal (LSW). Votta and colleagues (2001) examined whether parental involvement in an LSW decision had an impact on the perceptions and adjustment of parents whose child died in a pediatric critical care unit. Responses of parents whose child died after an LSW decision was made were compared with responses of parents whose child died without an LSW decision. Findings revealed that compared with parents whose child died without an LSW decision, a significantly greater number of parents whose child died following an LSW decision were certain about their child's future health; believed that their child's quality of life would have been unacceptable; and reported less dissatisfaction with time spent with their child, fewer negative changes in family functioning, and more positive changes in feelings toward staff.

Certain strategies have been identified as helpful for parents. The first is providing an environment that may facilitate the family's ability to integrate information at this stressful time. Taking the family away from the noises of medical monitors and alarms can be helpful. Physicians should be unhurried and uninterrupted at this critical time, by not only providing clear and honest information but also listening and encouraging family members to ask questions. Asking the family to describe their perception of the present situation is helpful, and identifying the roles of various physicians involved in their child's care may reduce confusion. The longer a child stays in the ICU, the more opportunity there is for confusion as parents seek out information about their child's medical condition (Vose & Nelson, 1999). Providing continuity in caregivers, both nurses and primary physicians, will help families gather information while demonstrating clinical competencies, which helps in trust-building.

Enhancing communication, which helps families process information vital to decision-making, is the second strategy. Asking parents to share their goals and desires for their child, as well as their values related to life, death, disability, and suffering, will encourage shared decision-making (Rushton & Glover, 1990). Information should be provided about the details of the child's present condition, diagnosis, prognosis, risks, and benefits of further treatment. Nursing staff may play a critical role in helping present information clearly and objectively, yet with sensitivity. Often it is helpful to have several staff people hear the information with the family to enable clarification in areas of confusion. Providing written materials may help some families feel a greater sense of control.

Discussion of pain and suffering helps parents explore their beliefs and what they feel would be the wishes of their child. Clarifying misconceptions is always crucial. Explaining observable or expected responses of the child to medical interventions such as suctioning helps reduce anxiety. Perhaps parents' most important concern is the ability to keep their child comfortable and experiencing as little pain as possible.

In addition, assessment of the family's support systems and previous experiences with loss helps identify needs. Inadequate support systems may have a negative effect on family decision-making. Connecting at-risk families with hospital-based resources and supports should be a priority. Social services, child life, pastoral care, palliative care, and nursing bring different perspectives to total family-centered care and decision-making and should be incorporated when available. Professionals who have greater knowledge of ethics, policies, and legal issues often feel more empowered as advocates for patients and families. The process of decision-making may have multiple steps, and assisting families from one level to the next often takes time. Information about particular responses to treatments or observations of the child's responses may help parents think further about the implications of ongoing aggressive treatment.

Although the federal Patient Self-Determination Act (PSDA) supports the right of adults age 18 years and older to information regarding the execution of advanced directives, the spirit of PSDA creates opportunities for minors to participate in treatment decisions and the right to determine the circumstances of their death. Many children and teens do have the capacity to help in making decisions about what is in their best interests. Rushton and Lynch (1992) suggested that children by 11 or 12 years of age should be assessed by the same criteria as are used for adults as far as having the (a) ability to comprehend essential information about their diagnosis and prognosis, (b) ability to reason about their choices in accordance with their values and life goals, and (c) ability to make an informed decision based on recognizing the important consequences of various courses of action. Further, it is felt that in the case of chronic illness, parents need to be supported throughout the process of illness and treatment in exploring their child's wishes and beliefs related to life-supporting medical technology (Vose & Nelson, 1999).

The standard of care in the "best interests of the child" focuses on the presumption of life, and when life can be saved, it should be. But when life cannot be saved, or the chance of survival is minimal and treatment would include repeated pain and suffering; invasive procedures; immobilization; and prolonged hospitalization and isolation from parents, family, and friends, then the decision of treatment should focus on comfort care while dying.

Participation of Children at Funerals

One of the most frequently asked questions at the time of a child's death concerns the participation of siblings, cousins, and other children at funerals or memorial services. Because the experience of loss is overwhelming, concerned family members often want to protect children from these feelings of sadness and loss. Yet children and teens who are included in rituals following the death of a loved one often demonstrate better coping skills and more favorable adjustment. The health-care professional may be the first person that families turn to for advice as they begin the experience of mourning the loss of a member of the family.

Children who are invited to participate in funeral or memorial rituals require preparation. If parents are unable either physically or emotionally to provide such preparation, another trusted adult may do so. Children need to know what they will see, hear, feel, and be expected to do, as well as understand how adults may be expressing their feelings of loss. Attention to the physical presence of the body of the person who has died should address the state of being dead, the end of all physiological processes of life, opportunities to touch the body, and accepted ritual behaviors. A child should never be forced to attend a funeral or do anything that may be uncomfortable.

Many funeral directors are becoming more knowledgeable about the needs of surviving children and may offer opportunities for grieving family members to be together at the funeral home or church before the arrival of extended family and friends. While families experience intense sadness, children also need to grieve, but in manageable doses. It is also important to have appropriate play and art activities available for children during the long hours of visitation. Many families find that encouraging children to create memory photo displays, select favorite toys for the casket, or assume helpful roles during the public rituals also is supportive.

Assigning responsibility for young children to a trusted adult or family member other than a grieving parent also helps families. For older children and teens, actual participation in the rituals may be healing (i.e., reading scripture or original poetry, sharing an anecdote, or taking part in rituals of particular religious symbolism). Whatever roles families choose for incorporating children are good, as long as the children are prepared and supported throughout the experience. It is not essential or even developmentally possible for a child to understand exactly what is happening at every point. What is important is that the child is included in the family's expression of grief. Part of the healing process will be helping the child "grow into" understanding as they grow up with the loss within the context of their own family.

Bereavement Programming

The work of bereavement by definition begins at the moment of death. For health-care professionals, follow-up care constitutes bereavement programming. Goals of such programs are threefold: (a) to help families through the immediate crisis of their child's death, (b) to offer ongoing support and resources to bereaved families for a period of time after the death of a child, and (c) to provide support, education, and resources for staff (Brown & Sefansky, 1995).

In a synthesis of family experience with the death of a child in the PICU, the final role that parents identified, after being a parent in the PICU and being supported in the PICU, was "'Parenting After Death" (Butler et al., 2015). For parents, this represented ways they tried to reconstruct and maintain their parental role after their child died. Critical to this process was follow-up and support during the stages of their bereavement. Letters, cards, and funeral attendance were noted to be important to parents, as parents frequently said that saying good-bye to caregivers was very difficult. Parents described the importance of memorial programs, because returning to the hospital and honoring their child by saying good-bye in formal rituals, naming his or her name, and talking about their child with other bereaved parents gave them comfort and helped in healing (Butler et al., 2015). Parents also identified the use of social media to aid in their grief work. Online support groups, blogs, and websites validated the importance of a wide range of support. Sharing their story with strangers on social media was comforting and supported parents' belief that their baby's existence had value and touched others (Tan, Docherty, Barfield, & Brandon, 2012).

Although availability of services varies greatly in different settings in terms of how support is given and by whom, certain elements of programming are assumed. Initially a family may need resources to help arrange for their child's funeral, with questions arising related to expenses, legal requirements, transport of the body, autopsy, and burial. Referral to appropriate resources within the family's home community may help the family find local supportive services. Pastoral care and social workers may be most helpful in addressing these first concerns. Physicians and other medical staff may be able to expedite concerns related to autopsy or organ donation. Child life should be available to answer questions related to the involvement of children and adolescents in rituals following a death. In the absence of child life services, a nurse, social worker, or other member of the health-care team who is highly skilled in children's developmental and psychosocial needs should be available. Other members of the multidisciplinary bereavement committee may respond immediately or after initial plans are made. For some families with complicated grief or issues of violent and tragic death, mental health counselors may be especially helpful in the hours soon after death to help diffuse anger and address mental health needs.

In the days following the death, many health-care professionals support grieving families by their participation or presence in the planned funeral and memorial rituals. The presence of someone who cared for the child in the final hours of his or her life or of staff who knew the child for months or years during the struggle with a chronic life-threatening illness can be invaluable. It often helps families to find comfort in the realization that their child's life, however short or long, had importance to others. Many times, a family's hospital stay may have occurred a long distance from home, especially in these days of high-tech treatment at tertiary care centers of excellence. For families who have traveled great distances for a child to have a bone marrow or organ transplant, the details and intensity of the medical experience may be simply incomprehensible to those family and friends who were not able to share in the experience of hospital treatment or be present at the time of death. In addition, parents closely identify with staff members with whom they may have had a brief but intense encounter and consider it significant that this person was the last to see their child alive. Parents consider the overwhelmingly difficult time they shared with staff to be valuable and helpful in keeping the memory of their child alive.

Sympathy notes by caregivers, follow-up phone calls, and the opportunity for families to return to the medical setting after the death all help families begin their grief work. Many bereaved parents return on special days, such as birthdays or anniversaries, to visit with staff or to bring memorial gifts to other patients in honor of their child who died. These expressions of helping others are often healing to families and health-care professionals. Recently a man was found standing at the door to one of the empty rooms in an ICU. When asked whether he needed help to find the patient he had come to visit, he replied, "No, my son died in this room 6 years ago, and I just needed to come by."

Hospitals have different ways to accomplish the overwhelming task of keeping records on the dates of death, birthdays, and significant dates in the lives of all the children who have died within the year. In some instances, bereavement counselors are the sole handlers of these follow-up contacts. In other places, staff nurses and others may be enlisted to accomplish the task of remembering for those families with whom they worked. The number of years that a family is followed also may vary. Many health-care professionals form lasting friendships with certain families during the dying of a child, and the relationship with the family continues for a long time. The more challenging aspect of bereavement care is providing the same standard of caring for all families.

The ability to provide this sensitive care for all families who have experienced a death is affected by cultural practices of grief, geographical distances, nontraditional family relationships, and staff turnover.

Resources for grieving families include printed materials, which should be available in several languages, as well as lists of resources with the names of counselors and support groups within the family's community. Resources for parents to help siblings should also be included, with suggested activities and a bibliography of books for grieving children (see Appendix 6.1).

Hospitals with a pediatric trauma center may also provide resources particular to traumatic death for families and for schools. Including health-care personnel who were involved in the initial on-site treatment of a child or the transport to the hospital is often helpful for families, especially siblings who may have been present at the scene of the injury or accident but not able to accompany parents to the tertiary medical center. At one children's hospital in the Midwest, the Flight for Life crew welcomes the opportunity to take siblings and other family members up to the helicopter landing area. Talking with a flight crew nurse or helicopter pilot frequently helps siblings sequence the events of the trauma while reassuring family that the child was well cared for and supported during those first critical hours after the traumatic event. A photograph of a sibling sitting in the pilot's seat of the helicopter helps a child master feelings of insecurity and vulnerability in addition to being the source of much discussion when the child returns to school.

Support to communities may include visits by bereavement or trauma team members to help children who have experienced the death of a classmate, or children who have witnessed a traumatic injury or death. Helping children understand the death of another child caused by accidental injury may require the combined skills of social work, nursing, pastoral care, and child life as children struggle with the sudden nature of loss and with their own vulnerability and loss of feelings of safety. Injury prevention for school-age children may be an important part of integrating a death and moving forward with an increased sense of control and security. In one intervention in a local community, a nurse, chaplain, social worker, and child life specialist visited several classrooms after the preschool sister of one of the students was struck by a motor vehicle in the crosswalk in front of the school's entrance. Helping the children understand what they had seen, facilitating discussion of feelings related to the incident, reassuring children while reviewing issues of safety, and encouraging age-appropriate processing through art and journaling helped students and teachers cope. The school crossing guard, whose feelings of guilt were overwhelming, was a welcome participant in the debriefing process.

Support groups for parents, grandparents, and siblings are another important element of bereavement programming. For parents to work together with other parents who have experienced the untimely death of a child often is crucial to beginning grief work. Facilitated by bereavement counselors, these parent groups allow parents to express feelings, vent anger and frustration, share ideas for coping, and help reduce feelings of isolation and utter hopelessness.

Support groups for grieving children accomplish similar goals within the context of age-appropriate activities. For children, the opportunity to know other children who have experienced similar losses is significant to gain peer understanding and normalize experiences. It is estimated that in 2012 there were more than 300 nonprofit counseling centers, up almost a third since 2004 (Seligson, 2014). There are also 150 peer-to-peer programs nationally that serve a similar purpose. Groups provide a safe and appropriate place to express many scary issues and feelings. Because the grieving parent may be emotionally unavailable for the grieving child, a peer group may provide alternative ways to enhance a child's sense of competence and self-esteem. Children's support groups may include discussion of problem areas of coping, art activities to facilitate expression of feelings and concerns, and social time to reassure grieving children and teens that it is still OK to laugh and have fun. Grieving children often demonstrate less resistance to group work than to individual counseling. Participants are extensively screened to be certain that the work of a peer group program is appropriate for each child or teen. And the ongoing presence of a group helps children and teens continue to learn new coping styles as their developmental or family needs change. Many child life specialists are specially trained in the skills of supporting grieving children and are excellent facilitators of groups, incorporating familiarity with the normal developmental needs of children and teens, the impact of grief, and the therapeutic expression of feelings through play and art.

The rise of children's grief camps has also provided necessary support, with more than 200 bereavement camps in the United States (Schreiber & Spear, 2014). All have a similar purpose in providing grieving children and teens with an experience that makes them feel less alone in their grief. Because grief is isolating for children and teens, and children often hide their grief with school classmates in order not to be "different," camp programming integrates traditional camping activities with grief work-related interventions. These activities allow camp participants to engage with others who have had similar experiences of loss, to play and have fun, while accompanied by adults who have no other responsibilities except to engage the campers. (Schreiber & Spear, 2014). Whatever programming activities are included at camp, the significant events are the "Opening," when children share their loss experience within the group and a closing "Memorial" wherein campers participate in some ritual of remembering. For most children and teens attending "grief camp," the experience is powerful and healing in many ways.

Any discussion of grief support must now explore the concept of "Thana-technology" (Sofka, 2014). Defined as digital grieving, literally the study of death and technology, the concept refers to the way that grief work has changed for adolescents today. Described as "digital natives," 95% of adolescents spend time online, 74% have cell phones, and it is estimated that almost 50% of teens have at least one device with always-on connections (Madden, Lenhart, Duggan, Cortesi, & Gassert, 2013). All of this means that for teens who have never not had digital technologies, all of grief work is affected, from the speed at which teens learn of tragedies yet unfolding, to seeking peer support for the work of grief long after a loss has occurred. The immediacy of receiving news of a friend or loved one's death is striking, and negates the old phone chain to inform others of a loss with perhaps a bit of compassion or support. The response to Facebook or other media news is equally as swift and often overwhelmingly huge. People become part of a "community of bereavement" (Sofka, 2014). It is far easier to respond with a brief text, or "like," whereas the old-fashioned method of taking a casserole to the neighbor's is far more difficult, as people are unsure how to act and what to say in face-to-face encounters following a loss. Yet Rebecca Soffer, co-founder of Modern Loss, a website providing resources, essays, and articles on issues related to loss, comments that when people respond on Internet sites it is often not enough, and people need to follow up with real support to the grieving person (Olin, 2014).

For bereaved teens, although the memorials that are placed at the actual site of tragic accident or loss may continue, and gatherings of adolescents marking the loss through candlelight vigils still occur, these digital-savvy teens now also commemorate the loss in the form of Web Memorials. These memorials allow space for family and friends to post information, photos, and tributes as well as survivor advocacy efforts. Some of these sites are specifically designed for adolescents. (See Appendix 6.1: Resources for Grieving Family Members.) Web memorials meet several of the needs of grieving teens, including talking to the deceased and maintaining a continuing bond, acknowledging holidays and major life events, anniversaries of the death, and commentaries (Sofka, 2014). There are also professionally monitored online support groups, such as Griefnet.org and others, that use e-mail to connect members with one another. For parents and adults who live with or counsel grieving teens, there is a cautionary need to continually monitor what teens are posting and where, in order to be alert to deeply troubled teens or those who are seeking personal support. As is the case with online resources, some sites may be inappropriate or inaccurate. In summary, teens do find peer support in online groups, chat sites, Twitter, instant messaging, Facebook, and elsewhere. Sofka (2014) also comments that social media helps teens know that others share their thoughts and fears, sadness, and grief while also noting upsurges in activity at times of renewed acute feelings of loss.

Memorial Programs

Memorial programs may be sponsored by the hospital for children whose death affected many caregivers and other personnel. The death of one toddler who spent more than 2 years in a hospital touched many personnel, including housekeeping, maintenance staff, dietary aides, nurses, physicians, and parents of other patients. Holding a nonreligious memorial service in the hospital auditorium was significant to honor this patient and helped many hospital personnel recognize their loss.

Many hospitals also provide memorial programs for families during the year. These programs are designed to help families who have lost a child recognize their loss and share positive memories with other families who have had similar experiences. These programs usually include rituals to help with coping, such as reading the names of the children who have died, lighting candles, and encouraging conversation with health-care staff and other families. Particular challenges, such as coping with holidays and anniversaries, may be addressed in programming. The provision of age-appropriate activities for siblings should be part of memorial programming as families mourn the loss together. Allowing families to create a memory symbol, light a candle, plant a flower, or create a quilt square may help to acknowledge their participation and continue the healing process in the days, weeks, and months to come.

Disengagement Versus Continuing Bonds

The prevailing view of grief during the past century holds that for successful mourning to take place, the mourner must disengage from the deceased and let go of the past. It has been only in these past 100 years that continuing bonds have been denied as a normal part of bereavement behavior. Klass, Silverman, and Nickman (1996) suggested that bereavement needs to be considered a cognitive as well as an emotional process that takes place in a social context of which the deceased is a part. The process does not end, but bereavement affects the mourner in different ways for the rest of his or her life. People do not "get over" the experience; rather, they are changed by it. Part of the change is a transformed but continuing relationship with the deceased.

The deceased becomes part of a child's inner world. The child continues the relationship by dreaming, by talking to the deceased, by believing that the deceased is watching, by keeping things that belonged to the deceased, by visiting the grave, and by frequently thinking about the deceased. These connections are not static, but are developmentally appropriate to the child and to the child's present circumstances.

The concept of continuing bonds has been embraced in the loss of a parent but is now being studied as a powerful concept as it applies to the sibling relationship (Packman, Horsley, Davies, & Kramer, 2006). Sibling relationships last a lifetime, and sibling identities are intimately connected because of similar histories. Therefore, it is understood that when one sibling dies, the surviving sibling loses a part of him- or herself (DeVita-Raeburn, 2004). In her book *The Empty Room: Surviving the Loss of a Brother or Sister at Any Age*, Elizabeth DeVita-Raeburn refers to the concept of continuing bonds as "carrying" and describes it in her research as the manner in which surviving siblings are able to carry forward their lost sibling without replacing them, thus continuing the bonds of siblings long after the loss. For the grieving child, maintaining bonds of connectedness means being able to talk about the sibling, share feelings of loss, and have such feelings acknowledged by others. All of this may be difficult for the child if others are advising the child to be "strong for the parents," or if the parents themselves are limited in their ability to support the child's expressions of continuing bonds (Packman et al., 2006). In addition, the child's need to talk about his or her experience continues beyond the time immediately after the loss, as the child enters each new developmental stage.

Bereaved parents undergo a similar process to develop a set of memories, feelings, and actions to keep them connected to the deceased child (Klass et al., 1996). A study of a self-help group of bereaved parents revealed that the processes by which parents resolved their grief involved intense interaction with their dead children. They sustained these interactions using similar means to those of the bereaved children. It is important for the family as a whole to acknowledge the concept of continuing bonds and for parents to use continuing bonds adaptively, role-modeling these activities for the child as well. For parents and surviving children, the task of mourning "successfully" "is linked to the ability to use continuing bonds in adaptive ways, figuring out how to preserve and continue a connection to the love that existed prior to the death" (Packman et al., 2006, p. 832).

These findings cause us to rethink the way we talk about the resolution of grief. The concept of a continuing relationship presents a challenge to the idea that the purpose of grief is to sever the bonds with the deceased in order for the survivor to be free to make new attachments and to construct a new identity. According to Klass et al. (1996), these bonds do not end, they simply change.

Conclusion

Working with families during the death of a child can be an overwhelming and emotionally exhausting task for any health-care professional. Research in recent years has identified the effects of a child's death on a family system, including parents, siblings, grandparents, and other extended family members. Long-term studies have demonstrated both the struggles and the resiliency of individuals affected by the loss of a child, sibling, or grandchild. Knowing the enormity of the issues facing the grieving family, researchers have also helped identify those areas where the skills and expertise of health-care professionals may be supportive to families anticipating the death, experiencing the death, and facing the changed future. The ability to provide family-centered care in the midst of great sadness is a challenging but necessary role. Encouraging family participation in end-of-life cares and choices, preparing family members of all ages for imminent death at home or in the hospital, and fostering open communication within families and between families and medical staff have documented value for a family's ability to live beyond the loss.

Developing the professional skills and confidence to provide specific interventions to address the unique needs of each family when a child is dying is a challenging task. When asked what he would teach all new medical students and residents about caring for families at the time of death, one pediatric physician responded that it is a true privilege to be present at the time of a child's death. Another described that moment as a gift. Both went on to say that parents want to know that you knew what to do medically, but more importantly, that you cared about their child. Years after the death, families may not remember what medical interventions were used in an attempt to save their child, but they remember those health-care staff who were supportive by their presence at the time of death and afterward. "The way a child dies will remain in the memory of his parents forever" (Postovsky & Arush, 2004, p. 67). It is also important to remember that there are critical roles for each member of the health-care team. As important as the respirator or the administration of pain-relieving medications is the placement of a beloved teddy bear in the dying child's hand.

Study Guide

1. Describe the effects of a child's death on parents, siblings, and other family members.

2. What are the phases of grief that parents experience?

3. How does grief affect marital and other relationships?

4. What factors influence children's understanding of death?

5. Describe responses of children to death and dying at various stages of development.

6. Why should death and dying be discussed with children?

7. What are some interventions health-care providers can use to help parents and siblings?

8. Describe four areas for intervention in sudden-death situations.

9. Define the concept of palliative care and how it would apply to a family who learn that their unborn child has a lethal anomaly.

10. Describe various forms of end-of-life care and their functions and usefulness for children.

Appendix 6.1

Resources for Grieving Family Members

Organizations

The Dougy Center, The National Center for Grieving Children and Families
www.dougy.org
Provides support in a safe place where children, teens, young adults, and their families grieving a death can share their experience. Located in Portland, Oregon, the center provides support and training locally, nationally, and internationally to individuals and organizations seeking to assist children in grief. Has a wealth of resources online.

The Center for Loss and Transition
www.centerforloss.com
The center for Dr. Alan Wolfelt, a leading grief expert in the United States, located in Fort Collins, Colorado

The Centering Corporation for Grief and Bereavement
www.centering.org
Offers many grief resources for all kinds of loss

Children's Hospice International
www.chionline.org
An award-winning nonprofit that has pioneered and promoted the idea that critically ill children should have access to hospice/palliative care along with curative care from the time their life-threatening illness is diagnosed. Offers a number of publications devoted to home care, palliative pain and symptom management, the development of hospice care services, and related subjects.

National Hospice and Palliative Care Organization
www.nhpco.org/pediatric
Committed to improving access to hospice and palliative care for children and their families, nationally and internationally. Offers resources for professionals and families.

Initiative for Pediatric Palliative Care (IPPC)
www.ippcweb.org
A curriculum to help pediatric health-care professionals in their mission of providing the highest quality of care to children and their families

The Compassionate Friends
www.compassionatefriends.org
A national organization providing grief support after the death of a child; has many local chapters throughout the United States

Resolve Through Sharing Bereavement Services
www.bereavementservicesoline.org
A comprehensive bereavement service for families whose baby died during pregnancy or shortly after birth. Provides local chapters of trained professionals for grief support

Share Pregnancy and Infant Loss Support
www.nationalshare.org
A national organization with more than 75 chapters in 29 states that serves anyone who experiences the tragic death of a baby. Share serves parents, grandparents, siblings, and others in the family unit, as well as the professionals who care for grieving families. Services include bedside companions, phone counseling, face-to-face support group meetings, resource packets, private online communities, memorial events, and training for caregivers.

National Alliance for Grieving Children
www.childrengrieve.org
Provides a network for nationwide communication between hundreds of professionals and volunteers who want to share ideas, information, and resources with one another to better support the grieving children and families they serve in their own communities. Offers online education, hosts an annual symposium on children's grief, maintains a national database of children's bereavement support programs, and promotes national awareness to enhance public sensitivity to the issues that have an impact on grieving children and teens.

Online Grief Support for Teens

Hello Grief
www.hellogrief.org
A place to share and learn about grief and loss

Teen Memory Wall
www.teenmemorywall.com
A place where friends and family can remember, share, and celebrate the life of a loved one; the site stands as a permanent, ever-evolving commemoration.

Decision-Making Resource for Parents

Wilkinson, D., Gillam, L., Hynson, J., Sullivan, J., & Xafis, V. (2013). *Caring decisions: A handbook for parents facing end of life decisions for their child.* Melbourne, Australia: The Royal Children's Hospital.
www.rch.org.au/.../130890 Caring Decisions book_v1.pdf
This handbook has been written to help families who are facing decisions about life support for their seriously ill child. The handbook is based on the authors' own experience of caring for families and of the ethical and practical questions that families face, and is based on research with parents who have been through such decisions. The aim of the handbook is not to tell parents what to do, but to help them think through questions that they may be facing.

Books for Young Children

Clifton, L. (1982). *Everett Anderson's goodbye.* New York, NY: Henry Holt.
Everett has a difficult time coming to terms with his grief after his father dies.

Cobb, Rebecca. (2013). *Missing Mommy: A book about bereavement.* New York, NY: Henry Holt and Company, LLC.
Explores the many emotions a bereaved child may experience.

DePaola, T. (1973). *Nana upstairs and Nana downstairs.* New York, NY: Putnam.
A small boy enjoys his relationship with his grandmother and great-grandmother but learns to face their inevitable death.

Douglas, E. (1990). *Rachel and the upside down heart.* Los Angeles: Price, Stern, Slogan.

The death of a little girl's father causes her to draw all her hearts upside down, but as she grows, she finds joy in her father's memory and begins to draw her hearts right-side up.

Kerner, S. (2013). *Always by my side.* Cambridge, MA: Star Bright Books.
A rhyming story that helps children understand that a father's presence is always with them

Johnson, J., & Johnson, M. (1982). *Where's Jesse?* Omaha, NE: Centering Corp.
A very young child tries to understand the death of his baby brother.

Lawton, S. (1990). *Daddy's chair.* Rockville, MD: Ken-Ben Copies.
When Michael's father dies, his family sits shivah, observing the Jewish week of mourning, and remembers the good things about him.

Melanie, B., & Kingpin, R. (1983). *Lifetimes: A beautiful way to explain death to children.* New York, NY: Bantam Books.
Explains life and death through plants, animals, and people living and dying in their time

Miller, M. (1987). *My grandmother's cookie jar.* Los Angeles: Price, Stern, Sloan.
Grandma passes on stories of their Native American ancestors to her grandchild as they eat cookies from the cookie jar.

Samuel-Traisman, E. (2015). *Remember … A child remembers.* Omaha, NE: The Centering Corporation.
A write-in memory book for children

Silverman, J. (1999). *Help me say goodbye.* Minneapolis: Fairview Press.
Activities for helping children when a special person dies

Tangvald, C. (2012). *Someone I love died.* Colorado Springs: David C. Cook.
Gently leads children through grief with age-appropriate words and solid biblical truth. The added interactive resources help the child create a memory book of the loved one's life.

Thomas, P. (2001). *I'll miss you: A first look at death.* Hauppauge, NY: Barron's Educational Services, Inc.
Offers a simple explanatory account of what

a child might feel and think when a loved one dies without subscribing to a certain spiritual belief system

Viorst, J. (1971). *The tenth good thing about Barney*. New York, NY: Athenaeum.
Young children learn about funeral rituals after the death of their cat named Barney.

Wilhelm, H. (1985). *I'll always love you*. New York, NY: Athenaeum, Crown.
A child's sadness at the death of a beloved dog is tempered by the remembrance of saying every night, "I'll always love you."

Wolfelt, Alan. (2002). *Healing your grieving heart for kids: 100 practical ideas*. Fort Collins, CO: Companion Press.
Offers suggestions for healing activities that can help survivors learn to express their grief and mourn naturally

Books for Older Children and Teens

Blackburn, L. B. (1991). *The class in room 44: When a classmate dies*. Omaha, NE: Centering Corporation.
A story to help children understand their feelings related to the death of a classmate

Bunting, E. (1990). *The wall*. New York, NY: Clarion Books.
A boy and his father come from far away to visit the Vietnam Veteran's Memorial in Washington, DC, and find the name of the boy's grandfather, who was killed in the conflict.

Fitzgerald, H. (2000). *The grieving teen: A guide for teenagers and their friends*. New York, NY: Fireside Publishing.
Addresses the special needs of teens struggling with loss

Grollman, E. (1993). *Straight talk about death for teenagers*. Boston, MA: Beacon Press.
Offers advice and answers the kinds of questions that teens are likely to ask themselves when grieving the death of someone close.

Hanson, W. (1997). *The next place*. Minneapolis, MN: Waldman House Press.
An inspirational journey of light and hope to a place where earthly hurts are left behind. Suitable for all ages.

Hughes, L. (2005). *You are not alone: Teens talk about life after the death of a parent*. New York, NY: Scholastic Paperbacks.
Words of reassurance and strategies for coping with the loss of a parent, by the director of the nation's largest bereavement camp for children

Krementz, J. (1988). *How it feels when a parent dies*. New York, NY: Macmillan.
Eighteen children ages 7 to 16 years speak openly, honestly, and unreservedly of their experiences and feelings after a parent has died.

Rubel, B. (2009). *But I didn't say goodbye: Helping children and families after a suicide*. Kendall Park, NJ: Grief Center, Inc.
A book seen through the eyes of Alex, an 11-year-old boy, whose father has died by suicide. This story is a glimpse into a child's traumatic and life-changing personal experience.

Rylant, C. (2004). *Missing May*. New York, NY: Doubleday/Dell.
For older readers; winner of the 1993 Newbery Medal. A 12-year-old girl and her uncle struggle to accept the death of Aunt May, who raised her.

Schwiebert, P., & DeKlyen, C. (2005). *Tear soup: A recipe for healing after loss*. Portland, OR: Grief Watch.
A complex story for older children, teens, and adults

The Dougy Center. (2001). *After a suicide: An activity book for grieving kids*. Portland, OR: Author.
In this hands-on, interactive workbook, children who have been exposed to a suicide can learn from other grieving kids. The workbook includes drawing activities, puzzles, stories, advice from other kids, and helpful suggestions for how to navigate the grief process after a suicide death.

The Dougy Center. (2011). *Helping teens cope with death*. Portland, OR: Author.
This practical guide covers the unique grief responses of teenagers and the specific challenges they face when grieving a death. Offers advice from parents and caregivers of bereaved teens on how to support adolescents and how to determine when professional help is needed.

The Dougy Center. (2012). *After a murder: A workbook for grieving kids.* Portland, OR: Author.
Through the stories, thoughts, and feelings of other kids who have experienced a loss through murder, this hands-on workbook allows children to see that they are not alone in their feelings and experiences. The workbook includes drawing activities, puzzles, and word games to help explain confusing elements specific to a murder, such as the police, media, and legal system.

Traisman, E. (1992). *Fire in my heart, ice in my veins: A journal for teenagers experiencing a loss.* Omaha, NE: Centering Corp.
A write-in journal for teenagers experiencing a loss

Wheeler, J. (2010). *Weird is normal when teenagers grieve.* Naples, FL: Quality of Life Publishing.
Written by a grieving teen for grieving teens

Wolfelt, A. (2001). *Healing your grieving heart for teens:* 100 practical ideas. Fort Collins, CO: Companion Press.
Offers suggestions for healing activities that can help survivors learn to express their grief and mourn naturally.

Wolfelt, A. (2002). *The healing your grieving heart journal for teens.* Fort Collins, CO: Companion Press.
This journal affirms the grieving teen's journey and offers gentle, healing guidance. Teens are encouraged to write what they miss about the person who died, the specific feelings that have been most difficult since the death, or the things they wish they had said to the person before his or her death.

Books for Parents and Caring Adults

Grollman, E. (2011). *Talking about death: A dialogue between parent and child.* Boston, MA: Beacon Press.
A read-along picture book explaining death to young children, with an extensive guide for parents; includes lists of pertinent organizations, books, tapes, and films

Silverman, P. and Kelly, M. (2009). *A parents guide to raising grieving children: Rebuilding your family after the loss of a loved one.* New York, NY: Oxford University Press.

Offers wise guidance on virtually every aspect of childhood loss, from living with someone who is dying to preparing the funeral; from explaining death to a 2-year-old to managing the moods of a grieving teenager; from dealing with people who don't understand to learning how and where to get help from friends, therapists, and bereavement groups; from developing a new sense of self to continuing a relationship with the person who died.

Wolfelt, A. (2001). *Healing a child's grieving heart: 100 practical ideas for families, friends and caregivers.* Fort Collins, CO: Companion Press.
A compassionate resource for friends, parents, relatives, teachers, volunteers, and caregivers that offers suggestions to help the grieving cope with the loss of a loved one

Warden, W. (1996). *Children and grief: When a parent dies.* New York, NY: Guilford Press.
Drawing on extensive interviews and assessments of school-age children who have lost a parent to death, this book offers a richly textured portrait of the mourning process in children. Presents major findings from the Harvard Child Bereavement Study and places them in the context of previous research, providing insights on both the wide range of normal variation in children's experience of grief and the factors that put bereaved children at risk.

References

Al-Gamal, E., & Long, T. (2010). Anticipatory grieving among parents living with a child with cancer. *Journal of Advanced Nursing, 66*(9), 1980–1990. doi: 10.1111/j.1365-2648.2010.05381.x

American Academy of Pediatrics Committee on Bioethics and Committee on Hospital Care. (2000). Palliative care for children. *Pediatrics, 106*(2), 351–355.

Attig, T. (1996). Beyond pain: The existential suffering of children. Journal of *Palliative Care, 12*(3), 20–30.

Back, K. J. (1991). Sudden, unexpected pediatric death: Caring for parents. *Pediatric Nursing, 17*(6), 571–575.

Bagatell, R., Meyer, R., Herron, S., Berger, A., & Villar, R. (2002). When children die: A seminar series for pediatric residents. *Pediatrics, 110*(2, Pt. 1), 348–353.

Bluebond-Langner, M. (1978). *The private worlds of dying children*. Princeton, NJ: Princeton University Press.

Bluebond-Langner, M., Beecham, E., Candy, B., Langner, R., & Jones, L. (2013). Preferred place of death for children and young people with life-limiting and life-threatening conditions: A systemic review of the literature and recommendations for future inquiry and policy. *Palliative Medicine, 27*(8), 705–713.

Bluebond-Langner, M., Belasco, J. B., & Wander, M. D. (2010). "I want to live, until I don't want to live anymore": Involving children with life-threatening and life-shortening illnesses in decision making about care and treatment. *Nursing Clinics of North America, 45*(3), 329–343.

Brown, P. S., & Sefansky, S. (1995). Enhancing bereavement care in the pediatric ICU. *Critical Care Nurse, 15*, 59–64.

Buckingham, R. W. (1983). *A special kind of love: Care of the dying child*. New York, NY: Continuum.

Butler, A., Hall, H., Willetts, G., & Copnell, B. (2015). Family experience and PICU death: A meta-synthesis. *Pediatrics, 136*(4), e910–e973.

Davies, B. (1999). *Shadows in the sun: The experience of sibling bereavement in childhood*. Philadelphia, PA: Taylor & Francis.

DeVita-Raeburn, E. (2004). *The empty room: Surviving the loss of a brother or sister at any age*. New York, NY: Scribner.

Doka, K. (1995). *Children mourning, mourning children*. Washington, DC: Hospice Foundation of America.

Doka, K. (2014). Living with life-threatening illness: An adolescent perspective. In K. Doka, (Ed.), *Helping adolescents cope with loss* (pp. 15–29). Washington, DC: Hospice Foundation of America.

Eilegard, A., Steineck, G., Nyberg, T., & Kreicbergs, U. (2013). Psychological health in siblings who lost a brother or sister to cancer 2 to 9 years earlier. *Psycho-Oncology, 22*, 683–691.

Feudtner, C., Kang, T., Hexem, K., Friedrichsdorf, S., Osenga, K., Siden, H., . . . Wolfe, J. (2011). Pediatric palliative care patients: A prospective multicenter cohort study. *Pediatrics, 127*, 1094–1101.

Foster, T., Dietrich, M., Friedman, D., Gordon, J., & Gilmer, M. (2012). National survey of children's hospitals on legacy-making activities. *Journal of Palliative Medicine, 15*(5), 573–578.

Frager, G. (1996). Pediatric palliative care: Building the model, bridging the gaps. *Journal of Palliative Care, 12*(3), 9–12.

Goldman, A. (1996). Home care of the dying child. *Journal of Palliative Care, 12*(3), 16–19.

Grollman, E. (1995). *Bereaved children and teens: A support guide for parents and professionals*. Boston, MA: Beacon Press.

Haas, F. (2003). Bereavement care: Seeing the body. *Nursing Standard, 17*(28), 33–37.

Himmelstein, B. P., Hilden, J. M., Boldt, A. M., & Weissman, D. (2004). Pediatric palliative care. *The New England Journal of Medicine, 350*, 1752.

Hogan, N. S., & DeSantis, L. (1994). Things that help and hinder adolescent sibling bereavement. *Western Journal of Nursing Research, 16*(2), 132–153.

Hooke, C., Hellsten, M., Stutzer, C., & Forte, K. (2002). Pain management for the child with cancer in end-of-life care: APON position paper. *Journal of Pediatric Oncology Nursing, 19*(2), 43–47.

Jones, W. H. (1978). Emergency room sudden death: What can be done for survivors? *Death Education, 2,* 231–245.

Klass, D., Silverman, P., & Nickman, S. (1996). *Continuing bonds: New understanding of grief.* Philadelphia, PA: Taylor & Francis.

Knopf, J. M., Hornung, R. W., & Slab, G. B. (2008). Views of treatment decision making from adolescents with chronic illnesses and their parents: A pilot study. *Health Expectations, 11,* 343–354.

Liben, S. (1996). Pediatric palliative medicine: Obstacles to overcome. *Journal of Palliative Care, 12*(3), 24–28.

Lowton, K. (2009). 'A bed in the middle of nowhere': Parents' meanings of place of death for adults with cystic fibrosis. *Social Science and Medicine, 69,* 1056–1062.

Machajewski, V., & Kronk, R. (2013). Childhood grief related to the death of a sibling. *Journal of the Nurse Practitioner, 9*(7), 443–448.

Madden, M. Lenhart, A., Duggan, M., Cortesi, S., & Gassert, U. (2013). *Teens and technology 2013.* Retrieved from http://www.pewinternet.org/files/old-media//Files/Reports/2013/PIP_Teen sandTechnology2013.pdf

Mathews. T. J., MacDorman, M., & Thoma, M. E. (2015). Infant mortality from 2013 period linked birth/infant death data set. *National Vital Statistics Reports, 64*(9), 1–29. http://www.cdc .gov/nchs/data/nvsr/nvsr64/nvsr64_09.pdf

Meeks, R. (2009). Parental presence in pediatric trauma resuscitation: One hospital's experience. *Pediatric Nursing, 35*(6), 376–380.

Munson, D., & Leuthner, S. R. (2007). Palliative care for the family carrying a fetus with a life-limiting diagnosis. *Pediatric Clinics of North America, 54,* 787–798

National Cancer Institute. (2013). *Grief, bereavement, and coping with loss.* Retrieved from http:// www.cancer.gov/about-cancer/advanced-cancer/caregivers/planning/bereavement-pd q#link/_65

O'Leary, J., Warland, J., & Parker, L. (2011). Bereaved parents' perception of the grandparents' reaction to perinatal loss and the pregnancy that follows. *Journal of Family Nursing, 17*(3), 330–356.

O'Malley, P., Barata, I., Snow, S., & American Academy of Pediatrics Committee on Pediatric Emergency Medicine, American College of Emergency Physicians Pediatric Emergency Medicine Committee Emergency Nurses Association Pediatric Committee. (2014). Joint Technical Report: Death of a child in the emergency department. *Pediatrics, 134*(1), e313–e330.

O'Quinn, L. P., & Giambra, B. K. (2014). Evidence of improved quality of life with pediatric palliative care. *Pediatric Nursing, 40*(6), 284–296.

Olin, R. (2014, November 1). A child's grief. *Brain, Child Magazine.* Retrieved from http://www .brainchildmag.com/2014/11/a-childs-grief/

Packman, W., Horsley, H., Davies, B., & Kramer, R. (2006). Sibling bereavement and continuing bonds. *Death Studies, 30,* 817–841.

Pearson, L. (1997). Family-centered care and the anticipated death of a newborn. *Pediatric Nursing, 23*(2), 178–182.

Pearson, L. (1999). Separation, loss and bereavement. In M. Broome & J. Rollins (Eds.), *Core curriculum for the nursing care of children and their families* (pp. 77–92). Pitman, NJ: Jannetti.

Piaget, J. (1960). *The child's concept of the world.* Patterson, NJ: Littlefield, Adams.

Postovsky, S., & Arush, M. (2004). Care of a child dying of cancer: The role of the palliative care team in pediatric oncology. *Pediatric Hematology Oncology, 21*(1), 67–76.

Price, J, Jordan, J., Prior, L., & Parkes, J. Living through the death of a child: A qualitative study of bereaved parents' experiences. *International Journal of Nursing Studies, 48,* 1384–1392.

Rando, T. (1986). *Parental loss of a child*. Champaign, IL: Research Press.

Rando, T. (2000). *Clinical dimensions of anticipatory mourning: Theory and practice in working with the dying, their loved ones, and their caregivers*. Champaign, IL: Research Press Company.

Rini, A., & Loriz, L. (2007). Anticipatory mourning in parents with a child who dies while hospitalized. *Journal of Pediatric Nursing, 22*(4), 272–282.

Roose, R. E., & Blanford, C. R. (2011). Perinatal grief and support spans the generations: Parents' and grandparents' evaluations of an intergenerational perinatal bereavement program. *Journal of Perinatal & Neonatal Nursing, 25*(1). 77–85.

Rosenberg, A. R., Postier, A., Osenga, K., Kreicbergs, U., Neville, B., Dussel, V., & Wolfe, J. (2015). Long-term psychosocial outcomes among bereaved siblings of children with cancer. *Journal of Pain and Symptom Management, 49*(1), 55–65.

Rushton, C., & Glover, J. (1990). Involving parents in decisions to forgo life-sustaining treatment for critically ill infants and children. *AACN Clinical Issues in Critical Care Nursing, 1*(1), 206–214.

Rushton, C. H., & Lynch, M. A. (1992). Dealing with advance directives for critically ill adolescents. *Critical Care Nurse, 12*(5), 31–37.

Schreiber, J. K., & Spear, C. (2014). The magic of grief camps: The impact on teens. In K. Doka, & A. Tucci (Eds.), *Helping adolescents cope with loss* (pp. 305–323). Washington, DC: Hospice Foundation of America.

Seligson, H. (2014, March 21). An online generation redefines mourning. *The New York Times*. Retrieved from http://nyti.ms/NAS9GI

Sellers, D., Dawson, R., Cohen-Bearak, A., Solomond, M., & Truog, R. (2015). Measuring the quality of dying and death in the pediatric intensive care setting: The clinician PICU-QUDD. *Journal of Pain & Symptom Management, 49*(1), 66–78.

Shapiro, E. R. (1994). *Grief as a family process: A developmental approach to clinical practice*. New York, NY: Guilford Press.

Sofka, C. (2014). Adolescent use of technology and social media to cope with grief. In Doka, K., & Tucci, A. (Eds.) *Helping adolescents cope with loss* (pp. 205–229). Washington, DC, Hospice Foundation of America.

Sourkes, B. M. (1995). *Armfuls of time: The psychological experience of the child with a life-threatening illness*. Pittsburgh, PA: University of Pittsburgh Press.

Speece, M. W., & Brent, S. B. (1996). The development of children's understanding of death. In C. A. Corr, & D. M. Corr (Eds.), *Helping children cope with death and bereavement* (pp. 29–51). New York, NY: Springer.

Stayer, D. (2012). Pediatric palliative care: A conceptual analysis for pediatric nursing practice. *Journal of Pediatrics Nursing, 27*, 350–356.

Steele, A. C., Kaal, J., Thompson, A. L., Barrera, M., Compas, B. E., Davies, B., . . . Gerhardt, C.A. (2013). Bereaved parents and siblings offer advice to health care providers and researchers. *Journal of Hematology Oncology, 35*(4), 253–259.

Sveen, J., Eilegard, A., Steineck, G., & Kreicbergs, U. (2014). They still grieve—A nationwide follow-up of young adults 2–9 years after losing a sibling to cancer. *Psycho-Oncology, 23*, 658–664.

Tan, J. S., Docherty, S. L., Barfield, R., & Brandon, D. H. (2012). Addressing parental bereavement support needs at the end of life for infants with complex conditions. *Journal of Palliative Medicine, 15*(5), 579–584.

Van der Geest, I., van den Heuvel-Eibrink, M. M., van Vliet, L. M., Pluijm, S., Streng, I., . . . Darlington, A. (2015). Talking about death with children with incurable cancer: Perspectives from parents. *The Journal of Pediatrics, 167*(6), 1320–1326.

Vose, L. A., & Nelson, R. M. (1999). Ethical issues surrounding limitation and withdrawal of support in the pediatric intensive care unit. *Journal of Intensive Care Medicine, 14*(5), 220–230.

Votta, E., Franche, R., Sim, D., Mitchell, B., Frewen, T., & Maan, C. (2001). Impact of parental involvement in life-support decisions: A qualitative analysis of parents' adjustment following their critically ill child's death. *Children's Health Care, 30*(1), 17–25.

Waechter, E. H. (1971). Children's awareness of fatal illness. *American Journal of Nursing, 71*(6), 1168–1172.

Wolfelt, A. D. (1994). *Creating meaningful funeral ceremonies: A guide for caregivers.* Fort Collins, CO: Companion Press.

Wolfelt, A. D. (1996). *Healing the bereaved child.* Fort Collins, CO: Companion Press.

World Health Organization & International Association for the Study of Pain. (1998). *Cancer pain relief and palliative care in children.* Geneva, Switzerland: WHO.

Xafis, V., Gillam, L., Hynson, J., Sullivan, J., Cossich, M., & Wilkinson, D. (2015). Caring decisions: The development of a written resource for parents facing end of life decisions. *Journal of Palliative Medicine, 18*(11), 945–955.

Youngblut, J. M., & Brooten, D. (2013). Parents' report of child's response to sibling's death in a neonatal or pediatric intensive care unit. *American Journal of Critical Care, 22*(6), 474–480.

7 Families in Children's Health-Care Settings

Judy A. Rollins

Objectives

At the conclusion of this chapter, the reader will be able to:

1. Discuss four theoretical perspectives on the family.
2. Compare and contrast a selection of types of families and the psychosocial challenges they face.
3. List three perspectives for effective practice when working with families.
4. Describe the skills essential to the effective provision of health care for families.

When thinking about a professional who works with families in pediatric health-care settings, the reader might first picture a health-care professional who works in a hospital. In this picture, the health-care professional is tending to a mother, a father, and a sick child. This traditional view is inadequate for at least three reasons: (1) the definition of family is more inclusive than mother, father, and child; (2) health-care settings are diverse, including many more places than hospitals; and (3) many health-care professionals intervene before families find themselves in crisis with sick family members.

This chapter will discuss theoretical perspectives on the family and the ways in which illness, injury, or disability disrupts the family system and its members. An overview of the many types of families is presented, along with the psychosocial challenges they face. The chapter concludes with descriptions of several perspectives that might be useful to health-care professionals who work with families and of the skills essential to effective health-care delivery.

Theoretical Perspectives on the Family

Every family is unique. However, family theories can help inform our understanding of families, reasons why family members may respond in a particular way, and how to best meet each family member's needs.

Family Systems Theory

Introduced by Murray Bowen in the 1950s, family systems theory has greatly influenced the ways in which families are viewed and services are developed and implemented. In the family-system model, the family is viewed as an interactive system of individuals and is based on four fundamental assumptions (White & Klein, 2008):

1. All parts of the system are interconnected, integrally linked with one another.
2. The family as a system can only be understood by viewing it as a whole rather than in terms of its individual parts.
3. The family system both is affected by and affects the environment.
4. Rather than being an actual physical phenomenon, the system is a way of knowing about the family and understanding its organization and experiences.

There are four major components to the family system (see Figure 7.1). These components and their relationship to the whole system are as follows:

1. *Family structure* consists of the descriptive characteristics of the family. This includes the nature of its membership and its cultural and ideological style. These characteristics are the input into the interactional system. They are the resources and the perception of the world that shape the way in which the family interacts.
2. *Family interactions* are the hub of the system. It is the process of interaction among family members that determines the rules by which the family is governed. This is the family's level of cohesion, its adaptability, and its communication style. Finally, these interactions work together to serve individual members and collective family needs.
3. *Family functions* represent the output of the interactional system. Using the resources available through its structure (input), the family interacts to produce responses that fulfill its needs.
4. *The family life cycle* (see below) introduces the element of change into the family system. As the family moves through time, developmental and non-developmental changes alter the family structure and/or the family's needs. These, in turn, produce change in the way the family interacts. (Missouri Department of Social Services, n.d.)

The family system is composed of subsystems that may include the parents, siblings, marital subsystems, parent–child subsystem, and extended family members. Meaningful support considers how family members affect one another and in turn are affected by outside forces. Health-care providers will likely have limited success in implementing any supportive intervention unless the whole family is considered (Hanson, 2013).

Family Development

Just as individuals enter different phases as they grow and develop, families, too, go through various challenges and conquer milestones unique to that phase. The family life cycle describes the series of developmental stages a family moves through over time. With each transition, the family system reorganizes, adapting the operating

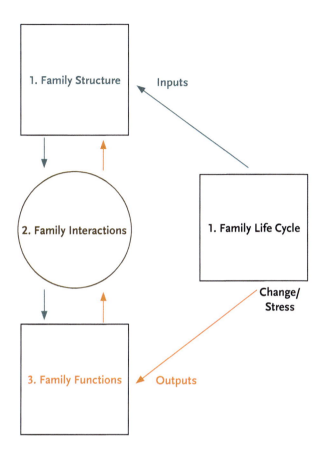

Figure 7.1. The family systems model. *Note.* From *Child Welfare Manual,* by Missouri Department of Social Services, n.d. Retrieved from http://dss.mo.gov/cd/info/cwmanual/section7/ch1_33/sec7ch1.htm

rules, roles, responsibilities, communications processes, and boundaries to meet the changing developmental needs of individual family members, family as a whole, and to adapt to the ever-changing community and larger sociocultural systems (Grossman & Okun, 2012).

In most models of the family life cycle, transitions from one stage to the next are based on the age of the oldest child (Duvall, 1977). Eight substages are embedded within three general categories of development (see Text Box 7.1: Family Life Cycle Stages).

A number of events may be happening in a family at the same time. For example, a new baby may arrive as an older child is entering elementary school. Many factors influence how a family navigates the family life cycle, which include the following (Grossman & Okun, 2012):

- Parents' stages of individual development
- Health
- Class
- Religion

Text Box 7.1
Family Life-Cycle Stages

- Foundling Family
  - Stage 1—Single married couple (no children)
- Expanding Family
  - Stage 2—Child-rearing families (children 0–30 months)
  - Stage 3—Families with preschoolers (children 2.5–6 years)
  - Stage 4—Families with school-agers (children 6–13 years)
  - Stage 5—Families with teenagers (children 13–20 years)
- Contracting Family
  - Stage 6—Families launching
  - Stage 7—Empty nest (middle-aged parents, time when all children leave home until retirement)
  - Stage 8—Retirement (retirement to death of both spouses)

Note. Adapted from *Marriage and Family Development* (6th ed.), by E. Duvall, 1977. Philadelphia, PA: J. B. Lippincott.

- Ethnicity
- Educational level
- Sexual orientation, generational, and geographical variables.

Having an understanding of the concept of the family life cycle can be important. It informs families about the tasks and concerns associated with different developmental phases and helps normalize behaviors such as teenage rebellion. As with individual development, the concept suggests that issues not dealt with successfully at one phase of development are likely to show up at later phases. For example, if an adult child has not individuated from his or her family of origin, difficulties may arise when the individual marries and becomes a parent.

Expected events frequently do not unfold in a typical sequence because other events occur, such as illness, death, or dislocation of the family unit. One factor in determining how a family is affected by such an event is the family's current phase in the family life cycle. For example, children with significant disabilities may need more time to launch or may even remain in the parental home.

Family Stress Theory

There are a number of theories about family stress. A commonly used theory in health care is the double ABCX model developed by McCubbin and Patterson (1983), which expands on Hill's (1949) ABCX model. In Hill's model, factor A (the stressor event) reacts with factor B (the family resources available to meet the stressor) and factor C (the family's appraisal or definition and interpretation of the event) to produce X (the response to the crisis). In the double ABCX model, more emphasis is placed on the family's appraisal of the event (C) and the interactive and additive nature of events (see Figure 7.2). In this model,

- A—the original stressor and the pileup of other stresses and strains
- B—the perception of resources
- C—the family's perception of the original stressor event and their appraisal of the demands and their own capacity for managing or meeting these challenges

Another feature of this model is the concept of sense of coherence—the family's ability to balance trust and control (i.e., their ability to know when to trust other authority figures versus when to take charge with their own resources) (Hanson, 2013). The concept of resiliency may also be applied to families, and its foundation lies in the understanding of family systems. Existing on a continuum from maladaption to positive adaption, the stresses of hospitalization, illness, or injury will determine whether the family faces a crisis with increased or decreased family functioning. A family's resiliency will be determined by the family's response to a given stressful event, such as a child in the hospital; their available resources; and the presence or absence of positive coping strategies. Each family, while nurturing individual members, also develops unique competencies, capabilities, and patterns of functioning that affect how the family reacts to and recovers from stressful events. A family's available resources, within themselves and the community, and their perception of the stressful event, will also affect how they respond and adapt. Family resiliency emerges from the family's adaptation and coping (Patterson, 2002).

Consider this scenario as we walk through the model. The Jefferson family faces a serious stressor. Their 5-year-old son, John, has been diagnosed with leukemia. They have two other children, an 8-year-old daughter, Maria, and another son, 2-month-old Max. The family unit goes through three stages during the time from a child's diagnosis of cancer: (1) role changes and relocation of family members and subsystems, (2) managing to maintain stability of the family unit, and (3) reuniting of family

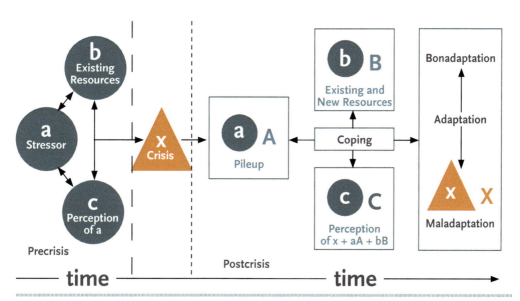

Figure 7.2. The double ABCX model. *Note.* From *Family Stress, Coping, and Social Support* (p. 44), by H. McCubbin, A. Cauble and J. Patterson, 1982, Springfield, IL: Charles C. Thomas. Copyright 1982 by Charles C. Thomas. Reprinted with permission.

members and subsystems into a unit (Kobayashi, Hayakawa, & Hohashi, 2015). The parents, Jim and Martha, both work outside the home, but Martha is still on maternity leave. The family is struggling to adjust to the new baby, with Martha, especially, being sleep deprived and the two older children growing accustomed to the altered routines a new and needy family member brings. Jim and Martha consider their resources. Both sets of grandparents live nearby and are always willing to help. The family is fortunate that Jim's employer provides excellent health insurance coverage. Martha teaches elementary school. The school year is ending soon, with the final month covered by her maternity leave, so she will not have to return to work until the fall. Jim and Martha gather information about John's condition, ask many questions, and believe they have a pretty good understanding of what lies ahead. They have worked successfully as a team to address past challenges, are confident in their health-care providers, and perceive that this event, as awful as it is, will be something they can cope with together by pulling on their own and outside resources.

Other families will have different circumstances. It is important to remember that regardless of circumstances, all families have strengths. Health-care providers can provide information and tools for coping and also help families discover the strengths that can help them traverse a crisis.

Illness/Disability as Disruption in the Family System

Although the impact of a child's illness, injury, or disability on family members has been addressed in other chapters, information here will focus on acute situations constituting a family crisis. In addition presenting the scenario of the child as the patient, the chapter will discuss the effects on a child when a parent is the ill or disabled family member.

When the Child Is the Patient

When a child is diagnosed with a serious illness or injury, the effects are felt throughout the family system. The situation affects each family member, and each family member's response affects all other family members in turn. Here we will look at the impact on parents and siblings.

Parents

The experience of a child's serious illness or injury can lead to significant and adverse psychological reactions in parents. Some studies report clinically significant acute traumatic stress reactions, involving symptoms of dissociation, re-experiencing, avoidance and arousal—all symptoms of acute stress disorder (ASD) (Muscari et al., 2015). Depression and anxiety have also been described (van Oers et al., 2014). These psychological reactions are not limited to one particular condition; they have been found in parents across a number of illness groups, for example, parents of children in pediatric intensive care (Bronner et al., 2010) or neonatal intensive care (van Oers et al.), parents of children with cardiac disease (Solberg et al., 2011), and parents of those newly diagnosed with cancer (McCarthy, Ashley, Lee, & Anderson, 2012). Research indicates that 60%–80% of individuals with ASD go on to meet diagnostic criteria for post-traumatic stress disorder (PTSD) or experience significant post-traumatic stress symptoms (PTSS) six months later (McCarthy et al.).

Parent functioning affects the psychological adjustment and recovery of the ill child, thus the need to explore these psychological reactions across different illness groups. Muscari and colleagues collected cross-sectional data from a prospective, longitudinal study of 194 parents of 145 children admitted to various hospital units for serious illnesses/injuries. Rates of acute traumatic stress, anxiety, and general stress symptoms were comparable across illness type, providing evidence that the child's medical condition is not associated with parents' experience of clinically significant psychological symptoms. Results emphasize the importance of health-care providers being aware of these potential psychological reactions in parents, regardless of the type of illness (Muscari et al., 2015).

From a family systems perspective, it is obvious that such psychological reactions in parents will in turn have an effect on other family members. So, although children and adolescents need support, it is necessary to support the parents as they provide stability for their children (Pakenham, Tilling, & Cretchley, 2012).

Siblings

Sometimes termed "the forgotten ones," siblings are likely the most left out and unattended to of all family members during the experience of a brother's or sister's serious childhood illness or injury. For example, at the time a brother's or sister is diagnosed with cancer, at least to some degree, all siblings feel left out. Family, friends—even health-care professionals—focus on the ill child and the parents. Siblings are frequently overlooked in the process.

Drastic changes may occur in the healthy siblings' relationships with parents and the ill sibling. Some of these changes result from the demands of the disease itself. The child who is sick becomes the focus of parental attention and concerns, resulting in a shift in family dynamics. For example, current protocols for cancer treatment typically require parents to spend extended time in the hospital or clinic (Long, Marsland, Wright, & Hinds, 2015). Day-to-day roles, responsibilities, and patterns of functioning change to accommodate treatment demands (Long & Marsland, 2011). Changes may interfere with holiday celebrations, vacations, and social interactions—intrusions that frequently demand self-sacrifice on the part of healthy siblings. Parents may be unable to attend siblings' school functions, ball games, or other activities and, in their own struggle to adapt, are often physically and emotionally unavailable.

Some of the difficulties siblings face can stem from the nature of the sibling relationship itself. It is within the sibling subsystem that children learn to share, compete, and compromise with others close to them in status. Healthy siblings lose their equal relationship with the brother or sister who has a serious illness or disability. A child's illness places constraints on siblings when love and competition have been part of their ongoing relationship. The siblings are no longer able to compete, at least temporarily. Furthermore, when siblings have a caring and loving relationship, the time apart can prove difficult, despite the many ways to stay in touch in today's digital world.

In recent years, with stem cell transplant becoming standard therapy for many life-threatening childhood disorders, many siblings are playing a more active role in their brother's or sister's treatment. Little attention has been focused on the psychosocial effects of the transplant process for siblings, whether they are donors or nondonors (see Text Box 7.2: Sibling Donors). Research shows that siblings are at risk for developing emotional reactions such as PTSD, anxiety, and overall low self-esteem (Packman, Gong, VanZutphen, Shaffer, & Crittenden, 2004). Interviews with siblings 11 to 24 years old have revealed "interruption" in the family as a main theme (Wilkins & Woodgate, 2007a). Basic everyday activities (e.g., going to school) were difficult. Schedules and roles changed dramatically; the family was no longer "normal." In another study, siblings told Wilkins and Woodgate (2007b) what kinds of support would be helpful during the transplant process: (1) Include me in the definition of *family*, (2) be caring, (3) share information with me, (4) give me choices, (5) help me share feelings, (6) provide opportunities for me to meet my peers, and (7) create a healthy hospital environment.

In an effort to identify the support that child life specialists provide to siblings, Schwartz (2013) conducted a survey of Certified Child Life Specialists across the United States and Canada through the Child Life Council's national Listserv. The

Text Box 7.2
Sibling Donors

The decision to donate stem cells to a brother or sister is a selfless gift, but the decision can be difficult. Siblings need to understand the process and what it involves, and to be aware of side effects that may affect their decision.

Some sibling donors report a lack of choice when asked to donate. They face a twofold dilemma: Their sibling is a chronically ill child, and they have been asked to take on the responsibility of serving as a donor (Weaver, Diekema, Carr, & Triplett, 2015). This overwhelming sense of responsibility for their sibling's survival often leads to psychological distress. In a study by MacLeod, Whitsett, Mash, and Pelletier (2003), 5 of the 15 siblings reported feeling as though their opportunity to say no was limited. They perceived having no choice because of expectations from doctors and family members. Nine of the participants felt that their own religious beliefs prevented them from declining to donate. Further, siblings stated that the informed consents involve no choice and the psychological aspects of the procedure significantly outweighed the physical aspects of the procedure.

Some medical centers are using child life specialists to educate, prepare, and lend support to sibling donors through counseling and therapeutic activities to address the emotional distress that accompanies their situation. Other centers have developed programs to assist sibling donors. At Hospital for Sick Children in Toronto, Canada, for example, siblings participate in age-appropriate medical play and discuss feelings and concerns. They receive a certificate for their donation. Evaluation findings indicate that the children and parents found the program very helpful and felt that it had a positive effect on the sibling donors' psychological health, with 97% rating the program as very helpful (Shama, 1998).

Sibling interventions are often limited to the donor sibling only. An early study suggests interventions are just as import for nondonor siblings. A study with 44 siblings of surviving pediatric bone-marrow transplant recipients—21 donors and 23 nondonors ages 6 to 18 years—reported significantly more school problems among nondonor siblings than for donor siblings (Packman, Crittenden, & Scheffer, 1998). A third of nondonor siblings reported a moderate level of post-traumatic stress reaction.

findings revealed a high prevalence of sibling programs, with 64% of medical institutions surveyed having programs focused specifically on siblings. Sibling programs featured education as well as emotional expression. Areas not commonly addressed by respondents but considered important include the use of support groups and activities to help children cope with disruption in daily activities.

When a Parent Is the Patient

In Western societies, it is estimated that 5% to 15% of children ages 4 to 18 years have a parent with a serious medical condition (Sieh, Visser-Meily, & Meijer, 2013). In a study that examined differences in adjustment between children from four groups: (1) a parent with illness, (2) another family member with illness, (3) both parental illness and other family member illness, and (4) "healthy" families, Pakenham and Cox (2014) reported that the presence of any family member with an illness was associated with greater risk of mental health difficulties for youths relative to peers from healthy families. This risk is elevated if the ill family member is a parent and has mental illness or substance misuse.

A parent's diagnosis of cancer triggers psychological and social pressure in children in all domains of child functioning, but particularly emotional well-being. Studies suggest that adolescents demonstrate greater anxiety, depression, and emotional distress than school-age children (Huizinga et al., 2011). However, in looking at risk behaviors and externalizing behaviors in adolescents dealing with parental cancer, Jantzer et al. (2013) concluded that for adolescents in their study, parental illness was not a developmental risk expressed in increased levels of risky behavior. Generally, the adolescents adjusted quite well, although some individuals did show signs of severe strain.

Pakenham and Cox (2015) point out that serious parental illness shifts family roles and is typically associated with more intense youth caregiving. Three interrelated components are involved: (1) behavioral caregiving tasks, (2) a psychological sense of caregiving responsibilities, and (3) broader psychosocial experiences associated with caregiving. Research has shown that higher youth caregiving is related to poorer mental health outcomes (Pakenham & Cox, 2012).

In a review of the literature on adolescents living with a parent with advanced cancer, Phillips (2014) found a consensus that parents did not receive guidance or support from health-care providers on how to talk to their children. In fact, parents felt that health-care providers avoided discussions about advanced cancer or death and they were left to deal with the issue alone. (See Appendix 7.1: Resources for helpful publications for parents and children.)

In her classic book, *How to Help Children Through a Parent's Serious Illness*, McCue (2011) emphasized that children must be told the truth about their parent because children are affected by everything that happens in the family; the more serious the situation, the more it will affect them; and lying to them, in any way, will inevitably make things worse. She cites three things that parents should tell their children, regardless of age:

1. Tell them you are seriously ill.
2. Tell them the name of your disease.
3. Tell them your best understanding of what may happen. (p. 18)

With some conditions, such as multiple sclerosis (MS), the inability to predict the course of the complex disease brings uncertainty to the whole family—uncertainty the children may live with throughout their childhood and beyond. The children's ability to cope with the chronic disease appears to be determined by how well the healthy parent copes (Ehrensperger et al., 2008). Communication is critical. If parents choose not to talk about it, the children may hesitate to ask questions, thus decreasing communication. How well children are able to cope also depends on their understanding of the disease. Finally, it is important to remember that all families have their own history and developmental phases, both as individuals and as families. A study that explored the perspectives of the parents with MS, the healthy parents, and the children found that healthy parents often took longer than their partner with MS to come to terms with the diagnosis (Bostrom & Nilsagard, 2016). Families tend to develop strategies for managing in everyday life over time.

Overview of Families

Over the past 50 years, the composition of families in the United States has changed significantly. According to Daugherty and Copen (2016), these changes have resulted from a delay in the age of first marriage, a steep rise and then decline in the divorce rate, a lower fertility rate, an increase in cohabitation, a higher proportion of births occurring outside of marriage and within cohabiting unions, and an increasing number of first births to older women. Studies have demonstrated that attitudes about family life, such as an increasing acceptance of premarital sex, cohabitation, and divorce, have changed not only by variation in age but also with the passage of time (England & Bearak, 2014; Twenge, Sherman, & Wells, 2015).

In 2014, 64% of children ages 0 to 17 years lived with two married parents, down from 77% in 1980 (Forum on Child and Family Statistics, 2015). Another 4% lived with two biological or adoptive cohabiting parents, and 24% lived with only their mothers, 4% with only their fathers, and 4% with no parent in the household. Of that 4% not living with a parent, 56% lived with grandparents (see Figure 7.3)

In addition to the nuclear family of married heterosexual mother and father and child(ren), a variety of other family configurations exist, each with its own psychosocial implications. A selection of these variations is described below.

Single-Parent Families

Single-parent families come about in several ways. The most common reason is parental divorce or separation. Research has shown that children whose parents divorce are more likely to show emotional and behavioral problems than are children in intact families (Coleman & Glen, 2009). Difficulties seem to be largely associated with aspects of the divorce, particularly conflict between parents, rather than single-parenthood itself (Golombok, Zadeh, Imrie, Smith, & Freeman, 2016). Other factors cited include the financial hardship often experienced by single-parent families following divorce, parental depression, and poor parenting quality (Golombock et al., 2016).

There has been a rise in the number of children born to single unmarried mothers as a result of unplanned pregnancies. Waldfogel, Craigie, and Brooks-Gunn (2010) found

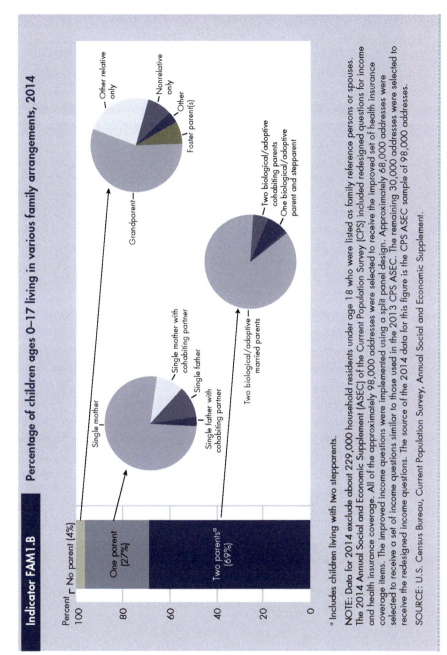

Figure 7.3. Percentage of children ages 0–17 living in various family arrangements, 2014. *Note.* U.S. Census Bureau, Current Population Survey, Annual Social and Economic Supplement.

more negative mental health outcomes for children born to single unmarried mothers than to married parents, even after controlling differences in parental resources. Some of the same factors associated with more negative outcomes for single-mother families formed by divorce—economic disadvantage, parental mental health problems, and poor parenting quality—have been cited as contributing factors (Kiernan & Mensah, 2010).

The newest type of single-mother family is the single heterosexual woman who has had a child through donor insemination and has chosen to parent alone, generally referred to as "mothers by choice" or "solo mothers" (Golombok et al., 2016). Even though these women have chosen to parent alone, the majority do so not from choice but because they do not have a current partner and feel that time is running out for them to have a child (Graham & Braverman, 2012). With the shift toward older first-time motherhood, the number of such families is expected to grow (Graham, 2012). In a study that compared 51 solo-mother families with 52 two-parent families, all with a child from 4 to 9 years of age conceived by donor insemination, Golombok and colleagues reported no differences in parenting quality between family types except for lower mother–child conflict in solo-mother families. No differences were found in child adjustment. Perceived financial difficulties, child's gender, and parenting stress were factors associated with children's adjustment problems in both family types. The researchers concluded that solo motherhood, in itself, does not result in psychological problems for children.

Golombok et al. (2016) remind us that a potential risk factor for the children of single mothers by choice that does not exist for children from other types of single-mother families is their donor conception. We know that adopted children show an increased interest in their biological parents at adolescence, which suggests that children of single mothers by choice may have the same experience. The absence of information about identity may produce challenges at that time. Further, in a study of 3- to 11-year-old donor-conceived children of solo mothers, Weissenberg and Landau (2012) reported that all the children expressed a wish for a father.

Fathers are increasingly heading single-parent households. In fact, the rate increased ninefold from 1960 to 2011 (Livingston, 2013a). This increase is likely attributable to a number of factors, most of which have contributed to the decline in two-married-parent and single-mother households:

- Marked increase in the share of nonmarital births
- Higher divorce rates than in the 1960s and 1970s
- Changes in the legal system giving more opportunities to fathers
- Acknowledgement of fathers' importance as caregivers (Livingston, 2013a, p. 3).

According to Pew Research surveys, the public believes that the father's greatest role is to provide values to his children, followed by emotional support, discipline, and income support. Of interest, the public ascribes roughly the same hierarchy of roles to mothers (Livingston, 2013a). As with single mothers, single fathers tend to be less educated and less well off than their married counterparts. However, households headed by single fathers appear to be much better off financially when compared to those headed by single mothers.

Contrary to findings in the general population that women are at greater risk for depression compared to men, Ayer, Woldetsadik, Malsberger, Burgette, and Kohl

(2016) found no significant differences in the prevalence of depression among male and female primary caregivers in the child welfare system. They also reported that fathers are less likely than mothers to seek medical care for themselves or for their children. Ayer et al. investigated the longitudinal effects of primary caregiving fathers' mental health and substance use on child mental health with a sample of 322 youths living with a male primary caregiver. They found that father depression at baseline consistently predicted child mental health outcomes three years later, even after accounting for demographics and baseline child mental health. Fathers' substance use was not a predictor, and interactions with child age and gender were not significant. Findings suggest that efforts to improve engagement of and attention to fathers with research, clinical, and policy efforts are likely to be worthwhile.

Blended Families

A blended or stepfamily is a family in which one or both parents have one or more children from a previous relationship that are not genetically related to the other parent. Blended families may come about following the death of a parent or from a divorce. In the case of divorce, children may live with one biological parent all the time or share time between biological parents.

In blended families, children often are grieving and may not be mature enough to explain their unhappiness (Forman, 2015). They may feel uprooted from their other biological parent and torn by the tension between them. They can feel alienated in the blended family and perhaps feel unwanted or disliked by their stepparent. Holidays and major events can be uncomfortable, and children may miss the parent–child traditions that existed before the new family. There may be the stress of a new house, school, friends, church, and so forth. And, with the remarriage, there's the loss of their dream or fantasy that their parents will reconcile.

A child's age is a factor in adjustment (Forman, 2015). Children 10 years old and younger may adjust the most easily because they have more daily caregiving needs and are more accepting of new adults in their life. Children age 11–14 years tend to have the most difficulty adjusting and move at a slow pace to bond with a new adult. Although they may not demonstrate their feelings openly, they may be more sensitive than a younger child. Children in this age range may find it very difficult to accept a stepparent's or new partner's discipline. Teenagers age 15 years and older may have less involvement with family life and may push away and separate from family to form their own identities. Although they may not express their feelings, they still crave approval and acceptance.

Papernow (1993) listed seven stages of stepfamily development that blended families move through in four to seven years:

1. *Fantasy*—Adults expect a smooth and quick adjustment, while children expect that the stepparent will disappear and their parents will be reunited.
2. *Immersion*—Tension-producing conflict emerges between the stepfamily's two biological subunits.
3. *Awareness*—Family members realize that their early fantasies are not becoming reality.

4. *Mobilization*—Family members initiate efforts toward change.
5. *Action*—Remarried adults decide to form a solid alliance, family boundaries are better clarified, and there is more positive stepparent–stepchild interaction.
6. *Contact*—The stepparent becomes a significant adult family figure, and the spouse assumes more control.
7. *Resolution*—The stepfamily achieves integration and appreciates its unique identity as a stepfamily.

According to the U.S. Bureau of the Census (2006), 60% of all remarriages eventually end in divorce. For stepfamilies, some never move through the seven stages of stepfamily development, often getting caught in a stage and unable to progress

Families With Multiples

A report from the Centers for Disease Control and Prevention (CDC) (2015) tells us that the twin birthrate in America is at an all-time high, almost doubling in the last 35 years. In 2014 there were 33.9 twins born for every 1,000 births, or from another perspective, 1 in every 29 babies is a twin. Two primary reasons are often credited with the increase (Martin et al., 2003). First, women are waiting until they are older to have children, and women in their 30s are more likely to have twins than young mothers. The report states that the average age at the time of her first child's birth is 26.3 years. Secondly, the increase in the use of assisted reproductive technology such as in-vitro fertilization often results in multiple children because its methodology prescribes the implantation of more than one egg per womb. However, guidelines now limit the number of embryos that can be inserted. The report added that the rates for triplets, quadruplets, and other multiple births (MB) have been steadily falling in the past few years, to the lowest levels in 20 years (CDC, 2015), likely a result of these guidelines.

Although the obstetric and neonatal risks of multiple births have been well described in the literature, psychosocial risks, quality of life, and other significant issues have received less attention. We do know that quality of life is compromised in parents of MB, especially triplets, as is maternal bonding in the first year of life; this can lead to emotional problems (Feldman & Eidelman, 2005). Further, research suggests that mothers of multiples have more problems related to parental stress than mothers of singletons (Golombok, Olivennes, Ramogida, Rust, & Freeman, 2007).

Examining mother–infant interaction variables, Feldman and Eidelman (2005) showed that there were more positive interactions in the singleton and twin groups than in the triplet group, and also that the maternal parenting style was less sensitive. They concluded that differences in cognitive scores at 24 months might be due, in part, to those effects. The higher incidence of maternal depression and child abuse in multiple-birth families are likely also the result of parental stress (Rand, Eddleman, & Sonte, 2005).

Impact of Multiples on Marriage

Haddon and Teschow (2008) surveyed 158 mothers and fathers of twins, triplets, and quadruplets from across Canada regarding how multiples can affect the marital relationship. Looking back at the pregnancy, 78% reported a strong relationship. By the end of the first year with their babies, 34% said their relationship got worse or much worse. However, nearly half of the parents experienced some improvement in their relationship *after* the first year and dramatic improvement after 3 to 5 years.

Respondents noted the lack of high-quality, early-onset relevant prenatal instruction. Almost half the parents took some kind of prenatal course together; however, only 23% of the courses were multiples specific. Also, classes reportedly did not address the effects of the multiples on marriage, or if so, did so only vaguely. Said one mother:

> I read several books, but I was still not quite prepared [for] the TOTAL EXHAUSTION after giving birth. People tended to talk a lot about pre-birth and then later (not the immediate few weeks after birth), which is tough when you have twins. Lack of sleep killed me and my husband (figuratively speaking, of course). (Haddon & Teschow, 2008, p. 2)

Multiples had both positive and negative effects on respondents' marriages. Positive effects included forcing teamwork and joint problem solving, developing strong family bonds, opening up new friendships through multiples support groups, and being able to really focus on one developmental stage at a time. They stated that the most difficult challenges are related to financial strain, lack of time (alone, for each other, and in general), and lack of sleep (Haddon & Teschow, 2008). The following are practices that help couples get through those first few difficult years:

- Being prepared
- Getting help for baby care, housecleaning, shopping, meal preparation
- Involving both partners with the care of the infants
- Using parental leave
- Connecting with other parents of multiples
- Setting aside regularly scheduled couples time
- Checking with each other and acting as a unified front
- Seeking professional help, if needed

The Twin Relationship

Being a twin is a unique experience. Unlike only children or nontwin siblings, twins are together from the time of conception through young adulthood and sometimes throughout their lifetime. Most of their time is spent together, and they share significant life events. These special environmental conditions have an effect on their psychosocial and social development and the relationships they form throughout their lives (see Figure 7.4).

For all children, forming an identity is important; however, forming an identity separate from the other twin is one of the biggest difficulties for twins. Twins often define themselves and are defined by others as a unit, part of a set. The "oneness" discussed by Erikson and Erikson (1982) is achieved not by one person but by two who share an identity. Separation from the parents and the home in late adolescence can be much more difficult for twins than for singletons. Lander (2008) pointed out that twins experience an extremely close bond with each other that compensates for difficulties parents may face in raising twins. In fact, parents may actively encourage one twin

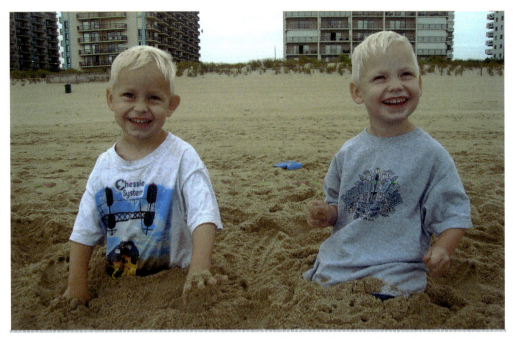

Figure 7.4. Being a twin is a unique experience. *Note.* Photograph used with permission of Milisa Rollins.

as a parent substitute for the other. Thus, given that twins often act as primary care-givers for each other, separation from the twin—not necessarily separation from the parent—could be the chief hurdle. Research indicates that separation from one's twin is extremely challenging and often comes with a great deal of conflict and hesitation (Cassell, 2011).

Twins also project the twinship onto other relationships, identified as "twin yearn-ing," or the apparent need to reestablish the twin relationship with other people in adult life (Jarrett & McGarty, 1980). Twins may consciously and unconsciously regress into thinking that they can expect the same intensity with new people in their lives as they had with their twin (Klein, 2003). Twin yearning is understandable, yet the con-tinuous longing for another twin can cause a strain on the twin relationship and is a hurdle for twins seeking their own identity to overcome.

Lesbian, Gay, Bisexual, and Transgender Families

Public opinion on same-sex marriage has progressed slowly for decades in the United States; only in the past 5 years did a majority of people come to approve of same-sex unions. Thus, on July 26, 2015, the U.S. Supreme Court redefined family, ruling in *Obergefell v. Hodges* that state laws prohibiting same-sex marriage are unconstitutional. The benefits of legally recognized marriage are now extended to sexual and gender minority couples.

According to the 2013 National Health Interview Survey, there are about 131,000 same-sex couples raising approximately 200,000 children in the United States (Gates, 2014). The bulk of the research on the well-being of children raised in same-gender households addresses lesbian parents. Findings taken together have confirmed that chil-dren are not disadvantaged as a result of being parented by lesbian women (Golombok

& Badger, 2010; Perrin & Siegel, 2013). There have been occasional challenges to this conclusion (e.g., Marks, 2012; Regnerus, 2012), but because of these studies' methodology or serious flaws in interpretation, much of the scientific community has discredited the conclusions (Cheng & Powell, 2015). The growing consensus is that

> children's well-being is affected much more by their relationships with their parents, their parents' sense of competence and security, and the presence of social and economic support for the family than by the gender or the sexual orientation of their parents. (Perrin & Siegel, 2013, p. e1378)

Most gay fathers through the mid-1990s were men who had parented children in heterosexual relationships and later came out as homosexual, and early research mainly documented the challenges presented to these families by social stigma surrounding divorce and homosexuality (Perrin, Pinderhughes, Mattern, Hurley, & Newman, 2016). With shifts in attitudes and social and legal changes, gay men now become parents through adoption or with the assistance of a lesbian couple or a surrogate carrier. Despite these breakthroughs, parenthood for gay men has challenges. People may criticize them and/or be suspicious about their motive to adopt and consider their family deficient because of the absence of a female parent. Their gay friends may be confused and critical about their choice to become parents (Goldberg, 2012).

Perrin and colleagues (2016) surveyed 61 gay fathers regarding their experiences. Findings revealed the experiences of stigma directed at them and their children, especially from family members, friends, and people in religious institutions. Nevertheless, the study reported gay fathers' active engagement in parenting activities and that their children's well-being was consistent with national samples.

Little is known about transgender parents, how they have negotiated their parental gender transition (PGT), and subsequent stressors. Family functioning is especially important for transgender parents because they often experience some form of familial rejection as a result of transition (Veldorale-Griffin & Darling, 2016). Furthermore, family acceptance has been shown to be a protective factor for a number of negative outcomes for transgender people, including substance abuse and suicide attempts (Grant et al., 2011). Veldorale-Griffin and Darling examined three stressors related to PGT (i.e., the impact of disclosure, the experience of stigma, and the presence of boundary ambiguity) with a sample of 73 transgender parents, ages 26–68 years. The researchers used a battery of eight quantitative measures. Results suggested that stigma, boundary ambiguity, and sense of coherence had the greatest effects on family functioning and that a strong sense of coherence may act as a protective factor against the effects of stigma. Greater experiences of stigma and boundary ambiguity were associated with lower satisfaction with family functioning, and a greater sense of coherence was linked to higher satisfaction with family functioning. The notion that viewing one's life as comprehensible and manageable can lead to better outcomes suggests that the extent to which a person's minority identity is an important, positive, and integrated part of him- or herself may alleviate the negative impact of minority stresses.

Children's Perceptions

In examining children's perceptions of being raised by same-sex parents, Farr, Crain, Oakley, Cashen, and Garber (2016) addressed feelings of differences, microaggressions (see Text Box 7.3), and resilience. They interviewed 49 adopted boys and girls ($M = 8$ years of age; 47% girls), 27 from two-father families and 22 from two-mother families. Over three-quarters of the children reported experiencing feelings of difference regarding being aware that their family was different from other families in some capacity, discomfort in telling others about having same-sex parents, having their guard up until establishing trust or security in their friendships before opening up about their families, having their own negative thoughts or feelings about their parents or families on the basis of parental sexual orientation, and fear of rejection. Over half of the children reported experiencing microaggressions. Heterosexism was the most common subtheme (e.g., "My friends sometimes they, like [say], then you tell your mom, then—but I'm like, dude, I have two dads" [p. 93]). Other microaggressions include having details about their family made public in school or other social situations, hearing derogatory comments about sexual-minority people and/or experiencing discrimination due to having same-sex parents, being teased or bullied, being the spokesperson and asked many questions about same-sex-parent families, and having others question the authenticity and legitimacy of their family on the basis of having same-sex parents.

In a recent study, children discussed an abundance of positive feelings regarding their families, with 71% reporting 92 total instances of resilience and positive feelings, and 25 of these children reporting more than one such instance (Farr et al., 2016). Children talked about how they coped with microaggressions or feeling different as a result of having same-sex parents (e.g., "One of my friends used to bully me because I had two moms, but I told him about how it [my family] is different and how it [my family] is the same and he changed his mind" [p. 94]). Many children termed their families special and talked about why they loved their parents (e.g., kind, awesome, nice to me, fun, exciting, energetic, making them feel special). The researchers concluded that with more reports of instances of resilience and positive family conceptualizations than microaggressions or feelings of difference, findings suggest that children develop positive perception of their family and navigate experiences of difference with resilience.

LGBT Families and the Health-Care System

According to Gulliford (2013), individuals and groups who are socially or culturally marginalized may face greater barriers to health care than others because of

Text Box 7.3
Microaggressions

Microaggressions are subtle ways in which others oppress individuals of marginalized groups (Sue et al., 2007), which includes non-heterosexual persons. There are three different categories of microaggressions based on severity (Sue, 2010).

- *Microinvalidations:* Communications that subtly exclude, negate, or nullify the experiences/thoughts/feelings of a marginalized group
- *Microinsults:* Verbal, nonverbal, and environmental communications that subtly convey insensitivity and rudeness that demeans another individual based on their minority status
- *Microassaults:* Conscious and intentional acts of name-calling, avoidance, or other derogatory behaviors toward a marginalized group

discrimination, difficulties with language, or anxiety about accessing services. Despite equity policies, other, less tangible barriers may remain, especially those related to cultural bias or lack of familiarity among staff with particular groups or cultures (Celik, Abma, Klinge, & Widdershoven, 2012).

Regarding same-sex parented families, a small body of research has identified the following barriers to health-care access:

- Intake or medical history forms often do not accommodate same-sex couples, thus providers may not have appropriate information and one parent may not be afforded decision-making power for the child's medical care (Hayman, Wilkes, Halcomb, & Jackson, 2013)
- Health providers' heterosexist assumptions may take the form of not recognizing a family as a family (e.g., assuming one parent is a friend or other relative (Hayman et al, 2013).
- Health providers may insist on information about children's genetic parentage even when it is irrelevant to the situation, which same-sex parents often experience as a lack of respect for their family makeup by not recognizing the parental role of nonbiological parents (Chapman et al., 2012).
- Health providers often engage with only one parent during the health-care consultations, usually excluding the nonbiological parent (Goldberg & Allen, 2012).
- Many health-care providers believe same-sex parents' disclosure of their sexuality is unimportant and has no bearing on the quality of care they deliver. Some parents do want to disclose this information, and this attitude places the onus on them to raise the topic (Chapman et al., 2012).

Von Doussa and colleagues (2016) held focus groups with 10 same-sex parents and 32 health providers regarding their perceptions of barriers for same-sex parents' engaging with health and welfare services. The findings revealed that the health-care providers lacked confidence and skills in working with same-sex parents. Although no parents in the study felt they had experienced direct discrimination or homophobia, they did mention encountering providers who, despite having an interest in offering an inclusive service, asked inappropriate questions or no questions at all, or did not offer appropriate acknowledgement of their family. The researchers concluded that professional training was needed, which should incorporate the following elements (p. 8):

1. Raise awareness and challenge attitudes among workers who currently hold negative attitudes towards same-sex parented families.
2. Provide information about issues regarding same-sex parents and their children and the opportunity to safely ask questions. This may include role-plays, which will allow providers to practice questions and help them develop language to have "at the ready" in consultations.
3. Encourage self-reflection on attitudes and assumptions and the implications for practice.
4. Include skill-based training in areas such as asking about sexuality or family makeup and opening discussions.

The aim of the study was the development of practice guidelines for health-care providers (von Doussa et al., 2016). See Text Box 7.4: Brief Guidelines for Working With Same-Sex-Parented Families in Health-Care Settings.

LGBT Children

LGBT individuals make up approximately 5% of the youth population (Morris, 2014). In 2012, the Human Rights Campaign conducted a groundbreaking study among more than 10,000 LGBT-identified youths ages 13 to 17 years to gain a better understanding of their experiences, needs, and concerns. Responses revealed that many LGBT youths are profoundly disconnected from their communities. Nevertheless, they often report resilience in facing challenges and a sense of optimism about future possibilities. Of interest, LGBT youths believe to a greater extent than their non-LGBT peers that they must leave their communities to make their hopes and dreams come true. For additional findings, see Text Box 7.5: Selected Findings From Growing Up LGBT in America.

Health-Care Services. Adolescents are known to have difficulty accessing health-care service for a variety of reasons, with lack of health insurance, poverty, and racial minority status predictors of the quality and quantity of health care received by adolescents in the United States (Williams & Chapman, 2012). For youths who identify as non-heterosexual or who report same-sex romantic attractions or relationships, concerns about stigmatization, marginalization, and mistreatment may be barriers to help seeking and service use. Youths may avoid discussing their sexuality out of concerns about privacy or fears of provider judgment or rejection, and thus preclude the delivery of needed services.

Williams and Chapman (2011) found that, as compared with heterosexual peers, sexual-minority youth (SMY) had significantly higher proportions of unmet health-care needs and unmet mental health needs. Regarding protective factors (i.e., child–parent connectedness, support of other caring adults, and school safety), Eisenberg and Resnick (2006) reported that SMYs have overall lower levels of protective factors compared with their heterosexual peers. Those SMYs with higher levels were less likely to report suicide ideation and attempts. Another study revealed that higher levels of family rejection based on adolescents' sexual orientation or gender identity were associated with health risk behaviors (i.e., increases rates of alcohol and drug use, unprotected sex) and negative mental health outcomes (i.e., higher rates of depression and suicidality) in young adulthood (Ryan, Heubner, Diaz, & Sanchez, 2009).

Using a representative national sample of adolescents ($N = 18,924$) from the national Longitudinal Study of Adolescent Health survey, Williams and Chapman (2012) explored sexual-minority status and child-parent connectedness in relation to the unmet needs for health or mental health care. They found that SMY had 31% higher odds of having an unmet health need compared with peers, but that youths who reported higher levels of child–parent connectedness had lower odds of having an unmet health need. As for mental health need, SMY had 48% higher odds of having an unmet need compared with peers. Significant predictors of unmet mental health needs were (a) child–parent connectedness, (b) youth health-insurance status, (c) parent disability status, and (d) family income level. As with health-care need, youths who reported higher levels of child–parent connectedness had significantly lower odds of having an unmet mental health need. Findings remind providers of the importance of family relationships in both health and mental health care for sexual-minority youth.

Text Box 7.4
Brief Guidelines for Working With Same-Sex-Parented Families in Health-Care Settings

What same-sex-parented families value when using health-care services:

- Accepting and affirming attitudes from service providers, with a welcoming and friendly approach
- Understanding from service providers that it is important that the role of both parents is openly acknowledged in consultations
- Inclusive language from service providers to indicate it is safe to "come out." This may include service providers asking directly whether a client identifies as LGB or same-sex attracted and/or the gender of their partner (see door-opening questions)
- Appropriate questions being asked about family makeup. Some questions about a child's biological heritage or conception can be intrusive and alienating (see door-opening questions)
- Knowledgeable service providers. Same-sex parents can become frustrated at having to educate service providers about their families, especially since useful information and resources are increasingly available online
- Trusted referrals. When referring same-sex parents to other providers, these should be to LGB-sensitive services where possible

Tips for creating a welcoming environment:

- Display LGB-inclusive signs, posters, and books in the waiting room
- Intake forms send a message about the inclusivity of the service as well as collecting important information. Review forms to ensure they use inclusive language and accommodate same-sex couples. Provide an opportunity for people to disclose their sexual orientation and the gender of their partner if relevant, or if the form is for a child, ask about the gender of each parent
- Make a habit of explicitly telling new clients that the service is welcoming of all types of families, including same-sex families. Communicate an inclusive message on all information and resources from the service
- Reflect on your own values and practices. Pay attention to times when you assume or take for granted that a client is heterosexual

Door-opening questions:

- Door-opening questions are designed to put clients at ease and invite them to talk about their family structure in a safe way. A simple and useful question is: "Tell me about your family." If a client is alone: "Tell me about yourself? Do you have a partner? How does your partner describe their gender?" If two clients present: "Tell me about yourselves—what is your relationship?" or, if there is a child: "Tell me about your family? Are you the parents?" Take care to acknowledge both adults when asking questions about children
- Pay attention to the language people use when they describe their family. Remember all same-sex families are not the same. When seeing a family in a counseling setting, for example, always ask about the language the family uses. You could ask: "So I can get a picture of your family, can you tell me what your kids call you at home? Is this different when you are away from home? Are there other people who play an important role in your family life?"
- Respect that the parent or parents who are caring for their child are, in fact, that child's parents. Asking questions about biology or conception out of curiosity can be alienating, so avoid doing this unless you know the clients well and are confident this will be OK for them. When information about a child's birth or biological parent is needed, ask sensitively. For instance, in a maternal/child-health nurse visit where the

(continues)

Text Box 7.4 (*continued*)

nurse needs to check the health of the birth mother, he or she could ask, "How are you both adjusting to parenthood? We like to check in on the mental well-being of both parents and the physical health of the birth mother. Who is the birth mother?"

Note. From "Building Healthcare Workers' Confidence to Work with Same-sex Parented Families," by H. von Soussa, J., Power, R. McNair, R. Brown M. Schofield, A. Perlesz, M. Pitts and A. Bickerdike, 2015, *Health Promotion International*. Advance online publication, p. 9. doi: 10.1093/heapro /dav010. By permission of Oxford University Press.

Text Box 7.5
Selected Findings From Growing Up LGBT in America

- Non-LGBT youths are nearly twice as likely as LGBT youths to say they are happy.
- LGBT youths are more likely than non-LGBT youths to report that they do not have an adult they can talk to about personal problems.
- LGBT youths are more than twice as likely as non-LGBT youths to experiment with alcohol and drugs.
- Roughly three-quarters (73%) of LGBT youths say they are more honest about themselves online than in the real world, compared to 43% of non-LGBT youths.
- LGBT youths described the most important problems they were currently facing as non-accepting families (26%), school/bullying problems (21%), and fear of being out or open (18%).
- LGBT youths are twice as likely as their peers to say they have been physically assaulted, kicked, or shoved at school.
- More than half of LGBT youths reported being out to their immediate family; a quarter are out to their extended family.
- Nearly half of LGBT youths chose their family among a list of places where they most often hear negative messages about being LGBT.
- 4 in 10 LGBT youths say the community in which they live is not accepting of LGBT people.
- Only 21% of LGBT youths say there is a place in their community that helps LGBT people; the same (21%) say there is a non-official place in their community where LGBT youths can go and be accepted.
- 18% of LGBT youths reported feeling out of place or lonely.
- LGBT youths are about twice as likely as non-LGBT youths to say they have been excluded by their peers because they are different; yet three-quarters of LGBT youths say that most of their peers do not have a problem with their identity as LGBT.

Note. Adapted from "Growing Up LGBT in America," by the Human Rights Campaign, 2012. Washington, DC: Author.

U.S. laws ensure that youths can seek health and mental health care without parental consent or knowledge, yet without parental assistance, many youths will not enter needed health or mental health treatment. Williams and Chapman (2012) suggested strategies such as building strong collaborations between health-care providers and parents; increasing parental awareness of the need for preventive health visits during adolescence; and involving school social workers, nurses, or guidance counselors in screening and facilitating needed treatment. They also suggested the need for services in places adolescents are likely to frequent, such as schools and other youth-serving agencies.

Transgender Children. Media has focused much attention in recent years on transgender children. Children with a diagnosis of gender dysphoria (GD), formerly known as gender identity disorder (GID), persistently, insistently, and consistently identify as the gender identity that is the "opposite" of their natal sex. Studies of children with GD have reported high rates of psychopathology, especially internalizing disorders such as anxiety and depression (Olson, Durwood, DeMeules, & McLaughlin, 2016). There is also evolving evidence that children and adolescents with gender dysphoria have a higher-than-expected rates of autism spectrum disorder (Shumer, Reisner, Edwards-Leeper, & Tishelmen, 2015). On the other hand, other studies suggest that children whose gender identities are affirmed and supported have relatively good mental health (Hill, Menvielle, Sica, & Johnson, 2010).

Increasing numbers of transgender children have socially transitioned: "They are being raised and are presenting to others as their gender identity rather than their natal sex, a reversible nonmedical intervention that involves changing the pronouns used to describe a child, as well as his or her name and (typically) hair length and clothing" Olson et al., 2016, p. 2). In a first study to examine mental health in socially transitioned transgender children, Olson et al. selected a community-based national sample of transgender prepubescent children ($n = 73$, ages 3–12 years), along with control groups of nontransgender children in the same age range ($n = 73$, age- and gender-matched community controls; ($n = 49$ siblings of transgender participants). Results indicated no elevations in depression and slightly elevated anxiety in the transgender children relative to population averages. The socially transitioned children did not differ from the control groups on depression symptoms and had only marginally higher anxiety symptoms. The researchers concluded that socially transitioned transgender children who are supported in their identity have developmentally normative levels of depression and only minimal elevation in anxiety, suggesting the psychopathology is not inevitable within this group. Especially notable, socially transitioned transgender children had notably lower rates of internalizing psychopathology than previously reported among children with GD living as their natal sex.

As transgender children reach puberty, the Endocrine Society and the World Professional Association for Transgender Health recommend the use of gonadotropin-releasing hormone agonists to suppress puberty, usually at about age 12. The purpose is to relieve suffering caused by the development of secondary sex characteristics, to provide time to make a balanced decision regarding the actual gender reassignment (by means of cross-sex hormones and surgery), and to make passing in the new gender role easier. The hormones may affect the normal pubertal increase in bone mineral density, and it is uncertain whether there is complete catch-up after treatment with cross-sex hormones. A major consequence of treatment is the loss of fertility. Further, as very early use of puberty suppression impairs penile growth, the fact that the penis and scrotum should be developed enough to be able to use this tissue to create a vagina later in life may be affected for boys wanting surgery. Despite guidelines, there is no consensus whether to use these early medical interventions. Vrouenraets, Fredriks, Hannema, Cohen-Kettenis, and de Vries (2015) called for more systematic interdisciplinary and worldwide multicenter research on the topic.

Cross-sex hormones are traditionally considered at age 16 years. There is a growing trend toward beginning this step as early as age 14 years (Chen, Fuqua, & Eugster, 2016). However, although puberty suppression is reversible, cross-sex hormones bring about partially irreversible physical changes.

Transgender individuals may consider sexual reassignment surgery, although very few transgender people have the surgery. Guidelines vary somewhat by country. However, in the United States, the person must be 18 years of age, have had 12 months of prior continuous hormone therapy, and 12 months of successful, continuous, full-time real-life experience (Swierzewski, 2015).

Overview of Practice With Families

Regardless of family type, when working with families, certain principles remain the same. Figure 7.5 provides an overview of the theory of family practice (Julian & Julian, 2005). Four major factors are represented. These factors in combination have the potential to make a significant impact on family health.

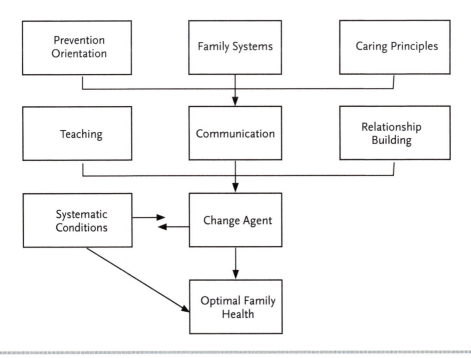

Figure 7.5. Interactions among perspectives, skills, roles, and systemic issues that influence partnerships for optimal family health. *Note.* Developed by Teresa W. Julian and David A. Julian.

Perspectives

The first factor involves three perspectives: (1) adopting prevention as a guiding principle, (2) viewing families as unique systems, and (3) using principles of caring practice to provide a strong basis for effective service delivery. Perspectives provide a system of values that guide professional practice.

Prevention

Problems addressed early reduce health-care costs and needless suffering. The U.S. health-care system traditionally has been crisis oriented rather than prevention oriented. However, through its Healthy People initiative, and more recently, Steps to a Healthier US, the U.S. Department of Health and Human Services has announced a bold shift in its approach from a disease-care system to a health-care system (U.S. Department of Health and Human Services, 2003).

The literature suggests some promising prevention strategies to assist families in maintaining optimal health. Giving parents information and education about postoperative care appears to be related to less pain and postoperative vomiting in children, which helps facilitate children's recovery time and decrease the number of days in the hospital setting (Kristensson-Hallstrom & Elander, 1997). Hovell et al. (1999) reported that counseling sessions with families are effective in preventing exposure to "environmental tobacco smoke" among asthmatic children. Heiberger (2004) described the key role that nurse practitioners can play in empowering parents to prevent sudden infant death syndrome (SIDS). Evaluators describe a host of programs that appear to be effective in preventing infectious disease, cardiovascular illnesses, drug abuse, and teen pregnancy. These examples provide evidence that well-conceived and evaluated prevention programs have the potential to reduce negative health outcomes.

Typically, the health-care professional will not have the opportunity to schedule appointments to discuss preventive strategies; such strategies must be communicated at opportune times. Consider a young boy or girl in the emergency department because of head trauma that might have been prevented by wearing a bicycle helmet. Appropriate counsel and education might prevent a brother or sister from suffering the same fate.

Family Systems

Thinking of families as systems may yield critical intervention points and opportunities to reinforce and enhance clinical treatment. As discussed earlier, the family systems perspective is based on the notion that the person or patient is embedded in a family system that, in turn, is embedded in a larger ecological system. According to Foster-Fishman, Salem, Allen, and Fahrbach (1999), the ecological view has several important features. First, people and contexts are interdependent; that is, individual actions are influenced by the characteristics of the settings that people occupy. Second, individuals are subjected to multiple contextual influences. People usually inhabit many different settings simultaneously, and each setting may have specific influences on behavior. Third, beliefs, values, and norms define what is acceptable in the various settings people occupy.

Strategies that view the family as part of a larger ecological system hold great promise for effectively addressing health-care issues for families in a holistic manner. Treatment of the individual or intervention at the individual level is conceptualized in terms of the influences of family and community variables. Thus, treatment of depression and antisocial behavior in children must address family issues, and effective interventions for HIV prevention must address community norms as well as individual behavior.

Situations in which children who are critically ill are hospitalized for extended periods of time are likely to precipitate a number of family issues such as care for siblings, financial concerns, transportation to and from the hospital, as well as needs for support and stress management. In turn, these factors are likely to influence the success of treatment and the length of time required for recovery. Patients and their families are greatly influenced by their own individual qualities as well as qualities of other significant individuals and outside environmental forces. To provide the most effective health care in a holistic manner, health-care professionals must adopt a family systems perspective and consider a variety of ecological factors and forces.

Caring

A caring orientation involves a host of behaviors that ensure competent and compassionate practice. Caring is a dynamic, multidimensional, and universal concept that enhances the preservation of human dignity. It is composed of nurturing activities, processes, and decisions that are essential for human birth, development, growth, and peaceful death. Caring behavior is manifested through attributes such as compassion, clinical competence and knowledge, confidence, conscience, and commitment. Caring professionals have control over their emotions and the clinical situation. They are self-reliant, and they anticipate problems and provide the highest-quality care. Caring arises out of a concern for and response to the patient or family.

Skills

The second tier of Figure 7.5 describes several skills essential to the effective provision of health care for families. The effects of skills such as teaching, communication, and relationship-building are likely to be enhanced to the extent that the perspectives discussed above influence the health-care professional. Whereas command of clinical skills is an obvious requirement for competent health-care practice, mastery of additional skills such as teaching, communication, and relationship-building will often facilitate the health-care professional's work with families.

Teaching Skills

Many teaching approaches are available to health-care professionals. Most teaching in health-care settings has as its goal the transfer of specific knowledge as a step in changing behavior. For example, teaching a family about proper dietary habits is an attempt to reinforce healthy behaviors and change unhealthy behaviors. Several principles may help health-care professionals to develop more effective teaching techniques. Research findings indicate that if a desired behavior change seems overwhelming or impossible to implement, patients or learners will not be likely to attempt to change their behavior. This is true even if the patient is capable of performing the required skills. Breaking a large goal or behavior change into smaller goals or tasks that can be readily mastered is a simple strategy that may enhance chances of success. The health-care professional also may provide aids to ensure success, such as allowing the child or parent to practice while providing feedback concerning progress. Other principles of effective teaching include making the information relevant to the family's lifestyle and health problems and providing rewards and feedback.

The concept of empowerment is now a well-established theoretical perspective in patient and parent education. Empowered families feel a sense of control and mastery over their situation as opposed to relying on professionals to meet their needs. For a comparison of traditional and empowering processes for asthma education, see Table 7.1. Although both traditional and empowering approaches to teaching parents can result in increased knowledge, McCarthy and colleagues (2002) reported significantly higher scores on measures of sense of control, ability to make decisions, and ability to provide care, for parents who participated in an empowerment approach to asthma education.

Table 7.1

Comparison of Traditional and Empowering Processes for Asthma Education		
Variable	**Traditional**	**Empowering**
Setting	Classroom setting: seats arranged in rows.	Classroom setting: seats arranged in a semicircle
Role of the professional	Professional lectures from the front of the class. Professional educator is portrayed as the expert.	Professional educator sits within semicircle Professional acts as a facilitator and resource person with emphasis on parent–professional partnerships
Role of the parents	Passive learners	Active learners Emphasis on parent–professional partnerships Parents recognized as experts who know their child best, have personal experience with child's illness, and can suggest how to adapt asthma management to fit family lifestyle
Teaching strategies	Primarily lectures	Interactive (e.g., parents share impressions, concerns) Emphasis on behavior change (e.g., learning to assess, interpret, and respond appropriately to changes in child's asthma; practicing proper use of asthma devices) Individualization and application of theory about each topic to own situation through use of common scenarios Emphasis on shared problem solving and learning from each other Repetition and review Monthly follow-up phone calls to family

Note. From "Empowering Parents Through Asthma Education," by M. McCarthy, J. Hansen, R. Herbert, D. Wong, M. Brimacombe, and M. Zelman, 2002, *Pediatric Nursing, 28*(5), p. 468. Copyright 2002 by Jannetti. Reprinted with permission.

Many critical implications of using teaching strategies exist in working with families. First, teaching is a primary prevention tool. Second, health-care professionals who work with families during an illness have unique opportunities to implement effective teaching that may enhance healing and wellness. In such situations, the health-care professional can observe family coping and adaptation to a disease. In the case of children, such awareness may transcend various developmental stages and needs and may require the health-care professional to act proactively to teach appropriate content and therapeutic strategies. For example, Eddy et al. (1998) found that preadolescent children with cystic fibrosis had greater stress and treatment problems when they had conflicts with parents. They suggested that when developing interventions, health-care professionals should consider key developmental transition points, children's and family members' perspectives about their illnesses, and family relationship patterns. Providing relevant teaching content for families can serve as a powerful preventive intervention and, in other cases, as an effective strategy to address illness.

Communication Skills

Research suggests that communication is often identified as an area in which health-care professionals need to improve. Horn, Feldman, and Ploof's (1995) research described stressors for families who have children with chronic illnesses that require lengthy hospitalizations. These researchers suggested that personal emotions and communication problems with the health-care team are predominant stressors. Similarly, Evans (1996) reported that mothers of children who are hospitalized state that they often feel stressed and out of control because of the impact of disease and treatment. To help these mothers, it is essential that health-care professionals communicate with families by negotiating and clarifying. Providing information about options parents have to help their children as well as creating a nonjudgmental atmosphere regarding their choices are other critical elements of good communication.

Empathetic, respectful, and genuine communication leads to trusting, empowering, therapeutic, and collaborative relationships. Three basic behaviors are associated with empathy: (1) awareness and acceptance of the self as a feeling person; (2) listening to messages and identifying the patient's or family members' feelings; and (3) responding to feelings exhibited in specific messages (e.g., using paraphrasing techniques). By exhibiting empathetic behaviors, the health-care professional will become aware of the child's uniqueness and individuality. The child or family member, in turn, will perceive the health-care professional as caring and feeling, which ultimately will facilitate open communication and trust.

Feelings of being respected are important for the child or family member to experience her or his right to exist as a unique human being. The health-care professional must exhibit a receptive attitude that demonstrates value for feelings, opinions, individuality, and uniqueness. Also, health-care professionals must show a high level of commitment to understanding through a willingness to explore subjects that are important to the family. Finally, they must convey acceptance and warmth by being nonjudgmental (free from prejudice) and must develop a high level of immunity to being embarrassed, shocked, dismayed, or overwhelmed by the child or family member's thoughts or behaviors. This requires appropriate verbal as well as nonverbal communication. Respect affirms the family's strengths and problem-solving capabilities.

Genuineness is synonymous with concepts such as authenticity, good faith, and sincerity. It is a sharing of self, exhibited by behaving in a natural, spontaneous, and non-defensive manner. However, the health-care professional must be sensitive to the family's readiness for specific messages. For example, self-disclosure is appropriate, but only when the family is ready to respond positively to the disclosure. As trust is established, the health-care professional can become more open and spontaneous, while adhering to the principles of empathy and respect.

Whether labeled as inadequate information, paternalism, limited negotiation, or lack of clarification, troubled communication is at the root of many problematic family and professional partnerships (Evans, 1996). Many problems in health-care settings can be traced to the way professionals talk to and otherwise interact with families. Most communication problems can be transcended if health-care professionals use empathy, respect, and genuineness along with basic therapeutic techniques.

Good communication skills are not innate. Health-care professionals must learn appropriate techniques to effectively communicate with families. By incorporating communication skills into their repertoires, health-care professionals can accurately gather information and understand the inner worlds and thoughts of the families they serve.

Relationship Building

A critical skill in working with families involves the need to facilitate parental and professional collaboration at all levels of health care. Eddy and colleagues (1998) claimed that forming supportive collaborative relationships with parents of children with a chronic illness such as cystic fibrosis should be an early intervention. Such partnerships increase the chances that parents will be open in sharing the stresses and hassles experienced in the daily care of their children. Some important steps in building collaborative relationships include (a) good communication with clarity of vision and a foundation for active involvement of all in goal setting, (b) use of educational materials and strategies that account for the psychological needs of the learner, and (c) development of relationships that build on the strengths of individuals and families (U.S. Department of Health and Human Services, 1996). In establishing collaborative relationships, it is important that common goals be developed and shared. The presence of a common goal that supersedes individual goals is a distinguishing characteristic of collaborative relationships (Julian, 1994). To develop common goals, health-care professionals need to continually investigate the needs of caretakers of critically ill patients, especially children (Scott, 1998). Consistent identification, prioritization, and incorporation of parental needs into a plan of care are important steps in building collaborative relationships. Interestingly, Scott suggested that parental needs usually revolve around

- knowing the expected outcome of medical treatment,
- being given honest answers,
- being assured that the best care is given,
- seeing and visiting children frequently, and
- being notified of any changes in the condition of their children.

Collaborative relationships between family members and health-care professionals may serve as a valuable tool in providing optimal health care. Parental participation has now become an accepted feature in the care of children in hospitals. Collaborative relationships can maximize family members' confidence and competence in caring for their children. This is an important element in family-centered care.

Systemic Conditions

The provision of health-care services to families is affected by a number of systemic conditions that describe the environment within which the health-care professional must operate. Systemic conditions represent social statuses, social states, or organizational practices and policies. This section identifies several features of the current environment.

Adherence to Scientific/Biomedical Beliefs About Health Care

Families have varied health beliefs. For the individual, beliefs are influenced by such things as (a) past experiences with the health-care system (e.g., degree of helpfulness, barriers to care), (b) family members' and influential others' experiences, (c) thoughts and cognition, (d) biochemical/structural strengths and weaknesses (e.g., level of wellness, perceptions related to disease), (e) culture, and (f) socioeconomic status.

The scientific/biomedical health paradigm is the dominant health belief system for the majority of families in the United States. The following are some of the values associated with the scientific/biomedical health paradigm:

- *Determinism*—Cause-and-effect relationships exist for all natural phenomena.
- *Mechanism*—Life is compared to the structure and function of machines.
- *Reductionism*—All life can be reduced or divided into smaller parts.
- *Dualism*—Mind and body are separated into two distinct entities.

Some serious weaknesses associated with the scientific/biomedical health paradigm include (a) the fragmentation of health-care services, (b) the lack of research and treatment that are holistic or preventive in nature, (c) the lack of health care that considers the mind–body connection, (d) the symptomatic treatment of diseases versus determining causation, and (e) "prescriptionism," or heavy reliance on pharmaceutical interventions.

Health-care professionals can reflect on the choices available to families. Most current treatment options are influenced by the scientific/biomedical health paradigm and are developed and provided by private-sector enterprises. It is reasonable to ask whether such treatments are always the best options for specific children and their families. Being aware of and understanding the strengths and weaknesses of the predominant health paradigm may lead to interventions based on alternative views of health and treatment for some children. Thus, health-care professionals might explore and incorporate practices from other health paradigms and cultures (e.g., holistic health, magic–religious health) into their interactions with families.

Poverty and Inadequate Access to Health-Care Resources

Several segments of the population struggle to acquire needed health-care services (e.g., homeless and low-income children and families, grandparents raising their children's children, foster children, the medically uninsured). Some of the reasons families are medically underserved involve individual factors, health-care professional factors, and system factors.

Many families who experience difficulty in accessing health-care services also are the most in need. For example, in 2011, 7.7 million children in the United States, or 1 in 10, were living with a grandparent, and approximately 3 million of these children were also being cared for primarily by that grandparent (Livingston, 2013b). Grandparents are raising children with special needs, including HIV, the effects of child abuse and neglect, and neurological deficits resulting from parental abuse of drugs. Research indicates that some of these grandparents suffer from significant financial burdens, feelings of anger and resentment toward their own children, and mental health problems (Kelley, Yorker, & Whitley, 1997).

Models designed to improve access to health-care resources usually involve case management strategies; family assessment models; and family advocacy, counseling, teaching, referral, and follow-up. Technology and the Internet may provide easy access to some types of health-care services. Advances in procedures, diagnostic tools, and innovations in how services are delivered may make health care more accessible to many consumers.

Same-day surgery or satellite health-care sites for minor surgical procedures are improving access to health-care resources. In these settings, families become important partners with the health-care team in the provision of care. Parents often are with their children during the preoperative and the postoperative phases. Parental presence for anesthesia induction is important for reducing stress in children and enhancing recovery. However, for this system to work effectively, parents must be viewed as major collaborators and educated about their role in caring for their children. There must be opportunities for parents to ask questions and discuss fears and concerns. Same-day surgery sites also seem to be user friendly (i.e., smaller facilities, greater availability of parking, and fewer personnel to get to know) and are frequently owned by small groups of physicians who have a vested interest in keeping their customers happy.

An added burden concerns the maze of procedures created by current health insurance practices. Families without health insurance or those that receive minimal support from the government often are forced to make difficult decisions concerning the quality of care their family receives. Inadequate access to health-care resources exacerbates existing health-care problems and affects individualized plans of care for children and their families

Proliferation of Technology and Widespread Access to Health-Care Information

Access to the Internet and technology has the potential to dramatically alter how health care is provided to families. There is little question that a vast amount of health-care information is currently available on the Internet. Websites that are devoted to specific diseases and conditions can provide families with access to expert medical opinions. In some cases, private companies will prepare reports about specific medical conditions and treatment options. Some hospital websites have extensive communications channels for patients and their parents.

Appropriate use of the Internet and other technological aids for information exchange seems to serve a useful function. Consumers appear positively disposed toward online solutions. Online services can offer a broad range of information at great levels of detail in a timely fashion. Further, communication with families via e-mail is one way to increase access to health-care resources. An e-mail delivery system might be used to confirm appointments, report information (e.g., "Your lab test is normal."), and answer questions. Some health-care agencies are already online and connect such interactions to electronic medical records. With many families online and many others having access through local schools and libraries, it is important that health-care professionals and policy makers adopt useful Internet strategies for sharing information and expanding access to health-care resources. It is also important that when strategies like those discussed above are implemented, health-care professionals develop and teach protocols for how to access the World Wide Web and pertinent Web-based resources.

Many strategies exist for using technology to increase access to health-care information. Families might be encouraged to bring digital voice recorders, smartphones, or tablets to the health-care setting. If families do not own such devices, some might be acquired and made available for loan. Simply recording a conversation with a health-care professional might help families share information with loved ones. Teaching receptionists and scheduling personnel how to schedule appointments so that children and their families are not burdened by long waits to see health-care professionals represents a simple technology. Telephones also are an effective means of communication. In many cases, telephone calls provide a continuum of care to postsurgical patients. Making follow-up phone calls to patients and family members can improve health-care outcomes

The Internet and a variety of electronic devices have the potential to make health-care information available to families and to increase access to health-care resources. The Internet is already a powerful communication tool that is readily available to many consumers. However, it will be necessary to educate consumers and to develop procedures to ensure that information obtained through the Internet and other channels is accurate and "user friendly." Although the Internet is a helpful tool for health-care professionals in their work with families, many challenges to responsible use must be addressed.

Home Care and Other Alternative Practice Settings

As the result of advances in scientific knowledge and technology, the number of patients—especially children—living with chronic illnesses is increasing. Some parents report that home-care options provide them with greater freedom, more privacy, and less disruption to family life. Families often express fears and concerns regarding symptomatic care of their children and other family members, and they need considerable support. For example, families may have insufficient knowledge of parenting skills and inadequate support systems, and they may be unable to help with vital childcare tasks. Managing the care of a medically fragile child at home often means finding unique solutions for the child's needs as well as providing emotional, educational, and financial support. For successful home care, parents need access to continuous supervision, help and support of well-trained personnel, and knowledge about respite care and quality day care services.

Formal home visitation programs provide the opportunity to help families with the care of loved ones at home. Visiting the child's nursery school and primary care physician can also be helpful. Home visitation offers an effective mechanism to ensure ongoing caretaker education and social support linkages with public and private community services. Health-care professionals can help families assess their ability to implement treatment regimens and to recognize signs of complications or symptoms in the child.

Not all home visiting programs are equal in effectiveness. The USDHHS launched the Home Visiting Evidence of Effectiveness (HomVEE) review to conduct a thorough and transparent review of the home visiting research literature. The report, released in 2016, provides an assessment of the effectiveness of home visiting program models that target families with pregnant women and children from birth to kindergarten entry (Avellar et al., 2016). Of the 18 home visiting program models with high- or moderate-quality studies that measure outcomes in child health, 8 had favorable effects on primary outcome measures (birth outcomes and counts of health-care service use extracted from medical records) and 8 had favorable effects on secondary outcome measures (parent reports about children's health and use of health-care services). The report also lists outcomes related to child development and school readiness, family economic self-sufficiency, linkages and referrals, maternal health, positive parenting practices, reductions in child maltreatment, reductions in juvenile delinquency, family violence, and crime.

Health-care professionals must also help families address their ability to manage disabilities and come to terms with their own psychosocial responses (e.g., management of social isolation, financial hardships, constriction of time, identity insults, profound sense of loss). Formal home visitation programs need to include physical and emotional support, as well as tangible ways to relieve parents and other caretakers of the continuous 24-hour care of their children and other family members. Further, in cases of life-threatening conditions, emotional support must continue after the child's death.

Home visitation programs provide many of the services necessary for sustained care of children with chronic conditions. These services included access to highly trained health-care professionals who provided advice and support.

Adopting the Role of Change Agent

To be a change agent means to facilitate or aid the process of change in a deliberate manner. Change can occur at a variety of levels. At the individual level, the health-care professional helps the individual define appropriate and healing behaviors and take action to ensure that such behaviors are adopted. Prochaska, Norcross, and DiClemente's (1994) transtheoretical model is a key tool for changing behavior at the individual level. Some strategies to effect change at the system level include (a) political action; (b) planning, needs analysis, and evaluation; and (c) grassroots movements. Each of these topics is addressed in detail in Chapter 13: Promoting Children's Well-Being in the Community.

Successful work with families is strongly related to the extent to which health-care professionals adopt the role of change agent. Historically, teaching, communication, relationship-building, and even medical treatment have represented significant health-care interventions. However, in the absence of deliberate action to change behavior, these strategies were insufficient to produce true health and wellness. For example, educational campaigns designed to promote the use of seat belts were only marginally successful. However, educational campaigns in combination with laws requiring seat belt use and enforcement of seat belt laws garnered more support.

It is imperative that health-care professionals perceive themselves as change agents and work at both the individual and system levels. To truly address the psychosocial needs of children in health-care settings requires a long-range perspective focused on the change agent role.

Conclusion

In pediatrics, the family is the unit of concern and intervention. A variety of family types have been described, with a focus on their challenges. When illness, injury, or disability occurs within the family system, every family member is affected in some way. In working with families, it is critical to remember that regardless of family composition or circumstances, every family has strengths. Embracing the perceptions for practice with families and implementing the strategies suggested can help families navigate crises as well as the everyday events of family life.

Study Guide

1. List four assumptions of family systems theory.

2. Describe the elements of McCubbin and Patterson's family stress theory.

3. Discuss a selection of family types and some of the important psychosocial issues they face.

4. What are some of the potential impacts of a child's illness or disability on his or her parents and siblings?

5. Which three pieces of information should children always be told when a parent is seriously ill?

6. Discuss the impact of the birth of multiples on the marriage relationship.

7. List three strategies health-care professionals can use to make health-care services more welcoming to LGBT families.

8. List the four major factors in the theory of family practice.

9. Discuss the skills essential to the effective provision of health care for families.

10. Define a *change agent*.

Appendix 7.1

Resources

Publications

Healthy People 2020
https://www.healthypeople.gov/sites/default
/files/HP2020_brochure_with_LHI_508
_FNL.pdf
Brochure updated with the leading health
indicators

**Helping Children When a Family Member
Has Cancer: Dealing with Treatment**
http://www.cancer.org/acs/groups/cid/docu
ments/webcontent/002605-pdf.pdf
A fact-filled 22-page publication from the
American Cancer Society with good information, advice, and recommended resources to
promote coping for children of parents with
cancer

**Helping Children When A Family Member
Has Cancer: Dealing With Recurrence or
Progressive Illness**
http://www.cancer.org/acs/groups/cid/docu
ments/webcontent/002603-pdf.pdf
An American Cancer Society publication that
provides information about what children
might be thinking and feeling and ideas on
how to help

**When Your Parent Has Cancer: A Guide for
Teens**
http://www.cancer.gov/publications/patient-
education/When-Your-Parent-Has-
Cancer.pdf
A National Cancer Institute publication for
young people who have a parent with cancer;
offers tips on what to say to friends, how to
deal with stress, and where to find support, as
well as information about cancer and cancer
treatments

Organizations

**Center for Excellence for Transgender
Health**
http://transhealth.ucsf.edu/trans?page=lib-pro
viders
An organization that combines the unique
strengths and resources of a nationally re-
nowned training and capacity-building institution, the Pacific AIDS Education and Training
Center (PAETC), and an internationally recognized leader in HIV prevention research, the
Center for AIDS Prevention Studies (CAPS),
both of which are housed at the University of
California San Francisco

LGBT Resources

General
**Schools in Transition: A Guide for Support-
ing Transgender Students in K–12 Schools**
http://hrc-assets.s3-website-us-east-1.ama-
zonaws.com//files/assets/resources
/Schools-In-Transition.pdf
This guide highlights best practices while offering strategies for building upon and aligning
them with each school's culture.

For Parents and Family Members
**Children's National Medical Center Gender
and Sexuality Psychosocial Programs**
www.childrensnational.org

Family Acceptance Project
http://familyproject.sfsu.edu

Gender Spectrum
www.genderspectrum.org

PFLAG's Transgender Network
http://community.pflag.org/transgender

Philadelphia Trans-Health Conference
www.trans-health.org

TransKids Purple Rainbow Foundation
www.transkidspurplerainbow.org

TransYouth Family Allies
www.imatyfa.org

For Youths
It Gets Better
www.itgetsbetter.org

Gender Spectrum Lounge
www.genderspectrum.org/join

The Trevor Project
www.thetrevorproject.org

Youth Pages
www.safeschoolscoalition.org/youth/index
.html

YouthResource by Advocates for Youth
www.youthresource.com

Program

Nurse-Family Partnership
http://www.nursefamilypartnership.org/
A free maternal-health visiting program that
introduces vulnerable first-time parents to
caring maternal and child health nurses. The
program allows nurses to deliver the support
first-time mothers need to have a healthy pregnancy, become knowledgeable and responsible
parents, and provide their babies with the best
possible start in life.

References

American Academy of Pediatrics. (2013). *Foster parents: FAQs.* Retrieved from https://www.healthy-children.org/English/family-life/family-dynamics/adoption-and-foster-care/Pages/Foster-Parents-FAQs.aspx

Avellar, S., Paulsell, D., Sama-Miller, E. Del Grosso, P., Akers, L., & Kleinman, R. (2016). *Home visiting evidence of effectiveness review: Executive summary.* Office of Planning, Research and Evaluation, Administration for Children and Families, U.S. Department of Health and Human Services. Washington, DC: USDHHS.

Ayer, L., Woldetsadik, M., Malsberger, R., Burgette, L. F., & Kohl, P. L. (2016). Who are the men caring for maltreated youth? Male caregivers in the child welfare system. *Child Maltreatment.* Advance online publication. doi: 10.1177/1077559516664985

Bostrom, K., & Nilsagard, Y. (2016). A family matter—When a parent is diagnosed with multiple sclerosis: A qualitative study. *Journal of Clinical Nursing, 25,* 1053–1061.

Bronner, M., Peek, N., Knoester, H., Bos, A., Last, B., & Grootenhuis, M. (2010). Course and predictors of posttraumatic stress disorder in parents after pediatric intensive care treatment of their child. *Journal of Pediatric Psychology, 35*(9), 966–974.

Cassell, S. (2011). *Examining the twin bond: A look at the psychological development of twins and the differences in individuality and identity differentiation between fraternal and identical same-sex twins.* Unpublished manuscript. Retrieved from http://aladinrc.wrlc.org/bitstream/handle/1961/9874/Cassell,%20Sophie%20-%20Spring%20'11.pdf?sequence=1

Celik H., Abma T. A., Klinge I., & Widdershoven G. A. M. (2012). Process evaluation of a diversity training program: The value of a mixed method strategy. *Evaluation and Program Planning, 35,* 54–65.

Centers for Disease Control and Prevention. (2015). *Multiple births.* Retrieved from http://www.cdc.gov/nchs/fastats/multiple.htm

Chapman, R., Wardrop, J., Freeman, P., Zappia, T., Watkins, R., & Shields, L. (2012). A descriptive study of the experiences of lesbian, gay and transgender parents accessing health services for their children. *Journal of Clinical Nursing, 21,* 1128–1135.

Chen, M., Fuqua, J., & Eugster, E. (2016). Characteristics of referrals for gender dysphoria over a 13-year period. *Journal of Adolescent Health, 58,* 369–371.

Cheng, S., & Powell, B. (2015). Measurement, methods, and divergent patterns: Reassessing the effects of same-sex parents. *Social Science Research, 52,* 615–626.

Coleman, L., & Glenn, F. (2009). *When couples part: Understanding the consequences for adults and children.* London, UK: One Plus One.

Daugherty, J., & Copen, C. (2016). Trends in attitudes about marriage, childbearing, and sexual behavior: United States, 2002, 2006, 2006–2010, and 2011–2013. *National Health Statistic Reports, 92.* Hyattsville, MD: National Center for Health Statistics.

Duvall, E. (1977). *Marriage and family development* (6th ed.). Philadelphia, PA: J. B. Lippincott.

Eddy, M., Carter, B., Kronenberger, W., Conradsen, S., Eid, N., Bourland, S., & Adams, G. (1998). Parent relationships and compliance in cystic fibrosis. *Journal of Pediatric Health Care, 12*(4), 196–202.

Ehrensperger, M., Grether, A., Romer, G., Berres, M., Monsch, A., Kappos, L, & Steck, B. (2008). Neuropsychological dysfunction, depression, physical disability, and coping processes in families with a parent affected by multiple sclerosis. *Multiple Sclerosis, 14,* 1106–1112.

Eisenberg, M., & Resnick, M. (2006). Suicidality among gay, lesbian and bisexual youth: The role of protective factors. *Journal of Adolescent Health, 39,* 662–668.

England, P., & Bearak, J. (2014). The sexual double standard and gender differences in attitudes toward casual sex among U.S. university students. *Demographic Research, 30,* 1327–1338.

Erikson, E., & Erikson, J. M. (1982). *The life cycle completed.* New York, NY: Norton.

Evans, M. (1996). A pilot study to evaluate in-hospital care by mothers. *Journal of Pediatric Oncology Nursing, 13*(3), 138–145.

Farr, R. H., Crain, E. E., Oakley, M. K., Cashen, K. K., & Garber, K. J. (2016). Microaggressions, feelings of difference, and resilience among adopted children with sexual minority parents. *Journal of Youth and Adolescence, 45,* 85–104. doi:10.1007/s10964-015-0353-6

Feldman, R., & Eidelman, A. I. (2005). Does a triplet birth pose a special risk for infant development? Assessing cognitive development in relation to intrauterine growth and mother-infant interaction across the first 2 years. *Pediatrics. 115,* 443–452.

Forman, K. (2015). *Multi-divorce & blended families.* Retrieved from http://www.formanmediation.com/articles/multi-divorce-blended-families/

Forum on Child and Family Statistics. (2015). America's children at a glance. *America's children: Key national indicators of well-being, 2015.* Retrieved from http://www.childstats.gov/americaschildren/glance.asp

Foster-Fishman, P. G., Salem, D. A., Allen, N. E., & Fahrbach, K. (1999). Ecological factors impacting provider attitudes towards human service delivery reform. *American Journal of Community Psychology, 27*(6), 785–816.

Gates, G. (2014). *LGB families and relationships: Analyses of the 2013 National Health Interview Survey.* The Williams Institute. Retrieved from http://williamsinstitute.law.ucla.edu/wp-content/uploads/lgb-familiesnhis-sep-2014.pdf

Goldberg A. (2012). *Gay dads: Transitions to adoptive fatherhood.* New York, NY: NYU Press.

Goldberg A. E., & Allen K. R. (2012). *LGBT-parent families: Innovations in research and implications for practice.* New York, NY: Springer-Verlag.

Golombok, S., & Badger, S. (2010). Children raised in mother-headed families from infancy: A follow-up of children of lesbian and single heterosexual mothers, at early adulthood. *Human Reproduction, 25,* 150–157.

Golombok, S., Olivennes G., Ramogida, C., Rust, J., & Freeman, T. (2007). Parenting and the psychological development of a representative sample of triplets conceived by assisted reproduction. *Human Reproduction, 22*(11), 2896–2902.

Golombok, S., Zadeh, S., Imrie, S., Smith, V., & Freeman, R. (2016). Single mothers by choice: Mother-child relationships and children's psychological adjustment. *Journal of Family Psychology.* Advance online publication. http://dx.doi.org/10.1037/fam0000188

Graham, S. (2012). Choosing single motherhood? Single women negotiating the nuclear family ideal. In D. Cutas, & S. Chan (Eds.), *Families: Beyond the nuclear ideal* (pp. 97–109). London, UK: Bloomsbury Academic.

Graham, S., & Braverman, A. (2012). ARTs and the single parent. In M. Richards, G. Pennings, & J. B. Appleby (Eds.), *Reproductive donation: Practice, policy and bioethics.* New York, NY: Cambridge University Press. http://dx.doi.org/10.1017/CBO9781139026390.011

Grant, J., Mottet, L., Tanis, J., Harrison, J., Herman, J., & Keisling, M. (2011). *Injustice at every turn: A report of the National Transgender Discrimination Survey, Executive Summary.* Washington, DC: National Center for Transgender Equality and the National Gay and Lesbian Taskforce.

Grossman, N., & Okun, B. (2012). Divorce and the family life cycle: Disruptions. *The Family Psychologist, 28*(1), 20–22.

Gulliford, M. (2013). Equity and access to health care. In M. Gulliford & M. Morgan (Eds.), *Access to health care* (pp. 36–60). London, UK: Routledge.

Haddon, L., & Teschow, V. (2008). Multiples and impact on couple relationship. *Multiple Births Canada.* Retrieved from http://multiplebirthscanada.org/mbc_documents/RelationshipSurveyreport-Final.pdf

Hanson, M. (2013). Families in context: Conceptual frameworks for understanding and supporting families. In M. Hanson, & E. Lynch (Eds.), *Understanding families: Supportive approaches to diversity, disability, and risk* (2nd ed., pp. 43–71). Baltimore, MD: Paul H. Brookes.

Hayman B., Wilkes L., Halcomb E. J., & Jackson, D. (2013) Marginalised mothers: Lesbian women negotiating heteronormative healthcare services. *Contemporary Nurse, 44*, 120–127.

Heiberger, G. (2004). Empowering parents for SIDS prevention: Nurse practitioners play a key role. *Advanced Nursing Practice, 12*(5), 57–58.

Hill, D., Menvielle, E., Sica, K., & Honson, A. (2010). An affirmative intervention for families with gender variant children: Parental ratings of child mental health and gender. *Journal of Sex & Marital Therapy, 36*(1), 6–23.

Horn, J., Feldman, H., & Ploof, D. (1995). Parent and professional perceptions about stress and coping strategies during a child's lengthy hospitalization. *Social Work Health Care, 21*(1), 107–127.

Hovell, M. F., Meltzer, S. B., Zakarian, J. M., Wahlgren, D. R., Emerson, J. A., Hofstetter, C. R. . . . Atkins, C. J. (1999). Reduction of environmental tobacco smoke exposure among asthmatic children: A controlled trial. *Chest, 106*(2), 440–446.

Huizinga, G., Visser A., Zelders-Steyn, Y., Teule, J., Reijneveld, S., & Roodbol, P. (2011). Psychological impact of having a parent with cancer. *European Journal of Cancer, 47*, Supplement 3(0), S239–S246.

Human Rights Campaign. (2012). *Growing up LGBT in America*. Washington, DC: Author.

Jantzer, V., Gros, J., Stute, F., Parzer, P., Brunner, R., Willig, K., … Resch, F. (2013). Risk behaviors and externalizing behaviors in adolescents dealing with parental cancer—a controlled longitudinal study. *Psycho-Oncology, 22*(1), 2611–2616.

Jarrett, D., & McGarty, M. (1980). Twin yearning. *The Hillside Journal of Clinical Psychiatry, 2*(2), 195–215.

Julian, T., & Julian, D. (2005). Families in children's health-care settings. In J. Rollins, R. Bolig, & C. Mahan (Eds.), *Meeting children's psychosocial needs across the health-care continuum* (pp. 277–312). Austin, TX: PRO-ED.

Kelley, S. J., Yorker, B. C., & Whitley, D. (1997). To grandmother's house we go . . . and stay: Children raised in intergenerational families. *Journal of Gerontological Nursing, 23*(9), 13–20.

Kiernan, K., & Mensah, F. K. (2010). *Unmarried parenthood, family trajectories, parent and child well-being*. Bristol, UK: The Policy Press.

Klein, B. (2003). *Not all twins are alike*. Westport, CT: Praeger.

Kobayashi, K., Hayakawa, A., & Hohashi, N. (2015). Interrelations between siblings and parents in families living with children with cancer. *Journal of Family Nursing, 21*(1), 119–148.

Kristensson-Hallstrom, I., & Elander, G. (1997). Parents' experience of hospitalization: Different strategies for feeling secure. *Pediatric Nursing, 23*, 361–367.

Lander, I. (2008). Using family attachment narrative therapy to heal the wounds of twinship: A case study of an 11-year-old boy. *Child Adolescence Social Work Journal, 25*, 367–383.

Livingston, G. (2013a). *The rise of single fathers*. Washington, DC: Pew Research Center.

Livingston, G. (2013b). *At grandmother's house we stay*. Pew Research Center. Retrieved from http://www.pewsocialtrends.org/2013/09/04/at-grandmothers-house-we-stay/

Long, K. A., & Marsland, M. A. (2011). Family adjustment to childhood cancer: A systematic review. *Clinical Child and Family Psychology Review, 14*, 57–88.

Long, K., Marsland, A., Wright, A., & Hinds, P. (2015). Creating a tenuous balance: Siblings' experience of a brother's or sister's childhood cancer diagnosis. *Journal of Pediatric Oncology Nursing, 32*(1), 21–31.

MacLeod, K., Whitsett, S., Mash, E., & Pelletier, W. (2003). Pediatric sibling donors of successful and unsuccessful hematopoetic stem cell transplants (HSCT): A qualitative study of their psychosocial experience. *Journal of Pediatric Psychology, 28*, 223–230.

Marks L. (2012). Same-sex parenting and children's outcomes: A closer examination of the American Psychological Association's brief on lesbian and gay parenting. *Social Science Research, 4*, 735–751.

Martin, J. A., Hamilton, B. E., Sutton, P. D., Ventura, S. J., Menacker, F., & Munson, M. L. (2003). Births: Final data for 2002. *National Vital Statistics Report, 52*, 1–102.

McCarthy, M., Ashley, D., Lee, K., & Anderson, B. (2012). Predictors of acute and posttraumatic stress symptoms in parents following their child's cancer diagnosis. *Journal of Traumatic Stress, 25*(5), 558–566.

McCarthy, M., Hansen, J., Herbert, R., Wong, D., Brimacombe, M., & Zelman, M. (2002). Empowering parents through asthma education. *Pediatric Nursing, 28*(5), 465–473, 504.

McCubbin, H., & Patterson, J. (1983). Family stress and adaptation to crises: A Double ABCX Model of family behavior. In D. H. Olson & R. C. Miller (Eds.), *Family studies review yearbook: Vol. 1* (pp. 87–106). Beverly Hills, CA: Sage.

McCue, K. (2011). *How to help children through a parent's serious illness*. New York, NY: St. Martin's Press.

Missouri Department of Social Services. (n.d.). *Child welfare manual*. Retrieved from https://dss.mo.gov/cd/info/cwmanual/section7/ch1_33/sec7ch1.htm

Morris, S. (2014, September 3). The forsaken: A rising number of homeless gay teens are being cast out by religious families. *Rolling Stone*. Retrieved from http://www.rollingstone.com/culture/features/the-forsaken-a-rising-number-of-homeless-gay-teens-are-being-cast-out-by-religious-families-20140903

Muscari, F., McCarthy, M., Woolf, C., Hearps, S., Burke, K., & Anderson, V. (2015). Early psychological reaction in parents of children with a life threatening illness within a pediatric hospital setting. *European Psychiatry, 30*, 555–561.

Olson, K., Durwood, L., DeMeules, M., & McLaughlin, K. (2016). Mental health of transgender children who are supported in their identities. *Pediatrics, 137*(3), e20123223.

Packman, W., Crittenden, M. R., Rieger Fischer, J. B., Schaffer, E., Bongar, B., & Cowan, M. J. (1997). Siblings' perceptions of the bone marrow transplantation process. *Journal of Psychosocial Oncology*.

Packman, W., Gong, K., VanZutphen, K., Shaffer, T., & Crittenden, M. (2004). Psychosocial adjustment of adolescent siblings of hematopoietic stem cell transplant patients. *Journal of Pediatric Oncology Nursing, 21*, 233–248.

Pakenham, K. I., & Cox, S. (2012). Test of a model of the effects of parental illness on youth and family functioning. *Health Psychology, 31*, 580–590.

Pakenham, K., & Cox, S. (2014). The effects of parental illness and other ill family members on the adjustment of children. *Annals of Behavioral Medicine, 48*(3), 424–437.

Pakenham, K., & Cox, S., (2015). The effects of parental illness and other ill family members on youth caregiving experiences. *Psychology & Health, 30*(7), 857–878.

Pakenham, K. I., Tilling, J., & Cretchley J. (2012). Parenting difficulties and resources: The perspectives of parents with multiple sclerosis and their partners. *Rehabilitation Psychology 57*, 52–60.

Papernow, P. (1993). *Becoming a stepfamily: Patterns of development in remarried families*. San Francisco, CA: Jossey-Bass.

Patterson, J. (2002). Integrating family resilience and family stress theory. *Journal of Marriage and Family, 64*, 349–360.

Perrin, E., Pinderhughes, E., Mattern, K., Hurley, S., & Newman, R. (2016, March 9). Experiences of children with gay fathers. *Clinical Pediatrics*. Published online before print. doi: 10.1177/0009922816632346

Perrin E., & Siegel, B. (2013). Promoting the well-being of children whose parents are gay or lesbian. *Pediatrics, 131*, e1374–e1383.

Phillips, F. (2014). Adolescents living with a parent with advanced cancer: A review of the literature. *Psycho-Oncology, 23*, 1323–1339.

Prochaska, J., Norcross, J., & DiClemente, C. (1994). *Changing for good*. New York, NY: Morrow.

Rand, L., Eddleman, K. A., & Stone, J. (2005). Long-term outcomes in multiple gestations. *Clinical Perinatology, 32*, 495–513.

Regnerus, M. (2012). How different are the adult children of parents who have same-sex relationships? Findings from the New Family Structures Study. *Social Science Research, 41*, 752–770.

Ryan, C., Huebner, D., Diaz, R., Sanchez, J. (2009). Family rejection as a predictor of negative health outcomes in white and Latino lesbian, gay, and bisexual young adults. *Pediatrics, 123*(1), 346–362.

Schwartz, L. (2013). *Sibling care in pediatric hospitals by certified child life specialist.* The Ohio State University. Retrieved from http://kb.osu.edu/dspace/handle/1811/54639?show=full

Scott, L. D. (1998). Perceived needs of parents of critically ill children. *Journal for the Society of Pediatric Nursing, 3*(1), 4–12.

Shama, W. (1998). The experience and preparation of pediatric sibling bone marrow donors. *Social Work in Health Care, 27*, 89–99.

Shumer, D., Reisner, S., Edwards-Leeper, L., & Tishelman, A. (2015, December 1). Evaluation of Asperger Syndrome in youth presenting to a gender dysphoria clinic. *LGBT Health.* Advanced online publication. doi: 10.1089/lgbt.2015.0070

Sieh, D. S., Visser-Meily, J. M. A., & Meijer, A. M. (2013). Differential outcomes of adolescents with chronically ill and healthy parents. *Journal of Child and Family Studies, 22*, 209–218.

Solberg, O., Gronning Dale, M., Holmstrom, H., Eskedal, L., Landolt, M., & Vollrath, M. (2011). Long-term symptoms of depression and anxiety in mothers of infants with congenital heart defects. *Journal of Pediatric Psychology, 3*(2), 179–187.

Swierzewski, S. (2015). *Transgender health and surgical guidelines.* Retrieved from http://www.health-communities.com/transgender-health/surgical-guidelines.shtml

Twenge, J. M., Sherman, R. A., & Wells, B. E. (2015). Changes in American adults' sexual behavior and attitudes, 1972–2012. *Archives of Sexual Behavior, 44*(8), 2273–2285.

U.S. Bureau of the Census. (2006). *Statistical abstract of the United States (122nd ed.).* Washington, DC: U.S. Government Printing Office.

U.S. Department of Health and Human Services. (1996). *Models that work: Compendium of innovative primary health-care programs for underserved and vulnerable populations.* Bethesda, MD: DHHHS/HRSA/BPHC.

U.S. Department of Health and Human Services. (2003). *Steps to a healthier US: A program and policy perspective—The power of prevention.* Washington, DC: Author.

van Oers, H. A., Haverman, L., Limperg, P. F., van Dijk-Lokkart, E. M., Maurice-Stam, H., & Grootenhuis, M. A. (2014). Anxiety and depression in mothers and fathers of a chronically ill child. *Maternal Child Health, 8*(8), 1993–2002.

Veldorale-Griffin, A., & Darling, C. (2016). Adaptation to parental gender transition: Stress and resilience among transgender parents. *Archives of Sexual Behavior, 45*, 607–617.

von Doussa, H., Power, J., McNair, R., Brown, R., Schofied, M., Perlesz, A., … Bickerdik, A. (2016). Building healthcare workers' confidence to work with same-sex parented families. *Health Promotion International.* Advance online publication. doi: 10.1093/heapro/dav010

Vrouenraets, L., Fredriks, A., Hannema, S., Cohen-Kettenis, P., & de Vries, M. (2015). Early medical treatment of children and adolescents with gender dysophoria: An empirical ethical study. *Journal of Adolescent Health, 57*, 367–373.

Waldfogel, J., Craigie, T.-A., & Brooks-Gunn, J. (2010). Fragile families and child wellbeing. *The Future of Children, 20*, 87–112. http://dx.doi.org/10.1353/foc.2010.0002

Weaver, M., Diekema, D., Carr, A., & Triplett, B. (2015). Matched marrow, sibling shadow: The epidemiology, experience, and ethics of sibling donors of stem cells. *Journal of Adolescent and Young Adult Oncology, 4*(3), 100–104.

Weissenberg, R., & Landau, R. (2012). Are two a family? Older single mothers assisted by sperm donation and their children revisited. *American Journal of Orthopsychiatry, 82*, 523–528. http://dx.doi.org/10 .1111/j.1939-0025.2012.01187.x

White, J., & Klein, D. (2008). *Family theories* (3rd ed.). Thousand Oaks, CA: Sage.

Wilkins, K., & Woodgate, R. (2007a). An interruption in family life: Siblings' lived experience as they transition through the pediatric bone marrow transplant trajectory. *Oncology Nursing Forum, 34*, E28–E35.

Wilkins, K., & Woodgate, R. (2007b). Supporting siblings through the pediatric bone marrow transplant trajectory: Perspectives of siblings of bone marrow transplant recipients. *Cancer Nursing, 30*(5), E29_E34.

Williams, K., & Chapman, M. (2011). Comparing health and mental health needs, service use, and barriers to services among sexual minority youth and their peers. *Health and Social Work, 36*, 197–206.

Williams, K., & Chapman, M. (2012). Unmet health and mental health need among adolescents: The roles of sexual minority status and child–parent connectedness. *American Journal of Orthopsychiatry, 82*(4), 473–481.

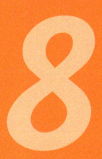

The Health-Care Environment

Mardelle McCuskey Shepley

Objectives

At the conclusion of this chapter, the reader will be able to:

1. Define *environment* in the context of health-care settings, and summarize the general impact of the physical environment on functioning, development, and behavior.
2. Discuss the aspects of the environment in health-care settings that may affect behavior, development, and recovery, highlighting those aspects that have research support.
3. Describe innovative approaches to designing children's health-care environments.
4. Discuss changes in health-care environments for children.

Design is a very broad-based discipline focused on issues of problem solving. Designers encompass a variety of professionals, including architects, interior designers, industrial designers, furniture and fabric designers, landscape architects, and urban designers. Although they are not primary caregivers, designers have an important role to play in health care.

The primary source of psychosocial support of children in the health-care continuum will always be caregivers and their programs. As a secondary source, conscientious designers attempt to provide spaces that will support the endeavors of these individuals. The physical setting of health-care domains can inspire the healing process and perceptions of well-being among patients (Dijkstra, Pieterse, & Pruyn, 2006). Excellent healing environments reinforce excellent clinical quality and, conversely, inferior environments can detract from fine clinical care (Fottler, Ford, Roberts, & Ford, 2000). Designers also aspire to create environments that will directly support the well-being of children and their families. These environments are intended to be inherently healing by reducing stress and providing appropriate settings for normalized activity. Upon accumulation of evidence about the benefits of healing environments, many organizations within health-care industry are integrating features into hospitals with stress reduction and healing promotion objectives (Zborowsky & Kreitzer, 2008).

An analysis of more than 400 research studies by the Center for Health Design shows a direct link between patient health and quality of care and the way a hospital is is designed (Center for Health Design, 2004). Although most researchers agree that the physical environment affects the healing process, patient and staff well-being, and quality of care, additional research is necessary to substantiate design recommendations (Huisman, Morales, Van Hoof, & Kort, 2012; Rollins, 2004; Ulrich et al., 2008; Ulrich, Berry, Quan, & Parish, 2010). A primary link between environment and healing is stress reduction. In this context researchers sometimes refer to psychoneuroimmunology (PNI), defined as "a transdisciplinary scientific field concerned with interactions among behaviors, the immune system, and the nervous system" (Solomon, 1996, p. 79). Proponents of PNI suggest that stress can compromise the immune system, thereby interfering with healing. Because research indicates that the environment can create stress, this theory supports the need for stress reduction in health-care settings.

Designers have an impact on many types of health-care settings. In the traditional context, building types might range from home-care settings to ambulatory care facilities, from day surgery to hospitals, and from skilled nursing facilities to hospices. Additionally, health care can be delivered in a variety of other environments, the primary purposes of which might focus on other services. Among these related building types are day care centers, halfway homes, schools, and community and recreational facilities. In addition to these specific spaces and buildings, designers who advocate a holistic healing process would argue that the health-care environment encompasses communities and regions. The healthy-communities movement is a grassroots effort that is gaining steam into the 21st century. However, while supporting this compelling holistic view of healthy environments, this chapter focuses on individual buildings and landscapes.

The following discussion will address the health-care environment from five perspectives: first, a summary of terms and objectives of *psychosocial issues*, as defined by environmental psychologists; second, examples of *health-care design philosophies* that support family and patient-centered care; third, general *design recommendations for pediatric hospital environments*; fourth, *recent trends in residential health-care settings*; and finally, *dimensions of healing environments*.

Psychosocial Issues

Environmental psychology, or "the study of transactions between individuals and their physical settings" (Gifford, 2014, p. 2), is a relatively new science, the basic tenets of which are steadily being formulated. "In these transactions, individuals change the environment, and their behavior and experience are changed by the environment. Environmental psychology includes theory, research, and practice aimed at improving our relationship with the natural environment and making buildings more humane" (Gifford, 2014, p. 2). Although few design professionals are trained as environmental psychologists, the more experienced design professionals are aware of some of the basic axioms and incorporate those into their design solutions. Many of these precepts are intuitively obvious, although, when not overtly identified, they can get easily lost in the morass of objectives that must be accommodated in a design project.

The importance of the environment in health care was eloquently articulated in the form of a theory proposed by Lawton and Nahemow (1973). Their theory, the press-competence model, suggests that the more compromised patients are with regard to their physical or emotional health, the more susceptible they may be to negative aspects of the physical environment. Environments with a high level of *press* (very challenging) are appropriate when the competence level of an individual is high. When competence is low, an overtaxing environment is not suitable. In these two conditions, adaptive behavior is most successful. The difficulty occurs when the environment is inappropriately matched with the individual's competence level. Hospitals, for example, which may be confusing or technologically overstimulating, can undermine a patient's self-confidence. However, gerontologists developed the press-competence model, and the place of children within this theory must be considered. Are children more vulnerable to the physical environment than adults? If we assume that adults, having more experience in the world, are more callused to environmental stimulation, then we should expect children to be more sensitive to it.

In spite of its youth, the field of environmental psychology deals with very important psychosocial issues. These include (a) control, (b) privacy and social interaction, (c) personal space, (d) territoriality, and (e) comfort and safety. All of these terms are interrelated, and it is often difficult to speak of one without incorporating the others into the definition.

Control

The concept of *locus of control* originated in personality theory and generally refers to the perceived seat of social control. When an individual's health or the health of a family member is compromised, the resultant mindset is one of disempowerment or lack of control. A physical environment that prohibits individuals from managing their space and thwarts opportunities for regulation of the environment can contribute to this disempowerment and helplessness. Several studies have directly linked the built environment to helplessness and shown that architecture may have an effect as well. Better feelings and improved mental health have been attributed to increased possibilities for control over one's surroundings (Evans, 1982, 2003). Roger Ulrich, an environmental psychologist, included the provision of a sense of control as one of his four primary health-facility design guidelines (see Ulrich, 1999, 2000, 2001; Ulrich et al., 2008; Ulrich et al., 2010) and a primary objective in patient-centered care (Devlin & Arneill, 2003).

A health-care environment can undermine control in many ways. A classic example is impeded *wayfinding*, the behavior an individual exhibits when attempting to locate or arrive at a destination. When a building design results in poor wayfinding, that individual may become frustrated and lost. People who have been lost as children recount that experience as among the most frightening of childhood and can find this experience very intimidating in adulthood, as well (Passini, 2002). Confusion over one's orientation and the impression of being lost can cause extreme emotional responses, including insecurity and anxiety as well as challenges with self-esteem and assessments of competence (Passini, 2002; Peponis, Zimring, & Choi, 1990). Regarding health-care settings, an individual may enter into a frustrating wayfinding situation in an already distracted state because of poor health or concern about the poor health of a friend or family member. The unpleasantness of this disorientation is exacerbated by these stresses.

Various techniques can be employed to mitigate the potentially confounding aspects of a building's configuration, including the location of landmarks (e.g., plants or paintings) at critical intersections of the building; placement of windows along circulation paths to orient individuals relative to the outside of the building; clear designation of building entries; and massing of buildings that suggest their interior use. Buildings with massing that supports wayfinding are buildings whose shape and size suggest the activity that takes place inside. For example, an auditorium might appear on the outside as a large windowless volume, and a corridor might be articulated as a long linear element. The objective is to allow the viewer to guess how the interior is organized by looking at the exterior envelope. Surprisingly, signage is not the primary means of providing wayfinding, although it can be very useful as a redundant system. There are several excellent articles and books on this topic, including Carpman and Grant's *Design That Cares* (2016).

In addition to wayfinding, other examples of how an environment can deprive a patient or family member of control include those that render patients and/or family unable to do the following:

- control room temperature,
- control lighting from bed,
- open or close window shades from bed,
- see out of a window because cubicle curtains, bed railings, or furniture block the view,
- open a door because of the strength required to overcome the door mechanism,
- turn a doorknob to open a door because of weakness associated with illness or medications,
- pass a wheelchair through a narrow entry,
- use a toilet because of lack of adjacent space to make a transfer off a wheelchair
- have privacy when needed,
- control noise, and
- accommodate the presence of family members.

An additional source of frustration for a child can be an environment that is designed at adult scale. Ergonometrically correct pediatric furniture and plumbing fixtures and conveniently placed door hardware and light switches are small gestures that can increase the accessibility of a child's environment. Appropriate healing environments should enhance feelings of efficacy rather than compromise them. The resultant sense of control helps reduce stress levels.

Privacy and Social Interaction

Health-care environments should provide opportunities for both privacy and social interaction. According to Altman (1975), privacy is directly related to control issues, in that privacy can be defined as the selective control of social interactions. Patients and families may wish to control access not only to themselves but also to groups with which they identify. The ability to control interactions is so important that these skills may be even more important than the interactions themselves.

In a health-care setting, privacy and social interaction can be accommodated through seating and furniture configuration, furniture and casework design, room configuration, and floor plan layout. Seating arrangements can directly support or undermine social interaction. *Sociopetal* seating, which orients chairs to enable conversation, has the opposite effect of *sociofugal* seating, which discourages interaction by orienting seats away from one another (see Figures 8.1 and 8.2).

Sociopetal seating is not always preferred over sociofugal seating (Nussbaumer, 2013). In a study of adult ICU waiting rooms, Fournier (1994) found that families sought both kinds of seating: those that allowed family members to be alone and those

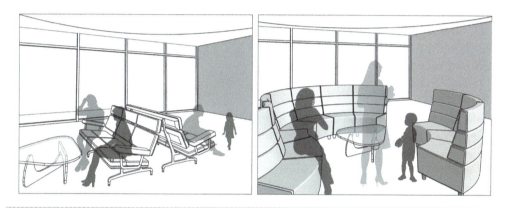

Figure 8.1. Sociopetal seating supports conversation, and sociofugal seating discourages social interaction.

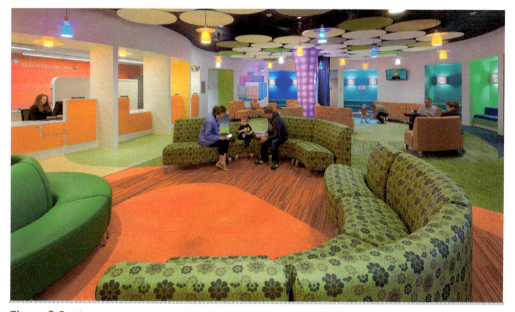

Figure 8.2. The seating arrangement in the waiting area allows for conversation and enables families to watch children while they play. *Note.* Photograph used with permission of Steffian Bradley Architects.

that allowed them to commiserate with other families visiting the ICU. The sharing of information that can take place in a sociopetal environment can support parents in coping with their crisis (Gooding, et al., 2011; Hughes, McCollum, Sheftel, & Sanchez, 1994). The quality of waiting time could be improved via combinations of sociopetal and sociofugal arrangements of seating; proximity and communication are improved in sociopetal arrangements, whereas sociofugal seating is more suited for patients who prefer solitude (Ibrahim, Harun, & Samad, 2010).

Furniture and casework (built-in counters and cabinets) also can be designed to encourage or discourage interaction. Highly elevated nurses' stations may intimidate children (and adults) who wish to interact with nursing staff. Similarly, room configuration can influence privacy. The placement of the restroom relative to the bed can be manipulated to allow nursing staff to observe activity once they enter the room but protect patient visibility from general passersby. Finally, the floor plans of nursing units should be flexible enough to accommodate a variety of activities along the private-to-socially interactive spectrum.

In addition to spatial and visual privacy, auditory privacy is an equally significant concern (Ulrich et al., 2008). When patients share rooms, they are privy to one another's personal phone conversations as well as their discussions with medical staff, family members, and visitors. Many prefer private rooms to reduce this intrusion. If grieving rooms are not provided for parents who have experienced the loss of a child, then grieving parents must withhold their response or demonstrate their loss publicly. Interestingly, outdoor space is sometimes used to provide privacy. The introduction of a fountain into a public area, either indoors or outdoors, will generate enough white noise to allow individuals to have a private conversation without being overheard. Designers can also enhance auditory privacy by using acoustical, maintainable materials to control sound.

Personal Space

Robert Sommer (2008) defined personal space as "an area with invisible boundaries surrounding a person's body into which intruders may not come." More colloquially, personal space is thought of as the imaginary bubble around oneself that defines one's relationships with others. Sommer noted,

> Hospital patients complain not only that their personal space and their very bodies are continually violated by nurses, interns, and physicians who do not bother to introduce themselves or explain their activities, but that their territories are violated by well-meaning visitors who will ignore "No Visitors" signs. Frequently patients are too sick or too sensitive to repel intruders. (p. 43)

An interesting aspect of personal-space behavior is that it may vary with age. This variation is particularly challenging in the design of pediatric units because the developmental age of the patients ranges dramatically. When recording the behavior of children ages 2 to 4 years, Okano (1985) found that the higher the mental age of the children, the farther away from themselves they would place a silhouette of someone they disliked. In a related study, Burgess and McMurphy (1982) observed the behavior of children 6 months to 5 years old and found that distance from adults increased with age, but distance to playmates decreased. Although infants (ages 6 to 18 months) stayed close to their adult caretakers, toddlers and preschoolers avoided the space around these adults.

Of the few studies examining the spatial behavior of children in health-care settings, one noted that hospitalized children participating in a program of planned play demonstrate more positive feelings in life-space drawings than those without a planned program (Gillis, 1989). In another study, Schoffstall (1984) examined how the stress of hospitalization affects children's personal space by comparing the distancing of stimulus figures by children 7 to 13 years of age who were hospitalized and nonhospitalized. The study measured stress levels and distancing patterns in response to figures representing mothers, fathers, nurses, doctors, strangers, and friends. The researcher predicted that hospitalized children would distance figures more than nonhospitalized children would; although the overall trend supported this prediction, the data were not statistically significant. The study indicated, however, that the increased stress associated with hospitalization was correlated with increased distances from nurses, doctors, and male strangers. Schoffstall concluded that personal space acts as a buffer to protect individuals from a perceived threat.

In a related study, Sanfilippo (1994) focused on the personal space and coping behaviors of terminally and chronically ill children with HIV and cancer. Three groups of children—HIV symptomatic, those diagnosed with cancer, and healthy children—were compared. Children who were HIV positive perceived their parents to distance themselves farther away from them than children with cancer did. All sick children reported greater distancing of parents than that perceived by their mothers.

A more recent study on Iranian and German children and adolescents' personal space preferences during their hospital stay revealed that spaces without physical barriers, which could increase chances of informal social interactions among individuals, were generally preferred. Separation of beds with curtains was among the least preferred options by the respondents (Litkouhi, Geramipour, & Litkouhi, 2012).

Proxemic behavior is integral to the concept of personal space. Hall (1990) described *proxemics* as "the interrelated observations and theories of man's use of space as a specialized elaboration of culture" (see Figure 8.3). Hall identified four types of psychological distance: public, social, personal, and intimate. Public distance in a hospital setting might be observed when a medical resident makes a presentation to interns. In this situation, the speaker generally stands at least 12 feet from an audience. Social distance is expressed frequently in health-care settings. This proxemic characteristic is the distance at which informal business takes place, such as asking questions at the information counter or making purchases at the gift shop. Social distance is thought to be between 4 and 12 feet. Individuals who know each another or who must share private information keep personal distance. Personal distance is often exercised in an exam room or inpatient room and, according to Hall, ranges from 18 inches to 4 feet. Intimate distance (less than 18 inches) is the distance at which caregiving might take place, particularly by friends or family members. Direct contact is not unusual. Natural conflicts, however, may take place when a caregiver who is unknown to the patient must trespass into the patient's intimate space to provide treatment or assess health.

Adult patients and staff in a critical-care setting were evaluated regarding their perceptions of the use of space and touch (Edwards, 1998). Using behavioral observation

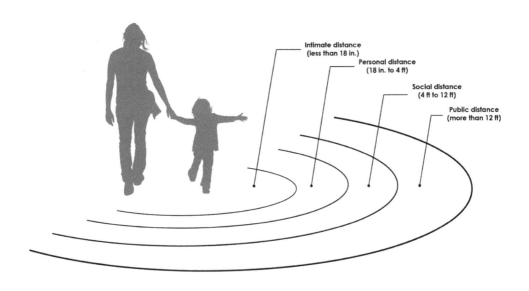

Figure 8.3. There are four types of psychological distance: public, social, personal, and intimate.

and interviews, the researcher found that normal spatial behavior was interrupted and that "rules" differed for patients and staff. Both staff and patients defined the patient's personal space as containing the curtain, bed, and adjacent furniture. Although patients accepted the intrusion of staff into this space, they did not accept intrusions by other patients.

Proponents of proxemic theory suggest that different cultures have different spatial behaviors. Awareness of these cultural differences is critical in contemporary health settings. Caregivers are serving multicultural communities, so awareness of differences between groups will enable them to increase their effectiveness. Researchers have proposed that people's sense of spatial distancing may vary depending on their cultural or ethnic background. Certain groups may have smaller personal space requirements and be more comfortable with physical contact. Olson (1999) identified those groups as Arabs (from Iraq, Kuwait, Saudi Arabia, Syria, United Arab Republic), Latin Americans (from Bolivia, Cuba, El Salvador, Mexico, Ecuador, Paraguay, Peru, Puerto Rico, Venezuela), and Southern Europeans (from France, Italy, Turkey). Noncontact groups may include Asians (from China, Indonesia, Japan, Philippines, Thailand), Northern Europeans (from Australia, England, Germany, the Netherlands, Norway, Scotland), and Indians and Pakistanis. North Americans have been described as falling into the noncontact group; however, our progressively multicultural composition may result in a behavioral shift. In 1998 Noyes reported that no studies examined different ethnic and cultural groups regarding parental health-care experience. However, two studies (i.e., Seid, Stevens, & Varni, 2003; Yeh, McCabe, Hough, Dupuis, & Hazen, 2003) discuss how access to health care is affected by race and ethnicity.

What are the environmental implications of proxemic behavior for children and their families? Because of the diversity of needs, designers should be careful to provide a variety of furniture arrangements and room activity densities to correspond to differing spatial perspectives.

Territoriality

The third commonly used term in environmental psychology is *territoriality*. Gifford (2014) defined territoriality as a pattern of "behavior and attributes" based on perceived, attempted, or actual control of a quantifiable physical space. Territoriality can be differentiated from privacy in that it addresses domain and ownership rather than sense of personal separation. As with privacy, there are multiple realms of territory, ranging from primary territory to public territory (Altman & Chemers, 1980). Primary territory in a hospital would be the patient's room. A hospital dining room is normally public territory. Lyman and Scott (1967) noted three ways in which a territory may be disturbed: (1) invasion (when a territory is physically entered by an outsider), (2) violation (when a territory is purposely modified by an outsider), and (3) contamination (in which something inappropriate is left behind in a territory). In the context of a hospital or clinic waiting room, territory would be invaded if a stranger sat between two family members having a conversation. The space would be violated if that stranger took a coat sitting on a chair in that conversational unit and moved it. It would be contaminated if the intruding individual spilled a cup of coffee and left it behind.

A single person may control a territory. In hospitals, territories controlled by individuals include patient rooms, nursing stations, and exam rooms. Groups can also control territories. A hospital billing office and the living room of a home are examples of territories under the control of several people. Subterritories can exist within the boundaries of public space: The corner of a waiting room that a family has been occupying for an extended period naturally evolves into its territory.

Spontaneous territorial gestures are evident throughout health-care environments. They include the following:

- photographs or drawings in a patient's room (see Figure 8.4),
- relocation of furniture by families in waiting rooms to accommodate their needs,
- advertisements for activities in a nursing station,
- placement of coats and belongings on furniture in a waiting room, and
- decorations on a playroom wall.
- Other more permanent territorial markers are signage, elevated nursing-station counters, and locked doors (see Figure 8.5).

Distinguishing between personal space and territory is important. Personal space is an invisible space that is "carried around" with an individual as he or she moves (Altman, 1975; Lane, 1990), whereas territory is associated with a particular physical environment (Altman, 1975; Leino-Kilpi et al., 2001). One of the few studies on territorial behavior in a health-care setting (Allekian, 1973) focused on adult patients and found that patients experienced anxiety when intrusions of territory took place, but when personal space was intruded, patients accepted the violation indifferently. Shepley, Fournier, and McDougal (1998) posited that "healthcare settings are effective socially when they have clear boundaries that create territories for people" (p. 163). Clarity of ownership helps deflect potential conflict. For a summary of the role of territoriality as it applies to health-care design for critical-care settings, see Hamilton and Shepley, 2010.

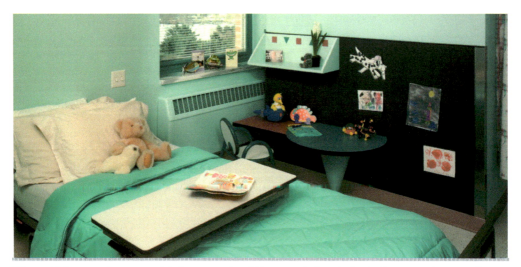

Figure 8.4. Space for personal belongings should be provided at the bedside. *Note.* Photograph used with permission of Newton-Wellesley.

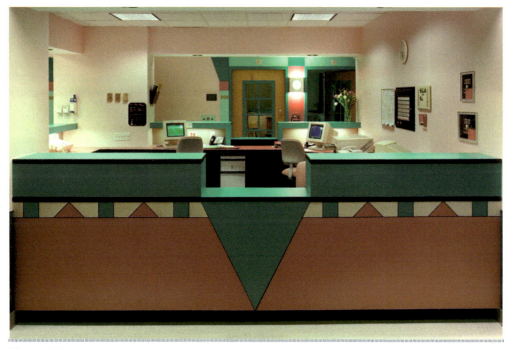

Figure 8.5. Nurses' stations can be barriers for children. Lowering the counter to child height will help eliminate unnecessary territorial markers. *Note.* Photograph used with permission of Newton-Wellesley.

When identifying the preference of health-care setting participants, Douglas and Douglas (2005) noted that a supportive environment and the space that fulfills public and private needs are key notions. The characteristics of a supportive physical space and social space were associated with negotiability and flexibility in space and having control and ownership over one's space by prior agreement (Douglas & Douglas, 2005).

The concepts of personal privacy in space and having control over one's space are important aspects of establishing a home environment in hospitals for patients (Burden, 1998). However, McLaughlin, Olson, and White (2008) suggest that patients are typically considered to be part of the hospital room by nurses and that the main control of the patient's room is maintained by nurses. For example, bedside tables are widely used as work spaces for the nurses and not considered to be part of the patient's space (McLaughlin et al., 2008). Meeting the privacy needs of all inhabitants in the constrained physical space of most hospital wards has led to considerable tension (Gilmour, 2006).

Comfort and Safety

Comfort and safety are critical aspects of psychosocial well-being and are related to issues of control and privacy. The majority of the studies on comfort needs in pediatric health environments focus on family members (e.g., Kasper & Nyamathi, 1988; Kirschbaum, 1990). Meyer, Snelling, and Myren-Manbeck (1998) noted that parents may be intimidated by the "unfamiliar physical surrounds, and the equipment." Farrell and Frost (1992) identified the following personal needs of parents related to the physical environment:

- a place to rest,
- a place to take care of personal needs,
- a nearby telephone,
- a nearby bathroom,
- available refreshments, and
- solitude (a place to be alone).

In a modified Delphi study, Endacott (1998) cited the following other areas of family need: physiological assessment, psychosocial needs, family-centered care, hygiene needs, nutrition needs, appropriate stimulation and rest, cultural needs, spiritual needs, specific interventions related to physiological needs, dependable equipment, safety needs, and collaboration with other professionals. Areas of need identified in the first round of the research were carried in the second round as "standard practices." For these items, 80% to 100% of the subjects agree that they should be routinely implemented. Standard-practice items relating to the physical environment included emergency equipment at the bedside, accommodation for parents, and refreshment facilities for parents.

Studies of environmental comfort needs, other than those of parents, have been limited but are increasing. In a review of the literature on children's needs (Price, 1994), the category of physical environmental needs was not included. However, in 1989 Oksala and Merenmies used nurse-administered questionnaires to determine child needs in an ICU during the first day, the middle day, and the last day in intensive care. The most clearly articulated need throughout all periods was the need for rest and leisure, both of which are dependent on the physical environment. The need for "beauty and aesthetic experiences, and sensory integrity" became more prevalent toward the end of the stay. Several subsequent publications (e.g., Shepley, 2014; Shepley, Fournier, & McDougal, 1998; Shultz, 2008) have focused specifically on the topic of health-care environments for children and their families.

Design professionals who are aware of all these psychosocial issues—privacy and social interaction, control, personal space, territoriality, and comfort and safety—will be better able to support caregivers' efforts and the well-being of patients and their families via the physical environment.

Health-Care Design Philosophies

Philosophies on healing environments generally address social ambience rather than physical space. A handful of philosophies, however, have evolved with a clear focus on the physical environment. The best known of these are patient-centered design, Easy Street and Rehab 1-2-3, anthroposophy, evidence-based design, generative design, and salutogenic design.

Planetree and the Institute for Patient-Centered Design

Barbara Cliff (2012), in an article on the evolution of patient-centered care, argued that under the Affordable Care Act, patient-centered care has evolved into a principal objective of the U.S. health-care system. By shifting the focus to the patient, considerable improvements in patient satisfaction, clinical outcomes, and cost reduction can occur (Cliff, 2012). As the reform in health care continues to direct hospitals toward achieving better patient outcomes using fewer sources and lower expenses, patient-centered care will continue its effective role by shortening length of stay, reducing visits to the emergency department and readmissions, and improving patient conformity with plans of care (Cliff, 2012). Two organizations have taken the lead regarding patient-centered design: Planetree and the Institute for Patient Centered Design.

Angela Thieriot founded Planetree in response to her personal unpleasant hospital experiences. Reacting in part to what she recognized as patients' need to become educated about their illness, she began by developing a health resource center where patients could access information. This concept eventually achieved its hospital incarnation in a 13-bed medical unit at a large San Francisco hospital (Frampton & Charmel, 2009; Orr, 1995).

According to Planetree's current website, Planetree's vision is the promotion of "the development and implementation of innovative models of health care that focus on healing and nurturing body, mind and spirit" (Planetree, 2014). The fact that Planetree is known for the physical environments that support its goals is unusual for a health-care philosophy, and therefore of particular interest to designers. Planetree environments are typically fully accessible and home-like, and include a variety of elements that support patients and their families, such as,

- resource libraries,
- kitchenettes,
- art carts,
- patient-welcoming nursing stations,
- lounges,
- activity rooms,

- chapels,
- gardens,
- overnight family sleep spaces,
- fountains, and
- healing gardens. (Planetree, n.d.)

Spaces are available for patient privacy as well as social opportunities. Break areas are provided for staff to allow them to reenergize.

Planetree supports values that most children's health organizations have adopted, although few children's facilities have fully incorporated its philosophies. One exception is the Wendy Paine O'Brien Adolescent Treatment Center (Samaritan Hospital) in Phoenix, Arizona. A recent remodeling of this facility involved taking the glass barriers out of the nurses' station and increasing the family visiting areas. Proposed projects for the Treatment Center include a patient-family resource center, healing garden, gift shop, and chapel (Planetree, n.d.). Planetree currently has affiliates around the United States and internationally. In 2002 Romano observed that Planetree's philosophy was on the health-care periphery; however, evidence has accumulated on its positive contributions to the lives of staff and improvements in clinicians' satisfaction levels (Stichler, 2008).

Another more recently founded organization, which aims to provide patients a voice in the development of the healing environment, is the Institute for Patient-Centered Design, Inc. (Institute for Patient-Centered Design, Inc., 2015). As a key component of developing a successful project, the Institute has adopted the objective of encouraging the participation of patients and families in the design process in addition to health-care providers, clinicians and design teams (Institute for Patient-Centered Design, Inc., 2015).

The Institute aims to enhance the environment of care by attending to the needs of patients and their families through design. Its mission is "to contribute to the quality of health-care delivery through patient-centered design advocacy, education and research" (Institute for Patient-Centered Design, Inc., 2015).

Easy Street and Rehab 1-2-3

Easy Street is a rehabilitative environment designed to simulate real-life experiences. Developed by David Guynes in 1985, the environment is used by adults who are attempting to reintegrate themselves into the mainstream by practicing on environments that more closely proximate what they will encounter in the real world (e.g., portions of checkout stands, turnstiles, cars and buses, restaurants, mailboxes). Guynes also developed an alternative for children. This alternative, Rehab 1-2-3, was designed around a gameboard concept that, like Easy Street, used the environment to support rehabilitation (Moore & Jordan, 1997; see Figure 8.6).

Providing inspiration for children to engage in rehabilitation activities can be a challenging task. However, through design it may be possible to change the objectives of completing rehabilitation exercises from the abstract (engagement in rehabilitation activities) to the concrete goals to which children strive: engaging in play activities with friends, returning to school, going back home after an injury or sickness (McClusky, 2008). Various components are intended to allow for improvements in children's cognitive and memory skills, dexterity, and range of motion as they develop their strength, balance, and memory (McClusky, 2008).

Anthroposophy

Founded by Rudolf Steiner in 1924, the Anthroposophical Society supports a philosophy focusing on "opening up to the various spiritual realms connected with human life through our conscious understanding" (Anthroposophical Society, 1999). The world-famous Vidarkliniken, in Jarna, Sweden, embodies these values in its architecture. The intent of this facility is to provide a "sense of living order" (Logsdon, 1995). Farms and a bakery provide activities on the site, in addition to a health facility for children and adults (Malkin, 1992). The philosophy reflected in the building assumes an evolution on the part of the healing patient from containment to exploration.

Evidence-Based Design

The Center for Health Design (CHD) defines evidence-based design as the "process of basing decisions about the built environment on credible research to achieve the best possible outcomes" (Goetz et al., 2010, p. 2). Stichler and Hamilton (2008) identified the objective for evidence-based design (EBD) as utilization of data from various creditable sources to inform design decisions, with the eventual objective of enhancing the patient care experience, the work environment for staff, and organizational performance.

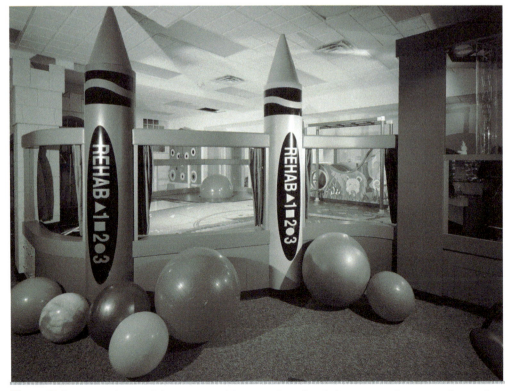

Figure 8.6. Designed around the concept of the game board, Rehab 1-2-3 simulates a nonhospital environment to support rehabilitation. *Note.* Photograph used with permission of Guynes Design.

Kirk Hamilton expanded the definition of evidence-based design in 1993 to include references to "critical decisions made with clients on the basis of the best available information." Later, the language of "conscientious, explicit, and judicious use" (Hamilton, 2006) was added to the description, building on David Sackett's definition of evidence-based medicine (see Sackett et al., 1996). Emphasizing process in the definition of evidence-based design was a response to those who anticipated a product. Hamilton's revised definition was: "Evidence-based design is a process for the conscientious, explicit, and judicious use of current best evidence from research and practice in making critical decisions, together with an informed client, about the design of each individual and unique project" (Hamilton & Watkins, 2009, p. 9). The definition has evolved to reflect the education obtained through the practice of the EBD process (Goetz et al., 2010). Research-informed design has enlivened this field through evidence-based health-care architecture, the creation of safe and healing environments for patient care, and enhancement of family engagement (Hamilton, 2003). EBD health-care architecture also encourages efficiency in staff performance, provides restorative experiences for clinicians under stress, and aims to improve the organization's clinical, economic, productivity, satisfaction, and cultural measures (Hamilton, 2003).

Generative Design

Generative space is among the emerging notions in designing for health-care environments (Ruga, 2008). Generative space addresses both physical space and social environment; experiencing interaction with other humans in the background of a physical environment substantially informs the patients' health outcomes (Ruga, 2008). Generative environments are described as the third kind of space, in addition to physical space and social environment (Ruga, 2008). By using both social and physical spaces for achieving improved experiences, generative space supports the "sustainability" of outcomes (Ruga, 2008). Tama Duffy Day, lead designer on the Arlington Free Clinic in Arlington, Virginia, viewed the project as a case study for generative design in its embrace of both evidence-based design and sustainable design, where the medical professional and the patient can engage in physical as well as the social space (The Caritas Project, 2015).

Salutogenic Design

The salutogenic approach to designing environments is based on eliminating features that generate negative stress and enriching the environment by adding factors that result in improvements in personal control, access to nature and daylight, inclusion of spaces for private and public relaxation, and spaces with aesthetically pleasing qualities (Heerwagen, Heubach, Montgomery, & Weimer, 1995).

Dilani (2008) asserted that the salutogenic approach creates a primary theoretical guideline for "psychosocially supportive design," which advocates for health and well-being. Heerwagen et al. (1995) provided a framework for a salutogenic design, emphasizing an ecological and holistic approach, which looks at interconnections among people, procedures, events, and places. This framework emphasizes the following factors: (1) social cohesion and providing opportunities for formal and informal interactions; (2) personal control and allowing for regulation of temperature, daylight, lighting, and sound, as well as access to private rooms; and (3) opportunities for relaxation and restoration via access to quiet rooms, nature, and soft lighting (Heerwagen et al., 1995). Also, in a psychologically supportive design, factors such as access to spiritual and symbolic features, access to ample lighting and art, an appealing environment for social interactions, spaces of solitude, and interior spaces affording positive experiences should be incorporated in design (Dilani, 2008). Psychosocially supportive design requires understanding of the meaning of "salutary management" by the entire organization; it is not the task of one individual (Dilani, 2008).

The salutogenic model of care requires a systematic investigation and verification of its principles through empirical studies identifying the range for well-being factors in psychosocially supportive design (Dilani, 2008). Empirical studies should encourage decision-makers to apply psychosocially supportive design and promote health and well-being (Dilani, 2008).

Most designers begin their projects by seeking goals that will help guide the design process. Evidence-based design, Planetree, Easy Street, anthroposophy, generative design, and salutogenic design provide philosophical approaches that can be readily embraced in the development of new facilities.

Design Recommendations for Pediatric Hospital Environments

Much has been written about traditional hospital and ambulatory care environments, and the reader is advised to consult these references for more detailed information (see Appendix 8.1). With regard to some of the specific psychosocial factors described above, the design guidelines summarized in *Healthcare Environments for Children and their Families* (Shepley et al., 1998), *Design for Pediatric and Neonatal Critical Care* (Shepley, 2014), and *Evidence for Innovation* (Shultz, 2008) are particularly relevant. Regarding the hospital environment as a whole, the authors make the following recommendations.

Access

A welcoming, accessible, clearly designated, and appropriately scaled entry and reception to the hospital will provide a supportive experience for children and their families. Consideration of such issues provides a "gentle" entry into an environment that may hold many unknowns for children and their families. The site of the facility should be designed to be psychologically supportive by clearly indicating destination locations, providing convenient access to buildings, and being safe. Having a drop-off area near the entrance, for example, accommodates individuals carrying belongings and equipment. The exterior of the building must also support accessibility and wayfinding through the message it communicates in its exterior massing and circulation systems (corridors and elevators). For example, the organization of the building should be evident and well marked, and separate corridors and elevators should be designated for the transport of critically ill patients.

Child Spaces

Spaces occupied by pediatric patients should be located near the services that hospital staff members are trying to provide. Psychological support can be communicated by the inclusion of spaces that allow for social interaction (e.g., lounges, large patient rooms), privacy (e.g., areas or wall spaces dedicated specifically to a patient), and access to nature (e.g., appropriately located gardens, outdoor play areas, windows). The environment should reflect child-centered care by providing areas such as playrooms or teen rooms for age-appropriate activities, adequately scaled furniture and light controls, and choices in types of space.

Family Spaces

Lack of dedicated space for family members may result in conflicts with staff, and opportunities for parents to care for their children may also be curtailed. Adequate space for guests within the patient room is essential, and the basic needs of a parent who might be confined to the hospital for an undetermined period of time must be taken into account. Such needs range from the basics (e.g., restrooms, showers, kitchenettes) to helping family members maintain their link to the outside world (e.g., computers, telephones, work spaces).

Staff Spaces

The needs of staff are often overlooked in hospital design. When staff needs are not considered, staff morale may be low, and existing patient spaces may have to be usurped for staff functions. Environments that support privacy (e.g., personal storage, staff lounges) and staff collaboration (e.g., conferences areas, large workstations) will indirectly benefit patients by supporting caregivers' psychological states.

Building Systems

Details such as lighting, acoustics, and ambience are important in hospital environments. If lighting is varied and flexible, then staff, patients, and families will have a greater sense of efficacy because a variety of tasks and activities will be supported. Natural light also should be considered because it clearly contributes to feelings of well-being. The detrimental effects of unwanted noise on sleep have been documented. Additionally, family and staff may wish to have private conversations and require spaces that are acoustically controlled. Sound-absorptive materials (e.g., carpet, acoustical ceiling tile) coupled with operational protocols involving noise control (e.g., beeper systems rather than public address systems) can go a long way toward eliminating noise problems. Lastly, aesthetics cannot be overlooked as an important factor in a supportive hospital stay. The application of trendy colors can be avoided if the designer seeks universal design solutions, such as the incorporation of nature elements and healing art.

Recent Trends in Residential Health-Care Settings

Innovations in hospital design reflect a growing awareness of and attention to the psychosocial needs of children and their families. Two trends include parent training spaces and single-room NICUs, and those will be discussed in the following section. This chapter also discusses the transition spaces outside hospital setting. The hospital room setting typically is the first to come to mind when considering pediatric health-care environments; however, there are other settings in the health-care continuum. Four of these settings—couplet care, rooming in, cooperative care, and home care—are gaining importance in children's health care. Rooming in and health system–sanctioned home care have been in existence long enough to confirm their usefulness in the spectrum of healing environments. Cooperative care is newer and represents the step between rooming in and home care.

Parent Training Spaces

Training spaces are critical to the psychological comfort of parents. One or more rooms are recommended in open-bay NICUs and PICUs where private spaces are required to simulate the home environment. When single family rooms (SFRs) are available, separate training rooms are not needed. Training rooms should be provisioned with the equipment that the child will be using at home, most typically ventilators, oxygen, or infusion therapy (Dittbrenner, 1999). Equipment and supplies should be in place at home prior to the child's arrival (Harris, 1988).

Single-Family-Room NICUs

One of the recent trends in the design of neonatal intensive care units has been the creation of single family rooms (Shepley, 2014). Traditionally, neonates have been placed in open rooms with 8 to 60 isolettes or smaller bays with 4 to 6 patient stations. SFRs are thought to be a better environment for infants because they enable customized light levels and control noise. Attendance to appropriate light and sound levels may positively influence a baby's ability to sleep and promote healing. Regarding families, individual rooms provide more privacy and the possibility of sleeping near one's child. Moreover, if a child dies or an emergency (code) takes place, other families do not have to be exposed to the incident. Studies of the impact of SFRs on staff suggest that they are thought to be more beneficial than open-bay arrangements (Shepley, Harris, & White, 2008).

In terms of potential shortcomings, some research suggests that separate rooms may reduce the opportunity for spontaneous communication between families and that some parents and staff may feel more confident when the babies are directly supervised and staff can respond quickly (Shepley, Harris, White, & Steinberg, 2006). Also, construction costs are higher because of expanded space requirements (Shepley et al., 2006). Overall, however, the research on SFRs suggests that they are of benefit to the infant, family, and staff (Shepley, 2014).

Couplet Care Environments

Couplet care allows a mother and her baby to stay together while they are both in the hospital. The physical environment plays a critical role because it creates the setting for their interaction. Spradlin (2009) cites facilitation of family bonding, support of successful breastfeeding, and increase in patient satisfaction among the goals for couplet care, especially after birth when mother and infant are kept together. In case of an unanticipated cesarean birth, providing safe and family-centered couplet care is a more complex challenge (Mahlmeister, 2005). Successfully maintaining a safe and supportive setting requires increased alertness from nurses with a comprehensive awareness of postoperative complications, which is most critical in the first 24 hours after birth (Mahlmeister, 2005).

Many research findings suggest the positive effects of couplet-centered maternity nursing on overall bonding and role attainment (Husmillo, 2013). Bystrova et al. (2009), as cited in Husmillo (2013), mentioned that a review of the literature on the influence of skin-to-skin contact between mother and baby in the first postbirth hour indicated multiple positive outcomes when compared with separation.

Rooming In

Similar to couplet care, rooming-in supports the presence of mother–child dyads during the traditional stay at a birthing facility but, unlike couplet care, the mother is not being detained due to her health status. Although the majority of children's hospitals have adopted rooming in, it is useful to summarize the design implications of this operational policy. Johnson, Jeppson, and Redburn (1992) recommended that in addition to sufficient space for sleeping and caregiving activities of families, space should be provided for a parent lounge, food preparation area, laundry, library, and consultation and teaching space. White (1993) also recommended dedicated storage and telephones. Another element of support for rooming in with a child would be Internet access. Although parents express a strong need to be near their child, parents should also have ready access to respite spaces such as outdoor seating areas, lounges, and cafeterias.

Jaafar, Lee, and Ho (2012) emphasized the importance of bed arrangement and mentioned that rooming in with the cot attached to the bed can be associated with greater frequency of breastfeeding. White (2003) also recommended telephone(s), restroom facilities, and lockable storage, as well as a separate and dedicated room in or immediately adjacent to the NICU for lactation support and consultation. A computer station in the parent lounge or at the infant's bedside will facilitate access to the educational materials and Internet.

Cooperative Care

Cooperative care involves the participation of a nonmedical care partner, but unlike couplet care or rooming in, the patient is not located in a full-fledged medical unit. The cooperative care center may be on another floor of the inpatient building or in an adjacent building. To qualify for this program, the patient must require acute hospitalization but not need continuous care. He or she must be capable, with the support of a care partner, of attending centralized eating facilities and clinical sessions (Grieco, Garnett, Glassman, Valoon, & McClure, 1990). Recruiting family and friends to provide for the basic needs of the patient, along with maximizing outpatient care are strategies behind this model (McCullough, 2009). Moreover, more responsibility for patient care is transferred from the staff to the care partner, and the increased control on the side of the patient and care partner makes the transition from hospital to home an easier process (McCullough, 2009).

According to Douglass (1994), the unique characteristics of a cooperative care unit are the separation between residential and support spaces, the hospitality ambience of the design, and the absence of nursing stations. Cooperative care has been used most frequently with geriatric patients, although the concept could be appropriate for children and their families if used as the transition between acute and home settings. McCullough (2009) noted that the cooperative model of care today is often used in caring for transplant, cancer, and rehabilitation patients. Also, it may be implemented in NICU settings to serve as a training room.

McLane, Jones, Lydiatt, Lydiatt, and Richards (2003) referred to the "homelike setting" of a cooperative-care room and its similarities to a hotel suite: the ability to lock doors from the inside for privacy, and a bedroom, bathroom, sitting area, and kitchenette. Additional amenities could be included such as TVs, newspapers, and laundry facilities. Rhode Island Hospital, University of Nebraska Medical Center, and the Tisch Hospital (NYU Medical Center), among others, have cooperative programs, although the author was unable to identify a program specifically dedicated to pediatrics. Shepley and colleagues (1998) suggested that the rarity of existing cooperative-care units for children may be the result of physician concern that children should be kept in acute-care settings until they can go home. They also suggested that the benefits of remaining in an acute-care setting may be outweighed by the stress of being in an institutional setting.

Home Care

The number of medically fragile children being cared for at home is increasing rapidly. Trends in health-care policy suggest a movement from long-term care (LTC) to care in the family home (Caicedo, 2015). Reasons cited for the increase in children being treated at home are (a) the development of ventilators and other sophisticated equipment for home use, (b) the recognition that hospitalization is stressful for children, and (c) the reimbursement structure. Because the pediatric market is linked to managed care and Medicaid, rather than Medicare (as with geriatric patients), it stands on firmer financial ground (Dittbrenner, 1999). Pediatric care also is one of the better sources of private pay (Dittbrenner, 1999). Concern about the susceptibility of children to nosocomial infections while in the hospital may be another reason home care has grown (Dittbrenner, 1999). Essentially, "pediatric homecare services have increased to support a nurturing environment in which families' needs for medical assistance and normal lifestyles combine to meet the comprehensive care needs of the medically fragile child" (Chapman, 1998, p. 12).

Although the medical and familial aspects of pediatric home care have been addressed in the literature, very little has been said about the physical environment needed to support children in these settings. However, Shepley and colleagues (1998) have suggested design criteria for generic home-care settings (see Text Box 8.1).

For successful home care, a candid evaluation of the family's willingness to provide complex home care, adequate experience, and availability of time and energy resources is vital (Elias et al., 2012). The home setting should be evaluated for compliance with safety and accessibility requirements; also, architectural barriers to the accommodation of wheelchairs, lift systems, medical supplies, and hospital beds must be evaluated (Elias et al., 2012). At the community level, local emergency services along with electrical and heating providers should be alerted for the best support for the child and family (Elias et al., 2012).

Text Box 8.1

Design Criteria for the Home-Care Environment

- Accessibility for emergency personnel
- Space for portable equipment
- Family sleep space
- Access to outdoors
- Emergency call system
- Patient-accessible communication systems
- Bedside control of lighting, television, and temperature
- Views outside
- Easy access to bathroom and snacks
- Sufficient space in family room for child in wheelchair or hospital bed
- Secure storage for medications

Note. Adapted from *Healthcare Environments for Children and Their Families,* by M. Shepley, M. A. Fournier, and K. McDougal, 1998, Dubuque, IA: Kendall-Hunt.

Visual impairment and limited mobility bring additional design considerations. Lang and Sullivan (1986) identified the following design guidelines to address the special needs of children who are visually impaired or blind:

- The colors in the room of a child who is visually impaired should be highly contrasting.
- Reflective materials and suspended objects can be used to attract the attention of a child who is visually impaired to the environment at large.
- Sound-making objects can be used in the room of a child who is blind to expand the environment.
- Floor textures can be used to define different spaces.
- Furniture should be located around the perimeter of the room.

Leibrock (1993) offered the following suggestions for children of limited mobility:

- Handrail heights should not exceed 26 inches.
- Lever handles should be used in showers to avoid accidental bumping, or an integral temperature control should be used to avoid scalding.
- Shower controls should be a maximum of 32 inches above the floor.
- Adjustable tables should be provided with sufficient clearance below to accommodate a wheelchair.

Additional factors particularly pertinent to pediatric home care that might be considered are (a) accommodations for siblings, (b) location of child's room near the entry to accommodate visitors, (c) opportunities for stimulation, (d) extension of home environment to school and day care, and (e) access to nature.

Accommodations for Siblings

According to Chapman (1998), siblings "are the least prepared members of the family to accept a medically frail child as part of the family unit" (p. 13). How can the physical environment support their needs? To some siblings, the introduction of home care may feel like an invasion of their private space. Families should recognize demonstration of behavioral problems or academic difficulties in the well sibling; pediatricians should pay close attention to the child–family interactions when family support and counseling might be necessary for the siblings' well-being (Elias et al., 2012). Home size permitting, siblings should be given a space of their own, even if just a study nook or a wall where they can hang posters. These gestures support the innate need for personal space and are a healthy expression of territoriality.

Room Near Entry

The presence of visiting caregivers in the home can feel like an intrusion (Chapman, 1998), in spite of the beneficial contributions they make. One way of reducing this intrusiveness is to select the room nearest the entry for the child's bedroom. This will eliminate the need for caregivers to pass through any more of the house or apartment than necessary. This lack of penetration into the household may also make the child's visitors feel more comfortable.

Opportunities for Stimulation

As Dittbrenner (1999) pointed out with regard to children, "the patients are not just ill; they are growing. They need stimulation in addition to health care, medication and feeding" (p. 13). One source of stimulation will be proximity to the heart of family life, perhaps the kitchen or family room. Another source should be a connection to the outside world. In an apartment, the connection might be a view of the street; in a home, a view of the street or yard.

As always, however, a balance must be struck between stimulation and a restful environment. Oksala and Merenmies (1989) found that the need for "rest and relaxation" was essential during the entire stay in a PICU, while the need for "beauty and aesthetic experiences" became more important during the latter portion of the stay. This latter need is probably similar to what might be appropriate for the home-care experience.

Extensions of Home

According to an interview with Jay A. Perman of the Virginia Commonwealth University Medical College of Virginia, it is important to stop thinking of home in the traditional sense. For most children, schools or day care centers have become an extension of home (Chapman, 1998). Ready accessibility to such facilities is necessary, and this need has been met more frequently since the passing of the Americans with Disabilities Act. Family-focused care incorporates "home care, school and community-based resources that will encourage the family's autonomy" (Chapman, 1998, p. 13).

Access to Nature

Access to nature is a critical component of home. Views of the outdoors support orientation through diurnal and seasonal clues. Access to nature has been associated with reduced stress and the resultant healing effects. Researchers at Johns Hopkins University found that 29% of patients who listened to nature sounds and viewed a nature mural during bronchoscopy found pain control to be good or excellent as opposed to 20.5% of patients in the control group (Diette, Lechtzin, Haponik, Devrotes, & Rubin, 2003). Regarding guidelines for children at home, a protected space where a child can be outdoors should be sought. This could be the stoop or roof of a multistory building or the yard or porch of a house.

Dimensions of Healing Environments

Caregiving environments, as discussed above, address specific settings. Dimensions of healing environments are not setting-specific. They can be applied to any health-care environment. Dimensions of healing environments can be defined as universal qualities of spatial experience that, when appropriately administered, contribute to the therapeutic process. Access to nature, the effects of light and color, and art, music, and sensory therapies are examples of healing dimensions about which studies have been conducted. Some cultures include geomancy as a cluster of therapeutic factors. The effectiveness of most of these proposed healing qualities has been scientifically substantiated, but some, such as geomancy, still require confirmation.

The notion that the physical environment influences healing is directly related to the concept of *psychoneuroimmunology*. Influences include geomancy, access to the outdoors, light and color, and art, music, and sensory therapies.

Geomancy

Geomancy, defined as "divination by means of figures, lines, or geographic features," is prevalent in Asian cultures, and feng shui is Chinese geomancy. *Feng shui* means "wind, water." Feng shui philosophy is used to evaluate the implications of certain spatial configurations and design for the purpose of enhancing energy flows and creating a positive space (Govert, 1993). Rossbach and Lin (1991) have applied the following feng shui guidelines to hospitals:

- Avoid long corridors leading directly from doors.
- Place the bed so that the patient can see the door from a kitty-corner perspective.
- Avoid heavy furniture or furniture behind the bed projecting into the space.
- Provide good views.
- Avoid adjacent beds.
- Do not place a bed directly between the door and the window.

Although feng shui may appear to be philosophical and abstract, many of its precepts are based on the practical experiences of observers. The author's experience with projects reviewed by professional feng shui experts confirms that many of their suggestions are compatible with the requirements of Western technology, particularly with regard to structure and safety.

Several other cultures have similar building philosophies, including the Indian *vastu*, described as "the art of correct setting in order to optimize the benefits of five basic elements of nature . . . and the influence of magnetic fields surrounding the earth" (Purush & Padam, 1998). There are five components of stable buildings: orientation, proportion, canons of Vedic (Hindu) architecture, and character (Purush & Padam, 1998). According to vastu philosophy, hospitals fall into the category of public buildings—one of five categories of architecture established in ancient texts. An example of a typical design guideline for hospitals would be that an L- or U-shaped building should be open to the northeast and heavy in the southwest (Panditji, 1999).

Access to the Outdoors

Nature is an important component in a child's life. Sebba (1991) found that being located in the outdoors is the most significant experience of childhood as identified by adults. Educators argue that being outside fosters all aspects of a child's development (Davies, 1996). Lack of access to the outdoors may be the single most unpleasantly institutional dimension of a hospital environment.

The affinity most children have for the outdoors is evident. Edward O. Wilson (1986) used the word *biofilia* to describe the innate affiliation humans have with other living things. Steve and Rachel Kaplan (1989) suggested that people's preference for the outdoors is the result of the critical contribution to our survival that is provided by an understanding of nature. According to their research, the nature scenes that have the most appeal are those that balance interest with understandability. Ulrich also has conducted studies demonstrating that views of nature may reduce stress and therefore support healing (Ulrich, 1984), as well as studies showing that driving through landscaped areas resulted in lower blood pressure and that such areas were preferred to urban areas with billboards (Parsons, Tassinary, Ulrich, Hebl, & Grossman-Alexander, 1998). Unfortunately, there have been no studies examining how views of the outdoors affect children in health-care settings, although designers have embraced access to nature in pediatric health-care facilities with a great deal of enthusiasm in recent years. (See Figures 8.7, 8.8, and 8.9.)

In a more quantitative study, Olds (1995) asked subjects to imagine where healing would take place. Participants, who included architects, designers, social workers, psychotherapists, nurses, parents, and students, responded with drawings. Seventy-five percent included the outdoors, nature elements, objects drawn with the suggestion of motion, and vistas. Light, animals, and beauty were also common components. Marcus and Barnes (1995) conducted research on the gardens in four hospitals. They found that people who used the gardens used them frequently and reported positive mood outcomes.

Gardens are also an essential part of the Planetree philosophy. "Bringing nature inside through the use of plants, fountains, and skylights as well as encouraging patients, families and staff to go outside into garden areas whenever possible can help transform institutions into healing environments" (Planetree, n.d.; see Figure 8.8). Several Planetree facilities incorporate significant nature components, including a three-story waterfall at Mid-Columbia Medical Center, a water sculpture in the ICU at Griffin Hospital, and a solarium in the rheumatology unit in Trondheim, Norway (Planetree, 2014).

Regarding selection of specific nature images, nonhospital-based studies on landscape preferences of children suggest that children prefer landscapes of the environ-

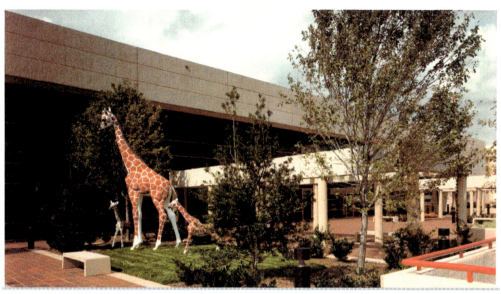

Figure 8.7. Views of nature and access to outdoor spaces are essential to stress reduction. *Note.* Photograph used with permission of Odell Associates.

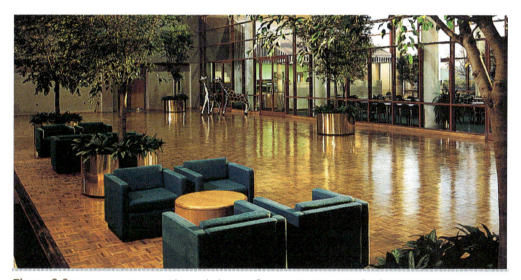

Figure 8.8. Bringing nature inside can help transform institutions into healing environments. *Note.* Photograph used with permission of Odell Associates.

ments with which they are most familiar (Lyons, 1983) and that younger children (11-year-olds) demonstrate less preference for landscapes suggesting risk than older children do (16-year-olds; Bernaldez, Gallardo, & Abello, 1987). This finding is sympathetic with the press-competence model discussed earlier, which suggested that the more competent the individual, the more adaptive the behavior in a challenging environment.

Hospital healing gardens, by providing access to nature and offering opportunities for playing, relaxing, and socializing, can improve health outcomes and benefit staff,

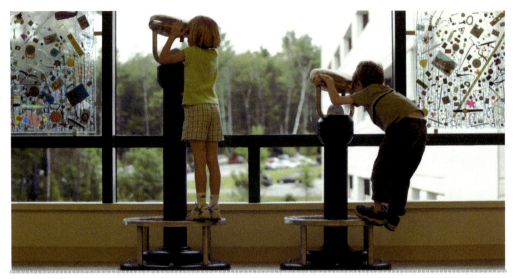

Figure 8.9. Window views and nature themes are powerful sources of positive distraction for children. *Note.* Photograph used with permission of Shepley Bulfinch Architects. Credit: Mark Washburn and Dartmouth-Hitchcock.

patients, and patients' families; they can reduce stress, provide positive distraction, and promote overall well-being (Pasha, 2013). Pasha (2013), in a study of five green outdoor spaces in three pediatric hospitals in East Texas, found that most visitors were not aware of presence of the gardens. This study also showed an association between certain design characteristics and the duration and frequency of garden visitation (Pasha, 2013). Uncomfortable seating and lack of shade resulted in decreased time of garden visitation by staff; lack of play features, scarcity of elements of landscape such as trees and flowers, and lack of design details in the outdoor spaces, negatively affected frequency of garden visitation (Pasha, 2013). Pasha and Shepley (2013) noted that design characteristics and quality of design of outdoor spaces in pediatric hospitals were associated with levels of physical activity in hospital gardens. Child-appropriate amenities, playful plan configurations and paths, varied planting, and shading are shown to increase levels of physical activity among visitors and children (Pasha & Shepley, 2013).

Publications on the effects of healing gardens have proliferated. In one of the more recent and thorough books, *Therapeutic Landscapes: An Evidence-Based Approach to Designing Healing Gardens and Restorative Outdoor Spaces* (Marcus & Sachs, 2013), the authors provide details on the appropriate design for gardens in health-care settings. Some of their design recommendations consider the following issues: (a) safety, security, and privacy; (b) accessibility; (c) physical and emotional comfort; (d) positive direction; (e) engagement with nature; (f) maintenance and aesthetics; and (g) sustainability.

With specific regard to children's hospital gardens they recommend the following:

- incorporating multiple gardens, such as an active play area for well children; a "quiet garden" with features that positively distract parents and sick children; a bereavement garden potentially attached to a chapel or meditation space; and gardens serving staff, which are best located near staff break rooms;
- employing the concepts of affordances (objects or spaces that suggest specific uses) or play opportunities while designing for active play;

- play features that engage children who are cautious, are shy, or have disabilities;
- clear expression of spatial boundaries;
- details that acknowledge that family and staff are usually the most frequent visitors to gardens in children's hospitals;
- early consultation with the therapists in the design process regarding elements that will facilitate their work with child-patients in the garden;
- pathways designed to entice a child-patient or a child with temporary disability to walk in the garden and to give them a sense of autonomy;
- seating that facilitates surveillance by parents and caregivers; seating in "private places of refuge; movable child-scale furniture; and a glider swing to accommodate a stroller or a wheelchair as well as accommodating parents with a small baby;
- avoiding poisonous or harmful plants and placing every plant with a purpose; and
- providing tools that allow a child to contribute to the upkeep of the garden, including a potting area for gardening and planting.

Light and Color

Literature relating to light and color includes three main topics: studies on chronobiology, studies on access to light, and studies on the impact of color.

Chronobiology

The relationship of light to biological and physical patterns of life is called *chronobiology*. Diurnal and season fluctuations are believed to affect the healing process, and a variety of studies confirm that adjusting light levels in nurseries to reflect diurnal variation has a positive effect on infants. As for seasonal variation, when the days are very short, some individuals are described as experiencing *seasonal affective disorder*, or SAD. Seasonal affective disorder can be defined as the negative psychological state associated with the lack of exposure to daylight during winter months. Although there are studies that support this concept, there is insufficient evidence to fully substantiate its scientific base. Preliminary studies on children that support the argument for a causal relationship between winter and depression include those of Rosenthal (1995) and Carskadon and Acebo (1993). Milman and Bennett (1996), however, reported that adolescent hospitalizations for suicide attempts are not related to time of year.

Access to Light

Studies on access to light generally focus on preferences expressed for daylight and window views. Previous efforts to eliminate windows in classrooms have been abandoned as a result of negative effects on academic performance and behavior. Research in work environments also demonstrates the preference of individuals for natural light in their work space.

Generally, it is recommended that lighting levels be reduced so that they do not exceed the required levels for performing care tasks. In a study by Walsh-Sukys et al. (2001) (cited in Sherman et al., 2005), it was shown that reducing NICU light levels from almost "200 lux to 15 lux for each individual patient" did not have any negative effect on patient safety or medical errors.

Studies have also investigated the question of cycled lighting to imitate day-night patterns (Sherman et al., 2005). Rivkees, Mayes, Jacobs, and Gross (2004) studied cycled lighting on infants and found that infants in diurnal conditions were more active during the day than at night, which indicates that circadian rhythms are in tune with common sleep-wake cycles. Also, the study suggested that two weeks prior to discharge, cycled lighting is preferred over continuous dim lighting in caring for premature infants (Rivkees et al., 2004).

Impact of Color

Research on the physical or psychological effects of color is limited. It is generally believed that soft colors are less stimulating than bright, saturated colors (Kleeman, 1981). The intention of chromotherapy is to cure illness through exposure to specific colors or color palettes. Documented research on the effectiveness of this technique is not available.

One of the most significant studies on how color affects children in hospital settings was conducted by Park (2009), who investigated the role of color as a component of a healing environment for pediatric inpatients. In his study, Park (2009) investigated color preference in three groups: pediatric inpatients, pediatric outpatients, and healthy children. One important conclusion of the study was that all three groups, regardless of gender, showed blue and green as the most preferred colors and white as the least preferred color (Park, 2009). With respect to gender, girls preferred red and purple more than boys did (Park, 2009).

There are several color theories that may be useful in the development of health-care facilities, including theories about lazure painting, full-spectrum palettes, and neutral backgrounds. Lazure painting, which is the multilayered, semitransparent technique used at Vidarkliniken, varies in tint from blue to rose depending on the health status of the patient (Marberry & Zagon, 1995). Marberry and Zagon recommended full-spectrum color, "a balanced mix of various proportions of tints and shades" from the seven colors of the spectrum. The intent of this approach is to provide a range of coordinated colors, as would appear in a natural environment. Planetree advocates a neutral background palette embellished by features selected by patients.

Most designers feel that children have different color requirements than adults and usually justify this position based on what are perceived to be developmental differences. Research indicates that strong colors may play a role in infant development and that toddlers express a preference for bright colors. However, the extension of this argument suggests that the palette must shift to accommodate children ages 2 to 18 years. Unless this population is separated spatially, it would be difficult to provide the implied universal palette.

Art

Almost all health-care facilities now advocate the integration of art into health-care environments. Many facilities also incorporate music therapy in their programs. Several studies that examine the art preferences of adult populations have been conducted in hospital environments and demonstrate patients' preference for realistic images to abstract art. McGhee and Dziuban (1993, 1994) also found preferences for realistic art among children, but these studies did not take place in pediatric health-care settings. Other issues that have been examined regarding children and art include the effect of previous exposure to art (Bowker & Sawyers, 1988), verbal responses to art (Ramsey, 1990), the effect of cognitive style (Salkind, 1993), and aesthetic perception (Winner, 1986). In one of the few more recent studies on art in pediatric hospitals, Eisen, Ulrich, Shepley, Varney, and Sherman (2008) investigated children's art preferences as well as the role of art in stress reduction for pediatric patients. The study indicated a preference for nature art among children and adolescents; however, pediatric patients in hospitals responded more to socially supportive imagery (Eisen et al., 2008).

One recommendation of the Eisen study was that children should have choices regarding the art hung in their hospital rooms. Eisen et al. (2008) suggested "an art cart" (see the discussion of Planetree) with the goal of giving pediatric patients options of different art images with multiple "nature-based images" (Eisen, et al., 2008).

Music

Music has been used for two purposes in health-care settings: to cover up unwanted noise and to act as a stress reducer. Parkin (1981) found that music reduced children's stress prior to examination in a dental clinic. The majority of pediatric studies, however, have taken place in neonatal intensive care unit settings. Collins and Kuck (1991) found an increase in oxygen saturation in neonates when uterine sounds were played. Standley and Moore (1995) had similar findings when babies listened to lullabies; however, oxygen saturation fell when the music stimulus was removed.

Elimination of patient sedation, reduction in procedural times, and a decrease in the number of medical staff required in procedures are all among consequences of music therapy–assisted procedures (Walworth, 2005). Standley and Walworth, as cited in Walworth (2005), noted that clinical music therapy services are provided as a response to medical referrals from many departments: NICUs, pediatrics/pediatric intensive care units, pediatric rehabilitation, oncology, heart and vascular institute, geriatric inpatient, extended care/long-term care, and labor and delivery. The present evidence on the exposure to music shows reductions in stress levels both for infants and pediatric patients, with important implications for systems and the promotion of healthy development (Sherman, Shepley, & Varney, 2005).

Sensory Therapies

Aroma has been evaluated in reducing psychological distress in clinical environments such as waiting rooms, dentistry, radiation endoscopy, and MRI (Schellhammer et al., 2013). Aroma has also been used as a distracting and soothing device in MRI rooms and as an orienting element in Alzheimer's units. The smell of cookies was released into an MRI unit to help calm a patient undergoing a test (Donnelly, 2007). In the Alzheimer's unit, baking smells have been used for redundant spatial cueing to help a resident locate the kitchen by smell (Nagy, 2002). There are no specific studies on the use of aromatherapy in children's environments, although such a study would be in order, because smell has been found to be effective in generating memories.

Conclusion

The field of environmental psychology is a new one, with discoveries being made every day. The range and exploratory nature of the material presented in this chapter suggest that more evidence is required on the relationship between the built environment and psychosocial factors influencing children and their families. The information contained herein should be applied judiciously until prototypes are fully tested and studies are corroborated. Regardless, consumers should demand that the designers who are developing projects base their decisions on the best information available. Designers should ask those who use or work in pediatric health-care environments—families, caregivers, and even the children themselves—to provide input regarding their needs. The informed decision-maker takes into account the role of environmental psychology, alternative design philosophies, alternative caregiving prototypes, and the potential healing contributions of specific environmental variables.

Study Guide

1. What types of (physical) environments best promote health and healing?

2. Describe the aspects of the environment that are particularly important to children's healing or continued developmental needs.

3. Compare and contrast psychosocial issues defined by environmental psychologists to those supportive of family- and patient-centered care.

4. List and discuss aspects of environmental design related to children's health care that are supported by research.

5. Discuss health design philosophies and draw implications for designing health-care environments for children.

6. Describe innovative environmental approaches in child health-care settings.

7. What are the dimensions of healing environments, and how can they be incorporated into child health-care settings?

8. Define *psychoneuroimmunology* and discuss its implications for children's health care design.

9. Discuss various therapies as related to children's health care and cite supportive research.

10. Suggest environmental changes essential to healing and normalization.

Appendix 8.1

Resources for Pediatric Health-Care Environments

Kobus, R. L. (2008). *Building type basics for healthcare facilities* (Vol. 13). Hoboken, NJ: John Wiley & Sons.

Malkin, J. (1992). *Hospital interior architecture.* New York, NY: Van Nostrand Reinhold.

Marcus, C. C., & Sachs, N. A. (2013). *Therapeutic landscapes: An evidence-based approach to designing healing gardens and restorative outdoor spaces.* Hoboken, NJ: John Wiley & Sons.

Shepley, M. M. (2014). *Design for pediatric and neonatal critical care.* New York, NY: Routledge.

Shepley, M. M., Fournier, M.-A., & McDougal, K. (1998). *Healthcare environments for children and their families.* Dubuque, IA: Kendall-Hunt.

Shultz, C. (2008). *Evidence for innovation: Transforming children's health through the built environment.* Alexandria, VA: National Association of Children's Hospitals and Related Institutions.

References

Allekian, C. (1973). Intrusions of territory and personal space. *Nursing Research*, *22*(3), 236–241.

Allgemeine Anthroposophische Gesellshaft. (n.d./1999). *Anthroposophical Society*. Retrieved February 6, 2006, from www.goetheanum.org/aag.html?&L51

Altman, I. (1975). *The environment and social behavior*. Monterey, CA: Brooks/Cole.

Altman, I., & Chemers, M. (1980). *Culture and environment*. Monterey, CA: Brooks/Cole.

Bernaldez, F. G., Gallardo, D., & Abello, R. P. (1987). Children's landscape preferences: From rejection to attraction. *Journal of Environmental Psychology*, *7*(2), 169–176.

Bowker, J. E., & Sawyers, J. K. (1988). Influence of exposure on preschooler's art preferences. *Early Childhood Research Quarterly*, *3*(1), 107–115.

Burgess, J. W., & McMurphy, D. (1982). The development of proxemic spacing behavior: Children's distances to surrounding playmates and adults change between 6 months and 5 years of age. *Developmental Psychobiology*, *15*(6), 557–567.

Caicedo, C. (2015). Health and functioning of families of children with special health care needs cared for in home care, long-term care, and medical day care settings. *Journal of Developmental and Behavioral Pediatrics*, *36*(5), 352–361.

Carpman, J., & Grant, M. (2016). *Design that cares* (3rd ed.). New York, NY: Wiley.

Carskadon, M., & Acebo, C. (1993). Parental reports of seasonal mood and behavior changes in children. *Journal of the American Academy of Child and Adolescent Psychiatry*, *32*, 264–269.

The Center for Health Design. (2004). *Evidence-based hospital design improves healthcare outcomes for patients, families, and staff*. Retrieved from www.healthdesign.org

Chapman, D. J. S. (1998). Family-focused pediatric home care. *CARING Magazine*, *17*(5), 12–15.

Cliff, B. (2012). The evolution of patient-centered care. *Journal of Healthcare Management*, *57*(2), 86–88.

Collins, S., & Kuck, K. (1991). Music therapy in the neonatal intensive care unit. *Neonatal Network*, *9*(6), 23–26.

Davies, M. (1996). Outdoors: An important context for young children's development. *Early Child Development and Care*, *115*, 37–49.

Devlin, A. S., & Arneill, A. B. (2003). Health care environments and patient outcomes: A review of the literature. *Environment and Behavior*, *35*(5), 665–694.

Diette, G., Lechtzin, N., Haponik, E., Devrotes, A., & Rubin, H. (2003). Distraction therapy with nature sights and sounds reduces pain during flexible bronchoscopy: A complementary approach to routine analgesia-bronchoscopy. *Chest*, *123*, 941–948.

Dijkstra, K., Pieterse, M., & Pruyn, A. (2006). Physical environmental stimuli that turn healthcare facilities into healing environments through psychologically mediated effects: Systematic review. *Journal of Advanced Nursing*, *56*(2), 166–181.

Dilani, A. (2008). Psychosocially supportive design: A salutogenic approach to the design of the physical environment. *Design and Health Scientific Review*, *1*(2), 47–55.

Dittbrenner, H. (1999). Pediatric homecare as a viable service. *CARING Magazine*, *18*(2), 12–13, 15.

Donnelly, G. F. (2007). Anxiety, aromas, and a trip into the MRI tube. *Holistic Nursing Practice*, *21*(1), 1.

Douglas, C. H., & Douglas, M. R. (2005). Patient centred improvements in health care built environments: Perspectives and design indicators. *Health Expectations*, *8*(3), 264–276.

Douglass, V. (1994). *Cooperative care study*. Unpublished manuscript, Texas A&M University, College of Architecture, College Station, TX.

Edwards, S. C. (1998). An anthropological interpretation of nurses' and patients' perceptions of the use of space and touch. *Journal of Advanced Nursing*, *28*(4), 809–817.

Eisen, S. L., Ulrich, R. S., Shepley, M. M., Varni, J. W., & Sherman, S. (2008). The stress-reducing effects of art in pediatric health care: Art preferences of healthy children and hospitalized children. *Journal of Child Health Care, 12*(3), 173–190.

Elias, E. R., Murphy, N. A., Liptak, G. S., Adams, R. C., Burke, R., Friedman, S. L., . . . & Wiley, S. E. (2012). Home care of children and youth with complex health care needs and technology dependencies. *Pediatrics, 129*(5), 996–1005.

Endacott, R. (1998). Needs of the critically ill child. *Intensive and Critical Care Nursing, 14*(2), 66–73.

Evans, G. (Ed.). (1982). *Environmental stress.* Cambridge, England: Cambridge University Press.

Evans, G. (2003). The built environment and mental health. *Journal of Urban Health, 80*(4), 536–555.

Farrell, M., & Frost, C. (1992). The most important needs of parents of critically ill children: Parents' perceptions. *Intensive and Critical Care Nursing, 8*, 130–139.

Fottler, M., Ford, R., Roberts, V., & Ford, E. (2000). Creating a healing environment: The importance of the service setting in the new consumer-oriented healthcare system. *Journal of Healthcare Management, 45*, 91–107.

Fournier, M.-A. (1994). *L'aménagement des aires d'attente dans les unités de soins intensifs pour adultes.* (The design of family waiting rooms in intensive care units for adults.) Unpublished master's thesis, Laval University, Quebec, Canada.

Frampton, S. B., & Charmel, P. A. (2009). *Putting patients first: Best practices in patient-centered care.* San Francisco, CA: Jossey-Bass.

Gifford, R. (2014). *Environmental psychology: Principles and practice* (5th ed.). Colville, WA: Optimal Books.

Gillis, A. J. (1989). The effect of play on immobilized children in hospital. *International Journal of Nursing Studies, 26*(3), 261–269.

Gilmour, J. A. (2006). Hybrid space: Constituting the hospital as a home space for patients. *Nursing Inquiry, 13*(1), 16–22.

Goetz, P., Malone, E., Harmsen, C., Reno, K., Edelstein, E., Hamilton, D., . . . Nanda, U. (2010). *An introduction to evidence-based design: Exploring health and design.* Concord, CA: The Center for Health Design.

Gooding, J. S., Cooper, L. G., Blaine, A. I., Franck, L. S., Howse, J. L., & Berns, S. D. (2011). Family support and family-centered care in the neonatal intensive care unit: origins, advances, impact. *Seminars in Perinatology, 35*(1), 20–28.

Govert, J. (1993). *Feng shui: Art and harmony of place.* Phoenix, AZ: Daikakuji.

Grieco, A., Garnett, S., Glassman, K., Valoon, P., & McClure, M. (1990). New York University Medical Center's cooperative care unit: Patient education and family participation during hospitalization—The first ten years. *Patient Education and Counseling, 15*, 3–15.

Hall, E. T. (1990). *The hidden dimension.* Garden City, NY: Doubleday.

Hamilton, D. K. (2003). The four levels of evidence-based practice. *Healthcare Design, 3*(4), 18–26.

Hamilton, D. K. (2006). Evidence-based design supports evidence-based medicine in the ICU. *ICU Management Journal (Belgium), 6*(3), 31.

Hamilton, D. K., & Shepley, M. M. (2010). *Design for critical care: An evidence-based approach.* Oxford, UK: Elsevier.

Hamilton, D. K., & Watkins, D. H. (2009). *Evidence-based design for multiple building types.* Hoboken, NJ: John Wiley & Sons.

Harris, P. (1988). Sometimes pediatric homecare doesn't work. *American Journal of Nursing, 88*(6), 851–854.

Heerwagen, J. H., Heubach, J. G., Montgomery, J., & Weimer, W. C. (1995). Environmental design, work, and well being: Managing occupational stress through changes in the workplace environment. *AAOHN Journal: Official Journal of the American Association of Occupational Health Nurses, 43*(9), 458–468.

Hughes, M., McCollum, J., Sheftel, D., & Sanchez, D. (1994). How parents cope with the experience of neonatal intensive care. *Children's Health Care, 23*(1), 1–14.

Huisman, E., Morales, E., Van Hoof, J., & Kort, H. (2012). Healing environment: A review of the impact of physical environmental factors on users. *Building and Environment, 58*, 70–80.

Husmillo, M. (2013). Maternal role attainment theory. *International Journal of Childbirth Education, 28*(2), 46–48.

Ibrahim, F., Harun, W. M. W., & Samad, M. H. A. (2010). The waiting space environment: Perception by design. *American Journal of Engineering and Applied Sciences, 3*(3), 569–575.

Institute for Patient-Centered Design, Inc. (2015). *History, mission and programs.* Retrieved from http://www.ifpcd.org/about

Jaafar, S. H., Lee, K. S., & Ho, J. J. (2012). Separate care for new mother and infant versus rooming-in for increasing the duration of breastfeeding. *Cochrane Database Systematic Reviews, 9:* CD006641. doi: 10.1002/14651858.CD006641.pub2

Johnson, B. H., Jeppson, E. S., & Redburn, L. (1992). *Caring for children and families: Guidelines for hospitals.* Bethesda, MD: Association for the Care of Children's Health.

Kaplan, S., & Kaplan, R. (1989). *The experience of nature.* New York, NY: Cambridge University Press.

Kasper, J. W., & Nyamathi, A. M. (1988). Parents of children in the pediatric intensive care unit: What are their needs? *Heart & Lung, 17*, 576–581.

Kirschbaum, M. (1990). Needs of parents of critically ill children. *Dimensions of Critical Care Nursing, 9*, 341–352.

Kleeman, W. (1981). *The challenge of interior design.* Boston, MA: CBI.

Lane, P. (1990). A measure of clients' perceptions about intrusions of territory and personal space by nurses. *Measurement of Nursing Outcomes, 4*, 199–218.

Lang, M. A., & Sullivan, C. (1986). Adapting home environments for visually impaired and blind children. *Children's Environments Quarterly, 3*(1), 50–54.

Lawton, M. P., & Nahemow, L. (1973). Ecology and the aging process. In C. Eisdorfer & M. Lawton (Eds.), *The psychology of adult development and aging* (pp. 619–674). Washington, DC: American Psychological Association.

Leibrock, C. (1993). *Beautiful barrier-free.* New York, NY: Van Nostrand Reinhold.

Leino-Kilpi, H., Välimäki, M., Dassen, T., Gasull, M., Lemonidou, C., Scott, A., & Arndt, M. (2001). Privacy: A review of the literature. *International Journal of Nursing Studies, 38*(6), 663–671.

Litkouhi, S., Geramipour, M., & Litkouhi, S. (2012). The effect of gender, age, and nationality on the personal space preferences in children's hospitals among Iranian and German children and adolescents. *Iranian Red Crescent Medical Journal, 14*(8), 460.

Logsdon, R. (1995). Understanding the application of Lazure painting techniques. *Journal of Healthcare Design, 7*, 205–212.

Lyman, S. M., & Scott, M. B. (1967). Territoriality: A neglected sociological dimension. *Social Problems, 15*, 235–249.

Lyons, E. (1983). Demographic correlates of landscape preference. *Environment & Behavior, 15*(4), 487–511.

Mahlmeister, L. R. (2005). Couplet care after cesarean delivery: Creating a safe environment for mother and baby. *The Journal of Perinatal & Neonatal Nursing, 19*(3), 212–214.

Malkin, J. (1992). *Hospital interior architecture.* New York, NY: Van Nostrand Reinhold.

Marberry, S., & Zagon, L. (1995). *The power of color: Creating healthy interior spaces.* New York, NY: Wiley.

Marcus, C. C., & Barnes, M. (1995). *Gardens in healthcare facilities: Uses, therapeutic benefits, and design recommendations.* Martinez, CA: The Center for Health Design.

Marcus, C. C., & Sachs, N. A. (2013). *Therapeutic landscapes: An evidence-based approach to designing healing gardens and restorative outdoor spaces.* Hoboken, NJ: John Wiley & Sons.

McClusky, J. F. (2008). Creating engaging experiences for rehabilitation. *Topics in Stroke Rehabilitation, 15*(2), 80–86.

McCullough, C. (2009). Family-centered care. In C. McCullough (Ed.), *Evidence-based design for healthcare facilities* (pp. 81–95). Indianapolis: Sigma Theta Tau.

McGhee, K., & Dziuban, C. D. (1993). Visual preferences of preschool children for abstract and realistic paintings. *Perceptual and Motor Skills, 76*(1), 155–158.

McGhee, K., & Dziuban, C. D. (1994). Visual preferences of Mexican preschool children for abstract and realistic paintings. *Perceptual and Motor Skills, 79*(1), 240–242.

McLane, L., Jones, K., Lydiatt, W., Lydiatt, D., & Richards, A. (2003). Taking away the fear: A grounded theory study of cooperative care in the treatment of head and neck cancer. *Psycho Oncology, 12*(5), 474–490.

McLaughlin, C., Olson, R., & White, M. J. (2008). Environmental issues in patient care management: Proxemics, personal space, and territoriality. *Rehabilitation Nursing, 33*(4), 143–147.

Meyer, E. D., Snelling, L. K., & Myren-Manbeck, L. K. (1998). Pediatric intensive care: The parents' experience. *AACN Clinical Issues, 9*(1), 64–74.

Milman, D., & Bennett, A. (1996). School and seasonal affective disorder. *The American Journal of Psychiatry, 153*, 849–850.

Moore, P., & Jordan, T. (1997). Children's health design: Improving child health outcomes with Rehab 1, 2, 3. *Journal of Healthcare Design, 9*, 137–140.

Nagy, J. W. (2002). Kitchens that help residents reestablish home. *Alzheimer's Care Today, 3*(1), 74–77.

Noyes, J. (1998). A critique of studies exploring the experiences and needs of parents of children admitted to pediatric intensive care units. *Journal of Advanced Nursing, 28*(1), 134–141.

Nussbaumer, L. L. (2013). *Human factors in the built environment.* New York, NY: Bloomsbury Publishing USA.

Okano, K. (1985). Development of personal space in 2- to 4-year-old children. *Journal of Human Development, 21*, 30–37.

Oksala, R., & Merenmies, J. (1989). Children's human needs in intensive care. *Intensive Care Nursing, 5*, 155–158.

Olds, A. (1995). Nature: The essential healing environment. *Child Health Design, 9*, 3–5.

Olson, T. (1999, October 11). *Analysis of cultural communication and proxemics.* Retrieved January 12, 2000, from www.unl.edu/casestudy/456/traci.htm

Orr, R. (1995). The Planetree philosophy. In S. Marberry (Ed.), *Innovations in healthcare design* (pp. 77–86). New York, NY: Van Nostrand Reinhold.

Park, J. G. (2009). Color perception in pediatric patient room design: Healthy children vs. pediatric patients. *HERD: Health Environments Research & Design Journal, 2*(3), 6–28.

Parkin, S. (1981). The effect of ambient music upon the reactions of children undergoing dental treatment. *Journal of Dentistry for Children, 48*(6), 430–432.

Parsons, R., Tassinary, L., Ulrich, R., Hebl, M., & Grossman-Alexander, M. (1998). The view from the road: Implications for stress recovery and immunization. *Journal of Environmental Psychology, 18*, 113–140.

Pasha, S. (2013). Barriers to garden visitation in children's hospitals. *HERD: Health Environments Research & Design Journal, 6*(4), 76–96.

Pasha, S., & Shepley, M. M. (2013). Research note: Physical activity in pediatric healing gardens. *Landscape and Urban Planning, 118*, 53–58.

Passini, R. (2002). Wayfinding research and design: An interdisciplinary approach in the development of design knowledge and its application. In J. Frascara (Ed.), *Design and the social sciences: Making connections* (pp. 97–102). London, UK: Taylor & Francis.

Peponis, J., Zimring, C., & Choi, Y. K. (1990). Finding the building in wayfinding. *Environment and Behavior, 22*(5), 555–590.

Planetree. (2014). *Planetree's vision.* Retrieved from http://planetree.org/reputation/

Planetree. (n.d.). *Planetree at Griffin Hospital.* Derby, CT: Griffin Hospital. Retrieved from http://www.griffinhealth.org/about-griffin/planetree.aspx

Price, S. (1994). The special needs of children. *Journal of Advanced Nursing, 20*, 227–232.

Purush, J., & Padam, A. (1998). *Vastu: Reinventing the architecture of fulfillment.* New Delhi, India: Vedams Books International.

Ramsey, I. L. (1990). An investigation of children's verbal responses to selected art styles. *Journal of Educational Research, 83*(1), 46–51.

Rivkees, S. A., Mayes, L., Jacobs, H., & Gross, I. (2004). Rest-activity patterns of premature infants are regulated by cycled lighting. *Pediatrics, 113*(4), 833–839.

Rollins, J. A. (2004). Evidence-based hospital design improves health care outcomes for patients, families, and staff. *Pediatric Nursing, 30*(4), 338.

Romano, M. (2002). Slow growing: Planetree philosophy sprouts new branches of support but remains on the healthcare periphery. *Modern Healthcare, 32*(32), 30–33.

Rosenthal, N. (1995). Syndrome triad in children and adolescents. *The American Journal of Psychiatry, 152*(9), 1402.

Rossbach, S., & Lin, T. (1991). Feng shui for healthcare design. *Journal of Health Care Interior Design, 3*, 17–25.

Ruga, W. (2008). Your general practice environment can improve your community's health. *British Journal of General Practice, 58*(552), 460–462.

Sackett, D. L., Rosenberg, W. M., Gray, J., Haynes, R. B., & Richardson, W. S. (1996). Evidence based medicine: What it is and what it isn't. *BMJ: British Medical Journal, 312*(7023), 71.

Salkind, L. W. (1993). The relationship of gender, age, and cognitive style to preference for works of art. *Dissertation Abstracts International, 53*(8-A), 2653.

Sanfilippo, M. D. (1994). Personal space and coping in terminal and chronically ill children. *Dissertation Abstracts International, 54*(8-B), 4406.

Schoffstall, M. C. (1984). The effect of the stress of hospitalization on the personal space of children. *Dissertation Abstracts International, 46*(5-B), 1717.

Sebba, R. (1991). The landscapes of childhood: The reflection of childhood's environment in adult memories and in children's attitudes. *Environment & Behavior, 23*(4), 395–422.

Seid, M., Stevens, G. D., & Varni, J. W. (2003). Parents' perceptions of pediatric primary care quality: effects of race/ethnicity, language, and access. *Health Services Research, 38*(4), 1009–1032.

Shepley, M. M. (2014). *Design for pediatric and neonatal critical care.* New York, NY: Routledge.

Shepley, M. M., Fournier, M.-A, & McDougal, K. (1998). *Healthcare environments for children and their families.* Dubuque, IA: Kendall-Hunt.

Shepley, M., Harris, D., & White, R. (2008). Open-bay and single family room neonatal intensive care units: Caregiver satisfaction and stress. *Environment & Behavior, 40*(2), 249–268.

Shepley, M., Harris, D., White, R., & Steinberg, F. (2006). Family behavior in a single-family room NICU. In *The AIA report on university research—Volume 3* (pp. 174–185). Washington, DC: The American Institute of Architects.

Sherman, S. A., Shepley, M. M., & Varni, J. W. (2005). Children's environments and health-related quality of life: Evidence informing pediatric healthcare environmental design. *Children Youth and Environments, 15*(1), 186–223.

Shultz, C. (2008). *Evidence for innovation: Transforming children's health through the built environment.* Washington, DC: NACHRI.

Solomon, G. (1996). Understanding psychoneuroimmunology (PNI) and its applications for healthcare. *Journal of Healthcare Design, 8*, 79–83.

Sommer, R. (2008). *Personal space: The behavioral basis of design.* Bristol, England: Bosko Books.

Spradlin, L. R. (2009). Implementation of a couplet care program for families after a Cesarean birth. *AORN Journal, 89*(3), 553–562.

Standley, J., & Moore, R. (1995). Therapeutic effects of music and mother's voice on premature infants. *Pediatric Nursing, 21*(6), 509–512.

Stichler, J. F. (2008). Healing by design. *Journal of Nursing Administration, 38*(12), 505–509.

Stichler, J. F., & Hamilton, D. K. (2008). Evidence-based design: What is it? *HERD: Health Environments Research & Design Journal, 1*(2), 3–4.

The Caritas Project. (2015). *The leading by design research project.* Retrieved from http://www.thecaritasproject.info/

Ulrich, R. (1984). View through window may influence recovery from surgery. *Science, 224,* 420–421.

Ulrich, R. (1999). Effects of gardens on health outcomes: Theory and research. In C. Cooper Marcus & M. Barnes (Eds.), *Healing gardens: Therapeutic benefits and design recommendations* (pp. 27–86). New York, NY: Wiley.

Ulrich, R. (2000). Environmental research and critical care. In D. Kirk Hamilton (Ed.), *ICU 2010: Design for the future* (pp. 195–207). Houston, TX: Center for Innovation in Health Facilities.

Ulrich, R. (2001). Effects of healthcare environmental design on medical outcomes. In A. Dilani (Ed.), *Design and health—The therapeutic benefits of design.* Proceedings of the Second International Conference on Design & Health, 2000, Stockholm, Sweden: Svenskbyggtjanst.

Ulrich, R. S., Berry, L. L., Quan, X., & Parish, J. T. (2010). A conceptual framework for the domain of evidence-based design. *HERD: Health Environments Research & Design Journal, 4*(1), 95–114.

Ulrich, R. S., Zimring, C., Zhu, X., DuBose, J., Seo, H.-B., Choi, Y.-S., . . . Joseph, A. (2008). A review of the research literature on evidence-based healthcare design. *HERD: Health Environments Research & Design Journal, 1*(3), 61–125.

Walworth, D. D. (2005). Procedural-support music therapy in the healthcare setting: A cost–effectiveness analysis. *Journal of Pediatric Nursing, 20*(4), 276–284.

White, R. (1993). *Recommended standards for newborn design.* South Bend, IN: Memorial Hospital.

White, R. D. (2003). Individual rooms in the NICU—an evolving concept. *Journal of Perinatology, 23,* S22–S24

Wilson, E. (1986). *Biofilia.* Cambridge, MA: Harvard University Press. (Reprint)

Winner, E. (1986). Children's perception of "aesthetic" properties of the arts. *British Journal of Developmental Psychology, 4*(2), 149–160.

Yeh, M., McCabe, K., Hough, R. L., Dupuis, D., & Hazen, A. (2003). Racial/ethnic differences in parental endorsement of barriers to mental health services for youth. *Mental Health Services Research, 5*(2), 65–77.

Zborowsky, T., & Kreitzer, M. J. (2008). Creating optimal healing environments in a health care setting. *Minnesota medicine, 91*(3), 35–38.

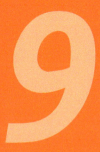

9 Spiritual Issues in Children's Health-Care Settings

Lynn B. Clutter

Objectives

At the conclusion of this chapter, the reader will be able to:

1. Define *spirituality* and discuss children's development of and understanding of spirituality.
2. Discuss ways in which spirituality may influence children's reactions to illness and health-care experiences.
3. Determine theories of spirituality, and draw implications for care of children in health-care settings.
4. Recommend various approaches to the use of spirituality with children in health care.

Many aspects of health care proceed with little thought of spiritual care. The spiritual aspect of life is often dealt with much like politics, with the perspective that "the less said the better" is the best policy. Most people, however, believe that there is a spiritual aspect of life and that God does exist. Health care of children usually involves times of crisis, illness, injury, or at the least, change. Any of these times can bring spiritual aspects into focus for the child, parent, or family member (Kloosterhouse & Ames, 2002). Health-care professionals can provide spiritual care in a way that offers comfort, hope, encouragement, and respect, and can use spiritual strength to better the outcome of overall care.

The goal of this chapter is to equip professionals with information useful for providing spiritual care to children and their families. Although a knowledge base in religion is valuable and having awareness of a religion in general can help with the care of specific children and families, this chapter does not include an in-depth discussion of religious beliefs. Instead, an annotated bibliography of selected references regarding religions is provided in Appendix 9.1: Resources for Religion. An overview of spirituality is followed by theoretical and developmental aspects of spirituality. Spiritual care will be described. Because literature specific to children's spirituality is limited, it is hoped that the strategies given will demonstrate the variety of spiritual-care options available to health-care providers. Barnes, Plotnikoff, Fox, and Pendleton (2000, p. 905) stated, "Spirituality and religion can serve as key organizing principles in the lives of children and their families, particularly in relation to children's illness, health, and healing."

The Importance of Spirituality

Spirituality is regarded as a basic characteristic of humanness important in human health and well-being. It is a fundamental element of human experience (Puchalski, Ferrell, Otis-Green, & Handzo, 2015). Qualitative data suggest that even children experience themselves as spiritual beings, and that taking that understanding and connecting with children around their spiritual lives can be an important adjunct to treatment (Houskamp, Fisher, & Stuber, 2004). Spirituality affects people's worldview and meaning in life. There is great diversity in spirituality, and yet spiritual strengths can be identified and may even ameliorate problems (Good & Willoughby, 2014). Many consider religious and spiritual orientations to be as significant as ethnicity, race, culture, social class, and gender because numerous fundamental beliefs are rooted in religion. People of all ages and circumstances have a spiritual dimension, even when disoriented, confused, emotionally ill, cognitively impaired, or delirious (Carpenito, 2012). A strong majority of Americans (74%) report that they believe in God, and 72% say they believe in miracles (The Harris Poll, 2013). To ignore individuals' spiritual needs denies them a holistic approach to care (March & Caple, 2015).

Spirituality has also been deemed important in health-care settings. Often as critical physical or mental health issues arise, spiritual needs may increase. One study of 120 inpatients with stomach cancer found that distress, anxiety, and depression correlated with spiritual needs ($p < .001$) (Sook & Yong, 2012). Research also supports benefits of spiritual strength (Bennett & Thompson, 2015). Standards of practice within health-care settings include spirituality; The Joint Commission (2009) recommend spiritual assessment with questions such as, "Does the patient use prayer in her life?" and "What type of spiritual/religious support does the patient desire?" Aspects of coping and hope are part of the spiritual assessment and involve questions, such as "What helps the patient get through this health-care experience?" and "How does your faith help the patient cope with illness?" Spiritual resources are also important, as is evident by the question, "What is the name of the patient's clergy, minister, imam, chaplain, pastor, rabbi?" (Costello, Atinaja-Faller, & Hedberg, 2012). Professionals, including nurses (Bennett & Thompson, 2015), nurse-practitioners (Haley, 2014), physicians (Dyer, 2011), educators (Miller, 2014; Zhang, 2012), psychologists (Ruddock & Cameron, 2010), social workers (Hodge, 2005), and child life specialists (Desai, Ng, & Bryant, 2002), are aware that spiritual assessment is part of their roles. Even the World Health Organization (WHO) considers spirituality an important aspect of quality of life (WHO, 2015).

Physical Health Benefits

A mounting body of evidence points to the power of the "faith factor." For example, deeply spiritual or religiously committed individuals experience less stress—cope better with it—have fewer drug and alcohol problems, less depression, lower rates of suicide, and enjoy their lives and marriages more than do the less religious (March &

Caple, 2015). Medical studies also have found measures of physical improvement with those having certain spiritual characteristics. Larson and Koenig (2000) reported that nearly every medical study that has considered religion has found it to be a positive factor; well-designed studies generally reveal a beneficial relationship between religious commitment, practices, and attitudes and patients' well-being.

People who report higher levels of strength of spirit tend to have higher measures of well-being. In a sample of Saudi Muslim children and adolescents (N = 7,211), Abdel-Khalek (2009) analyzed the relationship between religiosity, subjective well-being, and depression; among the 11- to 18-year-olds, religious individuals were happier, healthier, and less depressed. Holder, Coleman, and Wallace (2010) compared spirituality, religiousness, and happiness among 8- to 12-year-olds (N = 320) and found that spirituality but not religious activity was strongly linked to happiness. Spirituality was a significant predictor of happiness even after removing variance associated with temperament.

Desire for Spiritual Care

Findings indicate that people want spiritual care, especially when hospitalized (March & Caple, 2015). People do seem to perceive spirituality as something more than religion. Some individuals do not find religion important and do not want spirituality addressed in medical care; however, dissatisfaction with the impersonal nature of the U.S. medical system as well as awareness that medical science does not have all the answers regarding health and wellness may drive interest toward spiritual care. Spiritual care is increasingly considered an important aspect of health care (Bowers & Rieg, 2014).

Some studies show children need and value spiritual care (Carson & Koenig, 2008; Fosarelli, 2008; O'Brien, 2013) Spiritual care may be especially important to children during times of illness or injury when health-care professionals can have valuable input. Smith and McSherry (2004) contended that if children are to be given the opportunity to develop to their full potential, fostering spiritual growth must be a part of the process of caring for them. The International Association for Children's Spirituality recognizes the importance of addressing spiritual aspects of children and encourages interdisciplinary research and practice for children's holistic development (Willis, 2013). Further, interdisciplinary collaboration is important to address this dimension of patient care (Puchalski et al., 2015).

Unfortunately, some health-care providers may base their impressions regarding children's and families' desire for spiritual care on their own value systems or on what they see in the health-care setting, which can be significantly different from most people's reality. The underemphasis of spiritual care in the health-care professions is well known (Narayanasamy & Owens, 2001). Reasons include lack of education regarding its significance (Haley, 2014), inability to recognize signs of spiritual need, or a belief that addressing spiritual needs is not within the profession's scope of practice (Koenig, 2004). The trend of religious groups in the United States to unburden themselves of hospitals may further de-emphasize spiritual care in health-care settings. Until the early 20th century, almost all hospital development was the result of private donations motivated by Judeo-Christian ideals of "charity, love for one's neighbors, and dedication to a ministry of healing" (Bilchik, 1998, p. 38). Now, both Christian- and Jewish-owned centers are selling ownership and are merging with secular facilities. At the same time that U.S. consumers want more humanity, touching, healing, and listening, health care is becoming less personal and more mechanized. Many people want to be helped to mobilize their personal faith to get well or stay well, but that resource may not be available.

Children's Spiritual Care in Health-Care Settings

If spirituality is one of people's defining aspects and if it affects the other aspects of life (e.g., physical, mental, social), then consideration of children's spirituality is an important part of children's health care (Roehlkepartain, King, Wagener, & Benson, 2006). Further, when spirituality is viewed as a concept distinct from religion (March & Caple, 2015), it can be inclusive of all people—including children. Spiritual care too often is viewed as optional, yet often spiritual needs hold the key for appropriate intervention. Blockley (1998) provided an example of a 7-year-old boy, Cory, who sustained a fractured femur in a motor vehicle accident that killed his younger sister and left his mother in critical condition in the ICU. Cory was restless in a way that could not be accounted for by fear or pain. He could not get to sleep. His nurse closed the curtain and asked what he did at home before he went to sleep. Cory outlined the routine and added in a whisper, "and then I would sit on Mummy's knee and we would say the 'Our Father' together" (Blockley, 1998, p. 56). The nurse was able to provide pre-sleep spiritual and emotional care, having found the "key to his restlessness," and medication was never needed.

The writings of people such as Robert Coles (1990) created greater awareness that children do have their own spiritual lives and, when we are willing to listen, they will tell us about their spiritual ideas and experiences. This is especially true of children who are ill or grieving—sometimes their hurt makes them very willing to express themselves. In Kamper, Van Cleave, and Savedra's (2010) study, children with cancer reported what they do to feel closer to God (or a Higher Power). Prayer or talking to God was listed by 64%, going to church (17%), reading the Bible/devotions (7%), performing other spiritual acts (7%), and nothing (5%).

Parents and health-care professionals may tend to think that it is better to spare children from discussions of spirituality. This is not often in the child's best interest:

> Children do much better physically, emotionally and spiritually when their ideas are sought and they are included in important discussions. . . . Even though we may be uncomfortable with their questions and their emotions, we must not shy away from hearing them out and wondering with them. (Fosarelli, 2000, p. 7)

Children typically know when they need to talk. Spirituality, and often religion, is part of the human experience, and it is definitely a part of the experience when we are ill. Children are often ready to talk about spirituality during times of illness. According to Coles (2000),

> We should give children the permission to share with us what is on their minds, and so, my advice is to ask directly about the role of spirituality and religion in their lives and listen for the enormous insight you will hear. (p. 6)

Definition of Terms

A foundation for providing spiritual care begins with an understanding of terms. For example, the *spiritual* aspect of an individual is not equivalent to the *religious* aspect (March & Caple, 2015). Many patients are excluded from spiritual care when spirituality is confined in that way. See Text Box 9.1: Definitions of Terms Related to Spirituality.

Theoretical Underpinnings of Spirituality

Various writers have used developmental theories to deduce spiritual-care strategies. For example, in her classic book *The Spiritual Needs of Children* (1982), Judith Shelly took Erikson's Eight Ages of Man (Erikson, 1963) and explained the spiritual care appropriate for each stage (Shelly, 2000). Carson and Koenig (2008) provided an overview of three faith-development theories, including Aden's eight stages of faith, Westerhoff's four stages of faith, and Fowler's seven stages of faith. James Fowler's widely used work (Fowler, 1981, 1996; Fowler & Dell, 2006; Fowler & Keen, 1978) is influenced by the theoretical work of Erik Erikson, Jean Piaget, and Lawrence Kohlberg. These stages of faith apply to people of any or no religion because faith is viewed as being universally present (see Table 9.1).

Other spiritual-care authors have analyzed the theoretical underpinnings of spirituality (Barnum, 2010; Boynton, 2011; Carson & Koenig, 2008; Mueller, 2010). Piaget's stages of cognitive development have been related to spiritual development (Mueller, 2010). Discussions of Kohlberg's work on moral development (Fowler, 1981; Kohlberg, 1981, 1984; Mueller, 2010) and Maslow's theory of human motivation (Carson & Koenig, 2008) have shed light on spirituality in children.

Nursing theories are mixed in content and depth regarding spirituality (Bennett & Thompson, 2015; Barnum, 2010; O'Brien, 2013). However, nursing has gained much ground in the area of addressing spiritual issues by developing nursing diagnoses concerning spiritual well-being and spiritual distress (Cavendish et al., 2001). *Spiritual anguish* has also been described and validated (Chaves, Carvalho, & Hass, 2010). North American Nursing Diagnosis International (NANDA) lists spiritually related diagnoses under Domain 10—Life Principles (Herdman & Kamitsuru, 2014). These include diagnoses such as "readiness for enhanced spiritual well-being" and "moral distress" (Caldeira, Carvalho, & Vieira, 2013). National and international codes of ethics include language that recognizes the importance of spiritual care. Boynton (2011) acknowledges that current research is often underpinned by constructivist child development based theory and that considerable room exists for expansion in research on children's spirituality and theory development.

Assessment of Spirituality

Health-care providers work diligently to anticipate care needs before they are crying out to be heard. The same should be true when it comes to children's spiritual needs. Anticipation of needs happens through building one's professional knowledge base and

Text Box 9.1
Definitions of Terms Related to Spirituality

Belief—the holding of certain ideas; to hold dear, love, cherish (Fowler, 1981).

Faith—a confidence or trust in a person or thing (Hart & Schneider, 1997); an orientation of the whole person, giving purpose and goal to one's hopes and strivings, thoughts and actions (Fowler, 1981).

Faith communities or religious communities—congregations such as churches, synagogues, mosques, temples, or cathedrals where religion is practiced.

God—supreme presence, divine power, supernatural power, Divine, Ultimate Other, Great Mystery, Spring, Source, Spirit, and Divine Consciousness, supreme being, higher power, energy, force, power within, your personal definition of transcendence; a source of love, creativity, a social transformation.

Human spirit—the dimension of any individual that is distinct from physical, psychological, or social dimensions; the aspect of self that gives meaning and purpose to life (Espeland, 1999).

Religion—a set of cumulative traditions, symbols, rituals; service and worship of a god or supernatural power; a set of beliefs about God upon which practices are based (Fowler, 1981).

Spiritual care—activities that assist individuals to find meaning and purpose in life, to continue relationships, and to transcend beyond the self (Fulton & Moore, 1995); may include activities such as holding, comforting, play therapy, providing pain control, and fostering of parental participation in the child's care (Hart & Schneider, 1997).

Spiritual development—a dynamic process that differs from physical, emotional, or social development, in which a person becomes increasingly aware of the meaning, purpose, and values in life (Carson, 1989).

Spiritual distress—the state in which the individual experiences or is at risk of experiencing a disturbance in his or her belief or value system that is a source of strength and hope (Carpenito, 1997).

Spiritual health or well-being—one's views and behaviors related to the search for hope and meaning in life, which express a relationship with a higher power or some meaning to a transient dimension (Carpenito, 1997), and vary according to the child's age, religious tradition, and the severity of the illness (O'Brien, 1999); the integrating aspect of human wholeness characterized by meaning and hope (Clark, Cross, Deane, & Lowry, 1991); the center of a healthy lifestyle, which enables holistic integration of one's inner resources (Clark & Heidenreich, 1995).

Spiritual needs—meaning and purpose, love, trust, hope, forgiveness, and creativity (Carson, 1989).

Spiritual pain—the loss of or separation from God or institutionalized religion; the experience of evil or disillusionment; a sense of failing God; the recognition of one's own sinfulness; lack of reconciliation with God; a perceived loneliness of spirit (O'Brien, 1999).

Spirituality—dynamic principles developed throughout the lifespan that guide an individual's view of the world; influence his or her interpretation of a higher power, hope, morals, loss, faith, love, and trust; and provide structure and meaning to everyday activities (Hicks, 1999).

Table 9.1

Fowler's Seven Stages of Faith		
Stage	**Age**	**Characteristics**
1. Primal faith	Infancy	A pre-language disposition of trust forms the mutuality of one's relationships with parents and others to offset the anxiety that results from separations that occur during infancy.
2. Intuitive–projective faith	Early childhood	Imagination, stimulated by stories, gestures, and symbols and not yet controlled by logical thinking combines with perception and feelings to create long-lasting images that represent both the protective and threatening powers surrounding one's life.
3. Mythic–literal faith	Childhood and beyond	The developing ability to think logically helps one order the world with categories of causality, space, and time; to enter into the perspectives of others; and to capture life meaning in stories.
4. Synthetic–conventional faith	Adolescence and beyond	New cognitive abilities make mutual perspective-taking possible and require one to integrate diverse self-images into a coherent identity. A personal and largely unreflective synthesis of beliefs and values evolves to support identity and to unite one in emotional solidarity with others.
5. Individuative–reflective faith	Young adult-hood and beyond	Critical reflection on one's beliefs and values, understanding of the self and others as part of a social system, and the assumption of responsibility for making choices of ideology and lifestyle open the way for commitments in relationships and vocation.
6. Conjunctive faith	Midlife and beyond	The embrace of polarities in one's life, alertness to paradox, and the need for multiple interpretations of reality mark this stage. Symbol and story, metaphor and myth (from one's own traditions and those of others), are newly appreciated as vehicles for grasping truth.
7. Universalizing faith	Midlife or beyond	Beyond paradox and polarities, persons in this stage are grounded in a oneness with the power of being. Their visions and commitments free them for a passionate yet detached spending of the self in love, devoted to overcoming division, oppression, and brutality.

Note. From *Spiritual Dimensions of Nursing Practice* (p. 29), by V. B. Carson, 1989, Philadelphia, PA: Saunders. Copyright 1989 by Saunders. Reprinted with permission.

then adequately assessing the child and family. The first step is up to the caregiver. Leaving it to vulnerable patients to raise questions risks ignoring some of their most devastating concerns and most powerful resources.

How the health-care provider views spirituality affects his or her own ability to assess spiritual needs and give care. If there is openness or even a welcoming viewpoint toward encounters of a spiritual nature, care will be strengthened. Providers should be theologically honest, speak the language of children, enter into the child's world, be sensitive to nonverbal and verbal information, respect privacy, and let the child take the lead (O'Brien, 2013). Personal beliefs, feelings, perceptions, and experiences regarding spirituality are important. Basic questions for examining one's own beliefs include "How do I define the meaning of life?" "What is my relationship with a higher power?" and "How are my spiritual beliefs incorporated into my practice?" (Hicks, 1999). If we have struggled and come to a place of peace regarding spiritual aspects of life, we are free to help others and are not bound up in our own bewilderment. We have a base or core of spiritual belief.

Health-care professionals must avoid imposing their own ideas on the child or family while encouraging patients to voice their spiritual needs and questions. Aggressively passing on one's own beliefs without adequate assessment or a direct request can cause needless spiritual distress. Spiritual interactions should be about the child and family.

Assessment of Family Spirituality

A child comes to a health-care situation with the backdrop of family life and experiences that will radically affect the care experience. A child learns about health and illness, right and wrong, life and death, and faith in God within the context of a family. After assessing the parents' spiritual needs, it is often easier to understand their child's needs.

During a crisis, children easily sense their parents' fear and anxiety. If parents are supported in their coping efforts, children are better able to handle the ups and downs of hospitalization. Parents are better able to support their child if health-care professionals provide adequate information and incorporate them into the child's care. Parents may well be experiencing spiritual distress with the hospitalization of a child and may express this distress through anxiety, hostility, and blaming (Hart & Schneider, 1997). Parents are often at the bedside, but other family members may be in a waiting room. It may be helpful for the health-care professional to go to the waiting room or even on a break to the cafeteria to talk with family members. Once away from the child, a parent may have much to share. This type of break from the monotony-with-intensity can be a spiritual assessment opportunity. Parents may share valuable pieces of information about the child or family. On the other hand, they may say nothing but feel a burden lifted. They may let go of some grief.

Particularly with critical illness and the death of a child, families face one of the most difficult experiences of their lives. Sensitive communication is critical. The following are recommendations for end-of-life communication with parents:

- It may seem natural to ask, "How are you feeling?" However, when a family is obviously experiencing loss and emotional pain, this question could be considered insensitive. Better to simply ask how might be the best way support them at this time (Mullen, Reynolds, & Larson, 2015).
- Saying "I know how you feel" or "I understand how you feel" makes it more about how the speaker feels rather than the bereaved family and its unique experience. No one truly knows or understands another's experience. An honest, "I can only imagine how you are feeling right now" acknowledges the pain and often encourages dialogue (National Hospice and Palliative Care Organization [NHPCO], 2009).
- Statements such as, "You have other people to live for" or "Count your blessings" seem dismissive and minimize a family's pain at a time of devastating loss (Mullen et al., 2015).

- Reminding parents that they have other children or that they are young and can have more children ignores the uniqueness of the child (NHPCO, 2009); children cannot be replaced.

- "Your child is in a better place" or "He/she is better off now" may also be perceived as diminishing the child's value (NHPCO, 2009). Moving on to the future with "Time heals all wounds" disregards the crisis of the present moment; better to validate what the family is feeling in the present with "This is tough, isn't it?" (Bonifazi, 2004).

- Attempting to justify a child death with statements such as "There is a reason for everything" or "It's God's plan" can be disturbing because a grieving family would find no reason to be enough to justify their child's death. Communication can support the family's worldview by asking questions such as "What role does faith play in your life?" (Wender, 2012).

Spiritual Assessment of Children

An assessment may be structured or unstructured, brief or comprehensive. Sound assessment is more important for children than for adults. Children have a limited ability to communicate, particularly about abstract concepts. Sources for data collection include direct observations, a patient's chart, doctors, referral sheets, and observations of other health team members .

Much of spiritual assessment can be done through simple observation of people, interactions, and environment (see Figure 9.1). Look around the room for religious

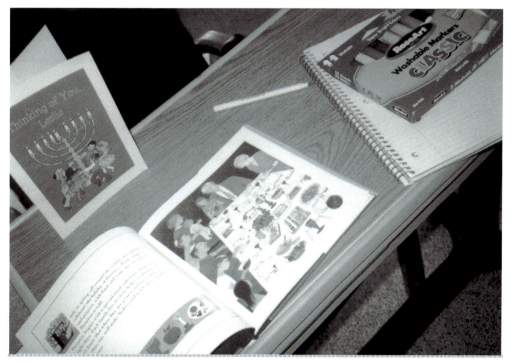

Figure 9.1. The presence of spiritual materials can indicate the importance of spiritual aspects to a particular child and family. *Note.* Photograph by Lynn Clutter. Used with permission.

objects or materials. Sacred books; religiously based storybooks, cards, or gifts; music or videotapes; or even the child's own artwork reflect spiritual beliefs. Observe the child's behavior, spiritual practices, those who provide spiritual support, and what support is provided.

Often, children do not use religious words. Observe for anxiety, stalling, nightmares, regression, loneliness, parents' perceptions of the child's subtle behavior changes, hostility, blaming, or expressed spiritual needs. Other emotions to observe for include despair, anger, frustration, guilt, or shame (March & Caple, 2015). Does the child mention God? If so, what is said? These sorts of observations make a significant difference in objectifying beliefs and differentiating those of child versus parent. These observations are noninvasive and useful.

In the spiritual-care literature, structured spiritual assessments have various categories. Stoll (1979) referred to four areas of spiritual assessment: concept of God, sources of hope and strength, religious practices, and relation between beliefs and health. Anderson and Steen (1995) adapted Stoll's four areas of assessment for use with children and parents (see Table 9.2). The assessment's strength is in the questions linked with particular aspects of spiritual concern that are directed toward the child or parent/adult caregiver.

Categorizing spiritual assessment questions according to developmental stage can be useful. Clutter (1991) offered an extensive list of age-appropriate questions categorized for use with preschoolers, school-age children, or adolescents, as well as questions for adults/parents.

Taking a child's faith or spiritual history is another way to categorize spiritual assessment information. The purpose of this type of history is to gather baseline background information, make careful observations, listen carefully, and note any cues that are spiritual in nature. The faith history enhances knowledge of sources of strength and identifies spiritual challenges for child and parent, and major life or faith change points. Spiritual history-taking is valuable but rarely done (Koenig, 2004).

Puchalski (2000a) developed a simple spiritual history tool that is represented by the acronym FICA. An explanation and questions suitable for children are listed below:

- F—Faith or beliefs; what the individual believes; "Do you believe in God?"
- I—Importance and influence; how important spiritual issues are in the person's health and life; "Do you think about God a lot or a little?"
- C—Community; the religious community involvement of the person; "Do you worship God somewhere with other people?"
- A—Address; how the person would like his or her health-care provider to address these issues in their care; "Do you want to talk about this kind of thing with me?"

The strengths of a tool such as FICA are that it is simple and quick to administer but can be applied broadly and yield in-depth information from patients. Phrasing questions with "Tell me about your . . ." may yield longer answers to the FICA. Children are often very willing to give honest answers to these types of questions.

The mnemonic B-E-L-I-E-F is the basis of McEvoy's (2000) spiritual history questionnaire. This history can be incorporated into the pediatric health-maintenance visit. Categories are B—belief systems, E—ethics, L—lifestyle, I—involvement in a

Table 9.2

Spiritual Assessment Questions for Parents and Children		
Area of Spiritual Concern	**Person to Answer Question**	**Faith Assessment Question**
Concept of God	Parent/ adult caregiver	Is faith or God important to you? How? How is God involved in your life? How is God involved in the life of your child? How would you describe God? Does your child have an interest in faith or God? How do you answer your child's questions about God? Does your child have a favorite Bible story? What is it? Why does he (or she) like it?
Concept of God	Child	Have you thought about God during this time? What is God like? How does God work? Does God make everything happen? Do you believe God causes ___? How do you see God acting or not acting now? Do you have a favorite Bible story or character? What do you like about this story?
Sources of strength and hope	Parent/ adult caregiver	Who do you turn to when you need help? How do they help? Is your faith important to you now? How is it important right now? What helps you when you feel afraid or alone? What gives you strength during difficult times? Are your beliefs a source of strength and support during hard times?
Sources of strength and hope	Child	How do you feel when you are in trouble? Who do you tell when you feel afraid (or sad, scared, alone, happy)? Who do you like to talk to when you feel that way? Who else? What makes you feel afraid (or sad, scared, lonely)? What helps you feel better?
Faith practices	Parent/ adult caregiver	Is your faith important to you now? How is it important? Are there faith practices that are important to you or your child now? What practices are important? Has having a sick child made a difference in your faith practices? Is prayer important to you? In what ways? Is the Bible or another book or symbol helpful to you? How? Are there any other helpful faith practices that we should be aware of?
Faith practices	Child	Have you thought about God? Are there things that you do that help you feel closer to God? What are they? Do you ever pray or talk to God?

Note. From "Spiritual Care: Reflecting God's Love to Children," by B. Anderson and S. Steen, 1995, *Journal of Christian Nursing, 12*(2), p. 15. Copyright 1995 by Journal of Christian Nursing. Reprinted with permission.

spiritual community, E—education, and F—future events. McEvoy provides specific spiritual-history questions and summaries of categories.

Spirituality-focused genograms can be useful, including in cases where religion has been used to commit abuse (Simonič, Mandelj, & Novasak, 2013). Untapped spiritual or religious resources for care or client coping may be revealed. Sample questions to consider when constructing a spirituality-focused genogram (Dunn & Dawes, 1999) include the following:

- What are the first religious or spiritual experiences you can remember?
- What role does religion or spirituality have in your everyday life or in times of crisis?
- What defining experiences or individuals have influenced the development of your sense of spirituality or religion?
- What were significant transitions and/or critical life events in the history of your family?
- What impact, if any, did religion or spirituality have in making sense of or coping with those life events? (p. 254)

Elkins and Cavendish's (2004) compilation of tools includes those listed above and Highfield's (2000) "SPIRITual" interview: S—spiritual belief system, P—personal spirituality, I—integration with a spiritual community, R—ritualized practices and restrictions, I—implications for medical care, and T—terminal-event planning. Blaber, Jones, and Willis (2015) explored various tools, with specific attention to those whose qualities are best for palliative care.

Highfield (2000) pointed to the importance of focusing the assessment on strengths. The child and family can rely on these strengths through illness and crisis. They will buoy the child and allow others to provide support by encouraging the use of his or her own strengths. Therefore, strengths should be identified and documented for further use. For example, if a child listens to spiritual music, later sings one of the songs and has a brighter outlook, and the mother states, "She really loves that song," the notation "Gains strength from use of spiritual music" could be charted for future intervention.

The use of known tools may bring a formality that yields valuable data but is less threatening for both client and health-care provider. Some formal spiritual assessment tools for adults may apply to children. Certain tools can be completed by the patient or a parent alone and then discussed later. Some tools are formatted as spiritual interviews with questions. Appendix 9.2 is an annotated bibliography of spiritual-care tools for use with children, adults, research, practice, and chart documentation.

Spiritual Distress and Spiritual Pain

Sometimes people are "cut off from their spiritual roots in facing the crisis of illness, dying, and death. Even people who are religious may lack the spiritual energy to cope with crisis situations" (Bailey, 1997, p. 242). Though spiritual distress may not be discernable biologically, it is accepted in society as real and must be dealt with by health professionals (Mullen et al., 2015; Prado Simão, Lopes Chaves, & Hollanda Iunes, 2015). Learning to identify spiritual distress is an important first step.

Indicators of spiritual distress include a loss of meaning and purpose in life, a diminished sense of love and relatedness, and a lack of forgiveness (Georgesen & Dungan, 1996). McHolm (1991) listed 13 indicators of spiritual distress:

1. inability to accept self,
2. description of somatic complaints,

3. cues about relationships with others,
4. cues about guilt and forgiveness,
5. cues about religious or spiritual needs,
6. inadequate coping,
7. despair or hopelessness,
8. fear,
9. depression,
10. helplessness,
11. anorexia,
12. silence, and
13. bitterness.

Another validation study (Twibell, Wieseke, Marine, & Schoger, 1996) identified the following as defining characteristics of spiritual distress:

- spiritual emptiness,
- disturbance in beliefs,
- no reason for living,
- request for spiritual assistance,
- concern over meaning in life,
- questioning of beliefs,
- doubt over beliefs,
- inability to practice rituals, and
- detachment from self or others.

Sometimes children express spiritual distress as anger, resentment, exaggerated fear, self-blame, questioning the meaning of one's own existence, or questioning the moral and ethical implications of the therapeutic regime (Feudtner, Haney, & Dimmers, 2003). Additional cues include crying, nightmares, asking many questions, and regressive behavior. Often this distress is expressed at nighttime or bedtime hours. Repeated questions or resistant behavior can occur as well. Caldeira and colleagues (2013) conducted an extensive review of this nursing diagnosis with detailed lists of assessment criteria, and Ku, Kuo, and Yao (2010) established content and construct validity measures with the four-factor, 30-item spiritual distress scale.

An international integrative review of the literature revealed many differences in the definition of spiritual distress (Prado Simão et al., 2015). The authors added that chronic illnesses such as cancer can trigger spiritual distress, which can impair physical and mental aspects of health. Two tools assessing spiritual distress were reviewed in the article.

Spiritual pain is similar to spiritual distress. McGrath (2002) indicated that demands of aggressive and invasive treatment lead to a need for a stronger sense of meaning-making and connection with life. Further, the disconnection resulting from disease and treatment can cause questioning of the meaning of life and a sense of void. Then, with varying degrees of intensity, there is the subjective experience of spiritual pain that leads to actual spiritual pain.

When Children Are Dying

Experiences of grief, loss, and death can be powerful times for children to experience spiritual growth, wholeness, and holiness. Dying is a spiritual event. Palliative care aims to improve the quality of life of patients facing problems associated with life-threatening illness and that of their families. Palliative care is designed to prevent and relieve suffering through early identification, and the correct assessment and treatment of pain and other problems that can be physical, psychosocial, or spiritual (WHO, 2015). A structured bereavement program can support families and children at the point of death (Mullen et al., 2015). Individuals who are dying can have quite a different spiritual reality, especially if they are suffering. Suffering is defined as "a loss of wholeness and the distress and anguish that accompany it." It is also the "experience of brokenness" (Attig, 1996, p. 20). Table 9.3 identifies ways of caring for children with spiritual anguish.

Attig (1996) explained that "terminal illness interrupts the ongoing stories of children's lives . . . it truncates their future and changes utterly both the shape and content of the remaining pages and chapters of their lives and the character of their biographies as wholes" (p. 20). Similarly, terminal illness (in the form of cancer) "intrudes on patients' lives, pulling the rug out from under them, and handing them a new script for life" (p. 20).

Illness seems to set children apart, and they often find it difficult to participate in or to feel "at home" in their families, friendships, and communities. They can also lose their sense of spiritual place or have fears of what lies beyond the boundaries of this life. Feeling disconnected from that which once brought value, hope, and meaning, and distant from what brings consolation and comfort leaves children or adolescents with "soul pain" (Attig, 1996). They long for the embrace of those who share their life and yearn to feel at home in the world. Listening is vital: "Careful and sensitive listening to patients who have spiritual beliefs, regardless of our own personal beliefs, can ease the pain of dying" (Lyon, Townsend-Akpan, & Thompson, 2001, p. 559). Many children are filled with questions that cry for honesty. Health-care providers can present clear, honest answers that orient children to present realities and what lies ahead.

Giving honesty in the face of death is not always easy. In the following example, Dr. Christina Puchalski recounts that as hard as honesty can be (for adults), children have the capacity to astonish:

> Sara was a nine-year old girl dying of metastatic cancer with an estimated few months to live. Both the doctor and mother wondered how (or if or when) they should tell Sara that she was dying. "Sara's mother and I were so caught up in the tragedy of a young child's shortened life that we could not see that Sara was at peace with herself." One evening after drawing another blood sample, Sara looked up at her doctor and asked if she ever knew anyone close to her who died. The doctor shared that her fiancé, Eric, had died two years before. Sara teased her with an impish grin and the childhood rhyme: "Eric and Christina sitting in a tree, K-I-S-S-I-N-G." With many giggles, then very seriously said, "a tree in heaven and when you die you'll see him again. Since I am going to die soon, I'll give him a hug for you." Sara turned to her mother and said, "I'll be okay, Mommy." (Puchalski, 2000b, p. 3)

Table 9.3

Characteristics and Care of Children With Spiritual Anguish

Characteristics

Young Children	• Uninhibited • Persistent in questioning • Open about what frightens them • Read well the anxieties of caregivers • Sense caregiver anguish • Express anguish nonverbally in play, through images in drawing or painting, or in behaviors that signal distress, such as tears, agitation, outbursts of anger or hostility, refusal to eat or to cooperate with treatment • Lethargic, withdrawn, have prolonged silences, turn toward the wall, hold themselves in fetal position, have clinging behaviors
6- to 12-Year-Olds	• Candid in revealing concerns when they feel safe • Reluctant to ask questions or show fright for fear of discouraging response • Read well the anxieties of caregivers • Sense caregiver anguish • Hold concerns inward to please, protect, or hold close their anxious caregiver • Focus on present with hopes focused on immediate future
Adolescents	• Fear exposure and rejection • Hold questions back for fear of embarrassment • Shield their privacy • Find more comfort in communication with peers • Express themselves (share with those they select) through poetry, diaries, journals, art, and music • Focus on future (that their meaningful lives lie ahead) so they feel deep deprivation, resent unfairness of their condition, and anguish over unrealized potential • Long for but realize that they will not fully have adult experiences • Struggle with hopelessness • Dread the return to greater dependence

Care

How to Help	1. Create a safe, secure place permeated with trust. 2. Allow and welcome expression of anguish. 3. Recognize the need for comfort. 4. Overcome own fears of being overwhelmed by the pain and anguish that might be expressed. 5. Avoid signaling in word or deed lack of receptivity to expressions of anguish. 6. Remember that symptom control cannot replace intimacy with child or mute expression of suffering. 7. Offer presence free of agenda (be a companion as they suffer). 8. Learn the power of special interventions such as image or dream work, art or music therapy. 9. Support prayer or meditation to express and process spiritual anguish. 10. Minister to fears (e.g., separation, abandonment). 11. Assure that they need not be alone unless they choose to be so. 12. Believe and state that they will always be worthy of caring attention.

(continues)

Table 9.3 (*continued*)

Characteristics	
How to Help (*continued*)	13. Address helplessness and powerlessness by including children in decision making for treatment, symptom control, where they live, and choices in shaping their daily lives.
	14. Remind them that they had no choice about their condition but can choose how they live in response to its intrusion and death's shadow.
	15. Encourage them to believe that their remaining life can be precious; then focus on opportunities for meaningful experiences, achievements, and expressions.
	16. Help them face the spiritual challenges of leaving this life.
	17. Assure them that they will always be in the hearts of those who love them, that we won't forget them.
	18. Be honest.
	19. Invite them to tell what they believe and hope about life beyond.

Note. Adapted from "Beyond Pain: The Existential Suffering of Children," by T. Attig, 1996, *Journal of Palliative Care, 12*(3), pp. 20–23. Copyright 1996 by T. Attig. Adapted with permission.

Puchalski (2000b) pointed out that adults can complicate things with intellectual and rational thinking: "In many ways, children are more in touch with their spirituality because of their innate sense of wonder and imagination. They can often 'see' a reality beyond the everyday, physical world most people live in" (p. 3). Their perceptions are unfettered and unencumbered.

Puchalski's sharing opened the door for the child to share. Traditionally, the "therapeutic relationship" has been described as only including talk of the *patient's* life. However, in times of crisis or critical need, adults and children are looking for authentic communication. Mullen and colleagues (2015) provide valuable examples of wording that can be used with patients and parents, such as, "I can only imagine how you are feeling right now" (p.48). Particularly with end-of-life bereavement, supportive communication is a skill and art that has lasting effect. On occasion and with careful consideration, authentic communication can include personal examples. Maugans (1996) wrote,

> At times, revealing one's own personal spirituality may be appropriate if it helps in building the patient–physician relationship [or that of patient with other health-care provider] or in breaking down barriers that have developed over conflictual belief systems. Generally this is done at the request of the patient and only if the physician [or other health-care provider] feels capable. (p. 15)

Immanent Justice

One common type of spiritual distress that occurs with children is termed *immanent justice*. This is the belief that illness is a punishment for wrongdoing. Children can think that misdeeds have caused the illness. These beliefs are primarily but not exclusively found in children under 7 years of age. Children may voice these perceptions, or perceptions may remain as internal concerns, which can be spiritually damaging. When voiced, however, misperceptions can be corrected. Health-care providers can offer different viewpoints. Statements such as, "I imagine it can feel like that. I wonder how much ＿＿ has to do with it also" can redirect thinking and feeling to consider other perspectives. Upadhaya and Kautz (2012) described ways that nurses can assist when a patient says something like, "God is punishing me" or "This disability is karma," including listening, exploring family or religious support, and finding means of adaptive transformation.

Distorted Images of God

Children and adolescents can have distorted images of God. Because of developmental-level differences, children may have unexplored feelings that cause negative reactions to God or others. These images may be of an angry, demanding, "scowl on his face" God rather than a kind comforter, counselor, and healer image of God. The child may think one way but feel another; that is, images of God are not the same as ideas of God. Parents, early caretakers, or spiritual community members can affect these images. The distortions of God, such as one who is abusive, a bully, unreliable, weak, or one who abandons can sometimes be changed through new examples of caring others, prayer, or through talk. Providing a competing image (such as God with a loving smile looking at and holding the child) can push away the painful image (Ryan, 1996).

Sommer (1989), a chaplain, spoke of the dying child and stated,

> It is helpful to share with children that God loves all people—especially little children—so they will not fear the prospect of going to be with an angry or mean God after they have died. Second, children need to be given a positive image of what lies beyond death. Because children have vivid imaginations, unless we fill the void of afterlife with positive images they may fill it with monsters and images of separation and darkness. (p. 232)

Baring (2013) conducted a study of Filipino children's image of God in relationship to their perception of father and mother qualities. Findings from fifth graders ($N = 241$) revealed that children found a focused image of God to be one of comforting attention of love and care. Additionally, there were qualitative differences noted between children's image of God and of their own parents.

Intense Spiritual Experiences

Sometimes, religious beliefs, particularly those of ultrareligious sects, or various spiritual experiences can be very intense. When are these normal, and when are they psychotic episodes? The following criteria are helpful for identifying when referral is needed. According to Greenberg and Witztum (1991), psychotic episodes

- are more intense than normative religious experiences in their religious community;
- are often terrifying for the individual;
- are often preoccupying and the individual can think of little else;
- are associated with deterioration of social skills and personal hygiene; and
- often involve special messages from religious figures. (p. 554)

When intense but not distorted, some spiritual experiences may be awe-inspiring and preoccupying. The difference is that these experiences are strengthening in nature. It can be difficult for mental health therapists who lack knowledge of the basic tenets of a particular religion to differentiate religious beliefs and rituals from delusions and compulsions (Greenberg & Witztum, 1991). Additionally, a lack of cultural awareness regarding cultural and spiritual perspectives of specific groups of people can lead to misconceptions. Non-therapists should document any signs of mental instability, seek out interdisciplinary communication, and refer to clergy or mental health specialists when applicable. Pre-episode functioning, stressful precipitants, onset of any new symptoms, and post-episode functioning should be noted if a child has an intense religious experience (Lukoff, Lu, & Turner, 1995).

Perceived Lack of Spiritual Support

Another facet of spiritual distress can be within the spiritual support system itself. Parents—especially those of children with disabilities—have sometimes experienced support from their spiritual community that is limited, insubstantial, or not comprehensive enough to meet the many strains of long-term disability. People with disabling conditions may be angry at their church for what feels like a lack of caring support, which can carry over to their relationship with God. The health-care team can assist parents and children in realizing that a local church or religious structure may not have enough resources or drive to meet the multiple spiritual needs that are present. Parents can be encouraged to explore widening their support systems to avoid cutting off valuable, though limited, support from their usual spiritual communities. Connecting with other parents of children with disabilities who have similar faith persuasions may be beneficial. Online support groups where parents can connect are available at specific disability websites. Children can connect to support groups or group blogs that may be of significant worth. Reliable Internet links can offer valuable "screen to screen" support or information.

Religious-Related Abuse or Spiritually Motivated Alteration of Care

Religion is nearly always positive toward children. However, religious beliefs can sometimes justify destructive behaviors (Simonič et al., 2013). On occasion these abuses become evident in health-care settings. Typically, referral is required. Accommodating parental and children's spiritual beliefs and practices is a directive in health care (The Joint Commission, 2010, p. 21). In situations where parents refuse treatment for their children, spiritual and legal knowledge is beneficial for health-care providers (see Chapter 11: Ethical, Moral, and Legal Issues in Children's Health Care).

A Developmental Approach

Interventions with children differ, depending on the age of the child (see Table 9.4). Health-care professionals should know basic developmental-stage aspects of care prior

Table 9.4

Developmentally Specific Spiritual-Care Interventions	
Developmental Staging	**Interventions**
Infants	
Erikson: *Trust versus mistrust* Requires sensitivity and consistency in meeting needs. Basis of self-identity and hope established. **Piaget:** *Sensorimotor* Uses senses, motor skills, reflexes to explore. Trial and error and "insight" problem-solving. **Fowler:** Stage 0: *Undifferentiated* No concept of right or wrong; no apparent religious beliefs or convictions to guide behavior. However, beginnings of faith are established with the development of basic trust through developing a relationship with their primary caregiver.	1. Actively listen to parental concerns. Be alert to the possibility that they may perceive their child's illness as some kind of religious omen or punishment. 2. Build self-worth by reassuring parents about the adequacy of their parenting skills. 3. Attend to emotional and physical needs of infants. Encourage parental presence. Provide safe, consistent care that is loving and accepting. 4. Encourage and facilitate the continued use of a religious support system for the family. Suggest to caregivers the possibility of using a religious-based support system. If desired, assist them in finding an appropriate support system.
Toddlers and Preschoolers	
Erikson: *Autonomy versus shame* (1–3 years) Limits (firm and consistent) lead to security. Acquires "will," feeling of self-control basis for self-esteem. *Initiative versus guilt* (3–5 years) Energy used in problem-solving. "Conscience" develops. Begins cooperation. Beginning of purpose. **Piaget:** *Preoperational* Self-centered; perception from own point of view; literal interpretation of works and actions; judges things for outcome, consequence to self. **Fowler:** Stage 1: *Intuitive–projective* Imitates the behavior of others; imitates religious gestures and behaviors of others with very limited comprehension of any meaning or significance of activity. Follows parental beliefs as part of daily life, but without an understanding of their basic concepts.	1. Teach and coach the parents to assist the child in positive coping behaviors. 2. Reassure the child that she or he is not being punished (by God or other authority figures) for the disease or hospitalization. 3. Using the information gained in the assessment, continue with routines from home, such as daily activities, limit setting, and religious rituals. 4. Appropriately initiate discussion of love and caring from a Higher Power, using developmentally correct language to relieve anxiety and loneliness. 5. Show the child behavioral qualities of love, acceptance, trust, respect, caring, setting of firm limits, and disciplining without anger. 6. Don't underestimate the child's level of comprehension. Respond to questions in an understandable, concrete manner. Give logical reasons for religious behavior.
School-Age Children	
Erikson: *Industry versus inferiority* Wins recognition by producing things, solving problems, and finishing tasks.	1. Be alert to anxiety about being punished by a deity.

(continues)

Table 9.4 (*continued*)

School-Age Children (*continued*)	
Piaget: *Concrete operations* Interpersonal collaboration and competition. Social reciprocity and sense of fairness. Uses elementary logic and manipulation of actual objects and experiences. **Fowler:** Stage 2: *Mythical–literal* Spiritual development closely related to experiences and social interactions. Usually has a strong interest in religion and is able to articulate his or her faith. Conscience is developing.	2. Provide appropriate, concrete explanations in response to questions regarding spiritual beliefs. 3. Continue with religious rituals. When appropriate, promote the use of prayer. 4. Encourage the child's personal relationship with his or her God. 5. Model behaviors that show forgiveness and acceptance. 6. Promote continued contact with school or church peers.
Adolescents	
Erikson: *Identity versus role confusion* Searches for self-identity. Begins socially responsible behavior and coping with emotions. Develops ideology and philosophy of life. Looks for powers and limits. **Piaget:** *Formal operations* Sees world from many and different perspectives. Thought is independent of concrete reality; is flexible; and manipulates symbols, forms hypotheses, and theories. **Fowler:** Stage 3: *Synthetic–conventional* (preadolescent) Becomes increasingly aware of spiritual disappointments. Begins to reason and question some of established parental religious standards. May drop or modify some religious practices. Stage 4: *Individuative–reflective (adolescent)* Becomes more skeptical and begins to compare religious standards of family with standards of others. A time of asking questions and searching for answers.	1. Provide an open, accepting attitude. Provide an atmosphere for the adolescent to discuss the implications of this illness in terms of philosophical and religious beliefs. 2. Encourage continued contact with friends and classmates. Use support groups with which the youth feels comfortable. Some may seek religious support groups from members of their peer groups. 3. Encourage the use of religious rituals if the adolescent desires to continue using them. 4. Provide answers to questions in an unbiased manner that encourages participation and stimulates his or her personal thinking. 5. Take the time to develop an honest, trusting relationship with the teen. 6. Assess and document verbalizations of the teen's values and beliefs.

Note. Adapted from *Seminars in Oncology Nursing, 13*(4), D. Hart and D. Schneider, "Spiritual Care of Children with Cancer," pp. 266, 268, 269. Copyright 1997 with permission from Elsevier.

to any care of children. Major illness or injury can alter spiritual development with the possibility of regression; however, an understanding of developmental concepts enhances spiritual care of children.

Below are concepts associated with each general developmental stage of childhood. This information is summarized and linked with age-specific interventions for infants, toddlers and preschoolers, school-age children, and adolescents in Table 9.4.

Newborns and Infants

Hall (2006), a midwife, views the unborn as having a spiritual nature. She explored spirituality and birth, various religious perspectives about the beginning of life, and implications of care at the point of birth. Most faith traditions acknowledge newborn spirituality. For example, a newborn has spirituality well established at birth in the Jewish tradition; Hindu and Buddhist traditions have the dharma of spirituality that abides through the karma of life, death, and reincarnation; and African animists celebrate spirituality in each newborn child (Surr, 2012).

Trust-building is an especially important spiritual support for a baby. Infants develop a sense of trust, belonging, and self-worth through consistent, loving care of their needs, which are prerequisites for the development of a relationship with a "Higher Being" (Hart & Schneider, 1997). Infants need predictable routines, normalcy, and a consistent nurturing caregiver. Parental comfort, such as holding, rocking, singing, and talking to the infant, develops trust. Surr (2011) explored research about early attachment experiences related to spirituality, describing differences between infants with different attachment relationships (securely, avoidant, resistant, ambivalently, or disorganized attachment). Early attachment experiences were found to be spiritually significant.

Mangini, Confessore, Girard, and Spadola (1995) described 6-month-old-Jason, a previously healthy infant, who was admitted for failure to thrive. Jason's father had died in a plane crash two months earlier. His mother was exhausted and tearful. She reported that the baby had been vomiting, was disinterested in feeding, and needed to be held constantly. Interventions included physical care for Jason (allowing his mother to rest), supportive listening by staff to Jason's mother, an opportunity for her to attend an in-hospital parent coffee hour, and an outside referral to a support group for grieving spouses. Jason and his mother responded well. Consistency of schedule and meeting Jason's basic needs diminished the negative effects of loss. The supportive listening allowed for spiritual and emotional support of his mother, helped increase her coping skills, and thus made her better able to help her baby.

Toddlers and Preschoolers

Any concrete approach that builds comfort is helpful for toddlers, such as (a) the thought that God is their protector; (b) simple prayers; (c) having religious stories read to them; (d) having picture discussions with comforting pictures or images such as those in picture Bibles; (e) participating in spiritual activities of normal living, such as mealtime grace or bedtime prayers; and (f) activities of religious holidays or rituals (see Figure 9.2).

Toddlers are beginning to develop a conscience and perceptions of right and wrong (Erikson, 1963). "Concrete cognitive thinking with beginning conscience can lead preschoolers to believing that an illness is a punishment for a 'bad' thought or action" (Hart & Schneider, 1997, p. 267). This concrete thinking can also lead to literal spiritual interpretations. For example, Amy, a 3-year-old, asked her mother to sing "Turn Your Eyes Upon Jesus" at bedtime. Amy kept lifting her head and looking around to "turn her eyes on Jesus" instead of being lulled to sleep (Steen & Anderson, 1995).

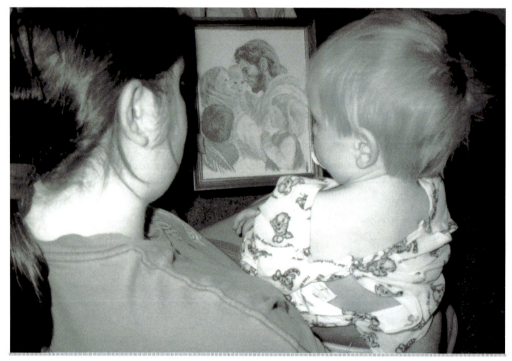

Figure 9.2. Spiritual pictures that portray caring or comfort can evoke pleasure, even with very young children. *Note*. Photograph by Lynn Clutter. Used with permission.

Toddlers need predictability in the daily schedule, clear expectations from consistent caregivers, clear structure yet the ability to explore within the structure, and opportunities to exert their independence and to develop their self-worth. Jegatheesan (2013) indicated that Muslim parents of toddlers allow their children to observe prayers as early as 3 years of age.

Preschoolers require self-assertion and self-discipline, consistent expectations, and appropriate discipline. They need to feel loved and secure, maintain a regular schedule and religious practices or rituals, and be surrounded by familiar objects, even in healthcare settings.

School-Age Children

Young school-age children have a limited ability to communicate needs or feelings. They may give no verbal hints about spiritual needs yet may give cues about their own religious beliefs. However, inner pain or distress is most often inferred by behaviors.

School-age children lack abstract thinking, so concrete interventions are appropriate. Reading spiritual passages or prayer books, saying learned or spontaneous prayers, and discussing meaning of prayers, sacraments, or family worship rituals may be parts of their lives. However, they may just as easily indicate needs by what they do not say or do. For example, they may avoid eye contact, display anger, frustration, or manipulative behaviors, or resist the plan of care (Fulton & Moore, 1995). Rev. Handzo of Memorial Sloan-Kettering Cancer Center indicated that children may tend to attribute Bible characters with what they themselves are feeling. A skilled listener can sometimes take a comment like, "I wonder if God forgot Jesus on the cross" and deepen the conversation with a follow up comment like, "Does it ever feel as if God forgets about you?" (Handzo, 1990).

Providing a supportive environment, trusting relationship, time, and opportunity to unlock spirituality will enhance spiritual well-being and help to identify any distress. Care will offer a developmentally appropriate means to gain control over their situation. Active involvement in spiritual intervention choices (e.g., drawing, listening to music) can help as the decision-making gives control.

School-age children are "learning and growing through producing and accomplishing things. They begin to feel competent and successful through mastery of knowledge and skills" (Hart & Schneider, 1997, p. 266). They may ponder the cause and require assurance of causes—not their own—for their illness, and may require explanations for their illness. They are exploring new awareness of forgiveness, acceptance, guilt, and the differences between supernatural and natural.

Religious concepts are still concrete. Talking with their God in prayer can nurture their spiritual relationship (Hart & Schneider, 1997). School-age children may think about what God does and how He does it. They may believe in good and evil, which can lead to feelings of fear and guilt (Steen & Anderson, 1995). Because they have a limited tolerance for acute sadness, they may be upset one moment and asking to go out to play the next.

Pre-adolescents

Pre-adolescent children, ages 9 to 12 years, are developing their sense of right and wrong behavior on a moral level. They understand time, space, quality, and causality. They are growing in their understanding of life and death. They have interest in biological details and need to have their questions answered accurately and honestly (Mangini et al., 1995). A broad question about spirituality and availability to hear their responses may focus the pre-adolescent enough to promote growth. Scott (2004) indicated that children and youth have experiences uniquely their own that they identify as spiritual. The effect on their own lives over time range from favorable effects, such as peacefulness or a sense of being cared for by the Divine or some "other," to uncertainty or fear.

Adolescents

Spirituality among adolescents involves ideological concerns more than rituals or religious customs. This developmental change is largely due to the advancement of abstract thinking. They focus more on internal aspects of religious commitment and of developing a strong personal relationship with a Higher Power. The search for identity may involve exploring spiritual belief systems to discover meaning, purpose, life direction, and hope in life (Hyde, 2008). They need to find meaning in suffering and illness (Hart & Schneider, 1997). In this population, meeting spiritual needs is especially important in the healing process to decrease stress and improve coping skills (Chapman & Grossoehme, 2002).

Teens are open to spiritual counsel at times. They are sometimes willing to talk with health-care providers about how the current health issue affects beliefs or meaning in life, and to deal with questions such as, "Why me?" Teenagers may participate in spiritual activities, receive visits from peers, cherish some privacy, talk on the phone about spiritual matters, or worship privately in their room. Adolescents may find strength by creating new religious rituals in the sickroom. They want a sense of normalcy, and desire some sense of control over decision-making in their plan of care. Spirituality may protect them from negative health influences (Good & Willoughby, 2014; Spurr, Berry, & Walker, 2013).

Adolescents may demonstrate spiritual strength in the midst of crisis or challenges (Cavendish et al., 2001). O'Brien cites the win-win words of Anna, a 13-year-old diagnosed with escalating Ewing's sarcoma with metastasis who said, "If God heals my body, then it will be wonderful and I can be a missionary and tell people about Him, but if He doesn't then I will die and be with Jesus, so there's no way I can lose" (O'Brien, 2013, p. 217).

Open and accepting attitudes help adolescents discuss spiritual beliefs. Providing answers to questions and encouraging their involvement is appreciated. Having visits from peers can provide youth support. However, teens may be very concerned with their image and not want peers or others to see them as weak.

General Concepts of Spiritual Intervention

In general, health-care providers should support children's existing faith. Inner resources or individualized spiritual expression can be supported in ways that continue their meaningful influence in the life of the child. Sometimes, especially during pivotal life events, such as the diagnosis of cancer, completion of treatment, or return of disease progression, children and adults experience severe spiritual disequilibrium. Supporting their existing spiritual strength and helping them identify, clarify, and deepen what is meaningful in their lives can be helpful.

Health-care providers can also support the family's faith (Wilson & Miles, 2001). Supporting existing faith does not require expertise in religion, and in many care situations, sensitive support is key in the presence of suffering. Some children and family members will simply want to discuss their beliefs. Health challenges can bring spiritual questions or conflicts to the forefront of a person's thinking. It may be much easier to discuss problems with health-care providers who are not in the person's spiritual sphere of involvement. In addition to listening, a health-care provider can locate significant resources after identifying the patient's or family member's formal religious belief system. For example, the teachings of spiritual leaders can be very health promoting. Written resources or suggestions of compatible spiritual practices that will help the child's physical and emotional situation may then be offered.

Religions have rituals, various spiritual practices, sacraments such as communion or anointing with oil, baptism, circumcision, or various traditions surrounding care of the sick. Because religion holds pervasive life value to the patient, and health-care intervention is superimposed on that life, health-care providers have a responsibility to make room for the beliefs and practices that the patient holds dear. Children who are involved with a church or spiritual group may benefit from ongoing involvement with members while they are receiving health care. Regular participation in healthy religious activities (e.g., prayer, scripture reading, worship attendance, healing ceremonies, community service, referral to and collaboration with clergy) has been shown to have health benefits (Matthews, 2000).

Having fun linked with spiritual life often is powerfully effective. For example, "the making of 'spiritual bracelets' (akin to friendship bracelets, except that the colors of threads represent different spiritual values) can both prompt discussions about faith and other values and allow the child to create a gift" (Thayer, 2001, p. 180).

Fostering spiritual growth is another important principle. Illness can be viewed as an opportunity or occasion to redefine values, to encounter uncertainty, and to seek out greater purpose and connectedness. The child may have an ability greater than adults have to express spiritual concerns when facing physical or emotional challenges. The health-care provider can maintain a readiness to hear and truly be with a child during this time. Spiritual growth is fostered through comfort, companionship, conversation, and consolation measures. Accepting, reassuring, caring, visiting, listening, concrete communications being "real" (not contrived), and sharing "straight" answers are valuable in care. Identifying helpful ways to make sense of what is happening to children is important in the plan of care (Mueller, 2010). The health-care provider can intervene with these measures or link others with the child. Spiritual or religious coping strategies are nearly always associated with adaptive health outcomes (Pendleton, Cavalli, Pargament, & Nasr, 2002).

Health-care providers can also promote the use of spiritual strength. Many children with life-threatening illnesses have phenomenal courage that is grounded in their spirituality, empowering them to life with deepened faith, hope, love, peace, and joy. The ability to transcend the crisis with this strength is exactly what health-care providers need to support (Carson & Koenig, 2008; March & Caple, 2015). Additionally, Clark, Cross, Deane, and Lowry (1991) mentioned the notion of the spirit-to-spirit encounter between caregiver and patient that includes the patient's acknowledgment of trust in the caregiver. Quality care, in their view, must include this spirit-to-spirit encounter.

Direct Spiritual Practices or Interventions

A myriad of options are available for spiritual work with children. Familiarity with strategies gives professionals an internal "toolbox" that will be useful at the moment of planned or spontaneous spiritual care.

The Ministry of Presence

Authentic human presence, being there, being with, and *caring presence* all refer to the same aspect (Gallia, 1996). Presence has been described as foundational for compassion. In fact, Carson (2011) identifies "ministry of presence," "ministry of word," and "ministry of action" as three primary modalities of providing spiritual care. Kendall (1999) indicated that aspects of bedside nursing such as "hands on" care, "accompanying," and "watching" give "presence" to the vulnerable patient. Zerwekh (1997, p. 260) uniquely described this quality as "presencing," converting *presence,* a noun describing a quality, into a verb expressing action. Kenny (1999) stated,

> The ability to be with children in this way confirms their uniqueness and offers acceptance of them and their experience. Out of this trusting contact, avenues of communication can open that are unique to the child and his/her developmental stage. (p. 32)

Within the concept of the ministry of presence, the professional must be committed and devoted to the child's growth. Just as our authentic presence can bring a measure of settling or healing to the child and family, we must be able to be truly present in the face of suffering, pain, sorrow, and grief. Shelly and Fish (1988) and Fulton and Moore (1995) called it the therapeutic use of self with empathy, vulnerability, humility, and commitment. Mullen et al. (2015) called it the capacity to be fully there with a quality of attention and authenticity—fully engaged, not distracted by personal bias or other obligations but with an aspect of compassionate intention.

So very often, talk is not needed—especially with children. Being there makes the difference. Nurses are at the bedside around the clock in many health-care situations. This is a wonderful advantage because presence alone can build trust and strengthen relationships. Sterling-Fisher shared some gracious wording that a health-care provider may use that sets a time limit but conveys authentic presence: "I need to be leaving in about 20 minutes, but I'm not in a hurry. I'm here to be with you" (Sterling-Fisher, 1998, p. 247).

Conveying Acceptance

Having true regard and respect for a person conveys acceptance and invites children to open their lives to us. Shelly (1995) described the importance of "unconditionally welcoming a child." Having unconditional acceptance and love allows the child to feel safe, secure, and able to express his or her real self. *Empathetic regard* is another descriptive phrase that implies acceptance.

Active Listening

Active listening is a means to assure caring, confirm a child's uniqueness, confirm acceptance, and tell the child that the listener is open or trustworthy to listening to their history and spiritual stories. Active listening can allow children to be the center of our attention for the time we are with them. This forum is powerful in touching the being of a child and allowing the child to lead us to the areas of greatest spiritual need. Burkhardt and Nagai-Jacobson (2015) encourage listening specifically for what is important to individuals, what gives meaning to their life, what gives them strength and hope, and what fears and concerns they have.

O'Brien talked about listening with a loving heart (O'Brien, 2013), to what is shared and to what is not said. Children will usually not express their needs in spiritual terms. Thus, it is up to the health-care provider to listen for the needs or for the strengths. Comments such as, "It isn't fair to have asthma," may be a lead to broad opening questions. However, before asking any questions, listening is necessary. Listening may lead to discovery of the "gift" to be affirmed or the needs to be met (Hungelmann, Kenkel-Ross, Klassen, & Stollenwerk, 1996).

In his culminating work of research, *The Spiritual Life of Children*, Robert Coles (1990) communicated a marvelous insight gleaned from William Carlos Williams:

I am with a child, and I want some information—and he'll clam up, or she'll stare at me stonily. I'll get impatient. I'll get angry. On a good day, though, I'll remember what I shouldn't have forgotten—what I've learned after hundreds and hundreds of house calls: When a kid falls silent I should keep my eyes open. . . . Pay attention to the wordless narration that can take place as a child uses his or her face, arms, or legs, or, as child psychiatrists have learned, a paintbrush, [or] some crayons. (p. 167)

Crisis situations warrant private listening without interruption. Mangini and colleagues (1995) explained,

You can create the sense of a timeless space in which you are fully present and focused on the situation. The other person should sense that you are fully there for them and have all the time they need for you to be with them. (p. 562)

Therapeutic Spiritual Communication

Talking with a child or family member about spiritual matters is, in itself, an intervention that can bring strength. Sometimes therapeutic listening will give way to spiritual discussions. During these discussions, health-care providers can employ communication methods such as facilitating, clarifying, validating feelings and thoughts, or identifying sources of strength and hope. Simply by using the content of the person's own words and adding therapeutic, supportive communication skills, much can be accomplished.

Reflective Communications or Further Questions

A question such as, "To whom do you turn when you need help?" lets clients clarify spiritual values, resources, and experiences (Sellers & Haag, 1998). "What are some of the lessons you've learned from this experience?" is an example of a question that can be fairly easy to ask but can yield meaningful spiritual answers. Other helpful questions are, "What aspects of spirituality would you like me to keep in mind as I care for you?" and "How has your spiritual history been helpful in coping with your illness?" (McBride, Arthur, Brooks, & Pilkington, 1998).

Prayer

Prayer is the main spiritual tool for seeking God's help. It is a common practice among a large percentage of the population and is relevant to health in addition to being supported as a beneficial practice by nursing evidence (Kim-Goodwin, 2013). Prayer is reaching out beyond ourselves for some and looking inward for others. Patients use prayer for themselves in times of crisis. Parents commonly pray for their children who face a crisis.

Prayer seems to benefit the doer and the receiver. Those who pray may feel less burdened because they have been able to do something about the problem. There may be a feeling of relaxation, release of endorphins, and release of other natural "tranquilizers." Physical, emotional, social, and spiritual strengths have been described as being associated with noncontact intercessory prayer, personal private prayer, or face-to-face joint prayer (Matthews, 2000; Roberts, Ahmed, & Hall, 2002). Finding meaning in suffering, coping, and perceptions of well-being for patients are recurrent results of prayer.

Prayer can be a petition, request, adoration, reparation, meditation, or contemplation; it can be thanksgiving, vocal, mental, discursive, affective, centering, mystical, private, or communal (O'Brien, 2013, 105; see Figure 9.3). Harmon and Myers (1999) identified petition, intercession, confession, lamentation, adoration, invocation, and

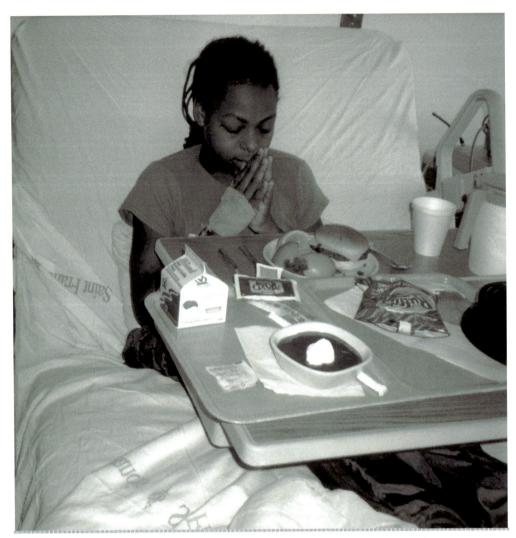

Figure 9.3. Spiritual routines, such as saying grace before meals, can be maintained in various health-care settings. *Note.* Photograph by Lynn Clutter. Used with permission.

Table 9.5

Four Dimensions of Prayer	
Dimensions of Prayer	**Examples of Prayer**
Ritual/recitational	Readings, reciting of prayers
Conversational/colloquial	Conversing with God in a less formal way
Petitionary/intercessory	Requesting something specific from God
Meditative	Reflective, listening, experiencing, and worshipping God

Note. From "Replenishing the Spirit by Meditative Prayer and Guided Imagery," by K. Brown-Saltzman, 1997, *Seminars in Oncology Nursing, 13*(4), pp. 255–259. Copyright 1997 by Saunders. Reprinted with permission.

thanksgiving as forms of prayer. In short, there are many types of prayer. Levin (1996) reviewed four dimensions of prayer, which are listed in Table 9.5 with examples.

Being aware of different dimensions or types of prayer is valuable for the health-care provider. Different types of prayer may bring different results for children. Variety in prayer may prove helpful. O'Hara (2002) pointed out that how a person prays and what happens when he or she prays is more important information than frequency of prayer. Prayer can happen anywhere. No special place is needed.

Hart and Schneider (1997, p. 269) offered the following guidelines for initiating and intervening through prayer if prayer seems suitable:

- Be prepared to offer the prayer—"Would you appreciate prayer at this time?"
- Allow the child or family to make the choice—"Yes, it couldn't hurt!"
- Pray . . . blessing, petition, formal prayer, and so on. If the nurse is praying, the prayer should be kept short and simple, endeavoring to reflect the child's feelings, fears, and concerns.

Wording must be comfortable for the health-care provider. Often, however, at the point when initiation of prayer is appropriate, the health-care provider may not come up with ready words. See Text Box 9.2: Ten Different Wording Styles for Initiating the Offer of Prayer, which presents different ways to word the same offer for prayer and demonstrates that there are many ways to word things well.

Text Box 9.2
Ten Different Wording Styles for Initiating the Offer of Prayer

1. "Would you like me or a spiritual advisor to pray with you now?"

2. "Would you appreciate prayer at this time?" or " . . . about the things we've discussed?"

3. "Would saying a prayer be helpful for you?"

4. "I would be happy to (honored to, able to, most willing to) say a prayer with you if that would help."

5. "Some people find prayer valuable at times like this. Would that be the case with you?"

6. "Do you ever say prayers at times like this?"

7. "I know a couple of children who have had a special prayer written on a paper or index card and it has helped them. Do you think something like that would be good for you?"

8. "Did you know you could write (or make a song out of) a special prayer that is your very own to God? I'd pray it with you if you ever did that."

9. "I like to pray about things like that. Do you?"

10. "This card of yours says 'God meets us when we pray.' What do you think about that? Would that help now?"

Prayers can be short and simple, reflecting the child's feelings, fears, and concerns, and "opening the lines of communication between the child and God" (Anderson & Steen, 1995, p. 16). Prayers may change with developmental stage. The earliest prayers of young children are vague because children have an indistinct understanding of prayer. In the next stage, children view prayer as a routine external activity. In the third stage, children view prayer as a private conversation with God with less egocentricism (Steen & Anderson, 1995).

It is important to distinguish prayer as an adjunct to care and not an alternative. The medical literature has mixed viewpoints on initiation of prayer, as does the nursing literature. Although physicians and nurse-practitioners—responsible for diagnosing and treating illness—may have a greater concern over any hint of religious coercion than other health-care providers, some degree of their caution is held by other providers as well. Patients should have the choice of having verbal prayer or not. Wellinghausen (2015) indicated that nurses must follow the patient's lead and pray when given explicit permission. Schoonover-Shoffner (2013) acknowledged the challenges of integrating prayer in nursing practice but gives an excellent example of effective spontaneous prayer with the patient's permission.

Proclaiming a Blessing

In many ways, people rely on the strength, hope, belief, and faith of others to get through difficult times. The assistance of a clergy member (priest, rabbi, minister) for spiritual blessing is common at times of need (March & Caple, 2015). It is possible for others to bestow a blessing upon an individual as an "intentional act of speaking God's favor and power into someone's life" (Anderson & Steen, 1995, p. 16). The Book of Psalms and various other sacred writings in the Bible, Torah, or Quran have many written blessings. Even for those living in death's shadow, health-care providers can foster strength where there was helplessness and powerlessness:

> Our confidence and affirmation that the life remaining can be precious can encourage the same appreciation in them and counter feelings that they are burdens upon others or failures. We can help them to focus upon remaining opportunities for meaningful experiences, achievements, and expressions. (Attig, 1996, p. 23)

Meditation

A wide variety of meditation practices are used throughout the world. Both Eastern and Western religions include meditation, as do Native American religions. Simkin and Black (2014) report data suggestive of the possible value of mediation and mindfulness techniques for treating symptomatic anxiety depression and pain in youths. In one study, children with neuroblastoma who used meditation required fewer analgesic doses to manage antibody infusion therapy induced pain (Ahmed, Modak, & Sequeira, 2014).

Children can be encouraged to use prayer and meditation to express and process spiritual anguish. Of course, if children indicate that meditation is part of their lives, health-care providers should facilitate its practice in the health-care setting through means such as helping in providing privacy.

Touch

Human touch can convey spiritual compassion in a way that words cannot. Children are especially responsive to touch. Referred to in religious literature (Mark 10:13, the *Bible*), human touch is important from birth to death, and is a powerful means of uniting people. Many types of touch are suitable for spiritual intervention with children. Patting, stroking, tussling of the hair, touching or holding a hand, patting or gently grasping a forearm or shoulder, patting a back, putting an arm around, rocking, soothing, holding, or even nestling can have their place with babies or children (see Figure 9.4). Of course, the type of touch by parents and family members is different from that of caregivers. Caregivers need to closely attune to cultural considerations as well as family norms but can be willing to use touch with children. Asking permission before hugging children or spouses/partners is appropriate (Mullen et al., 2015).

Anderson, and Steen (1995) described John, an 18-year-old boy who was hospitalized and in the terminal stages of leukemia. He was depressed and hopeless. His nurse offered a back rub, which was readily accepted. John said that she was the first person who had touched him during the month he had been hospitalized. Claassen (1998) demonstrated the value and communication benefit of touch toward children with multiple disabilities. Empathy, being vulnerable, humility, and commitment to being present through the time of support are qualities that can be expressed through touch. Spiritual communication often comes with close proximity and healthy types of compassionate touch.

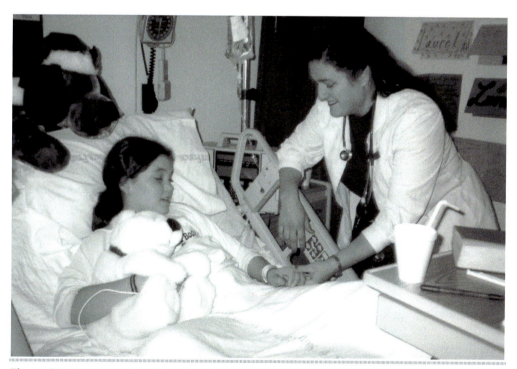

Figure 9.4. Empathy, vulnerability, humility, and commitment to being present can all be conveyed through touch. *Note.* Photograph by Lynn Clutter. Used with permission.

Therapies of Non-Western Origin

A variety of philosophical beliefs or cultural principles use complementary and alternative medicines (CAMs). Movement therapies and relaxation techniques are included in these types of CAM and have differing degrees of relationship to the spiritual. A holistic approach, as described by Thornton (2013), involves caring for each person as a whole, with an awareness of his or her physical, mental, emotional, and spiritual dimensions and needs. Holistic nursing, which emphasizes self-organizing, self-renewal, and self-transcendence with the ability to be self-assertive, does not imply complementary therapies but may use them.

Ancient Eastern philosophy, quantum theory, and the interconnectedness of all energies seem to have a strong link. Buddhism aims to alleviate suffering and teach enlightening through mindfulness, acceptance, cognitive defusion, emotional defusion, and balancing the functional alternative beliefs (Swart, 2014). These approaches are being used in health-care situations.

An array of other spiritually linked therapies or practices are derived largely from Chinese medicine, the Aborigines of Australia, American Indians, and ancient Eastern or ancient Indian spiritual traditions, many of which involve the flow of energy. Spiritual healing is connected with energy fields or centers and is not linked with religion or God or a higher power. Spiritual healers work with universal energy fields, human energy fields, laws of energy, energy systems, and the interconnectedness of energy or the flow of energy that happens when people become "well balanced" (Patterson, 1998). American Indian spirituality across tribal nations has many aspects that foster strength and resilience for youths in the face of adversity (Garrett et al., 2014).

Therapies that have New Age origins may be herbal, aroma, chanting, and prayer rituals with tefillins, chakras, or dantians. Healing through various therapies or channeling energies from one to another are aspects of New Age, American Indian, Aboriginal, or Chinese beliefs. One study found that the majority of parents of hospitalized Taiwanese children could be expected to use folk remedies for the purpose of psychological and spiritual support (Chen, Huang, Lin, Smith, & Liu, 2009).

Guided Imagery

Brown-Saltzman (1997) described the use of imagination, thoughts, senses, position, and internal images that create positive messages. The new images create new patterns or ways of seeing things. Imagery is used to reframe experiences and perceptions, facilitate problem-solving, and increase a client's sense of control. Glickman-Simon and Tessier (2014) described the effectiveness of guided imagery for postoperative pain.

Children are very able to use imagery. Computer programs have been developed to help children have positive health images (e.g., a computer game that has Pac-Man-type "body cells" that "eat" cancer cells). One can use spiritual images as well, for example, Psalms 91:4: "He will cover you with his feathers, and under his wings you will find refuge" (New International Version, the Bible). This evokes an image of a comforting, protecting God that children understand and can mentally picture.

Spiritual References, Bibliotherapy

Bibliotherapy tools can be sacred scriptures, devotional materials, written reflections on beliefs, poems, spiritual teaching tapes (audio, video), or sacred stories. With children and adolescents, the written word can draw on the imagination of hearts and minds. Certain materials, such as a Bible storybook, may be beloved and much read. Books can provide support and motivation because readers can identify emotionally with characters to gain understanding.

Health-care providers can observe a child's belief system and then identify books that may be useful. Timing and appropriateness are important in determining a book's acceptability to the child and parent. Often spiritual books will be brought from home to the health-care setting.

Cress-Ingebo and Chrisagis (1998) described two types of bibliotherapy: (a) finding the right fit of literature for readers to use by themselves, and (b) having an interactive, discussion approach. With the latter approach, the health-care provider must be prepared to discuss the material when the patient is ready to process content. Reading to the child allows opportunity for a private or discussive approach. Often with an interactive processing, the child may benefit from emotion clarification as emotions emerge. Betzalel and Shechtman (2010) identify types of affective and cognitive bibliotherapy for children with adjustment difficulties.

Anderson and Steen (1995) provided an example of bibliotherapy with a parent. The nurse preparing a 4-year-old child for surgery observed the child's mother reading the Bible. The nurse offered to share one of her favorite passages. The child's mother not only accepted the offer but also asked the nurse to pray with them for strength. Later, at a time of fear and apprehension for the family, the nurse was able to share a scripture—a welcomed encouragement.

Autobiographical scrapbooks and literature are comforting and reassuring, promote insight and reflection, and improve communication. These, in turn, empower the spirit of the child to find meaning and purpose in life.

Adults read sacred scriptures to feel closer to God, find peace, have meaning in life, stand against wrongs in society, be open and honest with self, and gain love toward others (Gallup & Lindsay, 1999). Children may or may not read for the same reasons. Before initiating the sharing of scripture with patients, the health-care provider should have some sense of when this would be an appropriate intervention.

Reassurance or Encouragement

Spiritual encouragement can take many forms. Support of the belief in God's caring presence, care notes, prayers that are written, and visits by trusted friends are examples of reassurance Even a visit from a pet can convey acceptance and encourage a child. A comment such as, "Blackie loves you in bed or outside . . . just like God," can offer a concrete symbol of reassurance. The Bible teaches Christians to encourage one another every day (Hebrews 3:13). Some children in health-care facilities may go days without encouraging words. With keen assessment and descriptive skills, nurses can regularly share specific encouragement with children and their families. Seeing the day-to-day progress gives nurses a position to share the parameters that demonstrate growth, which can be reassuring and foster hope.

Adapting the Physical Environment

Advocating for spiritual comfort or modifying the physical surroundings are two avenues for creating spiritually supportive environments. Posting notes on doors to maintain privacy at times can allow for spirituality. Providing a private area is a valuable intervention, especially with pastoral visits or meditations. Having a hospital chapel with beepers available for parents to use allows a parent of a child in surgery some freedom of space. Other physical environmental adaptations, including regulating crowding, lighting, minimizing unpleasant smells, regulating noise, preparing children for tactile sensations, and positioning children comfortably, can enhance environments in hospital settings to promote comfort (Desai et al., 2002). Fina (1995) stated,

> Orthodox Jewish parents may wish to chant, pray, or use tefillins (i.e., leather thongs used in prayer rituals) or prayer shawls. Islamic families may need a private place in which to wash and lay out their prayer rugs. Christian families may desire a private area in which to hold hands and pray aloud or to say a rosary. Prayer rituals and meditations may last for many hours. It is not unusual for family members to tell me that their prayers are for physicians and staff members caring for their child. (pp. 558, 560)

Instilling Hope

Hope can be a curative element or a preventive intervention. Health-care providers can themselves have hope, foster hope in others, or discourage feelings of hopelessness. Reed (1992) stated, "Hope, which in part represents a connectedness to possibilities and powers beyond the current situation, is frequently cited [in the literature] as the factor that can make a critical difference in the healing process" (p. 354).

Hope can be for life, recovery, and well-being. Hope can also exist for death and the hereafter. Health-care providers can assess the hope level of patients and families then support or influence accordingly. Hopelessness, the lack of hope, can hinder well-being. When the family places trust in their higher power, hope can rekindle. Hope in the capacity of the health-care team can be reassuring as well.

Porter (1995) described one parent's hope of life for her baby in the midst of staff having given up on the possibility. After the newborn survived her birth defect of gastroschisis, subsequent multiple complications and surgeries, and went on to live to adulthood, her nurse reflectively commented, "Perhaps the most valuable lesson I've learned is to listen to parents, get a feel for their instincts, show them how much I care and, most of all, never to say 'never'" (p. 26).

O'Brien (2014) explored expressions of hope in PICU settings, describing hope as a personal concept with different meanings for different people. Yet, even with clear understandings of the prognosis of a child's condition, expressions of hope can be meaningful. Expressions of hope can enhance end-of-life care as well.

Children Giving Back

An example of someone who has given back may be the best way to share the value of this intervention. Fina (1995) described Matthew, who at 12 years of age had a near-total amputation of his hand, with seven surgeries and a month of hospitalization. The experience pushed the family's coping strategies to the limit. Matthew received spiritual care from the chaplaincy department and often from the family's rabbi. Later, at the time of Matthew's bar mitzvah, part of Matthew's rite of passage was to donate the silk-flower centerpieces from the celebration to the surgical family waiting area where they often had prayed together. This act took the experiences at the children's hospital and placed a positive, lasting memory of a gift there. The gift probably served as a healing act related to this chapter of Matthew's life.

Children who are chronically ill or hospitalized or who have experienced critical illness or injuries are very able—at some point in time—to help other children. They can have very meaningful messages that benefit adults and children. One question for a child is "Do you spread love to others?" (Sterling-Fisher, 1998).

Nearly every religion encourages love and giving, both as actions and as noble character qualities. Health-care providers may facilitate "giving back" or simply allow it to happen. Health-care providers who value the belief that giving back helps children spiritually will be attuned to opportunities such as identifying a child who is struggling, a child who may be strong, and a means of connecting the two. They will foster outlets for individual children, and will encourage family members to find outlets for giving.

Journaling and the Use of Diaries

Writing can be useful (Blinne, 2010), particularly for children with spiritual concerns surrounding chronic or terminal illness, and especially for adolescents. Although adolescents may be as verbally articulate or as sophisticated in their thinking as adults, they tend to fear exposure and rejection more, and may hold back for fear of embarrassment. Journaling allows youths to explain themselves privately and without time or interactive pressure. For example, an individual experiencing a crisis of faith went to the ocean, discussed the crisis, and then wrote an essay full of water-related images. This process helped her move through spiritual pain to deepened faith, hope, and courage (Bailey, 1997).

Picture Therapy

Using pictures can encourage children to talk about topics that might evoke inner spiritual beliefs. Having a picture such as a sick child in someone's arms or care can simply be shown to a child. Usually children will offer comments or questions. The health-care provider can guide the comments once a child's voluntary comments fall silent. Questions such as, "What do you think this child is wondering?" can give way to comments that reflect the child's inner concerns. Answers can also be followed by more self-reflective comments such as, "He's lucky. His mom holds him." Even simple pictures of children out of magazines can be useful for particular aspects of spiritual care. Some children respond more readily to pictures than words. Adolescents can be prompted with questions such as, "If you were this person, what would you be thinking?"

Use of Memory, Reminiscence

Memories can bring to the forefront meaning, purpose, and satisfaction with life. For young children, memories of fun, special times, happy family moments, or closeness to God can be enjoyable, encouraging, and healing. Health-care providers can use reminiscence for assessment and trust-building. A concrete and creative approach is creating a "memory island," which involves having the child or family bring pictures and memorabilia. The island could be a poster board, scrapbook, or basket. This strategy allows others to visually join in the celebration of the person's life. Another approach is having the child, or the child and family members, share memories of "I remember when . . ." Spiritual themes are often present.

Forgiving Self or Others

Forgiveness can be an act, a process, and an attitude. Giving and receiving forgiveness brings healing and peace. Children can have powerful experiences of forgiveness. One young child said he "felt lighter or something" after he had forgiven his father for leaving him. A 6-year-old girl reported that she no longer got that "tight neck where I can't swallow when I think of her" after she forgave a particular person. An adolescent athlete was furious at the "guy who gave me this broken foot that makes me be out of basketball the whole season." Once he chose to forgive, he was able to say, "It wasn't really his fault anyway." His affect changed, and he felt he could better handle the problem.

One helpful method of helping children to forgive is the use of poetry. The poem "Wild Geese" (Oliver, 1992) begins with, "You do not have to be good. You do not have to walk on your knees for a hundred miles through the desert, repenting." Gustavson (2000, p. 329) stated, "You can easily see that this poem might be used in sessions with persons who are struggling to forgive themselves, or who may be having a hard time forgiving another person." The poem can spark a conversation on a topic that the child may have been reluctant to talk about.

Much of the 12-step materials first developed by Alcoholics Anonymous include information on forgiveness. Children can experience the same freeing from bitterness and hostility that adults experience once they decide to let go of the pain and forgive the offender. On the other hand, when a child has experienced abuse, too much willingness to forgive can be a red flag for psychosocial distress (McCullough, 2000). Forgiveness, love, and trust result in meaning, purpose, and hope in life (Carson & Koenig, 2008). With five systematic meta-analyses, Recine (2015) found strong evidence that forgiveness interventions are effective in promoting actual forgiveness.

Humor

Humor can relieve emotional tension and grief, bring health-care providers and families closer together, and allow people to stand back from the difficult situations and see other sides. Although humor cannot eliminate suffering, it can momentarily relieve the pain. Children with spiritual resilience often exhibit humor or a "lighter" perspective. Humor and pleasure can be important parts of a child's spiritual experience. Humor and laughter is important to bring as a health-care provider (Burkhardt & Nagai-Jacobson, 2015).

Play

The health-care provider can observe what gives a child pleasure, find favorite types of play, and then let the child have ample opportunities to have fun without the thought of illness. For example, the father of a girl with multiple disabilities and hospitalizations was in the room with his daughter. A nurse brought three finger puppets and said, "Would you like to see these? Here is the dad; here are the other two puppets." Her dad put one on, and the daughter had the others. They started playing and soon were lost in play, talking with "puppet voices" to each other for about 10 minutes. Their voices were animated and they laughed. They were unaware of anything else. Health-care providers can enter the child's world of play rather than forcing the child to enter theirs. Spiritual care can occur in the context of that play.

Spiritual play is especially therapeutic because it opens the spiritual dimension indirectly using the natural mode of communication. Points of pleasure can give way to trust and spontaneous comments. Child-centered play therapy allows the child to "talk" through the process of play, without requiring the child to be cognitive and verbal.

Children's anxiety may paralyze their imaginations and inhibit their capacity to play. What helps anxious children is opportunity to play, the safety of symbolic play, and play therapy. Play therapy provides the environmental situation to grow, to change, and to heal, a spiritual process. Our role is to communicate four messages: "I'm here, I hear you, I understand, and I care" (Landreth, 1991, p. 182).

Using stuffed dolls or animals, puppets, or simple finger puppets (easy to keep in the pocket) is perfect. Talking with transitional objects like this is appropriate, especially with young children, who can easily give these toys human qualities and will sometimes open up more readily than with a person they do not know well. Using a third-person technique (e.g., "Some children tell me that they worry when they have to go for tests. I wonder how it is for you") and identifying a change that would facilitate spiritual well-being can be helpful.

The Arts and Imagination

Music, visual arts, storytelling, poetry, and other expressive arts can be used to address spiritual issues. Lorrie's story is an example of the strength of spirituality and music. Lorrie had cancer. Her favorite song was "Jesus Loves Me." While in the hospital, she was asked to compose another verse to the song, the singing of which was very meaningful. Later, while Lorrie was in a coma, her music therapist visited and sang the song with Lorrie's verse, and then said, "Isn't that beautiful, Lorrie?" Lorrie woke up from her coma and nodded. She soon returned home, and before her death, was calmed regularly through her mother's singing of her verse (Lane, 1994, p. 28).

Children may be receptive to music or music therapy, such as hearing spiritually based or sacred songs, and active singing or playing instruments (O'Brien, 2013; Weitzel et al., 2011). Music is a part of all cultures and religions in some way, and especially in association with worship.

Art and art therapy are valuable tools with children who have spiritually linked issues (Koepfer, 2000). Working through these problems somehow happens as a by-product of working with media. Hyde (2008) pointed out that the use of tactile activities and sensory materials furthers religious education and creates space to nurture spirituality. Feelings can be expressed during the process or in the created outcome. For example, constructing and decorating a prayer or meditation pillow not only offers opportunities for activity, creativity, and discussion but also leaves the child with a physical object that may be used in meditation or prayer. Drawing and painting are discussed in general terms in Chapter 4: The Arts in Children's Health-Care Settings.

However, in a spiritually directed art session, requests for certain pictures can be given such as, "Will you please draw a picture of . . ."

- Anything at this time [Note: Sometimes this brings to paper and discussion what is foremost on the child's mind]
- How you feel now
- God or a specific spiritual leader, such as Jesus, Moses, higher power [Note: Islam prohibits depictions of Allah and Muhammed]
- A story from a sacred book
- A place of worship, such as synagogue, mosque, Mecca, temple, church, home
- A place where you feel close to God
- A time when you felt close to God
- You with people who help you be close to God

Spiritually related developmental changes in children's drawings have been noted. Anderson and Steen (1995) cited a study from 1944 that found that (a) children ages 3 to 6 years drew God as a king living in clouds, (b) children ages 7 to 12 years drew faith symbols (Jewish Star of David or Christian cross), and (c) youths ages 13 to 18 years drew diverse things, from conventional views of God to abstract depictions such as rainbows or sunrises (Pendleton et al., 2002).

Coles (1990) used the viewing of works of art to inspire spiritual discussions among school-age children. For example, when showing the painting *The Doctor* by the English artist Luke Fildes, which depicts a sick girl with a doctor, Coles wrote, "I have learned to ask nothing, to say nothing. Eventually the questions always come—inquiries that, of course, make their own statements" (Coles, 1990, p. 110). This approach of letting the artwork evoke the thoughts is fairly nonthreatening, can be directed by the choice of picture offered, and can reveal aspects of children's perceptions that may not otherwise emerge.

Telling stories that are spiritual in nature or those that encourage positive spiritual qualities such as courage can be excellent in use with children. The stories need to be consistent with the child's beliefs. "What makes one a Christian, a Jew, a Hindu, or a Muslim, is the sacred, master story of the religious community that shapes and nurtures each person's identity" (Webb-Mitchell, 1993, p. 148). These are the Old and New Testaments, the Hebrew Bible, and the Quran. Parts of the child's master story can be comforting to hear. The narrative approach can be a valuable tool for distraction and for incorporating spiritual content that can make a difference in health-care situations. Stories shape children's understanding of life, who they are, their faith, family, and the world around them. The telling or hearing of a story can be an act of care. A concept embedded in a story can bring lasting meaning for a child.

Sometimes writing poetry is of great value. Children may capture and identify a spiritual, emotional, physical, or social need in their poem. This is valuable because professionals seek to locate areas of needed healing and offer interventions accordingly. Merely the process of writing the poetry is therapeutic (Blinne, 2010). The sharing with others can strengthen, as well.

In her book *In-Versing Your Life: A Poetry Workbook for Self-Discovery and Healing*, Cynthia Gustavson (1995) used a procedure of pairing poems with exercises for personal growth. This process can be exemplified by having people write, "I used to be . . . but now I am. . . ." Once, an adolescent who recently gave birth filled in the metaphor with, "I used to be a beautiful flower, but now I am a stem, because I am broken" (Gustavson, 2000, p. 329). Though the girl had returned to her support group, and her baby was 2 weeks old, this was the first time she had spoken to anyone.

Another example of a verse is, "I am . . . but I will be . . ." Sometimes filling in the blanks can pull inner feelings out into the open in a way that talking never can. It is important that the poem match the person's developmental level, but poetry therapy can be used with children as young as 4 years of age. There are four stages in the process of using poetry for therapy. The individual

- identifies with the poem and feels it has something to say to him or her,
- examines the poem and discusses its meaning,
- thinks about other meanings to compare and contrast understandings (not necessarily those that the author intended but what the individual feels), and
- integrates the perceptions of meaning into his or her own self-understanding (Gustavson, 2000).

Much could be said about children's wonderful capacity to imagine, and the use of the imagination for spiritual care. Even very young children can abandon themselves to positive imaginations. For example, children who know they are dying find strength in imagining what heaven is like. Some caregivers use a "magic carpet" to help children imagine trips to heaven or a land of no pain so that children may then talk about their hopes, wants, or worries (Field & Behrman, 2003). Parents of dying children find security in the belief that they will see their child again. Sometimes parents imagine, with pleasure, that reunion in heaven. Imagination can be used as a distraction, as when undergoing a painful procedure (Glickman-Simon & Tessier, 2014). Imagination can soften a willful perspective or change a mood. Imagining the great stories of sacred books can bring a role model to one's recollection or can be applied to the current situation.

Horticultural or Pet Therapy

Horticultural therapy combines physical, mental, and emotional involvement and stimulates an interest in the future. It uses a living medium and requires someone with responsibility, time, energy, and care. Plants are responsive to care and do not discriminate. Spiritual growth can happen tangentially.

The unconditional love of a pet can comfort and give spiritual peace (Chu, Liu, Sun, & Lin, 2009). An increasing number of hospitals have pet therapy programs where specially trained dogs and other animals visit children in a group or at the bedside. Proximity, caretaking, and nurturing are valuable and can help to "reach the core" of a child. After playing with a pet, children are noticeably calmed and often more receptive to spiritual care.

Critical Moments for Spiritual Interventions

Often in life there are vulnerable times when spiritual care—that otherwise would not be possible—is welcomed with open arms. Health-care professionals can be sensitive to cues and structure time or interventions accordingly when possible. Making use of these "open windows" can dramatically change the course of care.

A clinical nurse specialist (CNS) shared such a moment with parents who had experienced the sudden infant death of their third child while overseas. The parents scheduled an appointment with the CNS to learn how to deal with their other children's grief. Knowing that this family had much grief, and being willing to take additional personal time if necessary, the CNS arranged an appointment at the end of a workday. Her broad opening comment to the parents was, "I never really heard how everything happened that day. Will you share that with me?" This comment alone gave way to five hours of the spilling of grief. The intensity of sharing was so great that there was not a thought of stopping. The CNS spoke very little and engaged in active listening to the talk and grief of each parent. At the end, the parents were exhausted but settled in a way that was lasting. There was prayer and the provision of literature on children's grief. Every "critical moment" experience is certainly not this long. Some can be very brief but with equally lasting results.

Often children open up just before bedtime. This is a valuable time to unlock spiritual and emotional issues. The wise health-care provider will set aside time at the child's bedtime to use for this purpose. Nighttime can also be that settling time when the provider can provide extra physical touch and special care, such as combing hair or giving extra pillows. These special ministrations open doors for critical moments and allow the provider to demonstrate value of the child, unconditional acceptance, and love without words.

Baptism

Baptism is a Christian practice. Infant baptism is important for the Roman, Byzantine, and Coptic branches of Catholicism, and the Greek Orthodox, Episcopal, Lutheran, Methodist, and Presbyterian churches. For members of these denominations, additional grief can occur if the newborn has not been baptized. Baptist, Assembly of God, Charismatic, Disciples of Christ, Church of Christ, Mennonite, and Pentecostal denominations practice baptism not in infancy but at older ages (Reeb & McFarland, 1995).

When a baby is critically ill, those of certain religions may desire infant baptism. See Text Box 9.3, which describes procedures for emergency infant baptism.

Referrals to Providers of Spiritual Care

Who should provide spiritual care? The range in health-care settings is broad. Sometimes a formal clergy member (priest, rabbi, minister) or chaplain is appropriate; other times, family members do a fine job with children, and sometimes friends offer welcome care. However, a multidisciplinary team approach is valuable for spiritual care (Desai et al., 2002). First, by using a team approach, more people can assess for spiritual distress or well-being. Second, the most appropriate person on the team can plan and intervene. Third, a coordinated effort of care for the whole person can happen. Barnes and colleagues (2000) offered some excellent general guidelines for integrating spiritual and religious resources into pediatric practice. Additionally, the book *Health Care and Spirituality: Listening, Assessing, Caring* (Gilbert, 2002) describes various patient

> ### Text Box 9.3
> ## Emergency Baptism
>
> If death seems inevitable and imminent:
> 1. Take the initiative and determine parental wishes.
> 2. Notify the chaplain or social service department of the parents' desire, and provide the name and phone number of the desired minister or priest.
> 3. If a spiritual care provider is not available at time of imminent death, perform the baptismal rite:
>   - Call the infant by name (or "child of God" if not named)
>   - Pour less than 30 cc tap or sterile water or even D5W on the baby's head and say, "(Name), I baptize you in the name of the Father and of the Son and of the Holy Spirit." (Note that the Methodist rite involves putting hands in water and then placing wet hands on the baby's head. The Lutheran rite has the water poured on the head three times.)
> 4. Give the parents or family members documentation of
>   - name of the nurse who baptized (with permission)
>   - date
>   - time
>   - place
>   - name given to the infant
> 5. If the parents wish, notify their church or a local church (of the family's denomination) and request that the baptism be recorded in that church's registry. Give the same documentation as in Item 4 above.
>
> *Note.* From "Emergency Baptism," by R. M. Reeb and S. T. McFarland, 1995, *Journal of Christian Nursing, 12*(2), pp. 26–27. Copyright 1995 by *Journal of Christian Nursing.* Reprinted with permission.

experiences with multidisciplinary spiritual care. Certain members of the health-care team or community have specific expertise that other members can call upon in times of need. These members include chaplains, pastoral caregivers, community ministers, spiritual advisors, parish nurses, and other community resources.

Chaplains and Pastoral Caregivers

Many hospitals and hospices have a pastoral care or chaplaincy department (see Figure 9.5). Hospitalized children's specific spiritual needs are listed in Text Box 9.4. LaRocca-Pitts (2015) described a spiritual assessment tool designed to help beginning chaplains. It may also help other professionals in use in acute care settings.

Chaplains frequently rely on health-care providers' referrals concerning patient emergencies and whom they should visit. With changes in health care, chaplains are feeling the impact of dwindling resources and are focusing on coordination with other disciplines. Before or after surgery is a time when children commonly wish to talk with clergy members or participate in a religious ritual such as prayer or blessing. Often they will see their minister or cleric before coming to the hospital, but they may have last-minute "crises of confidence or faith." It is important for health-care providers to arrange for a quiet, private space suitable for the visit.

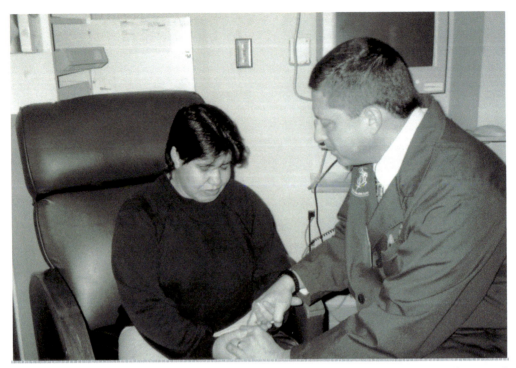

Figure 9.5. Visits and prayer from a hospital chaplain can bring support in the midst of suffering, and hope and encouragement to a weary parent. *Note.* Photograph by Lynn Clutter. Used with permission.

Text Box 9.4
Hospitalized Children's Spiritual Needs

Specific spiritual needs of hospitalized children as perceived by pastoral care workers and pediatricians in children's hospitals in the United States:
- Feeling fearful or anxious
- Difficulty with relationship between parents
- Difficulty coping with pain or other symptoms
- Difficulty with relationship between children and parent
- Why me?
- Feeling angry, bitter, or hostile
- Feeling happy, relieved, excited, or celebratory
- What is the meaning or purpose of suffering?
- Feeling helpless or hopeless or worthless
- When or how will death occur?
- What is the meaning or purpose of life?
- Feeling guilty

Note. Adapted from Figure 2 of "Spiritual Care Needs of Hospitalized Children and Their Families: A National Survey of Pastoral Care Providers' Perceptions," by C. Feudtner, J. Haney, and M. A. Dimmers, 2003, *Pediatrics, 111*(1), e67–e72.

Chaplains are formally designated pastoral caregivers (O'Brien, 2013). According to Burke and Matsumoto (1999), a chaplain functions with patients, families, or others by creating meaning or theological reflection and serving as

- a trustworthy listener,
- a pastor away from home,
- a calming presence,
- a fellow sojourner among the bereaved,
- a generator of ethical concerns, and
- an educator in using spiritual resources to cope.

Children or family members will often give cues indicating the need for a chaplain. Also, health-care providers may ask directly (e.g., "Zoey, would a visit from the hospital chaplain be helpful for you at this time?"). The chaplain can also be alerted that a family is having a particularly difficult time or has a child with a difficult diagnosis. A visit by the chaplain early in the child's hospital stay can open doors of communication and lay the groundwork for future support that can be vital to the family. Chaplains can participate in confidential discussions about helping the patient if the patient gives permission and the consent is written in the "progress note" section of the medical record.

Often the nurse at the bedside is able to give ample spiritual comfort. However, as with all interventions, individuals need to recognize limitations and determine when referral is needed. For example,

> A youth has sustained a gunshot wound to the head and is in surgery. Family members are in the waiting room sobbing with uncontrolled grief. The nurse's words are helpful but do not change the situation. The nurse offers to call someone from the family's church. The pastor comes and enters the situation with physical presence during the crisis, with touch, spiritual care, words of counsel, words of comfort, prayers, scriptures, and love. The time factor alone is more than the nurse can offer. The depth of past relationship allows the pastor to uniquely know what will make a difference. The spiritual care—specific to the family's belief system—brings a settled calm to those who are waiting. The pastor is available to help after the surgery and to offer ministry to the family and to the youth. The nurse is able to observe and assess the changes while the pastor does the work of ministry.

Pastoral Counselors

Pastoral counselors are clergy and others who have received graduate training in both religion and behavioral science for a clinical practice that integrates psychological and theological disciplines (Jordan & Danielsen, 1997). Many pastoral counselors are certified by the American Association of Pastoral Counselors (Woodruff, 1995), which also accredits pastoral counseling centers and training programs. Pastoral counselors combine counseling and spiritual values using prayer, scripture, and participation in congregations. They often pay special attention to the religious history of a child and family, which is used for identifying pathology or resources for coping. Because of the emphasis on historical information, childhood images and experiences are important.

Faith Community Nurses or Parish Nurses

Faith community nursing or parish nursing is a specialized area of professional nursing that focuses on health promotion within the context of the beliefs, values, and practices of a faith community (Patterson, Wehling, & Mason, 2008). A Lutheran minister named Granger Westberg introduced the concept in the United States in 1982. As a hospital chaplain, Reverend Westberg realized that health care was more than diagnosing and treating illness. Parish nurses focus on health as wholeness to prevent or minimize illness and emphasize the role of faith in health, illness, and healing (Bay, 1997).

Faith community nurses (FCN) fill a need. The church is the best "health place" in the community for several reasons. It is the only agency that interacts with people from beginning of life to end. It has structure for education, encourages volunteerism, and offers opportunity for community involvement. The church's mission is one of health for the whole person. Also, new community members use it as a resource for services, and in rural areas, it may be the only health place available (Solari-Twadell & Westberg, 1991).

Individuals and families that do not use regular health care may have the church as their primary social link from week to week. An FCN may see and know families that have not received health care for reasons such as difficulties with time and transportation, fear, distrust, or lack of finances. The faith community nurse's overarching role is being an integrator of faith and health and helping members (a) discover and identify the spiritual beliefs and values that affect their health; (b) understand the relationship between their faith and their health; (c) comprehend the associations among body, mind, and spirit; (d) explore the connections among attitudes, lifestyle, faith, and well-being; and (e) achieve higher levels of wellness by improving members' spiritual, physical, and emotional health (Shores, 2014). Offerings to the congregation include screenings, health fairs, workshops, classes, individual and family appointments, referrals, and visits to home, extended-care facility, or hospital.

In a study of 40 parish nurses with 1,800 client interactions, Rydholm (1997) found that half of the parish nurses' activities dealt with physical problems and the other half with spiritual or psychosocial concerns. Shores's (2014) study of 112 faith community nurses identified the following spiritual interventions: (a) the provision of spiritual support and spiritual care, (b) spiritual growth facilitation, (c) coping enhancement, (d) grief work facilitation, (e) care for the dying, (f) presence, (g) touch, (h) humor, (i) instilling hope, and (j) religious ritual enhancement.

Parish nurses or FCNs are not in competition with public health or community health services, but work in collegial relationships to enhance health-care delivery. They do not provide home health-care services or perform invasive nursing procedures. Parish nurses are "advocates, educators, gatekeepers to community resources, informal counselors for life transitions, motivators for healthy living, spiritual nurturers, and coordinators of faith community volunteers" (Abbott, 1998, p. 265). The focus is on healing, nurturing, "being," rather than curing or "doing" (O'Brien, 2013). For example, for a family that is financially limited or without transportation, a parish nurse may conduct home visits for developmental issues, health concerns, parent education, and explanations of doctors' comments. If the child is hospitalized, the parish nurse may visit and work in coordination with the hospital nurse, providing an important and trusted resource for the child, family, and hospital staff.

In 2011, the International Parish Nurse Resource Center (IPNRC) estimated that there were about 15,000 parish nurses in the United States (IPNRC, 2011). The IP-NRC has many resources about faith community nursing including FCN Scope and Standards of practice, Code of Ethics for nurses, qualifications to become an FCN, and a mission to integrate the practices of faith and nursing to promote wholeness in the people served. There is a standardized core curriculum (Foundations for Faith Community Nursing, 2014). FCNs usually have a bachelor of science degree in nursing (BSN); however, nurse practitioners and those with PhDs function in the role as well. The American Nurses Association recognized parish nursing as a specialty practice in 1997 and published "The Standards and Scope of Parish Nursing" in 1998. Currently the American Nurses Credentialing Center (ANCC) awards a credential of RN-BC for faith community nursing (ANCC, nd). Basic preparation courses and coordinators of preparation courses are available in many U.S. locations.

Other Community or Health-Care Team Resources

The use of referrals can broaden the usual support system to include unique aspects of assistance. Health-care providers can benefit from "thinking outside the box" when it comes to gathering support through community resources. When considering spiritual care of children as well as physical care, a completely different set of referral possibilities exists. For example, after initial assessment at one trauma center, in addition to chaplains, nursing staff usually initiate referrals to other support team members such as physicians, child psychiatrists, child life specialists, hospital trauma support teams, specialty nurses, social workers, and translators (Mangini et al., 1995).

In a community setting, health-care providers may suggest referral to a parent or patient, or make a referral with the family's permission. This referral could be a spiritually strong friend for a specific aspect of support, a spiritual official (i.e., a minister, shaman, guru, spiritual advisor), a support group, or website links.

Spiritual Experiences

Children sometimes have experiences that relate to their spirituality, such as a specific experience of finding meaning in illness or injury. Parents often report that their child has a different attitude or perspective about life or toward them than they had before hospitalization. Sometimes children report experiences—such as dreams—or events that cause them to stop resenting their illness or being mad at God. Listening is usually an important way of encouraging children. Although they may lack the language capacity to fully explain the experience, being there to care and listen can foster growth.

Spiritual Healing

Many patients participate in religious healing activities and find them to be helpful. Studies of religious practices found that minorities and lower socioeconomic groups commonly use religious healing activities to complement traditional medical care (Matthews, 2000). Waldfogel (1997) identified various studies indicating not only belief in faith healing but attendance at services, and large percentages of people saying they had been cured.

Therapies of "spiritual healing by others," "energy healing," and "self-prayer" were significantly increased in use from 1990 to 1997 (Eisenberg et al., 1998). Another study, of 207 patients in a rural family practice, demonstrated that 58% believed faith healers to be quacks, 29% believed that faith healers could help some people whose physicians could not help, 21% had attended a faith-healing service, and 6% reported actually being healed (King, Sobal, & DeForge, 1988).

In 1999, 30% of people in the United States reported that they had experienced "at some point in their lives a 'remarkable healing' related to a physical, emotional, or psychological problem" (Gallup & Lindsay, 1999, p. 2). Seventy percent of respondents attributed the healing to supernatural forces, with 42% naming Jesus Christ, God, or a higher power, and 30% more citing their own or others' prayers. Further, of these people who received the remarkable healing, 89% believed that it made them more aware of the importance of their spiritual life, and 84% said that it deepened their religious faith.

Combining the strength of a patient's belief in spiritual healing with the commonly used health-care strategies can be beneficial for those who believe. For example, a child who believes that the laying on of hands and prayer can bring healing may want church elders or peers to visit the health-care setting to pray while holding one or both hands on the child. Facilitating an uninterrupted visit could yield positive results. Baverstock and Finlay (2011) encouraged health professionals to ask about complementary or alternative medicine use, including faith healing.

Mystical Experiences

A dramatic rise has occurred in the percentages of those who report mystical and near-death experiences, visions, and other unusual experiences (Lukoff, Provenzano, Lu, & Turner, 1999). Many believe in angels or angelic beings (see Case Study 9.1). There have been many positive aftereffects from people who have experienced near-death or other mystical experiences. Mystical experiences are generally characterized as transient, extraordinary experiences marked by feelings of unity and harmonious relationship to the divine and everything in existence. "In several studies, people reporting mystical experiences scored lower on psychopathology scales and higher on measures of psychological well-being than did controls" (Lukoff et al., 1995, p. 468).

It is estimated that near-death experiences (NDEs) occur in about one-third of individuals who have had close encounters with death. Further, many studies on the aftereffects of NDEs provide strong evidence of their nonpathological nature. There can, however, be difficulties or adjustments afterward (Lukoff et al., 1995, p. 476). Children report vivid experiences. One hospitalized patient stated, "I tried to tell my nurses what had happened when I woke up, but they told me not to talk about it, that I was just imagining things" (Lukoff et al., 1995, p. 477). This should not be the case. Health-care providers can encourage children to share with parents and others, as well as explaining that this type of experience is not unusual. The child and supportive parent can focus on how it changes feelings, outlook, attitudes, and spiritual growth.

Ethier (2005) described a death-related sensory experience (DRSE) as a spiritually transforming experience that can have a messenger beyond the visible observable universe to guide a dying person through a dying process. These experiences are accompanied by feelings of peace and comfort and have also been described as veridical

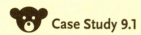 **Case Study 9.1**

Angels

According to Blanton (2004), 78% of adults in the United States believe in angels. Children do as well. Some children in hospital settings have claimed to "encounter an angel" (Hudson, 1996, p. 26) or to have "seen Jesus." For example,

> a 3-year-old child graphically told his mother and nurse that Jesus came and showed him how to take out the tube in his mouth. He had successfully extubated the endotracheal tube and, when found, did not require re-intubation because his condition had improved. He was soon released from the hospital.

This type of experience by a child usually brings comfort, but is also a critical moment for parents or health-care providers to listen and care. The physical care given must reflect the physical findings; however, often emotional settling and spiritual peace are evident. Anticipatory care is needed should the critical moment give rise to any difficulty or anxiety of the child or parent.

As many as 50% of individuals who have had near-death experiences have reported the presence of angels (Kennard, 1998). For example,

> Mallory was 9 years old and had been diagnosed with terminal cancer. She knew she was dying, and she was very afraid. One morning, she told her mother that three angels had come to her during the night. The angels had white wings and were very beautiful. They'd taken her on a trip to heaven. Mallory wasn't sick in the presence of the angels and even danced with them.
>
> Nine days before she died, Mallory made a videotape for other terminally ill children. She described the angels and heaven so that the children would not be afraid of death. She told them, "Believe what I say because it's true. It really is." (Kennard, 1998, p. 50)

Angels are seen in Judaism, the Talmud, the Kabbalah, the Bible, Islam, Mormonism, Buddhism, Hinduism, and Zoroastrianism (Kennard, 1998). Among other things, health-care providers should show spiritual respect by listening, remaining sensitive to the patient's interpretation, encouraging the patient to share with others, and documenting the event and any behavioral changes (i.e., from restlessness to calm alertness; Kennard, 1998).

hallucinations or predeath visions. Verifying the DRSE can be a means of opening a dialogue with the child.

Miracles

Gardner (1983) chronicled historical accounts of "miraculous" healings from the early 1900s with medical descriptions. Independent historical corroboration was cited for some of the cases of "almost inexplicable healing." Although no attempt was made to prove that miracles had occurred, historical written accounts were described.

Children can easily believe in miracles. They also can consider things to be miracles that are comprehensible or realistic to adults. Usually, children's beliefs and hopes are qualities of strength. Regarding miracles, it is important to ask, "What are you asking for?" It may be something simple, such as "another day together." Clarifying the language of miracles can allow for hope, as well as respectful and mutual accommodations between children, parents, and professionals (Rushton & Russell, 1996).

Religion-Motivated Medical-Care Avoidance

Spirituality and religion can have both constructive and destructive influences on individual and family development. In certain religious sects, some core values involve avoiding traditional means of health care. This can cause the most damaging aspects for children. Just as some cultures have their own healers and healing methods, some religious sects have a view of healing, and perhaps even of the value of human life, that differs significantly from the norm. Several of these sects will avoid medical services even to the point of death. Sects differ in reasons for what most would call medical neglect. For a listing of churches whose doctrines or teachings may refuse, limit, or have a preference for prayer over medical treatment for children, see Linnard-Palmer and Kools (2004).

Grievously, children can be the victims. In an overview of deaths of children between 1975 and 1995, Asser and Swan (1998) identified and studied 172 deaths of children from families that practiced faith healing *in lieu* of medical care. Of the children in this group, 145 died of conditions for which expected survival rates with medical care would have exceeded 90%. Eighteen more had conditions with typical survival rates greater than 50%, and all but 3 of the children would have had some benefit from clinical help. Their conclusions point to the strong danger of faith healing to the exclusion of medical treatment.

Protection laws for children differ from state to state, especially regarding religious exemptions. These laws may be inadequate to protect children from this form of medical neglect (Children's Healthcare Is a Legal Duty [CHILD], Inc., 2016). For example, 38 states and the District of Columbia have religious exemptions in their civil codes on child abuse or neglect, while 16 states extend religious defenses to felony crimes against children. In Florida, for example, a parent or legal custodian who, by reason of the legitimate practice of religious beliefs, does not provide specified medical treatment for a child, may not be considered abusive or neglectful for that reason alone. For additional information, see Chapter 11: Ethical, Moral, and Legal Issues in Children's Health Care.

Health-care providers are encouraged to work with children and families to intervene when religious values clash with traditional medical care (Baverstock & Finlay, 2011). Wagner and Higdon (1996) offered an example of an effective and supportive team approach: The father, a minister, was refusing treatment on "religious grounds" for his 13-year-old daughter, newly diagnosed with diabetes. The physician consulted the chaplain, who talked with the father. The chaplain asked the minister whether his daughter's illness might be an opportunity for his faith to grow, and also result in his providing a better model for his parishioners. The physician explained that medicine could not cure but that the treatment would only manage symptoms. If she was cured, the chaplain and the physician promised the father attendance at one of his church's Sunday services to support the testimony that God had healed his daughter. The father felt his basic faith had been affirmed and was willing to embrace a new perspective and accept treatment for his daughter.

In many—perhaps most—of the religious groups that believe in faith healing, medical care is not neglected or avoided at all. In fact, many leaders strongly encourage medical review even with healing results that are dramatically visible or evident to the "healed" person. The follow-up medical care is considered "confirmation" or "documentation" of the healing that occurs in a manner different from those medically treated. People believing in divine healing commonly feel that medical follow-up is a responsible action and not at all threatening to their faith or an act of doubt toward their healing.

Documentation

It is important to document the spiritual-care aspect of holistic nursing in patient records (Burkhardt & Nagai-Jacobson, 2015). Without documentation, an important aspect of patient care will not be communicated to other care providers to guide them in planning for holistic care. Individuals may avoid documentation of religious-sounding information and action out of fear of censure from superiors. Highfield recommended that nurses use accepted standards (i.e., the diagnoses of spiritual distress and potential for enhanced spiritual well-being) (Carpenito, 2012), and keep documentation focused on what patients find helpful or unhelpful (Highfield, 2000).

Professionals can identify actions and documentation strategies that help the agency meet the Joint Commission's requirements that spiritual care be provided to all patients (Joint Commission, 2008). Showing how spiritual care relates to the philosophy or mission statement of a facility aligns the health-care provider's patient care with overall standards or values. Meeting the Joint Commission's requirements does the same aligning, only with a strong benefit to the facility that may not have been considered.

Conclusion

Health-care providers are encouraged to first provide care that is spiritual. It is true that there are limits on time spent with patients. Also, there is a "difference between people who need just a little more and people who seem to never get enough" (Lane, 1994, p. 86). However, greater wholeness for children is marvelously possible when we provide whole person care that includes spiritual care.

Additionally, we have heard children and adults say things such as, "This illness has brought me closer to God," or "Knowing that people are praying for me really helps," and "Having this disease has made me a better person." These types of statements reflect the resources that come from spiritual strength and connectedness (Taylor & Mickley, 1997). Health-care providers have the opportunity to assist with spiritual coping strategies and, in so doing, buoy the spirit of each child and family we serve.

Study Guide

1. What are the aspects of children's health-care encounters that may bring spiritual issues into focus?

2. In what ways might spirituality affect children's responses to illness and health-care experiences?

3. Are children likely to express spirituality in the same manner as adults? What differences are there, and why?

4. How can health-care providers' spiritual beliefs have a positive or negative effect on the care of children and their families?

5. What are some of the current changes in health care that influence the spirituality of care?

6. Describe three theories of spirituality, and draw implications from each for spiritual care of children and their families.

7. List five things that health-care providers can do or say to assess children's spirituality.

8. How does spiritual distress differ from other forms of distress? What are the implications for intervention?

9. For each stage of children's development, discuss the critical issues of spirituality and cite appropriate interventions.

10. Outline direct spiritual practices and interventions that are useful in health-care settings.

Appendix 9.1

Resources for Religion

Carson, V. B., & Koenig, H. G. (Eds.). (2008). *Spiritual dimensions of nursing practice*. Philadelphia, PA: W. B. Saunders. First edition: Carson, V. B. (1989). *Spiritual dimensions of nursing practice*. Philadelphia, PA: W. B. Saunders. Carson and Koenig's text devotes an entire section on spirituality, religion, and health care with tables of the beliefs and practices of many religious groups (see pages 65–85). Many discussions of spirituality and health are included.

Coles, R. (1990). *The spiritual life of children*. Boston, MA: Houghton Mifflin. This text is the culmination of Robert Coles's career studying children all over the world. Coles conducted thousands of home and school visits with school-age children. He has written over 40 books about children. This 358-page book is insightful, with its many examples of children from Christian, Jewish, and Muslim families. Pictures drawn by children, and profound insights on children's spirituality, are included. One learns communicative techniques simply by reading the fascinating dialogues between Coles and the children.

Emblen, J. D. (1998). Suffering dialogues with five faiths. *Journal of Christian Nursing, 15(2)*, 27–29. This creative article uses a nursing, emergency-room case example of the death of a young man. The nursing-care approach is divided into care for those who are of different faiths. Humanist, Christian, Buddhist, Hindu, and Jewish beliefs are covered. Sensitive client care is encouraged.

Engebretson, J. (1996). Considerations in diagnosing in the spiritual domain. *Nursing Diagnosis, 7(3)*, 100–107. This article describes the traditions of Western and Eastern belief systems and compares Judeo-Christian thought with other perspectives. Monotheism is contrasted with pantheism and polytheism. Transcendence, dualism, humanism, and atheism are described. Trends in postmodern synthesis of beliefs are explained. The final pages overview patient, health care, and caregiver tendencies with an encouragement to foster active participation of the patient with either spiritual distress or spiritual growth.

Halstead, M. T., & Mickley, R. (1997). Attempting to fathom the unfathomable: Descriptive views of spirituality. *Seminars in Oncology Nursing, 13(4)*, 225–230. This article explores a brief history of human thought as it relates to truth, self, meaning, and purpose. Eastern philosophical traditions including Hinduism, Buddhism, Confucianism, and Taoism are described, and Eastern philosophies and attitudes are covered. Muhammad, Allah, and God as Creator are described. Philosophers such as Plato, Aristotle, Descartes, and Hegel are linked to current underpinnings of thinking. New Age philosophy is well described. Finally, definitions of religion and spirituality with nursing's view of spirituality are identified, along with research instruments for spirituality and spiritual well-being.

Hockenberry, M., & Wilson, D. (2015). *Wong's nursing care of infants and children* (10th ed.). St. Louis, MO: Elsevier Mosby. This text includes a discussion about the spiritual development of toddlers, preschoolers, school-age children, and adolescents. It also has segments on religion.

Minority Nurse. (2013, 30 March). Hindu dietary practices: Feeding the body, mind and soul. [Minority Nurse Blog Spot]. Retrieved from http://minoritynurse.com/hindu-dietary-practices-feeding-the-body-mind-and-soul/ This article reviews Hindu dietary codes, customs, and practices, including fasting and vegetarian diets.

Minority Nurse. (2013, 30 March). Meeting Jewish and Muslim patients' dietary needs, [Minority Nurse Blog Spot]. Retrieved from http://minoritynurse.com/meeting-jewish-and-muslim-patients-dietary-needs/ This article includes a review of Judaism and Islam religions. It has overviews of dietary aspects about Jewish and Muslim patients and about ancient foods.

O'Brien, M. E. (2013). *Spirituality in nursing.* Boston, MA: Jones and Bartlett Publishers. The section entitled Spiritual Care and Religious Tradition is an excellent, concise overview of world religions. Religions are categorized into Western spiritual philosophy and religions (such as Judaism, Christianity, and Islam) and Eastern religions and spirituality (such as Buddhism, Hinduism, and Confucianism).

Purnell, L. D. (2012). *Transcultural health care: A culturally competent approach* (4th ed.). Philadelphia, PA: F. A. Davis Co. The text's chapters have to do with culture groups with typical experiences and traditions through the lifespan. Each chapter has a section on spirituality with links to health behaviors.

Steen, S., & Anderson, B. (2002). Caring for children of other faiths. *Journal of Christian Nursing, 19*(1), 14–21. This article reviews care for those of the Jewish and Muslim faiths, Roman Catholic and Protestant denominations, and Hmong and Native American/traditional belief systems.

Websites:
www.adherents.com/
www.barna.org/
www.beliefnet.com/
www.religioustolerance.org/
www.ciolek.com/wwwvlpages/buddhpages/otherrelig.html
http://hubpages.com/religion-philosophy/The-Worlds-Top-10-Spirituality-Websites

Appendix 9.2

Resources for Spiritual Care Tools

Anderson, B., & Steen, S. (1995). Spiritual care: Reflecting God's love to children. *Journal of Christian Nursing, 12*(2), 12–17. Includes a list of spiritual-care questions specific to parents and children.

Barnes, L. L., Plotnikoff, G. A., Fox, K., & Pendleton, S. (2000, October). Spirituality, religion, and pediatrics: Intersecting worlds of healing. *Pediatrics, 106*(4 Suppl.), 899–908. Table 2, on Page 904, is "Seven questions for learning about connections families and children make among spirituality, religion, sickness, and healing." These questions are valuable for clinical, religious, spiritual, or cross-cultural encounters. This excellent article has 162 references.

Blaber, M., Jones, J., & Willis, D. (2015). Spiritual care: Which is the best assessment tool for palliative settings? *International Journal of Palliative Nursing, 21*(9), 430 –438. This reference reviews questions and various tools for palliative-care settings.

Cavendish, R., Luise, B. K., Bauer, M., Gallo, M. A., Horne, K., Medefindt, J., & Russo, D. (2001). Recognizing opportunities for spiritual enhancement in young adults. *Nursing Diagnosis, 12*(3), 77–91. Page 85 has an excellent tool of 14 open-ended questions or interview probes for assessing spiritual needs of young adults.

Clutter, L. B. (1991). Fostering spiritual care for the child and family. In D. Smith (Ed.), *Comprehensive child and family nursing skills* (pp. 263–270). St. Louis, MO: Mosby-Year Book. This includes a developmentally appropriate list of spiritual-care assessment questions. Nursing process is reviewed with rationale for each step. Information is specific to children and parents.

Dudley, J. R., Smith, C., & Millison, M. B. (1995). Unfinished business: Assessing the spiritual needs of hospice clients. *The American Journal of Hospice & Palliative Care, 12*(2), 30–37. This article contains lists of spiritual assessment topics, and includes an extensive list of open-ended spiritual questions.

Georgensen, J., & Dungan, J. M. (1996). Managing spiritual distress in patients with advanced cancer pain. *Cancer Nursing, 19*(5), 376–383.

This article describes the Dungan model of dynamic integration along with means to manage spiritual distress. Includes a table with six categories of nursing modalities of care.

Halstead, M. T., & Mickley, R. (1997). Attempting to fathom the unfathomable: Descriptive views of spirituality. *Seminars in Oncology Nursing, 13*(4), 225–230.
This article has a table of research instrumentation for spirituality and spiritual well-being.

Hart, D., & Schneider, D. (1997). Spiritual care for children with cancer. *Seminars in Oncology Nursing, 13*(4), 263–270.
This article includes child- and parent-specific assessment questions of religious preferences, activities, and use of support groups. Age- and stage-specific interventions are also included.

Hatch, R. L., Burg, M. A., Naberhaus, D. S., & Hellmich, L. K. (1998). The spiritual involvement and beliefs scale. *The Journal of Family Practice, 46*(6), 476–486.
This instrument is presented in full. It has 26 Likert-type format items. Validity and reliability information is presented along with comparison to other tools.

Hodge, D. R. (2001). Spiritual assessment: A review of major qualitative methods and a new framework for assessing spirituality. *Social Work, 46*(3), 203–214.
Table 1 of this reference has narrative questions and interpretive anthropological framework items.

Hungelmann, J., Kenkel-Ross, E., Klassen, L., & Stollenwerk, R. (1996). Focus on spiritual well-being: Harmonious interconnectedness of mind-body-spirit—Use of the JAREL spiritual well-being scale. *Geriatric Nursing, 17*(6), 262–266.
This instrument was developed as an assessment tool to establish a nursing diagnosis of spirituality. It has 21 Likert-type questions. Use of the instrument is demonstrated.

Kendall, M. L. (1999). A holistic nursing model for spiritual care of the terminally ill. *American Journal of Hospice & Palliative Care, 16*(2), 473–476.
Ten open-ended spiritual questions are presented in a table. The questions are designed for personal spiritual reflection.

Kerrigan, R., & Harkulich, J. T. (1993, May). A spiritual tool. *Health Progress, 74*(4), 46–49.
Chart documentation is the intent for the two tools presented. One is a checklist useful for quickly listing religious and spiritual care given. Another tool gathers spiritual belief and practice information about the patient. Each item has a detailed list of options to read and check.

Ku, Y., Kuo, S., & Yao, C. (2010). Establishing the validity of a spiritual distress scale for cancer patients hospitalized in southern Taiwan. *International Journal of Palliative Nursing, 16*(3), 133–137.
Table 4 of this source lists 30 items of a spiritual distress scale.

Maddox, M. (2001). Teaching spirituality to nurse practitioner students: The importance of the interconnection of mind, body, and spirit. *Journal of The American Academy of Nurse Practitioners, 13*(3), 134–139 6p. doi:10.1111/j.1745-7599.2001.tb00234.x
This includes a detailed Wellness Spiritual Protocol and the FICA approach (Faith, Influence, Community, and Address) in the two tables.

March, P., & Caple, C. (2015). Spiritual needs of hospitalized patients. *CINAHL Nursing Guide, Evidence-Based Care Sheet.*
This summary sheet identifies the HOPE model (sources of Hope, Organized religion, Personal spiritual practices, and Effects of these behaviors on health care), the BELIEF model (Belief system, Ethics of values, Lifestyle, Involvement in religious community, Education, and Future events), and Fowler's stages of faith.

Maugans, T. A. (1996). The SPIRITual history. *Archives of Family Medicine, 5*(1), 11–16.
This tool uses the mnemonic "SPIRIT" to list categories of questions. Details of the tool's use are presented.

McEvoy, M. (2000). An added dimension to the pediatric health maintenance visit: The spiritual history. *Journal of Pediatric Health Care, 14*(5), 216–220.
This tool uses the mnemonic B-E-L-I-E-F to categorize spiritual history, information for nurse-practitioners constructing initial pediatric health maintenance visits.

Monod, S. M., Rochat, E., Bula, C. J., Jobin, G., Martin, E., & Spencer, B. (2010). The Spiritual Distress Assessment Tool: An instrument to assess spiritual distress in hospitalised elderly persons. *BMC Geriatrics, 10.* doi:10.1186/1471-2318-10-88
This Spiritual Distress Assessment Tool (SDAT) assesses meaning, transcendence, values, and psychosocial identity yielding a score for unmet spiritual needs and spiritual distress.

Mueller, C. (2010). Spirituality in children: Understanding and developing interventions. *Pediatric Nursing, 36*(4), 197–208.
This article includes an overview of spirituality related to age and developmental stage specifics. Spiritual assessment (SPIRITual interview, FICA & questions), interventions, and ways to design interventions are also included. Case Studies with ways to support spirituality are given.

O'Brien, M. E. (2013). *Spirituality in nursing.* Boston, MA: Jones and Bartlett Publishers. The Spiritual Assessment Scale is presented along with validity and reliability. The 21-item tool has a Likert scale and is included in its entirety.

Piedmont, R. L. (2001, January–March) Spiritual transcendence and the scientific study of spirituality. *Journal of Rehabilitation, 67*(1), 4–14.
The psychometrical strength of the Spiritual Transcendence Scale is evaluated and compared with other scales. An overview of spirituality measurement is presented. Use of spiritual constructs is encouraged as part of a multidimensional assessment battery.

Puchalski, C. M., (2000). Taking a spiritual history allows clinicians to understand patients more fully. *Journal of Palliative Medicine, 3*(1), 129–137.
This tool uses the acronym FICA for a brief four-area method of spiritual assessment.
Rieg, L. S., Mason, C. H., & Preston, K. (2006). Spiritual care: Practical guidelines for rehabilitation nurses. *Rehabilitation Nursing, 6731*(6), 249–256.
Although not child specific, this gives an overview of spiritual care using the nursing process.

Soeken, J. (1989). Perspectives on research in the spiritual dimension of nursing care. In V. B. Carson (Ed.), *Spiritual dimensions of nursing practice* (pp. 354–378). Philadelphia, PA: Saunders.

An overview of the research process, tools, and measurement scales in spiritually related topics is given.

Stoll, R. I. (1979). Guidelines for spiritual assessment. *American Journal of Nursing, 79*(8), 1574–1577.
This classic spiritual assessment article lists sections of: the concept of God or Deity, sources of hope and strength, religious practices, and the relation between spiritual beliefs and health. Each section has a series of questions.

Swinton, J. (2001) *Spirituality and mental health care: Rediscovering a "forgotten" dimension.* Philadelphia, PA: Kingsley.
The appendix (pp. 179–190) of this book compiles various spiritual models for assessment and intervention.

Timmins, F., & Neill, F. (2013). Teaching nursing students about spiritual care—A review of the literature. *Nurse Education in Practice, 13*(6), 499–505. doi:10.1016/j.nepr.2013.01.011
This article summarizes mnemonic spiritual assessment devices in Table 1 and example questions in Table 2.

van Leeuwen, R., Tiesinga, L., Middel, B., Post, D., & Jochemsen, H. (2009). The validity and reliability of an instrument to assess nursing competencies in spiritual care. *Journal of Clinical Nursing, 18*(20), 2857–2869 13p. doi:10.1111/j.1365-2702.2008.02594.x
The Spiritual Care Competence Scale is presented and is designed to self-assess competency in providing spiritual care.

References

Abbott, B. (1998). Ask home healthcare nurse: Parish nursing. *Home Healthcare Nurse, 16*(4), 265–267.

Abdel-Khalek, A. M. (2009). Religiosity, subjective well-being, and depression in Saudi children and adolescents. *Mental Health, Religion & Culture, 12*(8), 803–815.

Ahmed, M., Modak, S., & Sequeira, S. (2014). Acute pain relief after Mantram meditation in children with neuroblastoma undergoing anti-GD2 monoclonal antibody therapy. *Journal of Pediatric Hematology Oncology, 36*, 152–155.

American Nurses Credentialing Center. (n.d.). *Faith community nursing.* Retrieved from http://www.nursecredentialing.org/FaithCommunityNursing

Anderson, B., & Steen, S. (1995). Spiritual care: Reflecting God's love to children. *Journal of Christian Nursing, 12*(2), 12–17.

Asser, S. M., & Swan, R. (1998). Child fatalities from religion-motivated medical neglect. *Pediatrics, 101*(4), 625–629.

Attig, T. J. (1996). Beyond pain: The existential suffering of children. *Journal of Palliative Care, 12*(3), 20–23.

Bailey, S. S. (1997). The arts in spiritual care. *Seminars in Oncology Nursing, 13*(4), 242–247.

Baring, R. (2013) Children's image of God and their parents: Explorations in children's spirituality. *International Journal of Children's Spirituality, 17*(4), 277–289.

Barnes, L. L., Plotnikoff, G. A., Fox, K., & Pendleton, S. (2000). Spirituality, religion, and pediatrics: Intersecting worlds of healing. *Pediatrics, 106*(4 Suppl.), 899–908.

Barnum, B. S. (2010). *Spirituality in nursing: The challenges of complexity.* New York, NY: Springer Publishing Company.

Bay, M. J. (1997). Healing partners: The oncology nurse and the parish nurse. *Seminars in Oncology Nursing, 13*(4), 275–278.

Baverstock, A., & Finlay, F. (2011). Faith healing in paediatrics: What do we know about its relevance to clinical practice? *Child: Care, Health & Development, 38*(3), 316–320.

Bennett, V., & Thompson, M. L. (2015). Teaching spirituality to student nurses. *Journal of Nursing Education and Practice, 5*(2), 26–33.

Betzalel, N., & Shechtman, Z. (2010). Bibliotherapy treatment for children with adjustment difficulties: A comparison of affective and cognitive bibliotherapy. *Journal of Creativity in Mental Health, 5*(4), 426–439.

Bilchik, G. S. (1998, May 20). When the saints go marching out. *Hospitals & Health Networks, 72*(10), 36–42.

Blaber, M., Jones, J., & Willis, D. (2015). Spiritual care: Which is the best assessment tool for palliative settings? *International Journal of Palliative Nursing, 21*(9), 430–438.

Blinne, K. C. (2010). Writing my life: A narrative and poetic-based autoethnography. *Journal of Poetry Therapy, 23*(3), 183–190.

Blockley, C. (1998). Children, too, have spiritual needs. *Nursing Praxis in New Zealand, 13*(3), 56–57.

Bonifazi, W. (2004). When a child dies. *Nursing Spectrum, 5*(8), 17–18.

Bowers, H., & Rieg, L. S. (2014). Reflections on spiritual care: Methods, barriers, recommendations. *Journal of Christian Nursing, 31*(1), 47–51.

Boynton, H. M. (2011). Children's spirituality: Epistemology and theory from various helping professions. *International Journal of Children's Spirituality, 16*(2), 109–127.

Brown-Saltzman, K. (1997). Replenishing the spirit by meditative prayer and guided imagery. *Seminars in Oncology Nursing, 13*(4), 255–259.

Burke, S. S., & Matsumoto, A. R. (1999). Pastoral care for perinatal and neonatal health care providers. *Journal of Gynecological and Neonatal Nursing, 28*(2), 137–141.

Burkhardt, P., & Nagai-Jacobson, M. G. (2015) Tips for spiritual care-giving. *Beginnings, 35*(5), 6–7.

Caldeira, S., Carvalho, E. C., & Vieira, M. (2013). Spiritual distress—Proposing a new definition and defining characteristics. *International Journal of Nursing Knowledge, 24*(2), 77–84. doi:10.1111/j.2047-3095.2013.01234.x

Carpenito, L. J. (2012). *Nursing diagnosis: Application to clinical practice* (14th ed.). Philadelphia, PA: Lippincott Williams & Wilkins.

Carson, V. B. (2011). What is the essence of spiritual care? *Journal of Christian Nursing, 28*(3), 173.

Carson, V. B., & Koenig, H. G. (Eds.). (2008). *Spiritual dimensions of nursing practice.* West Conshohocken, PA: Templeton Foundation Press.

Cavendish, R., Luise, B. K., Bauer, M., Gallo, M. A., Horne, K., Medefindt, J., & Russo, D. (2001). Recognizing opportunities for spiritual enhancement in young adults. *Nursing Diagnosis, 12*(3), 77–91.

Chapman, T. R., & Grossoehme, D. H. (2002). Adolescent patient and nurse referrals for pastoral care: A comparison of psychiatric vs. medical-surgical populations. *Journal of Child and Adolescent Psychiatric Nursing, 15*(3), 118–123.

Chaves, E. C. L., Carvalho, E. C., & Hass, V. J. (2010). Validation of the nursing diagnosis Spiritual Anguish: Analysis by experts. *Acta Paulista de Enfermagem, 23*(2), 264–270.

Chen, L., Huang, L., Lin, S., Smith, M., & Liu, S. (2009). Use of folk remedies among families of children hospitalised in Taiwan. *Journal of Clinical Nursing, 18*(15), 2162–2170 doi:10.1111/j.1365-2702.2008.02539.x

Children's Healthcare Is a Legal Duty, Inc. (CHILD, Inc.) (2016). *Religious exemptions from health care for children.* Retrieved from http://childrenshealthcare.org/?page_id=24#Exemptions

Chu, C., Liu, C., Sun, C., & Lin, J. (2009). The effect of animal-assisted activity on inpatients with schizophrenia. *Journal of Psychosocial Nursing & Mental Health Services, 47*(12), 42–48 doi:10.3928/02793695-20091103-96

Claassen, E. (1998). God's special children. *Journal of Christian Nursing, 15*(2), 21–23.

Clark, C. C., Cross, J. R., Deane, D. M., & Lowry, L. W. (1991). Spirituality: Integral to quality care. *Holistic Nursing Practice, 5*(3), 67–76.

Clutter L. B. (1991). Fostering spiritual care for the child and family. In D. Smith (Ed.), *Comprehensive child and family nursing skills* (pp. 263–270). St. Louis, MO: Mosby-Year Book.

Coles, R. (1990). *The spiritual life of children.* Boston, MA: Houghton Mifflin.

Coles, R. (2000). Face to face: Interview with Robert Coles, M.D. *Spirituality & Medicine Connection, 3*(4), 6–7.

Costello, M, Atinaja-Faller, J., & Hedberg, M. (2012). The use of simulation to instruct students on the provision of spiritual care: A pilot study. *Journal of Holistic Nursing, 30*(4), 277–281.

Cress-Ingebo, R., & Chrisagis, X. (1998). Try a good book: Bibliotherapy as spiritual care. *Journal of Christian Nursing, 15*(2), 14–17.

Desai, P. P., Ng, J. B., & Bryant, S. G. (2002). Care of children and families in the CICU: A focus on their developmental, psychosocial, and spiritual needs. *Critical Care Nursing Quarterly, 25*(3), 88–97.

Dunn, A. B., & Dawes, S. J. (1999). Spirituality-focused genograms: Keys to uncovering spiritual resources in African American families. *Journal of Multicultural Counseling and Development, 27*(4), 240–254.

Dyer, A. R. (2011). The need for a new "new medical model": A bio-psychosocial-spiritual model. *Southern Medical Journal, 104*(4), 297–298.

Eisenberg, D. M., Davis, R. B., Ettner, S. L., Appel, S., Wilkey, S., Van Rompay, M., & Kessier, R. C. (1998). Trends in alternative medicine use in the United States, 1990–1997. *Journal of the American Medical Association, 280*(18), 1569–1575.

Elkins, M., & Cavendish, R. (2004). Developing a plan for pediatric spiritual care. *Holistic Nursing Practice, 18*(4), 179–184.

Erikson, E. K. (1963). *Childhood and society* (2nd ed.). New York, NY: Norton.

Espeland, K. (1999). Achieving spiritual wellness: Using reflective questions. *Journal of Psychosocial Nursing, 37*(7), 36–40.

Ethier, A. (2005). Death-related sensory experiences. *Journal of Pediatric Oncology Nursing, 22*(2), 104–111.

Feudtner, C., Haney, J, & Dimmers, M. A. (2003). Spiritual care needs of hospitalized children and their families: A national survey of pastoral care providers' perceptions. *Pediatrics, 111*(1), e67–e72.

Field, M. J., & Behrman, R. E. (Eds.). (2003). *When children die: Improving palliative and end-of-life care for children and their families.* Washington, DC: The National Academies Press.

Fina, D. K. (1995). The spiritual needs of pediatric patients and their families. *AORN Journal, 62*(4), 556–564.

Fosarelli, P. (2008). The psychospiritual lives of ill or suffering children and adolescents: What we should know, what we should do. In V. B. Carson & H. G. Koenig (Eds.), *Spiritual dimensions of nursing practice* (pp. 154–192). West Conshohocken, PA: Templeton Foundation Press.

Fosarelli, P. (2000). The spiritual development of children. *Spirituality & Medicine Connection, 3*(4), 1, 7.

Foundations for Faith Community Nursing. (2014). *Fast facts.* Retrieved from http://churchhealth center.org/assets/1850/foundations_fact_sheet-lh.pdf

Fowler, J. W. (1981). *Stages of faith.* New York, NY: HarperCollins.

Fowler, J. W. (1996). *Faithful changes.* Nashville, TN: Abingdon.

Fowler, J. W., & Dell, M. L. (2006). Stages of faith from infancy through adolescence: Reflections on three decades of faith development theory. In E. C. Roehlkepartain, P. E. King, L. Wagener, & P. L. Benson (Eds.), *The handbook of spiritual development in childhood and adolescence* (pp. 34–45). Thousand Oaks, CA: SAGE Publications.

Fowler, J. W., & Keen, S. (1978). *Life maps: Conversations on the journey of faith.* Waco, TX: Word Books.

Fulton, R. A., & Moore, C. M. (1995). Spiritual care of the school-age child with a chronic condition. *Journal of Pediatric Nursing, 10*(4), 224–231.

Gallia, K. S. (1996). Teaching spiritual care: Beyond content. *NursingConnections, 9*(3), 29–35.

Gallup Jr., G., & Lindsay, D. M. (1999). *Surveying the religious landscape.* Harrisburg, PA: Morehouse.

Gardner, R. (1983). Miracles of healing in Anglo-Celtic Northumbria as recorded by the venerable Bede and his contemporaries: A reappraisal in the light of twentieth century experience. *British Medical Journal, 287*(6409), 1927–1933.

Garrett, M., Parrish, M., Williams, C., Grayshield, L., Portman, T., Torres Rivera, E., & Maynard, E. (2014). Invited commentary: Fostering resilience among Native American youth through therapeutic intervention. *Journal of Youth & Adolescence, 43*(3), 470–490 doi:10.1007/s10964-013-0020-8

Georgesen, J., & Dungan, J. M. (1996). Managing spiritual distress in patients with advanced cancer pain. *Cancer Nursing, 19*(5), 376–383.

Gilbert, R. B. (Ed.). (2002). *Health care & spirituality: Listening, assessing, caring.* Amityville, NY: Baywood.

Glickman-Simon, R., & Tessier, J. (2014). Guided imagery for postoperative pain, energy healing for quality of life, probiotics for acute diarrhea in children, acupuncture for postoperative nausea and vomiting, and animal-assisted therapy for mental disorders. Explore: *The Journal of Science & Healing, 10*(5), 326–329 doi:10.1016/j.explore.2014.06.012

Good, M., & Willoughby, T. (2014). Institutional and personal spirituality/religiosity and psychosocial adjustment in adolescence: Concurrent and longitudinal associations. *Journal of Youth and Adolescence, 43*(5), 757–774.

Greenberg, D., & Witztum, E. (1991). Problems in the treatment of religious patients. *American Journal of Psychotherapy, 45*(4), 554.

Gustavson, C. B. (1995). *In-versing your life: A poetry workbook for self-discovery and healing.* Lewiston, NY: Manticore.

Gustavson, C. B. (2000). In-versing your life: Using poetry as therapy. *Families in Society: The Journal of Contemporary Human Services, 81*(4), 328–331.

Haley, J. M. (2014). Incorporating adolescent spiritual/faith assessment into nurse practitioner education & practice. *Journal of Christian Nursing, 31*(4), 258–262.

Hall, J. (2006). Spirituality at the beginning of life. *Journal of Clinical Nursing, 15*(7), 804–810. doi:10.1111/j.1365-2702.2006.01650.x

Handzo, G. F. (1990). Talking about faith with children. *Journal of Christian Nursing, 7*(4), 17–20.

Harmon, R. L., & Myers, M. A. (1999). Prayer and meditation as medical therapies. *Physical Medicine and Rehabilitation Clinics of North America, 10*(3), 651–662.

Hart, D., & Schneider, D. (1997). Spiritual care for children with cancer. *Seminars in Oncology Nursing, 13*(4), 263–270.

Herdman, T. H., & Kamitsuru, S. (Eds.). (2014). *Nanda international nursing diagnoses: Definitions and classifications 2015–2017.* Oxford, England: Wiley-Blackwell.

Hicks Jr., T. J. (1999). Spirituality and the elderly: Nursing implications with nursing home residents. *Geriatric Nursing, 20*(3), 144–146.

Highfield, M. F. (2000). Providing spiritual care to patients with cancer. *Clinical Journal of Oncology Nursing, 4*(3), 115–120.

Hodge, D. R., (2005). Spirituality in social work education: A development and discussion of goals that flow from the profession's ethical mandates. *Social Work Education, 24*(1), 37–55.

Holder, M. D., Coleman, B. & Wallace, J. M. (2010). Spirituality, religiousness, and happiness in children aged 8–12 years. *Journal of Happiness Studies, 11*(2), 131–150.

Hungelmann, J., Kenkel-Ross, E., Klassen, L., & Stollenwerk, R. (1996). Focus on spiritual well-being: Harmonious interconnectedness of mind-body-spirit—Use of the JAREL spiritual well-being scale. *Geriatric Nursing, 17*(6), 262–266.

Hyde, B. (2008). The identification of four characteristics of children's spirituality in Australian Catholic primary schools. *International Journal of Children's Spirituality, 13*(2), 117-127. doi: 10.1080/13644360801965925

International Parish Nurse Resource Center. (n.d.). *Home page.* Retrieved from http://www.churchhealthcenter.org/fcnhome

International Parish Nurse Resource Center. (2011). *Parish nursing fact sheet.* Retrieved from http://www.queenscare.org/files/qc/pdfs/ParishNursingFactSheet0311.pdf

Jegatheesan, B. (2013). An ethnographic study on religion, spirituality, and maternal influence on sibling relationships in a Muslim family with a child with autism. *Review of Disability Studies: An International Journal, 9*(1), 5–19.

Jordan, M. R., & Danielsen, A. V. (1997, May). What is pastoral counseling? *The Harvard Mental Health Letter, 13*(11), 8.

Kamper, R., Van Cleve, L., & Savedra, M. (2010). Children with advanced cancer: Responses to a spiritual quality of life interview. *Journal for Specialists in Pediatric Nursing, 15*(4), 301–306.

Kendall, M. L. (1999). A holistic nursing model for spiritual care of the terminally ill. *American Journal of Hospice & Palliative Care, 16*(2), 473–476.

Kenny, G. (1999). Assessing children's spirituality: What is the way forward? *British Journal of Nursing, 8*(1), 28, 30–32.

Kim-Goodwin, Y. (2013). Prayer in clinical practice: What does evidence support? *Journal of Christian Nursing, 30*(4), 208–215.

King, D. E., Sobal, J., & DeForge, B. R. (1988). Family practice patients' experiences and beliefs in faith healing. *Journal of Family Practice, 27*(4), 505–508.

Kloosterhouse, V., & Ames, B. D. (2002). Families' use of religion/spirituality as a psychosocial resource. *Holistic Nursing Practice, 16*(5), 61–76.

Koenig, H. G. (2004). Taking a spiritual history. *JAMA, 291*(23), 2881.

Koepfer, S. R. (2000). Drawing on the spirit: Embracing spirituality in pediatrics and pediatric art therapy. *Art Therapy, 17*(3), 188–194.

Kohlberg, L. (1981). *The philosophy of moral development: Essays on moral development* (Vol. 1). San Francisco: Harper & Row.

Kohlberg, L. (1984). *The philosophy of moral development: Essays on moral development* (Vol. 2). San Francisco: Harper & Row.

Ku, Y., Kuo, S., & Yao, C. (2010). Establishing the validity of a spiritual distress scale for cancer patients hospitalized in southern Taiwan. *International Journal of Palliative Nursing, 16*(3), 133–137.

Landreth, G. (1991). *Play therapy: The art of the relationship.* Muncie, IN: Accelerated Development Press.

Lane, D. (1994). *Music as medicine.* Grand Rapids, MI: Zondervan.

LaRocca-Pitts, M. (2015). Four FACTs Spiritual Assessment Tool. *Journal of Health Care Chaplaincy, 21*(2), 51–59.

Larson, D. B., & Koenig, K. G. (2000). Is God good for your health? The role of spirituality in medical care. *Cleveland Clinic Journal of Medicine, 67*(2), 80–84.

Levin, J. S. (1996). How prayer heals: A theoretical model. *Alternative Therapies, 2*(1), 66–73.

Linnard-Palmer, L., & Kools, S. (2004). Parent's refusal of medical treatment based on religious and/or cultural beliefs: The law, ethical principles, and clinical implications. *Journal of Pediatric Nursing, 19*(5), 351–356.

Lukoff, D., Lu, F. G., & Turner, R. (1995). Cultural considerations in the assessment and treatment of religious and spiritual problems. *The Psychiatric Clinics of North America, 18*(3), 467–484.

Lukoff, D., Provenzano, R., Lu, F., & Turner R. (1999). Religious and spiritual case reports on Medline: A systematic analysis of records from 1980–1996. *Alternative Therapies, 5*(1), 64–70.

Lyon, M. E., Townsend-Akpan, C., & Thompson, A. (2001). Spirituality and end-of-life care for an adolescent with AIDS. *AIDS Patient Care and Standards, 15*(11), 555–560.

Mangini, L., Confessore, M. T., Girard, P., & Spadola, T. (1995). Pediatric trauma support program: Supporting children and families in emotional crisis. *Critical Care Nursing Clinics of North America, 7*(3), 557–567.

March, P., & Caple, C. (2015). Spiritual needs of hospitalized patients. CINAHL Nursing Guide, Evidence-Based Care Sheet. *Communicating Nursing Research, 34*(9), 333.

Matthews, D. A. (2000). Prayer and spirituality. *Rheumatic Disease Clinics of North America, 26*(1), 177–186.

Maugans, T. A. (1996). The SPIRITual history. *Archives of Family Medicine, 5*(1), 11–16.

McBride, J. L., Arthur, G., Brooks, R., & Pilkington, L. (1998). The relationship between a patient's spirituality and health experiences. *Family Medicine, 30*, 122–126.

McCullough, M. E. (2000). Forgiveness as human strength: Theory, measurement, and links to well-being. *Journal of Social and Clinical Psychology, 19*(1), 43–55.

McEvoy, M. (2000). An added dimension to the pediatric health maintenance visit: The spiritual history. *Journal of Pediatric Health Care, 14*(5), 216–220.

McGrath, P. (2002). Creating a language for "spiritual pain" through research: A beginning. *Supportive Care Cancer, 10*(8), 637–646.

McHolm, F. A. (1991). A nursing diagnosis validation study: Defining characteristics of spiritual distress. In R. M. Carroll-Johnson (Ed.), *Classification of nursing diagnoses: Proceedings of the ninth conference* (pp. 112–119). Philadelphia, PA: Lippincott.

Miller, D. F. (2014). Spiritually responsive education and care: Nurturing infants and toddlers in a changing society. *Montessori Life: A Publication of The American Montessori Society, 26*(2), 48–52.

Mueller, C. (2010). Spirituality in children: Understanding and developing interventions. *Pediatric Nursing, 36*(4), 197–208.

Mullen, J. E., Reynolds, M. R., & Larson, J. S. (2015). Caring for pediatric patients' families at the child's end of life. *Critical Care Nurse, 35*(6), 46–56.

Narayanasamy, A., & Owens J. (2001). A critical incident study of nurses' responses to the spiritual needs of their patients. *Journal of Advanced Nursing, 33*(4), 446–455.

National Hospice and Palliative Care Organization. (2009). *Partnering for children: Pediatric outreach guide*. Retrieved from http://www.caringinfo.org/files/public/outreach/Outreach_Guide_Pediatric.pdf

O'Brien, M. E. (2013). *Spirituality in nursing: Standing on holy ground*. Boston, MA: Jones & Bartlett.

O'Brien, R. (2014). Expressions of hope in paediatric intensive care: A reflection on their meaning. *Nursing in Critical Care, 19*(6), 316–321. doi:10.1111/nicc.12069

O'Hara, D. P. (2002). Is there a role for prayer and spirituality in health care? *Medical Clinics of North America, 86*(1), 33–46.

Oliver, M. (1992). *New and selected poems*. Boston, MA: Beacon Press.

Patterson, D., Wehling, B., & Mason, G. (2008). Parish nursing: Reclaiming the spiritual dimensions of care. *American Nurse Today, 3*(10), 38–40.

Patterson, E. F. (1998). The philosophy and physics of holistic health care: Spiritual healing as a workable interpretation. *Journal of Advanced Nursing, 27*(2), 287–293.

Pendleton, S. M., Cavalli, K. S., Pargament, K. I., & Nasr, S. Z. (2002). Religious/spiritual coping in childhood cystic fibrosis: A qualitative study. *Pediatrics, 109*(1), E8.

Porter, B. (1995). Joy comes in the morning: A newborn fights for life. *Journal of Christian Nursing, 12*(2), 23–26.

Prado Simão, T., Lopes Chaves, E. C., & Hollanda Iunes, D. (2015). Spiritual distress: The search for new evidence. *Revista De Pesquisa: Cuidado E Fundamental, 7*(2), 2592–2602. doi:10.9789/2175-5361.2015.v7i2.2591-2602

Puchalski, C. M., (2000a). Taking a spiritual history allows clinicians to understand patients more fully. *Journal of Palliative Medicine, 3*(1), 129–137.

Puchalski, C. M. (2000b). The gift of the child. *Spirituality & Medicine Connection, 3*(4), 3.

Puchalski, C. M., Ferrell, B., Otis-Green, S., & Handzo, G. (2015). Overview of spirituality in palliative care. *UpToDate*, topic 2198 Version 19.0.

Recine, A. C. (2015). Designing forgiveness interventions. *Journal of Holistic Nursing, 33*(2), 161–167. doi:10.1177/0898010114560571

Reeb, R. M., & McFarland, S. T. (1995). Emergency baptism. *Journal of Christian Nursing, 12*(2), 26–27.

Reed, P. G. (1992). An emerging paradigm for the investigation of spirituality in nursing. *Research in Nursing & Health, 15*, 349–357.

Roberts, L., Ahmed, I., & Hall, S. (2002). Intercessory prayer for the alleviation of ill health. *The Cochrane Library, 3*, Article CD000368. Retrieved from The Cochrane Library Web site, http://www.update-software.com

Roehlkepartain, E. C., King, P. E., Wagener, L., & Benson, P. L. (Eds.) (2006). *The handbook of spiritual development in childhood and adolescence*. Thousand Oaks, CA: SAGE Publications.

Ruddock, B., & Cameron, R. J. (2010). Spirituality in children and young people: A suitable topic for educational and child psychologists? *Educational Psychology In Practice, 26*(1), 25–34.

Rushton, C. H., & Russell, K. (1996). The language of miracles: Ethical challenges. *Pediatric Nursing, 22*(1), 64–67.

Ryan, J. R. (1996). Seeing God more clearly: Healing distorted images of God. *Journal of Christian Nursing, 13*(2), 23–28.

Rydholm, L. (1997). Patient-focused care in parish nursing. *Holistic Nursing Practice, 11*(3), 47–60.

Schoonover-Shoffner, K. (2013) Think about it: Praying with patients. *Journal of Christian Nursing, 30*(4), 197.

Scott, D. G. (2004). Retrospective spiritual narratives: Exploring recalled childhood and adolescent spiritual experiences. *International Journal of Children's Spirituality, 9*(1), 67–79.

Sellers, S. C., & Haag, B. A. (1998). Spiritual nursing interventions. *Journal of Holistic Nursing, 16*(3), 338–354.

Shelly, J. A. (1982). *The spiritual needs of children: A guide for nurses, parents and teachers*. Downers Grove, IL: InterVarsity Press.

Shelly, J. A. (1995). Welcoming children. *Journal of Christian Nursing, 12*(2), 3.

Shelly, J. A. (2000). *Spiritual care: A guide for caregivers*. Downers Grove, IL: InterVarsity Press.

Shelly, J. A., & Fish, S. (1988). *Spiritual care: The nurse's role* (3rd ed.). Downers Grove, IL: InterVarsity Press.

Shores, C. (2014). Spiritual interventions and the impact of a faith community nursing program. *Issues in Mental Health Nursing, 35*, 299–305.

Simkin, D., & Black, N. (2014). Meditation and mindfulness in clinical practice. *Child & Adolescent Psychiatric Clinics of North America, 23*(3), 487–534.

Simonič, B., Mandelj, T. R., & Novasak, R. (2013). Religious-related abuse in the family. *Journal of Family Violence, 28*(4), 339–349.

Smith, J., & McSherry, W. (2004). Spirituality and child development: A concept analysis. *Journal of Advanced Nursing, 45*, 307–315.

Solari-Twadell, P. A., & Westberg, G. (1991). Body, mind, and soul. *Health Progress, 72*(7), 24–28.

Sommer, D. R. (1989). The spiritual needs of dying children. *Issues in Comprehensive Pediatric Nursing, 12*(2/3), 225–233.

Sook, W. E., & Yong, J. (2012). Distress, depression, anxiety, and spiritual needs of patients with stomach cancer. *Asian Oncology Nursing, 12*(4), 314–322.

Spurr, S., Berry, L., & Walker, K. (2013). The meanings older adolescents attach to spirituality. *Journal for Specialists in Pediatric Nursing, 18*(3), 221–232.

Steen, S., & Anderson, B. (1995). Ages & stages of spiritual development. *Journal of Christian Nursing, 12*(2), 6–11.

Steen, S., & Anderson, B. (2002). Caring for children of other faiths. *Journal of Christian Nursing, 19*(1), 14–21.

Sterling-Fisher, C. E. (1998). Spiritual care and chronically ill clients. *Home Healthcare Nurse, 16*(4), 242–250.

Stoll, R. I. (1979). Guidelines for spiritual assessment. *American Journal of Nursing, 79*(8), 1574–1577.

Surr, J. (2011). Links between early attachment experiences and manifestations of spirituality. *International Journal of Children's Spirituality, 16*(2), 129–141.

Surr, J. (2012). Peering into the clouds of glory: Explorations of a newborn child's spirituality. *International Journal of Children's Spirituality, 17*(1), 77–87.

Swart, J. (2014). Applying Buddhist principles to mode deactivation theory and practice. *International Journal of Behavioral Consultation and Therapy, 9*(2), 26–30.

Taylor, E. J., & Mickley, J. R. (1997). Introduction. *Seminars in Oncology Nursing, 13*(4), 223–224.

Thayer, P. (2001). Spiritual care of children and parents. In A. Armstrong-Daley & S. Zarbock (Eds.), *Hospice care for children* (2nd ed.; pp. 172–189). Oxford, England: Oxford University Press.

The Harris Poll. (2013). *Americans' belief in God, miracles and heaven declines*. Retrieved from http://www.theharrispoll.com/health-and-life/Americans__Belief_in_God__Miracles_and_Heaven_Declines.html

The Joint Commission. (2008). *Spiritual assessment*. Retrieved from http://www.jointcommission.org/standards_information/jcfaqdetails.aspx?StandardsFaqId=290&ProgramId=47

The Joint Commission. (2010). *Advancing effective communication, cultural competence, and patient- and family-centered care: A roadmap for hospitals*. Oakbrook Terrace, IL: Author. Retrieved from http://www.jointcommission.org/assets/1/6/ARoadmapforHospitalsfinalversion727.pdf

The Joint Commission. (2009). *Requirements related to the provision of culturally competent client-centered care Behavioral Health Care Accreditation Program (BHC)*. Retrieved from http://www.jointcommission.org/assets/1/6/2009_CLASRelatedStandardsBHC.pdf

Thornton, L. (2013). *Whole person caring*. Indianapolis, IN: Sigma Theta Tau International.

Twibell, R. S., Wieseke, A. W., Marine, M., & Schoger, J. (1996). Spiritual and coping needs of critically ill patients: Validation of nursing diagnoses. *Dimensions of Critical Care Nursing, 15*(5), 245–253.

Upadhaya, R. C., & Kautz, D. D. (2012). God doesn't treat his children that way: How to care when faith interferes. *International Journal for Human Caring, 16*(4), 71–73.

Wagner, J. T., & Higdon, T. L. (1996). Spiritual issues and bioethics in the intensive care unit: The role of the chaplain. *Critical Care Clinics, 12*(1), 15–27.

Waldfogel, S. (1997). Spirituality in medicine. *Complementary and Alternative Therapies in Primary Care, 24*(4), 963–976.

Webb-Mitchell, B. (1993). *God plays piano, too: The spiritual lives of disabled children.* New York, NY: Crossroad.

Weitzel, T., Robinson, S., Barnes, M. R., Berry, T. A., Holmes, J. M., Mercer, S., . . . Kirkbride, G. (2011). The special needs of the hospitalized patient with dementia. *MedSurg Nursing, 20*(1). 13–19.

Wellinghausen, T. (2015). When is it right to pray with a patient? *Journal of Christian Nursing, 32*(4), 254.

Wender, E. (2012). The Committee on Psychosocial Aspects of Child and Family Health. Supporting the family after the death of a child. *Pediatrics, 130*(6), 1164–1169.

Willis, R. (2013). International Association for Children's Spirituality. *International Journal of Children's Spirituality, 18*(1), 131–132.

Wilson, S. M., & Miles, M. S. (2001). Spirituality in African-American mothers coping with a seriously ill infant. *Journal of the Society of Pediatric Nurses, 6*(3), 116–122.

Woodruff, C. R. (1995, Spring). Pastoral counselors and healthcare reform. *Treatment Today,* 31–32.

World Health Organization International Media Centre. (2015). *Palliative care fact sheet N 402, July 2015.* Retrieved from http://www.who.int/mediacentre/factsheets/fs402/en/

Zhang, K. (2012). Spirituality and early childhood special education: Exploring a 'forgotten' dimension. *International Journal of Children's Spirituality, 17*(41), 39–49.

10

Cultural Influences in Children's Health Care

Judy A. Rollins

Objectives

At the conclusion of this chapter, the reader will be able to:

1. Discuss culture and cultural identity and the implications for understanding the reactions of children and their families to health-care experiences.
2. Determine the barriers to understanding and communication among health-care professionals and parents and children of different cultures and outline approaches to improve understanding.
3. Delineate factors that have contributed to an increased awareness and concern for "cross-cultural competence" in health-care settings.
4. Outline "culturally competent" approaches to supporting children in health-care settings and encounters.

Each decade, our evolving society continues to grow more demographically complex. In 2011, the U.S. Census Bureau reported a historic tipping point, with Latino, Asian, mixed-race, and African American births constituting a majority of births (U.S. Census Bureau, 2012). By 2019, it is projected that fewer than half of all children will be White, non-Latino; by 2050, 36% will be White, non-Latino, and 36% will be Latino (Federal Interagency Forum on Child and Family Statistics, 2013). Conversely, the racial and ethnic composition of individuals in programs to train health-care practitioners to work with this diverse population does not mirror this racial and ethnic diversity found in the child and family (American Academy of Pediatrics [AAP], Committee on Pediatric Workforce, 2013). Moreover, according to the National Workforce Survey of Registered Nurses (Budden, Zhong, Moulton, & Cimiottti 2013), nurses from minority backgrounds represent only 19% of the registered nurse (RN) workforce. Approximately 83% of the RN population is White/Caucasian, 6% African American, 6% Asian, 3% Hispanic, 1% American Indian/Alaskan Native, 1% Native Hawaiian/Pacific Islander, and 1% other. Lack of diversity in language, socioeconomic status, and ethnicity may influence the provision of health services (AAP Committee on Pediatric Workforce, 2013).

This discrepancy between the diversity of the populations seeking health-care services and the diversity of the populations providing the services demonstrates the need for remedy on several levels. On one level, this disparity signals a greater need for organizational, systematic, and institutional solutions. A solution on this level may encompass having recruiting and hiring strategies that create a talented and diverse workforce to better serve a diverse family. However, the employment of minority ethnic workers, although desirable for many reasons, is not in itself a guarantee of improved service delivery. One cannot assume that minority ethnic health professionals trained in a traditional system will necessarily practice in less Eurocentric ways or possess the necessary skills to work in a culturally competent way with all minority groups.

On another level, there is a need to focus on the individual and thus to train and develop health-care practitioners to interact effectively and compassionately with people who may be culturally different from themselves. McEvoy (2003) recommended that rather than attempting to understand categories of culture, spirituality, and religion, perhaps more can be gained by focusing instead on understanding the individual child's or family's traditions, values, and beliefs and how these dimensions have an effect on the health of the child.

We each possess a cultural identity, and thus the situations in which a family and a practitioner of different cultures come together provide rich opportunities for challenge, growth, and personal and professional development for practitioners in the health-related professions.

This chapter presents the dimensions of culture, the within-group complexity found among members of any given culture, and information about developing cross-cultural competence. By providing information about terms and concepts related to culture, this chapter provides practitioners with a basic vocabulary for framing and discussing issues related to culture, as well as exposing practitioners to some of the complexity that is present in culture and is manifested in language and through experience. The knowledge and skills necessary for building cross-cultural competence are explored.

Culture

Culture is a powerful mechanism that guides our conscious and unconscious thoughts and activities; thus, culture influences the interactions between the practitioner, the family, and others who are a part of the support system and decision-making team for the child. We each belong to a culture and operate within one or more cultural frameworks. Culture is dynamic and evolving rather than static. All societies have cultural mores and practices that guide human behavior and provide a socialization framework that shapes interaction (Lynch & Hanson, 2011). It is difficult—if not impossible—to be knowledgeable about *all* aspects of many cultures or even one culture. However, if one is to effectively interact with those from a different culture, it is important to be familiar with—as well as sensitive to—the many aspects and dimensions of one's own culture and the cultures of one's family members.

Culture refers to "the integrated pattern of thoughts, communications, actions, customs, beliefs, values, and institutions associated, wholly or partially, with racial, ethnic, or linguistic groups, as well as with religious, spiritual, biological, geographical, or sociological characteristics" (Office of Minority Health, U.S. Department of Health and Human Services, 2013, p. 25). Culture can exist on several levels. For example, consider how a workplace or school encompasses several of the aforementioned components of culture. A person might also identify with a particular racial group or nationality. Although the concepts of race and ethnicity are linked, they are not synonymous terms. Race is a way of *socially* defining individuals or a group of people based on physical characteristics such as skin color, whereas ethnicity refers to one's membership in a group whose members identify with each other on the basis of common nationality or shared cultural traditions.

Culture involves the entire environment in which interactions among humans occur and is learned through instruction and imitation (Smith, 1995). More than just an abstract concept, culture helps shape how a person experiences and functions in different environments. Smith (1995), citing the work of Ali Mazrui, presented several functions of culture, including:

- how people view the world and construct reality through lenses of perception and cognition;
- how motivations for human behaviors are shaped, which may involve identical behaviors for two people, but because of different motivations, the behaviors hold different meanings;
- a basis for individual and group identity within a historical context encoded and described by oral, written, and social constructs;
- how value systems (e.g., beauty, morality, justice) are defined and described; and
- the modes of communication expressed through language, art, music, dance, cuisine, and other means.

As one begins to develop a greater understanding of the multiple functions of culture, one also may realize that in cross-cultural situations, there is an increased probability that conflicts might occur on the basis of differences in perceptions, values, communication styles, and motivations. Health-care practitioners may encounter families who speak a different language, cherish and operate from a different set of beliefs, or hold a different attitude about health and illness (Geissler, 1993). For example, the family may see illness as being connected to fate and thus feel that accepting the medical situation and providing comfort to manage the symptoms is more important than using an aggressive intervention to "cure" the body. When these differences are present, practitioners will need to work *with* the family to understand *their* desired outcome. This will enable the practitioner to develop an appropriate intervention and process.

The term *cross-cultural competence* appears throughout this chapter. Developing cultural competence is a multifaceted process. It requires us to cultivate an awareness of how culture shapes and influences our lives, how it plays a role in the lives of others who belong to a different culture, and how the interaction among people of different cultures affects all who are involved. But cultural competence also means cultivating a set of skills to help individuals manage cross-cultural interactions effectively and appropriately. Although being cross-culturally competent is an asset for individuals in all professions, it is a particularly important asset for those working in health-care settings in which practitioners often work directly with families in situations that are highly personal and emotionally intense. See Text Box 10.1 for definitions of cultural terms.

Text Box 10.1
Definitions of Cultural Terms

Cultural competence—a compilation of academic and interpersonal skills that allow individuals to increase their understanding and appreciation of cultural differences and similarities within, among, and between groups

Cultural imposition—the tendency of individuals to impose their beliefs, values, and patterns of behavior on other cultures

Culture—the shared values, norms, traditions, customs, arts, history, and institutions shared by a group of people

Ethnic—belonging to a common group—often linked by race, nationality, and language—with a common cultural heritage or derivation

Language—the form or pattern of speech—spoken or written—used by residents or descendants of a particular nation or geographic area or by any large body of people; can be formal or informal and include dialect, idiomatic speech, and slang

Mainstream—usually refers to a broad population that is primarily White and middle class

Nationality—the country where a person lives or identifies as a homeland

Race—a socially defined population that is derived from distinguishable physical characteristics that are genetically transmitted

Note. Adapted from *Cultural Competence for Evaluators: A Guide for Alcohol and Other Drug Abuse Prevention Practitioners Working with Ethnic/Racial Communities* (DHHS Publication No. 92-60067), by M. A. Orlandi (Ed.), 1992, Rockville, MD: U.S. Department of Health and Human Services.

The Culture of the Family

Human experience is contextual. We thus operate from and function as individuals within contexts that contain other people, rules, and norms for behavior. In these systems, we affect others and are affected by others. In the health-care setting, at least two types of culture are intertwined. The first is culture as it pertains to racial and ethnic groups; the second is the culture of the family. As we work with children, not only are we communicating and interacting with the child, but also we are interacting with family members, friends, and perhaps even clergy. These other people may be viewed as very important people in the child and family's "world."

Because children are members of a larger system, a family, acknowledging the role of this system and its members in the life of the child is important (see Chapter 7: Families in Children's Health-Care Settings). Practitioners also need to work closely with the parents or other designated decision makers. Part of effective work with families requires understanding the family's concerns, priorities, needs, strengths, and resources, which are shaped in part by their cultural background. The racial and ethnic group with which the family most strongly identifies significantly shapes the family's rituals, behaviors, dynamics, and approaches. Understanding how the family system works, in addition to how culture plays a role in shaping the family system, may present multiple challenges for the practitioner who strives not only to be knowledgeable in the technical aspects of the profession but also to be interpersonally effective.

Understanding the importance and centrality of the family is important in the health-care context and healing process. In addition to the child being affected by his or her health-care and healing experience, the family system is also affected by this experience. Parents, siblings, and others whom the family deems important are included in the process as participants and as witnesses. Much of what influences how the child and family experience the various aspects of the healing process and the health-care system is shaped by the assumptions and beliefs embedded in their cultural identity; just as the educator must be knowledgeable about a family's beliefs regarding child-rearing and developmental expectations, the health-care provider must be aware of the meaning that a family assigns to the use of surgery, drugs, and diagnostic procedures (Lynch & Hanson, 2011). The practitioner also needs to be aware of the differences in the ways people communicate, make decisions, and think about seeking outside assistance. McEvoy (2003) suggested three areas that can be used to broach culturally sensitive issues within the context of pediatric health care: (a) family beliefs and values, (b) family daily practices, and (c) community involvement. However, perhaps more basic is first understanding how families define their concept of family (e.g., immediate family, extended family, close family friends), the roles of the members of the family, and how the family makes decisions.

It may be tempting for a practitioner to want to help families *change* so that the family functions more like those in the mainstream culture. In a more cross-culturally appropriate approach, the practitioner assists families in functioning in a new environment by helping them navigate through the mainstream culture, rather than encouraging them to strip their cultural identity. A practitioner can help families by (a) serving as an interpreter of mainstream culture; (b) learning about the family's approach to child-rearing, health care, and socialization; and (c) helping to design a set of interventions that complement the family's preferences (Lynch & Hanson, 2011).

Cultural Assumptions, Biases, and Values

In addition to realizing the complexity and richness of culture, we must also realize that we not only emerge from and are products of a culture but also hold biases and make assumptions about those who have membership in a culture that is different from our own. Likewise, if a family is from a culture different from the practitioner's, family members may be cautious, anxious, or wonder whether the practitioner understands and respects their concerns, needs, and perspectives.

We each have biases as a product of living in a world that is rich with multiple perspectives, beliefs, and approaches. The world is complex, and thus it may be easier to manage this complexity by comparing other people, events, and phenomena to *our* reference points, ideas, and experiences, which serve as our anchors. Theorists as well as health professionals "sometimes show bias toward families who do not share their own personal values and view of effective family functioning" or other practices (Danielson, Hamel-Bissell, & Winstead-Fry, 1991, p. 143). Although bias is a reality in human existence, our biases may challenge our ability to function effectively in situations that bring less familiar cultures into our lives.

Eliminating all traces of bias in our lives is unrealistic, yet we can strive to work effectively with families with cultural perspectives different from our own. We each bring to and operate from a set of values and beliefs with every interaction and experience. This is true for a Latino practitioner working with an African American family, an African American practitioner working with a White family, a White practitioner working with a Native American family, and so on. Given the salience and presence of culture, we do not operate as a neutral party with a neutral perspective. However, if one happens to be a member of the dominant culture, this cultural perspective is likely to be reinforced by media images and political and educational institutions. Because of this institutional reinforcement of the dominant culture, people who hold membership in the dominant culture may not notice the absence of other perspectives and approaches. As a consequence, the practitioner may assume that his or her culture's perspective and approach is the most "normal," efficient, and appropriate.

Along with belonging to a culture, individuals hold a set of values and assumptions that are connected with a particular culture. Our values are indicative of the importance, desirability, worth, or usefulness we place on an object, behavior, or belief. Our assumptions are the ideas and actions that we hold as true without demanding proof or evidence.

Some may consider themselves members of the dominant culture of the United States in which certain values and assumptions permeate many aspects of mainstream life (e.g., television, film, music, and political, educational, and social institutions). Others consider themselves outside of the mainstream or dominant culture. Whether considering ourselves to be members of the dominant culture or not, it is valuable at least to be aware of the values, assumptions, and beliefs typically associated with the dominant culture in the United States and some of the ways these are reflected in cultural courtesies and customs:

- *The notion that all people are more or less equal.* Women and men are treated with equal respect. People providing daily services (cab drivers, waitresses, secretaries, salesclerks) are treated courteously.
- *People freely express their opinions.* Freedom of speech is a major characteristic of the culture. However, some topics (sex, politics, religion, personal characteristics such as body odors) typically are not openly discussed, particularly with strangers.
- *Persons are greeted openly, directly, and warmly.* Not many rituals are associated with greetings; maybe a handshake, particularly among men.
- *People usually greet each other and get to the point of the interaction.* Eye contact is maintained throughout the interaction. It is considered impolite to not look at the person to whom you are talking.
- *Social distance of about an arm's length is typically maintained in interactions.* People (men, in particular) do not expect to be touched except for greetings such as shaking hands. People walking down the street together typically do not hold hands or put their arms around each other unless they are involved in an intimate relationship.
- *Punctuality and responsibility in keeping appointments are valued.* Time is valued, and most people expect punctuality. It is considered rude to accept an

invitation to someone's home and not go, or to make an appointment with someone and not keep it.

These values and assumptions of the dominant U.S. culture are also those inherent in the U.S. health-care system and are reflected in ways institutions and those who work within them operate and interact with families. An awareness of some of the ways in which other cultures' values may contrast with dominant U.S. values can provide a helpful starting point for health-care providers (see Table 10.1). For example, a family from a culture in which human interaction holds a higher value than time may arrive late for a scheduled clinic appointment. This would likely cause friction in a system that is structured by and places a high value on time.

Because many cultures exist in the United States, our attempts to learn from and interact effectively with those who have different values and assumptions may be enriching yet challenging. One starting point, however, is to be aware of our operating values and assumptions, which have a role in constructing our ideas and beliefs about health care and how to interact with children. For example, U.S mainstream culture may place a high value on preventing disease and using the latest technological advances in medical practice. In this dominant culture, it common to see the latest diagnostic techniques and aggressive approaches used to manage illness (Lynch & Hanson, 2011).

Table 10.1

Contrasting Beliefs, Values, and Practices	
Anglo-American Values	**Some Other Cultures' Values**
Personal control over environment	Fate
Change	Tradition
Time dominates	Human interaction dominates
Human equality	Hierarchy/rank/status
Individualism/privacy	Group welfare
Self-help	Birthright inheritance
Competition	Cooperation
Future orientation	Past or present orientation
Action/goal/work orientation	"Being" orientation
Informality	Formality
Directness/openness/honesty	Indirectness/ritual/"face"
Practicality/efficiency	Idealism/theory
Materialism	Spiritualism/detachment

Note. Adapted from *Cross-Cultural Counseling: A Guide for Nutrition and Health Counselors*, by U.S. Department of Agriculture and U.S. Department of Health and Human Services, 1986, Washington, DC: Author.

There may also be an assumption that good health is a right and that medical science should be able to cure everything.

One should not assume, however, that certain cultures considered "less modern" would routinely reject these technological advances. Banks and Benchot (2001) reported that Amish people—who live in large multigenerational families on farms where hard work is valued and worldly conveniences such as electricity, telephones, and automobiles are usually shunned—are willing to accept and participate in modern health care if its value is clearly understood.

In terms of interacting with children, two central values in the mainstream U.S. culture are independence and privacy; thus, children are encouraged to be independent from an early age. An example of how this value is manifested is through a family having separate rooms for each child and infant so that they may sleep alone. In contrast, many families from cultures such as those from Mexico, Central America, South America, and Asia may view isolating young children in a dark room and having them sleep alone in a crib or bed as inappropriate (Lynch & Hanson, 2011).

Dimensions of Culture

There are several dimensions of culture (see Table 10.2). Rather than presenting a list of what aspects of the dimensions "typically" may be found in a given culture, Table 10.2 outlines the ways cultural groups and families can vary, thus presenting information about the dimensions without overgeneralizing.

The dimensions listed reflect many aspects of culture, with a particular focus on the dimensions that are relevant to health-care issues and contexts. For example, just as attitudes toward independence manifested through approaches to sleeping can vary, so too can approaches to feeding practices vary. For some cultural groups, mealtime may be highly structured, and for others, it is less defined. In some families, meals are served at the same time every day. In other families, a meal is prepared and then kept out so that the family members can take what they want when they want it (Lynch & Hanson, 2011). Thus, confusion can arise when a health-care professional instructs parents to give their child medication with meals without understanding what "mealtime" means to that family.

Cultural differences sometimes involve ethical issues. For example, some cultures consider it cruel to inform children as well as adults about life-threatening diagnoses or risks involved in procedures. An understanding of different approaches to truth-telling when seeking informed consent is critical. Crow, Matheson, and Steed (2000) presented an excellent illustration of approaches to truth-telling through Korean, Southeast Asian, and American Indian case studies.

Complexity in Culture

Although the dimensions of culture presented in Table 10.2 are not exhaustive, they do illustrate some of the complexity contained within culture. Additionally, it is essential to remember that although patterns of beliefs and practices are found among members of a culture, individual differences also exist within cultural groups. For example, two

Table 10.2

Dimensions of Culture	
Dimension	**Selected Considerations**
Approaches to family planning, pregnancy, and birth	• Contraception use • Attitudes toward abortion • Place of delivery (i.e., home, hospital, or birthing center) • Use of midwife or physician for delivery • Presence of the father and others (e.g., children, friends, other family) during delivery • Rituals after delivery
Beliefs about and attitudes toward death	• Acceptability of organ and tissue donation • Views on autopsy • Views on cremation • Preparation of the body after death • Time between death and funeral rites • Expression of grief
Child-rearing practices	• Response to a crying infant • Attitudes toward independence of children • Perspectives on and approaches to discipline • Use of cloth, disposable, or no diapers • Methods and timing of toilet training • Attitudes toward child labor
Communication	• Volume of voice • Acceptability of interruptions • Use of gestures • Body movements (e.g., bowing) • Touching (e.g., handshaking, hand-holding, hugging, kissing) • Cursing • Repetition • Boastfulness • Style (e.g., indirect, tactful, blunt) • Eye contact (e.g., direct, sustained, brief, looking away) • Comfort in discussing feelings
Food practices	• Fasting • Frequency of meals • Vegetarianism/veganism • Food preparation (e.g., kosher diet)
Gender and family roles	• Decision-making processes • Appropriate dress • Expectations for participation and involvement of family and others during hospitalization • Restrictions • Views toward elders
Infant feeding practices	• Breast or bottle feeding • Weaning (e.g., abrupt, gradual)

(continues)

Table 10.2 (*continued*)

Dimension	Selected Considerations
Language issues	• Oral and written proficiency in one's primary languages and in other languages • Number of languages spoken • Whether the language of the dominant culture is primary or secondary
Perceptions of time	• Attitudes toward punctuality (i.e., relaxed or strict observance) • Focus (i.e., present, past, immediate future, long-term future) • Taking medication (i.e., at scheduled times versus when one feels sick)
Reactions to pain	• Private or expressive reactions • Denial or acknowledgment of pain • Expectations for medical intervention
Religious and spiritual beliefs and practices	• Often intertwined with other dimensions of culture, such as beliefs about and attitudes toward death • Private or public uses of prayer and meditation • Presence of religious symbols and objects in room or on clothing • Observances of the Sabbath
Sick care, healing practices, and interventions	• Biomedical • Holistic • Magico-religious • Use of spiritual healers • Traditional
Views toward health-care professionals	• Attitudes toward doctors, nurses, and other members of the health-care team • Level of respect given and expected • Questioning and challenging diagnosis versus not questioning diagnosis • Views toward client being examined by a professional of a different sex • Level of formality expected in interactions
Other dimensions	• Attitudes toward transfusions and transplants • Attitudes toward surgery • Frequency of hand washing • Expectations for privacy • Discussion of outcomes (e.g., hope, optimism, fatalism) • Support systems (e.g., immediate family, extended family, friends, church) • Practice of regular physical examinations • Attitudes toward health, healing, disability, and help-seeking/intervention • Practice of male and female circumcision • Sleeping practices

Note. From "Home-Based Early Childhood Services: Cultural Sensitivity in a Family Systems Approach," by K. Wayman, E. Lynch, and M. Hanson, 1990, *Topics in Early Childhood Special Education*, *10*, pp. 65–66. Copyright 1990 by PRO-ED, Inc. Adapted with permission.

different families may be traced to a similar cultural background, but one child may be a visitor from another country and the other child may belong to a family that has been in the United States for several generations. Thus, the two different children may experience hospitalization and other health-care experiences in the United States differently. They may express themselves and their culture differently, for example, through dress and food choices. Culturally effective practitioners are aware not only of differences among cultures but also are open and curious about complexity *within* a cultural group (see Figure 10.1). Culturally aware practitioners realize that just because two children come from a similar cultural background does not mean that their experiences, values, and beliefs are identical.

Factors other than culture contribute to human behavior and mediate the impact of culture. Some common factors include socioeconomic status, sex, age, education, and length of residence in a locale (Lynch & Hanson, 2011). Additionally, individuals vary in how strongly they choose to adhere to cultural patterns and practices. Some individuals may identify strongly with one particular group, whereas others may embrace the practices of several groups simultaneously.

The degree of cultural identity falls along a continuum. Although individuals may identify with a given cultural group by way of birthplace, skin color, language, or religious practices, these factors will not determine the *degree* to which individuals see themselves as members of a group (Lynch & Hanson, 2011). On one end of the continuum, a person may try to assimilate or adopt fully the values accepted by the mainstream or dominant culture. In contrast, a person may choose to participate in both the dominant culture and their culture of origin. On the other end of the continuum, some individuals may choose to identify more closely with their culture of origin, rather than with the dominant culture.

Complexity of culture may increase when the family is bi- or multicultural or multiracial, and the number of such families is increasing. A 2010 survey revealed that

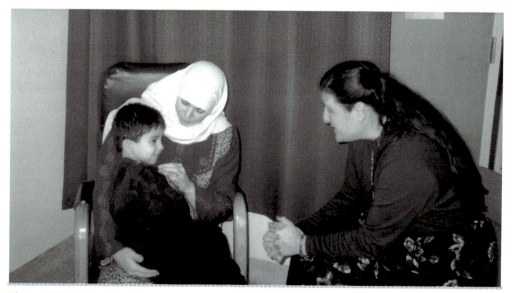

Figure 10.1. Culturally effective practitioners are open and curious about complexity within a cultural group. *Note.* Photograph by Lynn Clutter. Used with permission.

1 in 7 new U.S. marriages were between spouses of a different race or ethnicity from each other (Passel, Wang, & Taylor, 2010). Although some people have strong opposition regarding "marrying out" (see Case Study 10.1), overall, 63% of Americans say they approve of interracial or interethnic marriage, even in their own families (Pew Research Center, 2010). Important questions for the practitioner include (Lynch & Hanson, 2011, p. 465):

- How do individuals and the family members view themselves?
- With what cultural/ethnic/racial groups(s) do they most strongly identify?
- Are they dealing with issues of cultural identity, complementary or competing values, or differences in behaviors and beliefs, or are these nonissues for the family?
- Is the family accepted by parents, siblings, and other extended family members, or are there tensions related to differences in race, culture, or ethnicity?
- Are there issues that cause them to be marginalized in the neighborhood and community, or is the community supportive and accepting?

Cross-Cultural Competence

Becoming more cross-culturally competent is a process, rather than a destination, and it involves developing awareness, behaving with intention, and possessing a desire to grow and continually evaluate one's progress. Children learn and grow through this process. Although no human being is born with racist, sexist, or other oppressive attitudes, the very way that children learn to make sense of their world demands a focus on "differences." For example, early on, children notice differences and mentally organize these observations into categories. Attitudes about "us" and "them" are learned and

 Case Study 10.1

Cheerios

In 2013, General Mills ran a television ad for Cheerios cereal featuring an interracial couple and their child. In the commercial, a young biracial girl asks her White mother, "Mom, Dad told me Cheerios is good for your heart. Is that true?" The mother agrees, saying Cheerios are "heart healthy." The girl smirks and runs off. The next scene shows an African American man, presumably the girl's father, sleeping on a couch. He wakes up to find a pile of Cheerios all over his chest, right over his heart.

The ad sparked a backlash across social media, with people leaving racist and angry comments. Those comments were quickly countered by the many people who came to the defense of interracial families. General Mills requested the comments section to be turned off on YouTube but stood by its fictitious family, which reflected a Black–White couple uncommon in ads, especially on TV, at a time when interracial and interethnic couples are on the rise in real life.

reinforced in the home, school, and church, and through the media. By age 3 years, children have learned to categorize people into "good" or "bad" based on superficial traits such as race or gender (Derman-Sparks & A. B. C. Task Force, 1989). As they learn the names of colors, they apply these names to skin color. Even before the age of 3, children may show signs of being influenced by what they see and hear around them. By 4 or 5 years of age, children may use race as a basis for refusing to interact with others who are different from themselves, or they may exhibit discomfort around or even reject people with disabilities. By the time they enter elementary school, some children have developed prejudices built on stereotypes that persist until they have personal experiences that overturn these prejudices or someone attempts to correct them.

Regarding this process, Cross (1988) presented a 6-point continuum for cross-cultural competence ranging from cultural destructiveness to advanced cultural competence (see Figure 10.2). The points on the continuum can be described as follows:

1. *Cultural destructiveness*—actively carries out activities that destroy or disrupt cultural beliefs or practices.

2. *Cultural incapacity*—represents cross-cultural ignorance; often characterized by support of the status quo.

3. *Cultural blindness*—well-meaning but misguided "liberal" policies and practices based on the belief that if only the dominant cultural practices were working properly, they would be universally applicable and effective for everyone.

4. *Cultural precompetence*—reflects a movement toward the recognition that differences exist in individuals, families, and communities, and a willingness to begin to try different approaches to improve service delivery.

5. *Basic cultural competence*—acceptance and respect for difference, continuing self-assessment regarding culture, careful attention to the dynamics of difference, continuous expansion of cultural knowledge and resources, and a variety of adaptations to service models to better meet the needs of nondominant populations.

6. *Advanced cultural competence*—at the most positive end of the scale, characterized by actively seeking to add to the knowledge base of culturally competent practice by conducting research, developing new therapeutic approaches based on culture, publishing and disseminating the results of demonstration projects, and so on. In other words, advocates for cultural competence throughout the system and for improved relations between cultures throughout society.

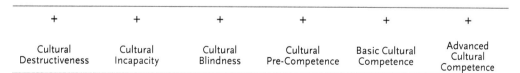

Figure 10.2. Cultural competence continuum. *Note.* From "Services to Minority Populations: Cultural Competence Continuum," by T. Cross, 1989, *Focal Point, 3*(2), pp. 1–5. Copyright 1989 by The Research and Training Center on Family Support and Children's Mental Health. Reprinted with permission.

In developing cross-cultural competence, the goal for practitioners should not be perfection. Rather, the goal could be to cultivate greater understanding, empathy, and sensitivity to those who have membership in cultures other than the practitioner's culture, as well as cultivating a set of skills to enable effective and productive interactions.

Cross-cultural competence is a multifaceted process. Lynch and Hanson (2011) outlined four aspects of cross-cultural competence:

1. The awareness of one's culture and limitations
2. An openness to and respect for cultural differences
3. A willingness to learn from intercultural interactions
4. An ability to use cultural resources during interventions

In contrast, cross-cultural competence does not mean adopting the values, beliefs, or behaviors of another culture, shedding one's cultural identity, or knowing everything about another culture. A culturally sensitive person recognizes that both differences and similarities exist between cultures. The culturally sensitive person strives to acquire knowledge about the cultural groups that live in one's region or state and thus knows the general parameters of those cultures. The culturally sensitive person also understands that culture affects families' participation in intervention programs (e.g., health, education, social services; Lynch & Hanson, 2011).

Although cultural sensitivity is an aspect of cross-cultural competence, merely being culturally sensitive does not make one cross-culturally competent. With cross-cultural competence, we must have an ongoing commitment to understanding ourselves, our culture, our biases and assumptions, as well as to actively cultivating a set of *skills* to help us function effectively in cross-cultural situations. Cross-culturally competent individuals are aware of how they are affected by, and how they affect, individuals of different cultures. Further, they possess a repertoire of skills to aid in effective cross-cultural interactions.

Lynch and Hanson (2011) reported that cross-culturally competent practitioners who work with culturally diverse families, are able to:

- feel comfortable and be effective in interactions with families;
- interact in ways that help families from different cultures feel positively about the interactions and practitioner; and
- accomplish the goals established by the family and practitioner.

In addition to the many benefits of being a more culturally aware and competent practitioner, one may encounter challenges that are a product of this journey. Perhaps one of the greatest challenges is developing a tolerance for ambiguity and contradiction. Challenges may manifest themselves through the experience of *culture shock*. "Every culture has subtle, if not unconscious, signs by which people evaluate what they say and do. Losing these cues produces strain, uneasiness, and even emotional maladjustment if the person is received badly" (Igoa, 1995, p. 39). Culture shock results when a series of disorienting encounters occur in which an individual's basic values, beliefs, and patterns of behavior are challenged by a different set of values, beliefs, and behaviors. When one is confronted with something that is unfamiliar (e.g., sounds, odors, sights, behaviors), one may experience interest, excitement, confusion, frustration, fear, anger, or disgust. Culture shock is particularly pronounced when individuals discover dramatic differences between their values and beliefs and the values and beliefs of the people around them. Although both the practitioner and the family can experience culture shock during interactions, the practitioner must remain effective and professional when working with the family. Developing cross-cultural competence is one way to manage culture shock.

The American Academy of Pediatrics uses the more inclusive term *culturally effective* care rather than *cultural competence* because it encompasses the values of competence and focuses on the outcomes of the physician–patient or physician–family interaction (AAP, 2013). *Culturally effective health care* (CEHC) is defined as "the delivery of care within the context of appropriate physician knowledge, understanding, and appreciation of all cultural distinctions, leading to optimal health outcomes, quality of life, and family situation" (AAP, 2013, p. e1106). The AAP presents a strong case for a diverse workforce and the promotion of CEHC through health policy and education at all levels, from premedical education and medical school through residency training and continuing medical education.

The U.S. Department of Health and Human Services Office of Minority Health (2013) has developed the National Standards for Culturally and Linguistically Appropriate Services in Health and Health Care (the National CLAS Standards), which are intended to advance health equity, improve quality, and help eliminate health-care disparities. The standards provide a blueprint for individuals and health and health-care organizations to implement culturally and linguistically appropriate services. See Appendix 10.1: Resources for details on how to obtain the blueprint.

Cross-Cultural Communication

In addition to remembering that individual differences and subgroup differences exist in all cultures, the practitioner should be mindful of differences in styles of communication. For example, some people from a particular cultural group may use a louder volume when talking, whereas others may tend to speak softly. A practitioner may mistakenly interpret a person who speaks more loudly as being angry, when actually that is not the case. Conversely, a practitioner may misinterpret a person who speaks in a softer voice as being timid, indecisive, or incompetent, which is also an inappropriate assumption (Davidhizar, Dowd, & Bowen, 1998).

A practitioner should also be aware of differences in the use of personal space and touching. Touching another person may be acceptable in some groups and taboo in others. For example, touching can convey caring and empathy, or in the case of touching someone of a different gender, it may be seen as extremely inappropriate (Davidhizar et al., 1998).

Culturally Sensitive Language and Terminology

Language is a powerful tool by which thoughts are conveyed and meaning is constructed. A culturally sensitive practitioner is intentional in and careful with how he or she uses language to reflect an understanding and desire to accurately communicate thoughts, as well as respectfully addressing members of communities that are culturally diverse, complex, and rich.

Just as sensitivity to language is an important component of cross-cultural competency, so is making a special effort to pronounce someone's name correctly. It may be tempting to try to reduce discomfort that sometimes accompanies cross-cultural interactions by avoiding contact with someone of a different cultural background or trying to avoid saying the name of someone who has a less familiar name to the practitioner. For many people, names are an important piece of how they identify themselves and are reflective of their culture. If in doubt on how to pronounce a name, asking for the correct pronunciation and making a note of it is a good step.

On one level, verbal communication consists of the terminology used to describe the people with whom we interact. People may have a preference for certain terms when referring to themselves as people with a racial, ethnic, and cultural identity. When practitioners are unaware of or lack precision with the language and terminology they use, they risk alienating the people they are charged with assisting.

Within any group of people, individuals may have preferences for terminology they use when referring to members of their racial and ethnic group; therefore, a practitioner needs to be careful not only in thinking about what terms to use but also how and why to use these terms to make a racial or ethnic distinction. Complicating this process is the fact that many people are bicultural or biracial and thus do not fit easily into one particular category. The National Conference for Community and Justice (1999) offers the following terminology commonly used to refer to racial and ethnic groups; these suggestions are merely a guide and should be used with caution:

- *African Americans.* The terms *African* and *African American* are not synonymous. African refers to the people or language of the continent of Africa, not a country. Some African Americans may prefer the term *black* (with a lowercase *b*) or *Black* (with an uppercase *B*) to the term *African American.*

- *Asian Pacific Americans.* Recent immigrants may have their names written in the style of their homeland. For example, most Chinese names have two parts, family name followed by a personal name. These names may be hyphenated or may run together. It is generally good practice to double-check individual preferences for listing names. The term *Asian* refers to someone of Asian ancestry, but the term *Asian American or Asian Pacific American* refers to an American citizen with Asian ancestry. Do not refer to Asians or Asian Pacific Americans as Orientals. Oriental is an adjective that is used to describe an object (e.g., Oriental rug). Refer to people by their national origins (e.g., Chinese, Filipino, Japanese, Korean, Burmese, Vietnamese) if you are aware of their background.

- *Caucasians or Whites.* Americans of European descent may be recent immigrants who prefer to be identified by their national origin (e.g., Irish, Polish). Do not refer to Caucasians or White people as Anglos or WASPs (White Anglo-Saxon Protestants). Other terms for Caucasian people are *white* (with a lowercase *w*), *White* (with an uppercase *W*), and *European Americans.*

- *Latino Americans.* Although Latino Americans are often portrayed as undocumented immigrants, many Latino American families have been U.S. citizens for hundreds of years. The terms *Latino* and *Latina* refer to people of Latin American ancestry and are generally the terms preferred by those in the community and by activists. *Latino* refers to men and *Latina* refers to women.

The term *Hispanic*, which refers in general to those with Latin American or Spanish roots, is rarely used by these members of the community. When possible, replace the terms *Latino* and *Latina* with a specific designation (e.g., Puerto Rican, Cuban, Mexican).

- *Native Americans.* Native Americans usually identify with a particular tribal nation (e.g., Cherokee). It is good practice to ask them their preferred tribal identification. Recognize that the terms *American Indian* and *Native American Indian* are used interchangeably; however, some individuals may have a preference.

Communication Styles

The first element of communication styles is nonverbal communication: such things as eye contact and facial expressions. Although a set of behaviors or gestures may look identical between two cultures, in different cultures these gestures can hold different meanings. For example, brief glances versus prolonged eye contact may be interpreted as sincerity, trustworthiness, and directness, or as disrespect and shame. Cultures also vary in the display of affect. Some cultures may demonstrate emotions through facial expressions, whereas others do not.

Another element is proximity and touching. Some cultures prefer communicating at an arm's length (approximately 3 feet) or closer, whereas people from other cultures prefer communicating from a greater distance. One way to tell a person's comfort with social distance is whether they back up during conversation (indicating discomfort with how close the other person is standing) or move closer. Interpreting touching is more complex because some of the factors that influence what is appropriate include gender, age, religion, and personal preference. For example, in some cultures, patting someone on the head is inappropriate, as is using the left hand to touch another person, since that hand is associated with bodily waste (Lynch & Hanson, 2011).

A final element of communication style is body language, which refers to various body positions and posture. Gestures are encompassed in body language and are used to supplement or substitute for verbal communication. Gestures include arm movements, head nodding, and pointing.

Effective Cross-Cultural Communication

Because cross-cultural interactions and communication are so complex and varied, it may be tempting to want to avoid engaging in such interactions. However, cultivating competence in cross-cultural situations requires a willingness to engage in such interactions and a willingness to explore differences with openness and respect, as well as using these interactions as opportunities to dispel myths and gain greater understanding. According to Lynch and Hanson (2011), some examples of effective cross-cultural communication include

- showing respect to individuals from other cultures,
- making multiple and sincere attempts to understand others' points of view,
- being open to learning new things;
- being flexible,
- having a sense of humor,

- possessing the ability to tolerate ambiguity,
- having an appreciation of other cultures, and
- having a desire to learn about those from other cultures.

Communication can take on increased importance in health-care settings in which comprehension may be critical to the health and welfare of a child or may have ethical implications. Text Box 10.2 offers some techniques to facilitate effective cross-cultural communication. However, hospitals and other health-care institutions and agencies that are committed to providing culturally competent care offer written materials and signage translated into the languages most common in the populations they serve, have interpreters available to families within a reasonable period of time, and keep resource lists of agencies and individuals who can help when serving families from cultures less common to the area.

Conclusion

Throughout this chapter, the saliency and complexity of culture are mentioned in terms of how humans perceive the world and behave in it. For a child, the role of culture may manifest itself in a number of ways. For example, depending on a child's culture and other factors, such as age and gender, children may exhibit different responses to pain or ways of relating to authorities. Some children may be very vocal when experiencing pain, while others may be more stoic. Some children may desire comfort from physical contact through hugs, while others may be less comfortable with initiating or receiving hugs. Some children may feel comfortable in making direct eye contact with those in authority positions, while other children may look away from an adult. By observing

Text Box 10.2
Techniques for Effective Cross-Cultural Communication

1. Speak slowly and clearly.
2. Pause more frequently.
3. Use simple sentences.
4. Use active verbs.
5. Repeat each important idea.
6. Use visual measurements such as graphs or pictures.
7. Act out and demonstrate.
8. Focus on nonverbal behavior.
9. Remember that silence is communication. Listen.
10. Check comprehension.

how the family interacts with the child, the practitioner can gain useful clues about what is culturally appropriate.

This chapter's main focus is on developing cross-cultural competence on an individual level. It can be argued that this is an appropriate focus for several reasons, particularly because we each possess the capacity to become more informed about ourselves and others and behave in a way that can help us work effectively and compassionately with others, especially if they come from a culture that is different from our primary cultural orientation.

Practitioners working in multicultural contexts should actively cultivate an awareness of self and others and develop the skills to facilitate interacting effectively with a variety of people. Essential to the development of cross-cultural competence is the integration of education and training in the process of lifelong learning (AAP Committee on Pediatric Workforce, 2013). See Appendix 10.1: Resources for a variety of tool kits designed to develop cultural competence. Increasingly, professional organizations such as the National Association for Social Workers, are developing standards for cultural competence. To complement individual efforts, it is also valuable to consider ways that the health-care industry or a particular organization can help create an environment that reflects the demographics of the child and family and employs professionals that come from diverse backgrounds, therefore reflecting a rich array of cultures, perspectives, experiences, and styles.

Three possibilities for developing cross-culturally competent organizations include (a) encouraging and recruiting people of color into the human service professions, (b) providing staff development sessions covering the topic of intercultural competence, and (c) actively working to change practices that discriminate against people of color (Lynch & Hanson, 2011). Some may think that only administrators at the uppermost ranks in the organization can institute these changes, but each person has the power and responsibility to raise questions or concerns about discriminatory practices. Speaking on behalf of cultural fairness takes courage, much in the same way becoming a member of the health-care field takes courage to confront issues of illness, injury, and death.

Study Guide

1. Define *culture* and *cultural identity*.

2. What purpose does culture serve?

3. How does culture influence children's perceptions of and reactions to health care?

4. How can lack of common cultural reference affect the health care of children and their families?

5. Discuss factors that mediate culture's effects and list two to three ways in which these factors may affect children's health care.

6. Describe "cross-cultural competence."

7. List several aspects of cultural sensitivity and competence that are particularly essential to the effective coping of children.

8. Does lack of diversity among health-care providers, such as nurses, affect quality of children's health care? If so, in what ways?

9. How can practitioners' cross-cultural competence enhance children's health care?

10. Discuss methods for improving cultural sensitivity and competence among health-care providers.

Appendix 10.1

Resources

American Academy of Pediatrics
https://www.aap.org/en-us/professional
-resources/practice-support/Patient-Manage
ment/Pages/Culturally-Effective-Care-Tool
kit.aspx
Offers an extensive resource, the *Culturally
Effective Care Toolkit*, a practical, hands-on
resource to help practicing pediatricians and
others provide culturally effective care to
patients and families

**American Association
of Colleges of Nursing**
http://www.aacn.nche.edu/education-resourc
es/cultural-competency
Offers two tool kits for culturally competent nursing education, one for baccalaureate
nursing education and one for graduate nursing
students

Child Life Resources
http://www.childliferesources.com/cultural
ly-competent-practice/

A user-generated resource site for child life
specialists and students; includes a section of
resources on cultural competency

Intercultural Engagement
http://iengage.multicultural.ufl.edu/resources
/campus_resources/cultural_competence
_resources/
Offers more than 30 tools to help people assess
their own cultural competence

**Videos on Cultural Competency in Health-
care**
What is Cultural Competency in Healthcare
https://www.youtube.com/watch?v=rEtZCh
Pb-6c

Cultural Competence for Healthcare Providers
https://www.youtube.com/watch?v=dNLtA
j0wy6I

References

American Academy of Pediatrics, Committee on Pediatric Workforce. (2013). Enhancing pediatric workforce diversity and providing culturally effective pediatric care: Implications for practice, education, and policy making. *Pediatrics, 132*(4), e1105–e116.

Banks, M., & Benchot, R. (2001). Unique aspects of nursing care for Amish children. *American Journal of Maternal and Child Nursing, 26*(4), 192–196.

Budden, J., Zhong, E., Moulton, P., & Cimiottti, J. (2013). *Highlights of the National Workforce Survey of Registered Nurses.* Retrieved from https://www.ncsbn.org/JNR0713_05-14.pdf

Cross, T. (1988). Services to minority populations: Cultural competence continuum. *Focal Point, 3*(2), 1–5.

Crow, K., Matheson, L., & Steed, A. (2000). Informed consent and truth-telling: Cultural directions for healthcare providers. *Journal of Nursing Administration, 30*(3), 148–152.

Danielson, C. B., Hamel-Bissell, B., & Winstead-Fry, P. (Eds.). (1991). *Families, health, and illness: Perspectives on coping and intervention.* Boston, MA: Mosby.

Davidhizar, R., Dowd, S. B., & Bowen, M. (1998). The educational role of the surgical nurse with the multicultural patient and family. *Today's Surgical Nurse, 20*(4), 20–24.

Derman-Sparks, L., & A. B. C. Task Force. (1989). *Anti-bias curriculum: Tools for empowering young children.* Washington, DC: National Association for the Education of Young Children.

Federal Interagency Forum on Child and Family Statistics. America's children in brief: Key national indicators of well-being, 2013. *Demographic background.* Retrieved from www.childstats.gov/americaschildren/demo.asp.

Geissler, E. M. (1993). *Pocket guide to cultural assessment.* St. Louis, MO: Mosby.

Igoa, C. (1995). *The inner world of the immigrant child.* Mahwah, NJ: Erlbaum.

Lynch, E. W., & Hanson, M. J. (Eds.). (2011). *Developing cross-cultural competence: A guide for working with young children and their families* (4th ed.). Baltimore, MD: Brookes.

McEvoy, M. (2003). Culture and spirituality as an integrated concept in pediatric care. *American Journal of Maternal and Child Nursing, 28*(1), 39–43.

National Conference for Community and Justice. (1999). *Building bridges with reliable information: A quick guide about our community's people.* Washington, DC: Author.

Office of Minority Health, U.S. Department of Health and Human Services. (2013). *A blueprint for advancing and sustaining CLAS policy and practice.* Washington, DC: Author.

Passel, J., Wang, W., & Taylor, P. (2010). *Marrying out: One-in-seven new U.S. marriages is interracial or interethnic.* Washington, DC: Pew Research Center. Retrieved from http://www.pewsocialtrends.org/files/2010/10/755-marrying-out.pdf

Pew Research Center. (2010). *A year after Obama's election.* Washington, DC: Author. Retrieved from http://www.pewsocialtrends.org/files/2010/10/blacks-upbeat-about-black-progress-prospects.pdf

Smith, D. (1995). The dynamics of culture. *Treatment Today, 7*(1), 15.

U.S. Census Bureau. (2012). Most children younger than age 1 are minorities, Census Bureau reports [press release]. Washington, DC: US Census Bureau; May 17, 2012. Retrieved from www.census.gov/newsroom/releases/archives/population/cb12-90.html

11

Ethical, Moral, and Legal Issues in Children's Health Care

Teresa A. Savage

Objectives

At the conclusion of this chapter, the reader will be able to:

1. Discuss the history of concern for, and identification of, ethical and legal issues in child health care.
2. Outline current legal, moral, and ethical issues in child health care, and draw implications for working with children in those settings.
3. Analyze the legal, moral, and ethical aspects of children making their own health-care decisions versus parents or health-care professionals making such decisions.
4. Discuss the emerging issues in children's health care and hypothesize future ethical, moral, and legal issues.

At the beginning of the new millennium, some ethical issues in children's health care persisted, and some new ones appeared. In the last 3 decades, health care for children has changed. Examples of changes include (a) improved neonatal and pediatric intensive care; (b) improved management of chronic illnesses; (c) recognition for improved communication during the dying process; (d) improvements in transplantation care; and (e) the emphasis on outpatient, home, and school settings, rather than the hospital, for delivery of health care. There has been, and continues to be, discussion of the child's rights, including the right to consent and the right to be included in clinical research. Violence perpetrated by children has been increasing, and in some cases society's response has been to hold children more responsible by treating them like adults in the criminal justice system. Violence and terrorism have also been an impetus for migration of thousands of displaced people. Often children cross borders without adults in order to escape violence, oppression, and poverty of their homeland. Unfortunately, these children are vulnerable to unscrupulous adults who may kidnap and force them into unpaid labor or sex trafficking (Greenbaum & Crawford-Jakubiak, 2015). One encouraging change has been the passage of the Affordable Care Act, which increased access to health care for millions of Americans and extended coverage of dependent children up to the age of 26 years (U.S. Department of Health and Human Services, 2015). This chapter will review some of the familiar issues—such as treatment decisions for very small or very sick newborns; ethical issues regarding children with disabilities, including neurobehavioral conditions; and research on children—but will also challenge conventional thinking on these issues and raise new questions to be faced.

Ethics and Ethical Decision-Making in Health Care

Since the birth of bioethics in the 1970s, a great deal has been written about ethics and ethical decision-making in health care. *How to decide* and *who should decide* are the central questions. For children, parents are the surrogate decision makers. Many of the ethical issues posed by various clinical situations revolve around the parents' responsibility to make treatment decisions for their children. The settings may be different, such as the neonatal intensive care unit, the outpatient clinic, the school, the research office, or the juvenile justice system, but parents or a legal guardian must decide what is in the child's best interests.

A number of approaches have been used for identifying and analyzing ethical issues in health care. The most popular approach is principlism, or the application of ethical principles. Autonomy, beneficence, nonmaleficence, and justice are the four primary principles most often mentioned in health-care ethics. In children's health care, autonomy is exercised by parents, but the child's developing autonomy is important, especially in light of chronic or terminal illness. Beneficence (doing good) and nonmaleficence (preventing harm) undergird decisions for children, such as mandatory immunization programs or the inclusion of children in clinical drug trials. Justice—how society allocates benefits and burdens—is seen in decisions regarding access to scarce resources, equitable selection in research, and supportive services for children with chronic illnesses or disabilities and their families. Application of principles sometimes falls short in facilitating decision-making but may help clarify the priorities and values of the parents and health-care providers.

Another approach is the ethics of care, which goes beyond applying principles to viewing the issue in its context. Gilligan (1982) first described this approach when studying women who were contemplating abortion. She found that the women considered the context of their situations, strove to preserve relationships, and made choices to relieve burdens, even if it meant self-sacrifice. The use of principles as a framework to unravel the complexities in clinical situations is helpful. Applying a principlism approach with an ethics of care approach, health-care providers can appreciate the values of the parents' and their own values in the context of a particular case. Combining both methods of analyzing a case is helpful in resolving the immediate clinical problems.

Health-care providers see similar scenarios in their specialties—the preterm newborn, the child who needs an organ transplant, the adolescent who refuses treatment, the parents who want extraordinary treatment for their child. How these cases are approached guides future decisions in a heuristic manner. Health-care providers learn from the application of ethical principles to specific cases, which then become instructive for future cases.

Decision-Making for Children

Parents are responsible for making decisions, including health-care decisions, for their minor children. It is presumed that the parents have their children's best interests at heart. Parents' decisions are challenged only on the rare occasion when a decision appears to be against the child's interests. A common example in the health-care setting is the use of blood in treating children whose parents are Jehovah's Witnesses. When a life-threatening condition exists and a blood transfusion is determined to be medically necessary to save the life of the child, parents are fully informed and asked for their consent. Parents who are Jehovah's Witnesses may refuse their consent because blood transfusions are forbidden by their religion. The physician has the option of seeking temporary custody for the purposes of consenting to the blood transfusion, and often this route is quickly accomplished through administrative channels in hospitals. The courts grant this shift of custody based on the belief that children should not forfeit their lives on the chance that they would choose their parents' religion upon reaching adulthood.

Another source of conflict between pediatric providers and parents is parents' refusal to immunize their children, based on either religious beliefs or concern for neurological complications from the immunization. In early 2015, there was a measles outbreak at Disneyland in California (Lin & McGreevy, 2015). It was estimated that 131 people from California and 26 out-of-state visitors became infected. At least 1 in 5 who were infected were hospitalized with complications, but there were no deaths. The public health department estimated that in some communities in California, 50% of the children have not been immunized. In response to the outbreak, legislators passed a law that requires a course of 10 immunizations before a child can attend public school, eliminating exemptions for religious or personal reasons (Seipel, 2015). Petition drives to get the issue on a referendum for a vote have failed thus far. The American Academy of Pediatrics (AAP) encourages pediatricians to address individual parents' concerns regarding vaccines. If counseling efforts have failed and parents decline immunizations, the AAP says pediatricians may request that parents sign a vaccine refusal form and/or seek care from a different health care provider (AAP, 2016). Further discussion of conflict between parents and health-care providers will occur later in the book.

Parents, as surrogate decision makers for their children, make health-care decisions based on the family's beliefs, values, and wishes. As children grow and mature, parents inculcate their beliefs and values. Although children may have specific preferences and wishes, parents are empowered to make the decisions regardless of a child's agreement or dissent. Not only is this paternalism acceptable, it is expected. In the case of an adult patient who is unable to make a health-care decision (lacks decisional capacity), a surrogate decision maker is expected to make decisions using the substituted judgment standard. The surrogate knows the wishes of the patient and, acting as the patient's substitute, relays those wishes as the patient would. The patient, having reached adulthood, had the capacity to make decisions and share beliefs, preferences, and wishes with the surrogate over time. Substituted judgment does not work with children because children are thought to lack decisional capacity until they reach adulthood. The age of majority, determined by state statute, is an arbitrary age, usually 18 or 21 years. Recognizing the arbitrariness of the age, health-care providers may wish to include the child in the decision-making process.

When a child requires a medical intervention, informed consent is sought from the parent or guardian. Additionally, the physician or nurse will discuss the proposed intervention in terms understandable to the child. Depending upon the intervention and its degree of necessity, the child's cooperation is sought, but the intervention may be performed without cooperation. Infants are given immunizations despite their crying, and older children are restrained to have blood drawn when they are unable to cooperate. Nurses and other pediatric health-care providers demonstrate respect for the child through various methods of soliciting cooperation, but at times realize that it may be necessary to "force" a child to accept an intervention.

In 1995, the American Academy of Pediatrics (AAP) Committee on Bioethics issued a position statement on informed consent, parental permission, and assent in pediatric practice. The Committee recognizes that consent involves making judgments for oneself and one's "unique personal beliefs, values, and goals" (AAP Committee on Bioethics, 1995, p. 315). Therefore, parents do not give "consent" but do give their informed permission. Three categories of consent were recommended. The first category relates to a child who lacks decisional capacity, and for whom parents make the decision unless there is evidence of parental abuse or neglect. The second category refers to the child whose capacity for decision-making is developing but not yet sufficient, and in these cases the parents give permission, but assent must be obtained from the child. The third category is for the child who has decisional capacity; he or she should be approached for consent. Parents would be consultants to the child, but the child's consent or refusal would be honored. No age level is assigned to the categories, nor is a method of assessment of decisional capacity presented. The assessment of decisional capacity is left to the health-care provider seeking consent.

It is generally accepted that capacity to consent is made by clinical assessment relative to the decision to be made. For example, assessing a child's capacity to decide which college to attend is different than assessing a child's capacity to decide whether to undergo an amputation for treatment of osteogenic sarcoma. Both decisions have long-ranging implications for the child's future. Although both decisions are very important, the decision regarding the amputation is irreversible and potentially lifesaving. Some children at age 10 or 11 years may make either decision; some children at age 17 years may not have the capacity. Grisso and Appelbaum (1998) have identified the following four elements as necessary for the capacity to consent:

1. Understanding of the treatment-related information
2. Appreciation of the significance of the information for the patient's situation
3. Reasoning, which involves comparing alternatives and projecting what the impact could be on the patient's life
4. Expressing a choice

The physician or health-care provider assesses the patient for these elements for informed consent in relation to the decision facing the patient. A formal assessment, however, is done only when the patient's capacity to consent is questioned. For children, because they are presumed to lack capacity and legally are considered incompetent before the age of majority, little attention has been given to assessing their capacity to consent.

Grisso and Vierling (1978) delineated the following abilities children should have in order to be considered capable of reasoning:

- the ability to sustain attention to the important issues under discussion
- the ability to deliberate the issues
- the ability to weigh the pros and cons of the options
- the ability to consider the possible risks and the alternatives
- the ability to use both inductive and deductive reasoning

Some children may possess these abilities; some may not. Flavell (1985) found that there was not much difference between early, middle, and late childhood in having cognitive functions to make decisions. The AAP's position statement reflects an attitude shift toward children as autonomous persons. Strongly influenced by Bartholome's work in the "experience, perspective and power of children" (AAP, Committee on Bioethics, 1995, p. 314), the statement pushes the issues of a child's capacity to consent. Some opponents see the statement as going too far.

Lainie Friedman Ross (1997), a pediatrician and bioethicist, believes that competency is not sufficient for a change in practice. She believes that the decisions children make are based on limited experience and subject to impetuosity. In those cases where the child is capable of making the decision and he or she disagrees with the parents' decision, mechanisms already exist to emancipate the child (if appropriate and by a court order) and honor the child's wishes. Any further government involvement in family decision-making is seen as inappropriate and unwanted. Ross challenges the movement to grant decision-making rights to children only in the health-care context. "Why," she asks, "can't a child buy cigarettes or elect to participate in school sports without parental consent?" (1997, p. 43). Child liberationists, by abandoning traditional paternalism, would allow children to make bad decisions. To honor only decisions with which the parents or health-care providers agree is not honoring the child's autonomy. Ross also disagrees with the recommendation that a third party become involved in the decision-making process. Parents should have the final decision-making authority. Again, mechanisms exist to challenge parents if health-care providers believe that parents are not making decisions in the child's best interests. The AAP recommendations and Ross's critique offer the health-care provider thoughtful arguments for approaching decision-making by children.

Both the AAP position and Ross's position use the best interest standard. How does one decide what is in a child's best interests? Kopelman (1997) described the standard in terms of identifying a *threshold*, the *ideal*, and as a *standard of reasonableness*. The issue of "best interests" is raised when parents decide against medical advice, when policymakers strive to improve laws to protect children, and in various court decisions bearing on a child's welfare. Threshold is a point in the process when a decision does not rise to the level of best interests. The level is usually a judgment call by the professionals involved. For example, a child who requires anticonvulsant medication does not bring the medication to school. When reached, the mother tells the school nurse that she has not had time to get the prescription refilled. Is this mother acting in the child's best interests? The threshold for best interests is that the child receives the medication without interruption. The ideal is the course of care that would be followed if there were no barriers (e.g., cost, time, distance). In another example, a child with cystic fibrosis has frequent visits to the emergency room. Parents are advised to put the child on a waiting list for a heart–lung transplant at a center several states away. The child is gravely ill, and the only hope for survival is a transplant. The ideal would be that the child would receive the transplant and recover to a healthy state. Using that same example, the standard of reasonableness hinges on *if* the child qualifies for the transplant and *if* the family can move to the distant state and afford to live there until the transplant takes place and the recovery period is over. How reasonable is it to assume that all parents could or should do this? Most parents may be willing, but do they have the means, and is it reasonable to expect parents to do the ideal? The standard of reasonableness allows the best interests standard to be interpreted as what is reasonable in the specific situation with the specific players. Buchanan and Brock (1990) extended the discussion of best interests and reasonableness to this conclusion:

> Not only should the best interest principle as a guidance principle for parents' decision not be understood as requiring literal *optimization* of the child's interests in all cases, but also suitable *intervention* principles will allow parents considerable leeway—tolerating departures from what would be best for the child—in order to protect the family from intrusions that would violate the privacy which it requires if it is to thrive as an intimate union whose value to those who participate in it depends in great part upon its intimacy. (p. 237)

Although parents are the legal decision makers for children, there are some conditions for which parental consent is not needed. Emergency treatment can be provided without parental consent if delay in seeking consent could result in loss of life or greater injury to the child. Each state has non-emergency conditions for which children can be treated without parental consent. State statutes delineate the condition, the age of the child, and in some cases, the duration of the treatment. Conditions may be pregnancy, sexually transmitted diseases, substance abuse, or mental health disorders.

The Emergency Medical Treatment and Active Labor Act (EMTALA) requires that treatment be provided without consideration of reimbursement issues; however, uncompensated charges may result from the EMTALA requirement of treatment for all without regard to payment. Health-care providers must ensure that the financial issues surrounding a patient's treatment do not result in a breach of patient confidentiality, especially if an unintended parental notification may result for the receipt of an itemized medical bill. The policy statement has been endorsed by the American College of Surgeons, the Society of Pediatric Nurses, the Society of Critical Care Medicine, the American College of Emergency Physicians, the Emergency Nurses Association, and the National Association of EMS Physicians. The Health Insurance Portability and Accountability Act (HIPAA, P.L. 104-191) Privacy Rule views parents as "personal representatives" of their children and allows them to access their children's medical records except under these three conditions:

1. When the minor is the one who consents to care and the consent of the parent is not required under State or other applicable law;

2. When the minor obtains care at the direction of a court or a person appointed by the court; and

3. When, and to the extent that, the parent agrees that the minor and the health-care provider may have a confidential relationship (U.S. Department of Health and Human Services, 2013).

Although confidentiality is critical in treating adolescents without parental consent, it is not absolute. When an adolescent's condition may lead to suicide (such as in depression) or death, or if a teenage girl refuses surgery for an ectopic pregnancy, confidentiality may be breached. In ambulatory settings, procedures can be established to inform both parents and adolescents of the parameters for treatment, confidentiality, and when confidentiality could be breached. Strasburger and Brown (1991) suggested a form letter be sent to parents upon a child's 12th birthday notifying the child and parents that the child now qualifies for confidential adolescent health care. In addition, the office will have procedures for alternative billing and dual record keeping to ensure privacy of the encounters when teens desire to see the provider for conditions covered in the state's statutes. Health-care providers for children should be aware of their state's statutes relating to mature and emancipated minors—a designation that means a child under the age of majority can be treated without parental consent—and those statutes that cover specific conditions for which underage children can consent to treatment.

Increasingly, consumer groups are demanding quality health care and are more knowledgeable regarding health-care practices (Williams, 2002). O'Neill (2002) proposed that in such an environment, children need information to enable them to participate in the medical decision-making process. Thus, health-care professionals need the ability to establish rapport and trust not only with the parents but also with the child, through effective communication techniques. Particularly with respect to sexuality and reproductive health care, substance abuse, and mental health issues, health-care providers should be cognizant of relevant laws and should educate the parents and adolescents in their practices about confidentiality policies.

Children With Chronic or Terminal Conditions

With chronic and terminal illness, children gain experience and a certain level of medical sophistication. If the condition is not addressed within the state statute, parental consent must be obtained for health-care decisions, and usually this does not pose a problem. Occasionally, there may be a disagreement, either between health-care providers and parents, or between parents and the child, about what the best course of care should be. For example, an adolescent who was treated for leukemia at a young age has now developed a secondary cancer. Recalling his experience, he refuses treatment and states that he prefers to die rather than undergoing surgery, chemotherapy, and radiation. His parents disagree and want him treated with maximal therapies. Health-care providers assess the teen's decisional capacity and are convinced that the teen is making an informed decision. Does it matter whether the teen is 13 or 17 years old? According to the AAP position, the decision of the teen should be respected. Ross (1997) would say the parents should have final authority. Should the teen be treated against his will? Are there control issues aside from the cancer treatment that are undercurrents in the family relationships? In difficult situations like this, family mediation through a family therapist and ethics consultation to the family and health-care team may help in resolving the conflict.

Adolescence is a time for rebellion and testing limits. Children with chronic conditions who have followed health maintenance practices may be less attentive to these practices, and may suffer complications as a result. Feeling different from peers, the adolescent may wish to deny the chronic condition exists, or may neglect certain habits, such as checking blood glucose or performing self-catheterization. Should adolescents have the freedom to abandon health-preserving, and sometimes lifesaving, practices? Are parents who do not "force" their children to take their medicine, test their blood, or self-catheterize being neglectful? While respecting the developing autonomy of the adolescent, parents are still considered responsible for their children's health care. The degree to which parents should intervene is related to the likely severity of the consequences of noncompliance. Renal failure from hydronephrosis and urinary tract infections may result from forgoing intermittent catheterization, but it may take several years before the damage results. Much like cigarette smoking, the results are not immediate and therefore seem too remote to imagine. Forgoing insulin may result in immediate and unpleasant consequences, serving to reinforce the wisdom of compliance. Allowing the teen to test the limits risks the teen befalling harm. The concept of "dignity of risk" applies to the decision to allow the teen to make choices, even potentially harmful choices, in an effort to develop and exercise decision-making abilities. Oberman (1996) would reject this analysis. She finds chronic illness to be an impediment to developing autonomy and is not surprised when adolescents with repeated hospitalizations regress developmentally. She has urged an increased skepticism regarding adolescents' abilities to make health-care decisions, especially regarding forgoing life-sustaining treatment. Out of respect for the child or adolescent's emerging autonomy, and with parental approval, there should be discussion of the degree of involvement the child should have in health-care decisions.

An international conference was held in 2014 to develop policy guidelines for assessing the capacity of an adolescent to make autonomous health-care decisions (Michaud, Blum, Benaroyo, Zermatten, & Baltag, 2014). Among the guidelines that emerged from the conference was the recommendation to assess adolescents by using the *MacArthur Competence Assessment Tool-Treatment* (Grisso, Appelbaum, & Hill-Fotouhi, 1997), which is widely used with adults but has not yet been adapted for use with adolescents. The MacCAT-T (and there is also a MacCAT-R for research) provides questions a provider can ask to determine a patient's understanding, ability to reason, deliberate, and express a choice. However, there is no "score" that indicates the patient has decision-making capacity; it is within the assessor's clinical judgment. So the authors caution that the assessor must be mindful of biases that can influence their assessment, and ideally, a team of assessors will see the patient. It is likely that most pediatric health-care providers use this type of approach when assessing decision-making capacity of children, but the MacCAT-T offers a structured, consistent approach in the interview process. The assessor must still use a developmentally appropriate communication style and consider the gravitas of the decision that needs to be made.

The most challenging situations in caring for a child with a terminal illness involve conflict over treatment considered futile. Often it is the health-care providers who believe continued treatment offers no benefit and desire to withhold further treatment or even withdraw current treatment and allow death to occur. Occasionally it is the parents who think treatment is futile and want only comfort care.

Palliative care has been available to adults for many years, and is becoming more available for children. One of the challenging issues is deciding at what point to involve palliative care providers in the child's care. There is the misconception that palliative care signals the abandonment of curative treatment and is introduced as the "last resort." It may require the child to be moved to a different setting than an acute care hospital's pediatric unit. Although some families want palliative care, they are unable to manage it at home. The American Academy of Pediatrics encourages the development of palliative care multidisciplinary teams that are capable of offering direct care to the child and support for families and siblings in a variety of settings—home, hospitals, and pediatric hospices (AAP, 2013). There are few pediatric hospices; most hospices are unable to provide care to infants, children, or adolescents. So palliative and hospice care are often delivered in the hospital or at home. When the decision is made to include palliative care during the treatment phase, it is useful to do advance care planning. Sometimes the primary care physicians or pediatric subspecialists avoid discussing advance care planning, but the palliative care providers have the expertise and comfort level to do this. Although advance care planning is often associated with documents such as a living will or durable power of attorney, the concept is to delineate plans for escalation of treatment, discern preferences, and identify areas of potential conflict. Parents may resist the discussion for fear that it suggests a lack of hope for cure; such a discussion, in fact, prepares them for crisis management prior to a crisis and facilitates communication as the child's course evolves.

For children who are in the dying process, parents may ask providers to "do everything" or alternatively, may ask that something be done to end the child's suffering. Ongoing discussions with parents, ideally started with the first advance care planning conversation, may help in preparing them for the dying process and the relative value of various interventions. An explicit discussion about resuscitative measures should occur, and is often mandatory when hospice providers are coming into the home. In many states, the Physician's (or Provider's, in some states) Order for Life-Sustaining Treatment (POLST) has become the legally recognized Do Not Resuscitate (DNR) order form, although it addresses treatment to be given as well as those to be withheld (www.polst.org). Completion of the form requires decisions about resuscitation, administration of blood products or certain medications, and methods for meeting nutrition and hydration needs. For states that do not recognize the POLST form, a home DNR order should be discussed, and if written, communicated to all providers.

Some parents may be aware of a practice of palliative sedation, in which the patient is sedated to the point of unconsciousness and remains sedated until death occurs. It is used when there is intractable suffering that cannot be relieved with maximal pain and symptom management. There may be a fine line between maximal pain and symptom management and palliative sedation. The practice is controversial and is not endorsed by the AAP and other professional societies (AAP, 2013). The doctrine of double effect permits an act that is intended to relieve pain and suffering but has a foreseeable consequence of hastening death as permissible if the actor's intention is to relieve suffering and not hasten death. Some reject this justification, and there is often reluctance on the part of parents and nurses to effectively medicate a child's pain for fear of hastening death. Advance care planning discussions can include the possibility of increasing medications in doses higher than usual to manage pain at this point.

In conclusion, parents are responsible for health-care decision-making for their children. How much to involve the child in the decision-making process is at the parents' discretion. Health-care providers can help parents understand their children's ability to reason, and should work with the parents in effectively communicating with their children, especially around sensitive topics such as sexual activity and terminal illness. Throughout the chapter, parental decision-making will be revisited in the context of treatment decisions for selected conditions affecting children's health.

Ethical Issues Involving Newborns

Some specific ethical issues may be encountered at the time of birth. Three—mandatory newborn screening, genetic testing of children for adult onset-conditions, and imperiled newborns—are explored here.

Mandatory Newborn Screening

Since 1962, mandatory newborn screening has been conducted in every state, and since then, has been expanded. Each state decides which conditions will be screened, and there still remains controversy over whether parental consent should be obtained prior to testing, rather than through an opt-out process.

Initially, newborn screening for phenylketonuria (PKU) involved testing the wet diaper of a baby who had ingested a protein-based formula or breast milk for 72 hours or more. A positive result meant further testing; a diagnosis of PKU meant a lifetime of special diet without phenylalanine. Best of all, it meant that an intellectual disability from a metabolic malfunction could be avoided. For other tests that were added to the screening profile, a therapy was available to ameliorate the condition, such as thyroid supplementation for hypothyroidism. Currently, there are 32 core conditions included in the Recommended Uniform Screening Panel (RUSP), as of March 2015, and 26 secondary conditions (U.S. Department of Health and Human Services, 2015). The process in adding tests to the RUSP is based on "evidence that supports the potential net benefit of screening, the ability of states to screen for the disorder, and the availability of effective treatments" (U.S. DHHS Advisory Committee on Heritable Disorders in Newborns and Children, 2015).

Does mass mandatory screening, on balance, provide a benefit to the newborn, parents, or public at large? Is the outcome of the newborn's condition improved by the screening? Do the benefits justify waiving parental consent? For adult-onset disorders, there are additional ethical concerns.

Genetic Testing for Adult-Onset Conditions

Because the technology is available for screening more and more conditions in a newborn, is it a benefit to do this? The American Academy of Pediatrics (AAP) issued a position statement limiting the use of genetic testing in children of late-onset conditions (2001), reaffirming it in 2013, as has the American College of Medical Genetics (ACMG) Report (Ross et al., 2013). Informed consent involves the weighing of the benefits or potential benefits against the harms or possible harms. Can the harms be known? Should an abnormality be discovered, this knowledge can affect the newborn who was tested, the parents, and possibly extended family who may be carriers of the abnormality. Will this knowledge affect the family relationships, the parent–infant attachment, and later, the child's self-image? Federal legislation prohibiting discrimination based on genetic test results was passed in 2008 (Genetic Information Nondiscrimination Act [GINA] of 2008), so the concern about discrimination in health insurance or employment may be reduced. However, there may be only a few instances where the value of obtaining the information when the child is a newborn justifies testing for an adult-onset condition. These instances are, if there is a treatment given in childhood that would reduce morbidity or mortality prior to the onset of the condition, or if the psychological burden of not knowing is so distressing to the parents and the child.

With direct-to-consumer (DTC) genetic testing available, questions arise as to the wisdom of doing an entire genome sequencing for newborns or older children. Current technology permits parents (or their children) to spit in a tube, mail it in, and get a report in 6–8 weeks (https://www.23andme.com/about/tos/) (23andMe, 2015). The DNA is genotyped for "important health conditions, ancestry, and traits" (http://www.23andme.com/genetic-science). Again, both the AAP and ACMG strongly discourage direct-to-consumer testing of children out of concern for quality of the test and interpretation of results. The American Society of Clinical Oncology (ASCO) revisited this issue and updated its 2003 ASCO Statement on Genetic Testing for Cancer Susceptibility (American Society of Clinical Oncology, 2015. Regarding testing of children for cancer susceptibility, ASCO recommended that the decision to offer testing to potentially affected children should consider the availability of evidence-based risk-reduction strategies and the probability of developing a malignancy during childhood. When risk-reduction strategies exist or the cancer predominantly develops in childhood, ASCO believes that the parents have the right to choose or reject testing. In situations where increased risk of a childhood malignancy is absent, ASCO recommended delaying genetic testing until the individual is of a sufficient age to make an informed decision regarding such tests. Current websites for ASCO discuss special issues in cancer risk counseling (2015) (http://www.asco.org/genetics-toolkit/special-issues-cancer-risk-counseling).

In addition to cancer susceptibility testing, direct-to-consumer testing may not have demonstrated clinical validity of the testing nor clinical utility. Professional genetic counseling is not provided with the testing kit and parents may be left with worries regarding results of unknown significance. Should whole exome/whole genome sequencing become available, it should be done for infants with "detectable anomalies," and not used as a screening test for infants without symptoms (Francescatto & Katsanis, 2015, p. 620). Even with a developmental disability diagnosis of unknown etiology, Janvier and Farlow (2014) question the value of doing a microarray-based comparative genomic hybridization test, and propose that it should only be done in a research context. Given the rapid developments in genetics and genomics, the pediatric health-care providers need to stay abreast and consider the evidence when weighing the pros and cons of genetic testing for newborns and children.

Imperiled Newborns

Neonates who require intensive care treatment following birth are often referred to as *imperiled newborns*. They are imperiled—in danger of dying or suffering injury—

because they are not able to live without specialized care. Such infants may have been born prematurely, experienced perinatal complications, or have problems with organs or organ systems interfering with normal functioning. Since the advent of neonatal care in the 1950s, infant mortality and morbidity have improved for imperiled newborns. Infants weighing less than 1 pound (450 grams) have survived; infants with previously lethal conditions, such as hypoplastic left ventricle, can be treated; and infants who are profoundly compromised at birth with an Apgar score of 0 can be successfully resuscitated. Some conditions remain untreatable. An infant born with anencephaly cannot survive an extended period without technological assistance; however, infants with anencephaly pose a unique ethical problem that will be addressed later in this chapter.

Neonatal care has improved survival for preterm infants. In the early 1970s, the threshold of viability was around 28 weeks' gestation. Today, infants born at 24 weeks' gestation are considered viable; those born between 22 and 23 weeks' are considered periviable. Neonatal care has become more sophisticated with the regionalization of neonatal care into perinatal centers; the proliferation of neonatal nurse practitioners; and research on neonatal medical treatment, nursing care, and the effect on the family. Widespread use of ventilators was just beginning in the 1970s, with the entire concomitant care of pulmonary toileting, blood testing, X-rays, and nasogastric feedings. Iatrogenic problems such as pneumothoraces, pulmonary hemorrhages, and Mikity–Wilson disease (later called bronchopulmonary dysplasia) soon became apparent. Necrotizing enterocolitis was common, as was intraventricular hemorrhage. Parents could visit 24 hours but could only touch their infants.

Also in the 1970s, Duff and Campbell (1973) published an article in which they acknowledged that 14% of the deaths in their Yale-New Haven Hospital nursery was the result of withholding or withdrawing treatment. The previously taboo subject of "letting babies die" was brought to public attention. The infants whose treatment was withheld or withdrawn were usually considered too small to save. The equipment and the skill of the staff limited the number of infants who could get a trial of neonatal intensive care. As the equipment became available and the skills of the physicians and nurses improved, smaller and sicker babies were treated in the neonatal intensive care unit (NICU). Infants who in the past were given oxygen via hood and were kept warm were now being aggressively treated with ventilators and medications such as epinephrine and sodium bicarbonate. Some would still die despite aggressive treatment, but others would survive. Those survivors might experience complications of ventilator dependency, malnutrition and rickets, necrotizing enterocolitis necessitating surgery (and resulting in short gut syndrome), and intraventricular hemorrhage resulting in seizures and hydrocephalus. Withdrawal of treatment was considered for infants who suffered short gut syndrome or intraventricular hemorrhage. Withholding of additional lifesaving measures was also discussed with the parents.

Because of Duff and Campbell's article, there was concern that the deliberate withdrawing of life-sustaining treatment, usually in terms of discontinuing intermittent mandatory ventilation or extubation, would be seen as euthanasia. Many hospitals did not have DNR policies; however, there were unit practices of "no codes" or "slow codes" in which resuscitative measures would be withheld or not effectively performed with the intent of resuscitating. Although outcomes could not be predicted, the fear was that infants who experienced a brain hemorrhage, short gut, or ventilator dependency would have a poor quality of life, and their parents were informed of the possibility.

With parents' agreement, treatment (i.e., the ventilator or cardiopulmonary resuscitation) would be withdrawn or withheld.

Infants who were born full term but experienced complications such as asphyxiation or had congenital problems such as diaphragmatic hernia also were treated, but might have had treatment withdrawn if the outcome looked poor. Criteria were published on selective treatment of infants with spina bifida, which recommended maximal treatment for low-level lesions and nontreatment for high-level lesions (Lorber, 1972). An infant with prolonged hypoglycemia who became flaccid and unresponsive or an infant with Down syndrome could be left unfed at parents' request. Fost (1999) referred to this period as the era of serious undertreatment of infants who might have survived. It was an infant with Down syndrome who provoked the end of the undertreatment period.

The Baby Doe regulations came about in response to the death of an infant with Down syndrome. Baby Doe was born in Bloomington, Indiana, in 1982. He had esophageal atresia, which prevented anything from passing from the esophagus into the stomach. A common complication of Down syndrome, the atresia could be repaired surgically. The parents opted not to treat; they worked in special education, and they were familiar with Down syndrome. A pediatrician thought the infant should be transferred to a neonatal intensive care unit where surgery could be performed, but the parents refused. The Indiana Supreme Court upheld the parents' right to make the decision when faced with two diverse medical opinions. The hospital and the state child welfare agency planned to appeal the Indiana Supreme Court decision to the U.S. Supreme Court, but the infant died at 6 days of age.

Margaret Heckler, the secretary of health, education, and welfare in the Reagan administration, orchestrated the Baby Doe regulations. Section 504 of the Rehabilitation Act of 1973 was invoked, and hospitals that were found to have discriminated against infants on the basis of their disabilities were in danger of losing federal funds. Signs in both English and Spanish urged anyone who suspected discrimination to call a toll-free number. After a court challenge, the signs were made smaller and placed in staff areas only, but the message was clear. The regulations became the Child Abuse Prevention and Treatment Act. The AAP (American Academy of Pediatrics, 1984) urged the use of pediatric review committees to avoid judicial intervention. Ethics committees proliferated in hospitals across the nation. Decisions to withhold or withdraw treatment were no longer simply between parents and physicians, but were considered in terms of whether they would hold up to public scrutiny. Very preterm infants, infants with severe asphyxiation, and infants with trisomies, such as trisomy 18, were aggressively treated. Some authors argued that the regulations changed practices related to spina bifida or Down syndrome (Carter, 1993), and others maintained that the regulations did not give enough consideration to parents' rights or to infant suffering (Kopelman, Irons, & Kopelman, 1988). Fost (1999) described this time as the era of serious overtreatment. There was probably some overlap between the eras of undertreatment and overtreatment, as evidenced by the publication of a book by parents of a preterm infant whose treatment was continued despite their requests for discontinuation (Stinson & Stinson, 1979).

Since the early 1980s, aggressive treatment became standard. A "wait until certainty" approach before discontinuing treatment was adopted, supplanting a statistical prognostic approach. In the latter approach, the decision to forgo treatment was made if there was a possibility that the child could be disabled. Follow-up data showed reduced mortality but did not always reflect the morbidity. Survivors had cerebral palsy, mental retardation, seizures, hydrocephalus requiring shunting, and a myriad of sensory deficits. For those who were less affected, attention problems and learning difficulties were reported. Early intervention programs flourished and targeted NICU graduates who were displaying developmental problems or were at risk for those problems. Legislation for integration and inclusion of children with disabilities was passed so that children could attend local schools and receive education as well as speech, occupational, and physical therapies if needed.

What impact does this history have on decision-making today? There is still a tension between parental rights to consent or refuse treatment as surrogates for their children and the rights of children to be treated. Although many NICUs will treat the smallest infants (those under 500 grams or 23 weeks' gestation), guidelines have been proposed for determining when treatment is obligatory and when its benefits may be ambiguous (AAP and American College of Obstetrics and Gynecology, 2007; Guillén et al., 2015). Despite significant reductions in mortality and morbidity of the tiniest infants from 1990 to 2000, there has not been much change from 2000 to 2010 (Malloy, 2015). Malloy attributes the lack of change since 2010 in morbidity and mortality in infants of 22–23 weeks gestation to the uncertainty about whether aggressive treatment is the right course. Carter, Rosenkrantz, Windle, and MacGilvray (2015) echo the angst felt by neonatal teams and provide a pro and con analysis of the use of guidelines. Guidelines recommend shared decision-making with parents, and the use of national data to aid in predicting possible outcomes from treatment. Both Carter et al. (2015) and Zayek et al. (2011) argue that parents should have current outcome data from the unit where their baby is, or will be born. Both groups believe data from a single unit can be more helpful to parents in their decision-making, rather than only relying on the statistical outcomes in national data. The goal of neonatal care is to have a child who survives without morbidity, although iatrogenic morbidity may be the cost of survival.

Some are even more critical of guidelines, believing them to be simplistic and ethically flawed (Dupont-Thibodeau, Barrington, Farlow, & Janvier, 2014). Because of the inability to predict disability with certainty, treatment is expected to continue. Some activists in the disability community believe that withholding treatment for a child with disabilities (or probable disabilities) demonstrates a lack of respect and devalues the lives of people with disabilities (Brennan, 1995; Charlton, 1998; Gallagher, 1995; Shapiro, 1994). Others suggest a specific process-based public policy approach to futility determinations on a case-by-case basis is overdue (Clark, 2002). Janvier, Barrington and Farlow (2014) recommend that uncertainty be acknowledged, but discussions on the parents' views of "regret, hope, quality of life, resilience and relationships" should be explored using the mnemonic "SOBPIE" (p. 38). The mnemonic stands for situation, opinions and options, basic human interactions, and for parents, their story, concerns, needs, and goals, information they need, and emotions related to coping, social supports, adaptation, and resilience.

Parents of children in NICUs need to know the likely course of their child's hospitalization. The "window of opportunity," a point in the course of a child's treatment in which withholding or withdrawal of treatment will result in death, is more difficult to defend. Quality-of-life determinations are subjective; no one can know the quality of life of another person. Saigal et al. (1999) found that health-care providers underestimate the quality of the lives of children with disabilities, and it is possible that they impart their bias to the parents (Asch, 1998). The disability rights movement celebrates progress since the passage of the American with Disabilities Act but argues that much more needs to be done other than structural changes like curb cuts and antidiscrimination in education, employment, housing, and insurance. The challenges that a family faces with a child with a disability are often presented to parents in the prenatal period, when delivery seems imminent, and after the birth of a preterm infant. At this very stressful and emotional time, parents are given the range of possibilities (no disability to multiple, severe lifelong disabilities), then are asked to imagine the worst possible scenario and decide if they can live with that outcome. They are reminded that obtaining services for a child with disabilities is a constant struggle throughout the life of the child; care for the child will mean the rest of the children will receive less attention; and parents with a disabled child often end up divorced. Some physicians see this frank approach as being honest and dispelling false hopes. Obstetricians and neonatologists, however, often do not provide care for infants post-discharge and may only see the tiniest and sickest infants who meet the follow-up criteria that focus on morbidity such as an abnormal head ultrasound. Their perspective may be skewed and their sense of responsibility in each infant's outcome may move them to counsel parents to forgo intervention if they believe disability is likely to result (Meadow & Lantos, 2009). Although there have been gains in societal changes for people with disabilities, much remains to be improved and parents should not be "held hostage to the revolution" (Kothari, personal communication, May 21, 2001).

When there is conflict between parents and the neonatology team on the best course to pursue, it may help to get outside advice. Ethics committees provide a forum for discussion, and ethics consultants can be a sounding board for health-care providers and parents. Often an ethics consultant can help focus the questions if communication between parents and the NICU staff breaks down. Kon (2015) cautions that, as with other aspects of pediatric care, specialized knowledge and expertise is required when conducting an ethics consultation in the neonatal and pediatric domains. Some institutions have separate pediatric ethics committees and others have pediatric practitioners as permanent members on their hospital-wide ethics committees. There may also be the need to include an ad hoc member with knowledge and expertise in certain conditions. In the Ashley X case, in which a child with multiple disabilities had high estrogen treatment to stunt her growth, her breast buds removed, and a hysterectomy, the ethics committee deliberated and supported her parents' request for these treatments (Kirschner, Brashler, & Savage, 2007; Shannon & Savage, 2007). Once the procedure was publicized on a national talk show, there was an outcry from disability associations and a review of the decision-making process by the state's disability advocacy agency. It determined that the hospital was at fault for not getting a court order for the hysterectomy (viewed as sterilization of an incompetent person) and for not including anyone from the disability community on the ethics committee when Ashley's case was discussed. There is no single disability perspective; views are as diverse as within the general population, however, someone from a disability advocacy organization can raise questions that may not otherwise be raised. The Ashley X case will be discussed in detail later in the chapter.

Another highly controversial issue is the active euthanasia of newborns. The Groningen Protocol, introduced in the Netherlands and first published in the medical literature in 2005, allows for intentional euthanasia of infants by physician-administered lethal injection. The infant would be eligible under these criteria: "(1) diagnosis and prognosis must be certain, (2) hopeless and unbearable suffering must be present; (3) a confirming second opinion by a second doctor, (4) both parents give informed consent, and (5) the procedure must be performed carefully, in accordance with medical standards" (Verhagen, 2013, p. 294). Since its inception, its use has decreased from 15 to 20 cases/year to 2 cases from 2008 to 2013. Verhagen attributes the decrease to a wider use of prenatal ultrasounds leading to pregnancy terminations and the possibility that not all cases are being reported or viewed as euthanasia. The use of paralytic drugs to stop the gasping of a dying infant may not be viewed as euthanasia but as symptom management (Verhagen, 2013). No other countries have adopted an infant euthanasia protocol, and professional societies oppose its practice.

Ethical Issues Involving Children

Other ethical issues surface after the newborn period. Those concerning children with disabilities, brain death, children with neurobehavioral disorders, and research on children are discussed here.

Children With Disabilities

A number of conditions in children beyond the newborn period pose similar ethical questions. When, if ever, is it justifiable to withhold or withdraw life-sustaining treatment? Children who have significant developmental disabilities, such as cerebral palsy or mental retardation, challenge society to question what is in these children's best interests. As stated above, much of the affective positions toward children with disabilities stem from the presumption that their quality of life is poor. Research has shown that both health-care providers (Saigal et al., 1999) and nondisabled laypeople underestimate the quality of life of people with disabilities (Albrecht & Devlieger, 1999). The question may be that the quality of the family life is profoundly affected, but not all families view the experience of having a child with significant disabilities as negative (Savage, 2000). Depending upon support for the family for round-the-clock care of the child with disabilities, families can be resilient. Singer et al. (1999) found that the resiliency of mothers of children with severe disabilities exacted a psychologic toll, mediated by feelings of mastery and satisfaction in parenting.

Since Baby Doe, there has been a growing ethical consensus toward treatment of imperiled newborns and children with disabilities (Shevell, 1998). Two major pieces of legislation support this movement—the Individuals with Disabilities Education Act and the Americans with Disabilities Act. Beyond the battles in the hospital, parents have had to fight for educational programs appropriate to their children's needs. In the 1970s, Public Law 94-142, the Education for All Handicapped Children's Act of 1975 was passed. It was renamed the Individuals with Disabilities Education Act (IDEA) in 1990 (Public Law 101-476) and was again amended in 2004 (http://idea.ed.gov/). The IDEA has provided the most sweeping protections of educational rights for children with disabilities than any prior legislation. The initial act had four main provisions:

- parental involvement in the educational plan,
- least restrictive environment,

- an individual education plan (IEP), and
- multidisciplinary assessment of needs.

Children with disabilities were to be included in classroom activities and other school activities and not segregated. One major advantage of this integration is the education of the nondisabled students about children with disabilities. Integration of children with disabilities into the community can have a favorable impact on nondisabled individuals' attitudes toward people with disabilities. Since then, the details of the IDEA are quite extensive. The Individualized Education Program (IEP) has been revised to become the Individualized Family Service Plan (IFSP), the least restrictive environment means that that the services may be delivered in the home for the early intervention (birth to 3 years and may be extended beyond three years depending upon the needs of the child). The child may begin early childhood education at age 3 and should be mainstreamed into the general classrooms as appropriate to fulfill the child's educational objectives. The IDEA provides detail regarding the identification of a child at risk, the process for a comprehensive evaluation, and determination of services, which do not have to be the "best" or "optimal" services. This determination can be a source of distress for families who may have received what they view as "optimal" services in early intervention programs. If there is a dispute between the school and parents, the parents may request "mediation, complaint investigation, and/or a due process hearing" (Lipkin, Okamoto, Council on Children with Disabilities, & Council on School Health, 2015). Parents need to be informed of their child's rights under the IDEA and also, for some students, under the ADA.

To facilitate the integration of people with disabilities into the community, the Americans with Disabilities Act (ADA) was passed in 1990 and amended in 2008 to broaden definitions and thus extend the law's protections. Its intent is to protect people with disabilities against discrimination in the workplace and in public. Access to public transportation, public buildings, movie theaters, restaurants, and physicians' offices were examples of the intent of the law. The amendments had an impact on education for children with learning disabilities, attention-deficit/hyperactivity disorder, and those who had been ineligible for services if their disability was mitigated by assistance, for example, reliance on hearing aids or the use of a tutor (Americans with Disabilities Act Amendments Act, 2008). These two laws pave the way for the child with disabilities to transition into adulthood and continue to get the services necessary to find employment, housing, and insurance. The IDEA requires a plan be developed for transition to adult services. In many areas of the country, particularly rural areas, it is difficult to find adult practitioners familiar with the care involved for adults with disabilities, such as Down syndrome, spina bifida, or cerebral palsy. Some practitioners may not be familiar with treating adults with cystic fibrosis or post-polio syndrome. The transition to adult services also focuses on preparation of the youth for autonomous decision-making to the extent possible (Racine et al., 2014).

Two ethical issues in caring for children with disabilities can often pose immense distress for families. The first is the decision to forgo oral feedings and place a feeding tube. The second is the decision to place the child outside of the home for residential care.

Children with congenital or acquired neurodevelopmental disability often have problems with oral intake. There may be a dysphagia or choking and aspiration, or an inability to take in enough nourishment necessary for growth and development.

Especially for children who have been eating orally, it is often difficult for parents to make the decision to forgo oral feedings and accept placement of a feeding tube. Some parents have related their sense of failure when their child can no longer be fed orally, or the concern that the inability to take oral feedings is a sign that the child's condition is deteriorating. Parents who have been told to expect a shorter life for their child may see a surgical procedure to insert a feeding tube as too painful for the child to endure, considering the risk/benefit analysis. Mahant, Jovcevska, and Cohen (2011) conducted a review of qualitative studies that examined the experiences of parents who faced such a decision. They concluded that parents viewed oral feedings as something their child enjoyed and it also represented a "normal" social process, so that tube feeding signified disability. The cultural and societal emphasis on eating as part of celebrations and religious rituals and as a sign of love and nurturing is involved in the parents' feelings of loss. Parents in these studies felt that the difficulty in making the decision to forgo oral feedings was not appreciated by the health-care providers, and some said they felt rushed and pressured to make a decision. For health-care providers, tube feedings are often seen as preferable to oral feedings, especially when the risk of aspiration is high. It has become common for children with disabilities to use feeding tubes as they age. For parents, though, this is a major decision and is often fraught with trepidation, sadness, and sometimes relief.

Another major decision for families is the decision to place a child with disabilities outside of the home. Since 1981, parents can apply for the Katie Beckett waiver that provides Medicaid coverage to eligible technology-dependent children who otherwise would remain in a hospital (http://mchb.hrsa.gov/about/katiebeckett.html). The majority of children with extensive and significant intellectual and developmental disabilities live at home. These children may be at home out of parental preference or because there may not be an available, suitable facility for which the parents can secure funding (Friedman, Kalichman, & the Council on Children with Disabilities, 2014). Parents seek out-of-home placement usually when the care needs of the child exceed the capacity of the parents to fill them. They may no longer feel safe to provide the physical care or may feel depleted in their energy to continue. Some families may tire of the problems associated with having staff coming into their home to provide care, or they may find that the increasing needs of other family members require more attention. For whatever reason, the decision can be heartrending. Overall, parents have reported that the decision to place was positive, but they still felt guilty (Friedman et al., 2014). See Case Study 11.1 for one parent's response to the increasing care needs of a child with extensive disabilities.

Children With Brain Death

With the ability to maintain cardiopulmonary function in the face of extensive brain damage, there was a need to define death. Speculation exists that the impetus for a brain-based definition of death was the increasing need for transplantable organs (Fox & Swazey, 1992), but the primary impetus was the desire to use resources appropriately. If there was no possibility of survival, use of technology to maintain cardiopulmonary function was inappropriate. The distinction between sustaining life and prolonging death needed to be made, and the diagnosis of brain death was useful to that end. The following Harvard Medical School criteria were proposed: unresponsiveness, lack of

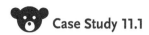

Case Study 11.1

Ashley X

The Ashley X case raised a myriad of ethical issues surrounding children with disabilities. Ashley X was a 6-year-old with static encephalopathy that resulted in tetraplegic cerebral palsy and significant intellectual disability. Her parents learned of a treatment used in the 1950s to stunt growth, and they believed that if Ashley remained smaller than the height and weight she might achieve without treatment, they could keep her at home and continue to provide her 24-hour-care themselves. The pediatric endocrinologist they consulted was willing to provide the high-dose estrogen treatments but wanted review by the hospital ethics committee. The parents also believed that removal of Ashley's breast buds and uterus would eliminate possible complications of large breasts and breast cancer (family history) and any problems once Ashley started menstruating. They also thought these surgeries would minimize the possibility of sexual abuse and pregnancy. The ethics committee approved the procedures, and the "Ashley X treatment," as the parents called it, was conducted.

The endocrinologist and pediatrician published an article about the high-dose estrogen treatment and hysterectomy (Gunther & Diekema, 2006). Ashley's parents blogged about the procedure and received only positive comments in support of their decision. When news outlets shared the story, it quickly became a national topic of discussion. Prominent disability groups considered the surgery "mutilation" and vehemently opposed the Ashley X treatment (American Association on Intellectual and Developmental Disabilities, 2006; Disability Rights Education & Research Fund, 2007; Stein, 2010). The groups viewed the Ashley X treatment as a medical solution to a social problem—the parents' perception that they could not keep Ashley at home and continue her care without limiting her size. Some disability groups believed that the interests of Ashley's parents in keeping her portable and easier to care for had prevailed over Ashley's best interests. For disability groups, ease of care was not a sufficient reason for surgically altering Ashley. Ashley's parents were devoted, well-meaning parents faced with the realities of 24-hour care for the rest of their child's life. They sought the advice and assistance of medical experts who have not publicly voiced any misgivings about having done the procedure. The pediatrician directly involved in the case and a medical ethicist revisited the case and concluded that despite the criticism, the treatment was consistent with Ashley's best interests (Diekema & Fost, 2010).

reflexes, lack of spontaneous breathing, and an isoelectric EEG (Ad Hoc Committee, 1968). If the examinations done 24 hours apart were essentially unchanged, the patient would be declared legally dead and treatment discontinued. For children, these criteria were inadequate. With technological advances, the techniques to assess brain function changed, but health-care providers were warned to use caution in applying these assessment techniques to infants under 7 days of age (Task Force for the Determination of Brain Death in Children, 1987). The guidelines offer specific criteria for assessing brain death in children between 7 days and 2 months, 2 months and 1 year, and over 1 year of age. In 2012, the American College of Critical Care Medicine formed a multidisciplinary committee of specialists from the Pediatric Section of the Society of Critical Care Medicine, the Section on Critical Care of the American Academy of Pediatrics, and the Child Neurology Society to review the 1987 Task Force Recommendations on guidelines for the determination of brain death in infants and children. They reaffirmed the definition from 1987: "An individual who has sustained either (1) irreversible cessation of circulatory and respiratory functions, or (2) irreversible cessation of all functions of the entire brain, including the brainstem, is dead. A determination of death must be made in accordance with accepted medical standards" (Nakagawa, Ashwal, Mathur, Mysore, & Committee for Determination of Brain Death in Infants Children, 2012, p. 574). Brain death remains a clinical diagnosis when the cause of the irreversible coma is known and there is absence of neurologic function (Nakagawa, Ashwal, Mathur, Mysore, & the Committee for Determination of Brain Death in Infants Children, 2012). The guidelines exclude preterm infants less than 37 weeks gestation because there are not enough data in the literature to support their application in this population. The difference between adult assessment and assessment of infants and children is the requirement for two separate assessments 24 hours apart or longer, performed by two different qualified attending physicians who are experienced in pediatrics, neonatology, neurology, neurosurgery, or anesthesia. All reversible conditions for the coma should be excluded prior to the assessment. Because there are differences in state laws pertaining to the declaration of brain death, providers should be aware of their applicable state statutes.

There have been a number of controversies surrounding the issue of brain death in children. Some cultures, as well as some religions, do not recognize brain death. Some Orthodox Jewish rabbis reject brain death and state that a Jew is obligated to accept life-sustaining treatment because "so long as it is possible for a Jew to live, he ought to want to live" (Bleich, 1998). Health-care providers who may wish to discontinue treatment after making a diagnosis of brain death in a child may encounter opposition from families whose religious or cultural values do not accept brain death. The health-care team may view continued treatment as futile and an inappropriate use of resources, while the family may view continued treatment as a religious mandate. Two states, New Jersey and New York, have statutes that specify the physician must consider the individual's preferences, as professed by the next-of-kin, be considered when declaring death by neurologic criteria (Burkle, Sharp, & Wijdicks, 2014). Recognizing that the decision to discontinue treatment is not just a medical one is a beginning in the dialogue with the parents. Rubin (1998) suggested that the concept of futility should be a negotiated reality. The health-care team's reasoning should be "transparent" to the parent; that is, it should be clearly explained how the team arrived at its diagnosis and why discontinuation of treatment is recommended. Rubin also accepts moral suasion, the health-care provider's encouragement of the patient or family to accept the provider's recommendation, as legitimate because the health-care team has greater experience and expertise in cases of brain death than the public. She acknowledged that the disagreement may not be reconcilable, so that ethics committee consultation or even judicial intervention may be needed if the heath-care team believes that continued treatment is not in the child's best interests, yet the parents insist on continued treatment. The case of Jahi McMath, however, may cast doubt in the public's view of the accuracy of the brain death diagnosis (see Case Study 11.2).

Wijdicks, Varelas, Gronseth and Greer (2010) maintain that there are no published reports of anyone recovering after a diagnosis of brain death. However, there is a public

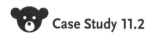

Case Study 11.2

Jahi McMath

Jahi McMath, a 13-year old-girl from Oakland, California, underwent a tonsillectomy, adenoidectomy, and redundant sinus tissue removal on December 9, 2013. After the procedures, Jahi developed complications that rendered her comatose. Two attending physicians conducted assessments of her condition, and she was declared brain-dead on December 12, 2013.

The McMath family did not accept the diagnosis and maintained that because her heart was beating and she moved when touched, she was alive. The hospital sought a court order to remove the ventilator, and a court issued a temporary restraining order (TRO) to permit a court-appointed physician from another institution to examine Jahi. This physician also concluded that Jahi was brain-dead. The family asked for time to find another institution to accept Jahi, and two more TROs were issued. During that time, the family also asked that a tracheostomy and gastrostomy tube be placed, which would be typical for comatose patients being transferred a long-term care facility. The hospital refused on the basis that Jahi was dead, and it would not permit these procedures to be performed on a dead body. The hospital also asked that the county coroner accept Jahi's body prior to its release to her mother. The coroner issued a death certificate indicating that Jahi died on December 12, 2013, and her mother had Jahi transferred to another facility January 6, 2014. She now resides at home in New Jersey, where there is a brain-death exemption (Proctor, 2015). Burkle et al. (2014) consider Jahi's case exceptional because most patients who are brain-dead have cardiac arrhythmias leading to cardiopulmonary arrest.

In 2015 Jahi's family sued the Oakland hospital and the surgeon for malpractice. The family also brought a federal suit alleging that Jahi's civil rights had been violated and asked to have her death certificate revoked. In July 2016, the McMath family cleared an important hurdle in its legal battle when a California appellate court denied appeals by the hospital and surgeon that claimed Jahi was declared legally dead in January 2014 and ruled that Jahi's mother could try to prove that her daughter is alive (Gafni, 2016). Determination of Jahi's status has financial implications for the family: "If the court rules Jahi is alive, the family could sue her surgeon and hospital for millions of dollars, however if the court rules she is dead, they would be limited to a wrongful-death lawsuit capped at $250,000" (Gafni, 2016, para. 6).

skepticism that the diagnosis may not be accurately applied. A cursory Internet search yielded a report from *The Washington Post* that in 2009, a Syracuse, NY, woman awoke in the operating room where she had been taken for organ retrieval (Kaplan, 2015). Her family was told she was brain-dead after she fell into a coma from ingesting a combination of drugs, and they consented to organ donation. The woman recovered and was discharged home two weeks later. An investigation revealed that a number of signs that the woman was not brain-dead were missed by her providers, and although the suspected cause of her coma was a combination of drugs, a toxicology screen to rule out the presence of drugs was not done (Proctor, 2015). The danger in having an accurate diagnosis of brain death rejected means continued distress for the family, inappropriate use of resources, and missed opportunity for organ donation, if that was the wish of the adult patient. Scrupulous adherence to the guidelines for determination of brain death and respectful, transparent, and compassionate communication with the family should occur.

Children With Neurobehavioral Disorders

As smaller and smaller infants were surviving and their development was being evaluated, a condition originally called MBD, or minimal brain dysfunction, was identified. These children were noted to be very active, distractible, and impulsive, and had difficulty with school performance. One theory was that they had been overprotected because of their fragile beginning (vulnerable child syndrome) and lacked discipline and limit-setting abilities. Over time, a condition known as attention-deficit/hyperactivity disorder (ADHD) was described, and both children born prematurely and those born at term were affected. The presentation was usually parental observation about the child's high activity level and his or her inability to attend to tasks, follow directions, or inhibit inappropriate responses.

The specialty of developmental pediatrics grew in the 1970s, and children with attention or behavioral problems were evaluated by this new specialty. Merging neurology, psychiatry, and education, this specialty views learning and development as an interweaving of processes that affect and influence each other. Children who may have an organic predisposition for inattention or impulsivity engender certain responses from their environment. The environmental responses (e.g., difficult relationships with parents, siblings, and peers) further shape the child's behavior. Academic performance may be poor although the child may test in a normal or high range of intelligence. The interplay between a child's intelligence, motor performance, interpersonal relationships, and self-esteem is not easily understood; often the child is identified as a "behavior problem" or the child's abilities are thought to be limited. Through evaluation, usually including neuropsychological testing and a neurologic examination, the child's strengths and weaknesses are discovered, and they may fall into a pattern characteristic of a neurobehavioral disorder. The rubric of "learning disabilities" captures a multitude of disorders from dyslexia, central processing disorder, or nonverbal learning disability to attention-deficit disorder with hyperactivity. The latter condition has created a furor over its alleged overdiagnosis.

The standard approach to diagnosing and managing ADHD requires information and cooperation from the child, the parents, and the school or other structured environment such as day care. The AAP guidelines have been updated (AAP, 2011), and the prevalence is considered to be 8% in children and teens (Harstad, Levy, & the Committee on Substance Abuse, 2014). Recommendations vary from previous guidelines in that the age range for evaluation and treatment of ADHD is 4 to 18 years of age, vs. 6 to 12 years. Evidence-based behavioral therapy is recommended as the first line of treatment for children ages 4–5 years, and consideration of using stimulant medication only if behavioral therapy is unavailable. For older children, stimulants and behavioral therapy at both home and school are recommended.

One of the ethical issues in treating ADHD is the possibility of misuse of stimulant medication. Some children may take more than prescribed, believing that if a little is helpful, more would be better. They also may be approached by friends, or family members to share their medication; the perception is that a controlled substance like methylphenidate or other stimulants can give the user a "high" or improve one's performance on academic papers or tests. The child may decide to sell the medication, or in some cases, a family member may sell the medication. Careful instruction should take place regarding the proper use, administration, and storage of the medication; students are usually required to get their midday dose from the nurse's office, but many schools do not have school nurses, or do not have them present on a daily basis. A process to secure the medication while making it available at the appropriate time should be arranged.

Another ethical issue with stimulant medication is neuroenhancement. Neuroenhancement in this context is when a healthy person takes a stimulant medication in order to improve performance. In one study, 25% of university students reported that diverted stimulant medication is easy to obtain (White, Becker-Blease, & Grace-Bishop, 2006). Stimulant medication is likely to improve attention in most people. Physicians and advanced practice nurses are the gatekeepers to prescription medications, and they have an ethical and fiduciary responsibility to act in their patients' best interests. Off-label use of stimulant medication would be inappropriate for healthy children and teens who do not have ADHD (Graf et al., 2013).

Another group of children who may or may not have ADHD but have a neurological diagnosis are children with autism spectrum disorder. The Centers for Disease Control and Prevention (2014) estimated the prevalence of autism disorders to be 1 in 68 children 8 years old based on data collected from the Autism and Developmental Disabilities Monitoring Network. This network is composed of 11 sites throughout the United States. Based on IQ scores, 46% of the children had average or above-average IQ scores, 31% had scores in the intellectual disability range (below 70), with the remaining 23% having scores between 71 and 85. The *Diagnostic and Statistical Manual of Mental Disorders (DSM)*, fifth edition (2013), has collapsed the categories of pervasive developmental disorder and Asperger's disorder into one category of autism spectrum disorder. The behavioral categories were also collapsed, making the diagnosis of autism spectrum disorder harder to apply. Opponents of these changes believe it will make services more difficult to obtain as fewer children will now be eligible for the services (Kulage, Smaldone, & Cohn, 20114). *Autists*, as some prefer to be called, would like to see autism considered a human variant, like homosexuality, and not as a psychiatric or pathological condition (Autistic Self Advocacy Network, 2015; Jaarsma & Welin, 2012). The neurodiversity movement views autism as a different way of being. They acknowledge that some differences may require some accommodations, much as someone who is deaf may require an accommodation. The Deaf culture also subscribes to the position that people who are deaf are different, not disabled. They function differently than the neurotypical, or "normal," dominant population. Jaarsma and Welin (2012) raise the question of vulnerability and argue that everyone may be vulnerable at one time or another, and autists who are low-functioning versus high-functioning are disabled and need a label to obtain services. They propose using "vulnerability" to indicate the degree of assistance one might need at any point in time. The approach of the autists, consistent with the disability rights movement, is a civil rights movement; their slogan is "Nothing About Us Without Us."

Research on Children

Willowbrook State School was the setting for one of the more infamous instances of unethical research on children. In the 1970s, children with significant developmental disabilities were enrolled in a hepatitis vaccine study; their parents were told that the children would not gain admission into the residential facility unless parents would consent for the children to be in the study. The children were inoculated with the experimental vaccine, gamma globulin, whose effectiveness the researchers wanted to gauge. The children were then exposed to the rest of the institution's population in order to contract hepatitis, which was thought be to inevitable. The parents were placed in the position of either keeping their children at home or submitting their children to an experiment regardless of the potential risks or benefits. Children in institutions were especially vulnerable to exploitation by researchers (Weisstub, 1998).

The Belmont Report (National Commission for the Protection of Human Subjects in Biomedical and Behavioral Research, 1978) was a presidential commission's report on biomedical and behavioral research on human subjects. Seventeen federal agencies adopted the recommendations as the Common Rule for regulation of human subjects research. Institutional review boards (IRB) were charged with oversight of research, using the Common Rule as a guide. The guidelines pertaining to children recognized that children are a vulnerable group who need special conditions to justify inclusion in research. Those conditions are divided into four categories (see Table 11.1). On September 8, 2015, a Notice of Proposed Rule-Making (NPRM) was issued in which the most sweeping changes to the Common Rule since 1981 are being proposed (http://www.hhs.gov/ohrp/humansubjects/regulations/nprmhome.html). There seems to be little change with recommendations related to research with children. Children are still considered a vulnerable group who need special protections. One of the changes requires that those who contributed a biospecimen as a child should be asked to provide informed consent to continue inclusion of the specimen in the study once reaching adulthood. The American Academy of Pediatrics policy statement "Guidelines for the Ethical Conduct of Studies to Evaluate Drugs in Pediatric Populations" (Shaddy, Denne, the Committee on Drugs, & the Committee on Pediatric Research, 2010) offers additional groups for which there should be special circumstances before they are included in research. These groups are children who are institutionalized, either in a facility where they require special care or under supervision of a court or social welfare agency; children with a life-threatening illness; and those who may be eligible for emergency research.

With changes in federal legislation since 1997, pediatric drug studies have markedly increased (Shaddy et al, 2010). As with consent for children in treatment decisions, parents are expected to weigh the risks and benefits to their child when considering the child's participation in research. In some areas, such as oncology, many of the treatments for childhood cancers are available only through enrollment in clinical trials. The newest drugs and drug combinations are presented as one arm of a study; the currently accepted standard drugs and drug combinations are the other arm. Many studies are very complex, involving varying drugs, dosages, and schedules of treatment. In the informed consent process, the oncologist explains the complex study to the parents and, depending on the age and developmental level of the child, may also include the child in these discussions, or may have a separate discussion with the child. The parents give or refuse consent for their child to participate in the research and may withdraw the child from the study. The child's assent, or affirmative agreement, to be a research participant is also sought. If the study is likely to provide a direct benefit to the child, such as most oncology studies, the parents may override the dissent of the

Table 11.1

Categories of Permissible Research on Children			
Level of Risk	Prospect of Direct Benefit	Child Assent Needed	Parental Permission Needed
No greater than minimal	N/A	Yes	Yes
More than minimal	Yes[a]	Yes[b]	Yes
Minor increase over minimal	No	Yes	Yes[c]
Same as the previous 3 categories	No	Yes	Yes[c]

[a]The relation of the anticipated benefit to the risk is at least as favorable to the subjects as that presented by available alternative approaches (45 CFR § 46.405). [b]Assent may be waived if the child is likely to directly benefit from inclusion in the research. [c]Consent from both parents is required unless one of the parents is deceased, incompetent, whereabouts are unknown or is not reasonably available, or when one parent is the custodial parent.

Note. From *Summary of Basic Protections for Human Subjects,* by the Office for Protection From Research Risks, 1997, Rockville, MD: Author.

child. In those instances where assent is desirable but not necessary, the child should not be asked for assent if the dissent will not be honored. The older or more mature the child, the more weight should be given to the child's preferences. Parents usually know their children best and gauge how and when to discuss the study protocol with the child. One of the more difficult situations for the health-care team is when there is disagreement between the professionals and the parents about discussing the diagnosis and treatment options with the child. In these instances the parents often want continued treatment, while the child may be indicating a desire to stop treatment. Although parents retain the legal right to consent, the team may wish to explore the disagreement further to ensure effective communication between the child and parents. The medical center's institutional review board (IRB), when reviewing the research projects for research on children, may stipulate when a child's assent is required, when it can be waived, and whether both parents, if reasonably available, must give informed consent.

For those conditions in which an adolescent can consent to treatment without parental permission, some authors believe that the adolescent should be able to consent to research (Leiken, 1993; Santelli et al., 1995). As discussed previously, state statutes specify conditions in which an adolescent may be treated without parental consent, and the statutes may address consent for research. However, the institution's IRB should ensure that their requirements for consent are consistent with state law.

Despite the surge in pediatric drug research, as much as 50% of drugs still do not have pediatric labeling (AAP, Committee on Drugs, 2014). There is sometimes confusion about off-label use of drugs with children, and such use can be perceived as unethical, illegal, or experimental. It is none of these if the decision to use the drug is made on the best available evidence and after a risk/benefit analysis for use with a specific child. For many years, when there had been no data on a drug's efficacy in children, pediatricians made clinical judgments to try a medication off-label with a particular child.

With more pediatric drug research, off-label use may dwindle, but until that time, it is essential in pediatric care.

Conclusion

This chapter has explored a myriad of ethical issues in children's health care. Many of these ethical problems occur within hospitals, but with health-care settings moving beyond hospital walls, health-care professionals need a broader appreciation of issues affecting children. The answers can be elusive, but it is worthwhile for health-care professionals to contemplate them.

Each setting should identify the current policies and guidelines for informing ethical decision-making relevant to that setting. For example, school personnel should examine policies on medication, including self-medication, use of psychotropic medications, and administration of medication in emergent situations. Additionally, school personnel should explore how they would respond to a request for withholding resuscitation on a student with a terminal illness who still is capable and willing to attend classes.

Not all settings have access to an ethics committee for assistance in analyzing ethical issues. However, there may be ethics consultants with expertise in pediatrics who can serve as ad hoc consultants. These consultants can perform case consultation and inservice education and may assist in the development of an ethics committee for the specific setting.

The Internet provides many ethics resources. E-mail provides almost instant access to colleagues and consultants who can provide information, support, and advice. One caveat is the issue of confidentiality when using electronic communication methods (e-mail, fax); communications must be HIPAA (Health Insurance Portability and Accountability Act of 1996) compliant (Centers for Medicare and Medicaid Services, n.d.). Using an encryption program provides some protection against breaches of confidentiality, and most institutions now have a plethora of security measures to be followed when dealing with electronic data. Another caveat is that the information available on some sites should be evaluated carefully, as there is no assurance that the information is correct or current.

Ethical issues will always be present in health care of children, so professionals should be prepared through education, networking, and accessing resources to face and resolve those issues in their setting. They should also participate in their professional organizations or other groups to share their experiences and expertise in shaping an ethically responsible and child-friendly society.

Study Guide

1. Discuss various approaches to identifying and analyzing ethical issues in children's health care.

2. List and discuss current ethical, moral, and legal issues in children's health care.

3. To what degree can and should children make decisions about their health care?

4. Compare current perspectives and issues on children's participation in decision-making with those of 25 years ago.

5. Describe psychosocial, economic, cultural, and medical changes related to current concerns on ethics, morals, and legal aspects of children's health care.

6. Discuss the implications for practice from "the best interests of the child."

7. In what situations are parents as decision makers for children appropriate? Inappropriate?

8. Describe children's ability to make health-care decisions at various stages of development, and draw implications for practice.

9. Discuss emerging issues in children's health care, and hypothesize future ethical, moral, and legal issues.

10. Outline situations in which a child can make health-care decisions, those in which parents can make decisions, and those in which surrogates must make decisions.

References

23andMe. (2015). *DNA genetic testing & analysis.* Retrieved from www.23andme.com

Ad Hoc Committee of the Harvard Medical School to Examine the Definition of Death. (1968). A definition of irreversible coma. *Journal of the American Medical Association, 205,* 337–340.

Albrecht, G. L., & Devlieger, P. L. (1999). The disability paradox: High quality of life against all odds. *Social Science & Medicine, 48,* 977–988.

American Academy of Pediatrics. (1984). Joint policy statement: Principles of treatment of disabled infants. *Pediatrics, 73,* 559–566.

American Academy of Pediatrics. (2016). American Academy of Pediatrics publishes new policies to boost children's immunization rates. Retrieved from https://www.aap.org/en-us /about-the-aap/aap-press-room/Pages/American-Academy-of-Pediatrics-Publishes-New-Poli cies-to-Boost-Child-Immunization-Rates.aspx

American Academy of Pediatrics and American College of Obstetrics and Gynecology. Obstetric and Medical Complications. (2007). *Guidelines for perinatal care.* (6th ed.). Elk Grove Village, IL: AAP.

American Academy of Pediatrics, Committee on Bioethics. (1995). Informed consent, parental permission, and assent in pediatric practice. *Pediatrics, 95,* 314–317.

American Academy of Pediatrics, Committee on Bioethics. (2001). Ethical issues with genetic testing in pediatrics. *Pediatrics, 197*(6), 1451–1455.

American Academy of Pediatrics, Committee on Drugs. (2014). Off-label use of drugs in children. *Pediatrics, 133,* 563–567.

American Academy of Pediatrics Section on Hospice and Palliative Medicine and Committee on Hospital Care. (2013). Pediatric palliative care and hospice care commitments, guidelines, and recommendations. *Pediatrics, 132,* 996–972. doi: 10.1542/peds.2013-2731

American Academy of Pediatrics Subcommittee on Attention-Deficit/Hyperactivity Disorder, Steering Committee on Quality Improvement and Management. (2011). ADHD: Clinical practice guideline for the diagnosis, evaluation, and treatment of attention-deficit/hyperactivity disorder in children and adolescents. *Pediatrics, 128*(5), 1–16.

American Association on Intellectual and Developmental Disabilities. (2012). *Growth attenuation: Position statement of AAIDD.* Retrieved from http://aaidd.org/news-policy/policy/position-statements/growth-attenuation#.Vog0k1IRrSg

American Psychiatric Association. (2013). *Diagnostic and statistical manual of mental disorders* (5th ed.). Washington, DC: Author.

Americans with Disabilities Act Amendments Act of 2008, Pub. L. No. 110–325, 122 Stat. 3553 (2008).

Asch, A. (1998). The "difference" of disability in the medical setting. *Cambridge Quarterly of Healthcare Ethics, 7,* 77–87.

Autistic Self Advocacy Network. (2015). *Position statements.* Retrieved from http://autisticadvocacy .org/policy-advocacy/position-statements/

Bleich, J. D. (1998). *Bioethical dilemmas: A Jewish perspective.* Hoboken, NJ: KTAV.

Brennan, W. (1995). *Dehumanizing the vulnerable: When word games take lives.* Chicago, IL: Loyola University Press.

Buchanan, A. E., & Brock, D. W. (1990). *Deciding for others: The ethics of surrogate decision making.* New York, NY: Cambridge University Press.

Burkle, C. M., Sharp, R. R., & Wijdicks, E. F. (2014). Why brain death is considered death and why there should be no confusion. *Neurology, 83,* 1464–1469.

Carter, B. S. (1993). Neonatologists and bioethics after Baby Doe. *Journal of Perinatology, 13*(2), 144–150.

Carter, B. S., Rosenkrantz, T., Windle, M. L., & MacGilvray, S. S. (2015). *Ethical issues in neonatal care.* Retrieved November 11, 2015 at http://emedicine.medscape.com/article/978997 -overview#a6

Centers for Disease Control and Prevention. (2014). *Prevalence of autism spectrum disorder among children aged 8 years—Autism and Developmental Disabilities Monitoring Network, 11 Sites, United State, 2010.* Retrieved from www.cdc.gov/mmwr/preview/mmwrhtml/ss6302a1.htm?s_cid=s -s6302a1_w

Centers for Medicare and Medicaid Services. (n.d.). *Health Insurance Portability and Accountability Act (HIPAA): Administrative simplification.* Retrieved from http://www.cms.hhs.gov/hipaa/hipaa2/

Charlton, J. I. (1998). *Nothing about us without us: Disability, oppression, and empowerment.* Berkeley, CA: University of California Press.

Clark, P. (2002). Medical futility in pediatrics: Is it time for a public policy? *Journal of Public Health Policy, 23*(1), 66–89.

Diekema, D. S., & Fost, N. (2010). Ashley revisited: A response to the critics. *American Journal of Bioethics, 10*(1), 30–44.

Disability Rights Education & Defense Fund. (2007). *Modify the system, not the person.* Retrieved from http://dredf.org/public-policy/medical-ethics/modify-the-system-not-the-person/

Duff, R. S., & Campbell, A. G. M. (1973). Moral and ethical dilemmas in special care nurseries. *New England Journal of Medicine, 289,* 890–894.

Dupont-Thibodeau, A., Barrington, K. J., Farlow, B., & Janvier, A. (2014). End-of-life decisions for extremely low-gestation-age infants: Why simple rules for complicated decisions should be avoided. *Seminars in Perinatology, 38,* 31–37. doi: 10.1053/j.semperi.2013.07.006

Flavell, J. (1985). *Cognitive development* (2nd ed.). Englewood Cliffs, NJ: Prentice Hall.

Fost, N. (1999). Decisions regarding treatment of seriously ill newborns. *Journal of the American Medical Association, 281*(21), 2041–2042.

Fox, R. C., & Swazey, J. P. (1992). *Spare parts: Organ replacement in American society.* New York, NY: Oxford University Press.

Francescatto, L., & Katsanis, N. (2015). Newborn screening and the era of medical genomics. *Seminars in Perinatology, 39,* 617–622. doi: http://dx.doi.org/10.1053/j.semperi.2015.09.010

Friedman, S. L., Kalichman, M. A., & the Council on Children with Disabilities. (2014). Out-of-home placement for children and adolescents with disabilities. *Pediatrics, 134,* 836–846. doi: 10.1542/peds.2014-2279

Gafni, M. (2016, July 13). Jahi McMath: Court says family can try to prove she's alive. *East Bay Times* Retrieved from http://www.eastbaytimes.com/2016/07/13/jahi-mcmath-court-says -family-can-try-to-prove-shes-alive/

Gallagher, H. G. (1995). "Slapping up spastics": The persistence of social attitudes toward people with disabilities. *Issues in Law & Medicine, 10*(4), 401–414.

Genetic Information Nondiscrimination Act of 2008. (2008). Retrieved from www.genome .gov/24519851

Gilligan, C. (1982). *In a different voice: Psychological theory and women's development.* Cambridge, MA: Harvard University Press.

Graf, W. D., Negal, S. K., Epstein, L. G., Miller, G., Nass, R., & Larriviere, D. (2013). Pediatric neuroenhancement: Ethical, legal, social, and neurodevelopmental implications. *Neurology, 80,* 1251–1260.

Greenbaum, J., & Crawford-Jakubiak, J. E. (2015). Child sex trafficking and commercial sexual exploitation: Health care needs of victims. *Pediatrics, 135*(3), 566–574. doi: 10.1542/peds.2014-4138

Grisso, T., & Appelbaum, P. S. (1998). *Assessing competence to consent to treatment: A guide for physicians and other health professionals.* New York, NY: Oxford University Press.

Grisso, T., Appelbaum, P. S., & Hill-Fitiuhi, C. (1997). The MacCAT-T: A clinical tool to assess patients' capabilities to make treatment decisions. *Psychiatric Services, 48*(11), 1415–1419.

Grisso, T., & Vierling, L. (1978). Minor's consent in treatment: A developmental perspective. *Professional Psychology, 9*(3), 412–427.

Guillén, Ú., Weiss, E. M., Munson, D., Maton, P., Jefferies, A., Norman, M., Naulaers, G., . . . Kirpalani, H. (2015). Guidelines for the management of extremely premature deliveries: A systematic review. *Pediatrics, 136*(2), 343–350. doi: 10.1542/peds.2015-0542

Gunther, D. F., & Diekema, D. S. (2006). Attenuating growth in children with profound developmental disabilities. *Archives of Pediatric and Adolescent Medicine, 160*(10), 1013–1017.

Harstad, E., Levy, S., & the Committee on Substance Abuse. (2014). Attention-deficit/hyperactivity disorder and substance abuse. *Pediatrics, 134,* e293–e301.

Jaarsma, P., & Welin, S., (2012). Autism as a natural human variation: Reflections on the claims of the neurodiversity movement. *Health Care Analysis, 20*(1), 20–30. doi: 10.1007/s10728-011-0169-9

Janvier, A., Barrington, K., & Farlow, B. (2014). Communication with parents concerning withholding or withdrawing of life-sustaining interventions in neonatology. *Seminars in Perinatology, 38*(1), 38–46. doi: 10.1053/j.semperi.2013.07.007

Janvier, A., & Farlow, B (2014). Arrogance-based medicine: Guidelines regarding genetic testing in children. *American Journal of Bioethics, 14*(3), 15–16.

Kaplan, S. (2015, Dec 29). When are you dead? It may depend on which hospital makes the call. *The Washington Post.* Retrieved from www.washingtonpost.com/news/morning-mix/wp/2015/12/29/when-are-you-dead-it-may-depend-on-which-hospital-makes-the-call/

Kirschner K. L., Brashler, R., & Savage, T. A. (2007). Ashley X. *American Journal of Physical Medicine and Rehabilitation, 86,* 1023–1029.

Kon, A. A. (2015). They're not just little adults: Special consideration in pediatric clinical ethics consultation. *American Journal of Bioethics, 15*(5), 30–32.

Kopelman, L. M. (1997). The best-interests standard as threshold, ideal, and standard of reasonableness. *Journal of Medicine and Philosophy, 22,* 271–289.

Kopelman, L. M., Irons, T. G., & Kopelman, A. E. (1988). Neonatologists judge the "Baby Doe" regulations. *New England Journal of Medicine, 318*(11), 677–683.

Kulage, K. M., Smaldone, A. M., & Cohn, E. G. (2014). How will DSM-5 affect autism diagnosis? A systematic literature review and meta-analysis. *Journal of Autism and Developmental Disorders, 44,* 1918–1932.

Leiken, S. (1993). Minors' assent, consent, or dissent to medical research. *IRB: A Review of Human Subjects Research, 15*(2), 1–7.

Lin, R.-G., & McGreevy, P. (2015, April 17). California measles outbreak is over, but vaccine fight continues. *L.A. Times.* Retrieved from http://www.latimes.com/local/california/la-me-measles-20150418-story.html

Lipkin, P.H., Okamoto, J., the Council on Children with Disabilities and Council on School Health. (2015). The Individuals with Disabilities Education Act (IDEA) for children with special education needs. *Pediatrics, 136,* e1650–e1661. doi: 10. 1542/peds.2015-3409

Lorber, J. (1972). Spina bifida cystica: Results of treatment of 270 consecutive cases with criteria for selection for the future. *Archives of Disease in Childhood, 47,* 856–867.

Mahant, S., Jovcevska, V., & Cohen, E. (2011). Decision-making around gastrostomy-feeding in children with neurologic disabilities. *Pediatrics, 127*(6), e1471–e1481. doi: 10.1542/peds.2010-3007

Meadow, W., & Lantos, J. (2009). Moral reflections on neonatal intensive care. *Pediatrics 123*(2), 595–597.

Michaud, P.-A., Blum, R. W., Benaroyo, L., Zermatten, J., & Baltag, V. (2014). Assessing an adolescent's capacity for autonomous decision-making in clinical care. *Journal of Adolescent Health, 57,* 361–366.

Nakagawa, T. A., Ashwal, S., Mathur, M., Mysore, M., & the Committee for Determination of Brain Death in Infants Children. (2012). Guidelines for the determination of brain death in infants and children: An update of the 1987 Task Force Recommendations—Executive Summary. *Annuals of Neurology, 71*(4), 573–585.

National Commission for the Protection of Human Subjects in Biomedical and Behavioral Research. (1978). *The Belmont Report: Ethical principles and guidelines for the protection of human subjects of research* (DHEW). Publication No. OS 78-0012. Washington, DC: U.S. Government Printing Office.

Oberman, M. (1996). Minor rights and wrongs. *Journal of Law, Medicine, and Ethics, 24,* 127–138.

O'Neill, K. (2002). Kids speak: Effective communication with the school-aged/adolescent patient. *Pediatric Emergency Care, 18*(2), 137–140.

Proctor, K. (2015, Dec 24). Family wants brain-dead girl declared alive. *Courthouse News Service.* Retrieved from www.courthouse news.com/2015/12/24/family-wants-brain-dead-girl-declared -alive.htm

Racine, E., Bell, E., Yan A., Andrew, G., Bell, L. E., Clarke, M., . . . Yager, J. Y. (2014). Ethics challenges of transition from paediatric to adult health care services for young adults with neurodevelopmental disabilities. *Paediatrics & Child Health, 19*(2), 65–68.

Ross, L. F. (1997). Health care decision making by children: Is it in their best interests? *Hasting Center Report, 27*(6), 41–45.

Ross, L. F., Saal, H. M., David, K. L., Anderson, R. R., the American Academy of Pediatrics, & the American College of Medical Genetics and Genomics. (2013). Technical report: Ethical and policy issues in genetic testing and screening of children. *Genetics in Medicine, 15*(3), 234–245. doi: 10.1038/gim.2012.176

Rubin, S. B. (1998). *When doctors say no: The battleground of medical futility.* Bloomington, IN: Indiana University Press.

Saigal, S., Stoskopf, B. L., Feeny, D., Furlong, W., Burrows, E., Rosenbaum, P., & Hoult, L. (1999). Differences in preferences for neonatal outcomes among health care professionals, parents, and adolescents. *Journal of the American Medical Association, 281*(21), 1991–1997.

Santelli, J. S., Rosenfeld, W. D., DuRant, R. H., Dubler, N., Morreale, M., English, A., & Rogers, A. S. (1995). A special issue of the *Journal of Adolescent Health* on guidelines for adolescent health research. *Journal of Adolescent Health, 19,* 262–269.

Savage, T. A. (2000, July). *Factors influencing parental decision-making regarding life-sustaining treatment for children with severe disabilities.* Paper presented at the 5th International Family Nursing Conference, Chicago, IL.

Seipel, T. (2015, October 8). California vaccine law: Opponents' repeal effort fails but fight goes on. *Mercurynews.com.* Retrieved from http://www.mercurynews.com/health/ci_28936729/cali fornia-vaccine-law-opponents-repeal-effort-fails-but

Shaddy, R. E., Denne, S. C., the Committee on Drugs and Committee on Pediatric Research. (2010). Clinical report—Guidelines for the ethical conduct of studies to evaluate drugs in pediatric populations. *Pediatrics, 125,* 850–860.

Shannon, S. E., & Savage, T. A. (2007). The Ashley treatment: Two viewpoints. *Pediatric Nursing, 33*(2), 175–178

Shapiro, J. P. (1994). *No pity: People with disabilities forging a new civil rights movement.* New York, NY: Times-Books, Random House.

Shevell, M. I. (1998). Clinical ethics and developmental delay. *Seminars in Pediatric Neurology, 5*(1), 70–75.

Singer, L. T., Salvator, A., Guo, S., Collin, M., Lilien, L., & Baley, J. (1999). Maternal psychological distress and parenting stress after the birth of a very low-birth-weight infant. *Journal of the American Medical Association, 281,* 799–805.

Stein, G. (2010). Ashley's case: The ethics of arresting the growth of children with serious disability. *Journal of Social Work in Disability and Rehabilitation, 9*(2), 99–109.

Stinson, R., & Stinson, P. (1979). *The long dying of baby Andrew.* Boston, MA: Little, Brown.

Strasburger, V. C., & Brown, R. T. (1991). *Adolescent medicine: A practical guide.* Boston, MA: Little, Brown.

Task Force for the Determination of Brain Death in Children. (1987). Guidelines for the determination of brain death in children, *Neurology, 37,* 1077–1078.

U.S. Department of Health and Human Services. (2013). *Health Insurance Portability and Accountability Act Combined Regulation Text of All Rules.* http://www.hhs.gov/hipaa/for-professionals/privacy/laws-regulations/combined-regulation-text/index.html

U.S. Department of Health and Human Services. (2015). *Affordable Care Act.* Retrieved from http://www.hhs.gov/healthcare/about-the-law/index.html

U.S. Department of Health and Human Services Advisory Committee on Heritable Disorders in Newborns and Children. (2015). *Recommended Uniform Screening Panel.* Retrieved from http://www.hrsa.gov/advisorycommittees/mchbadvisory/heritabledisorders/recommendedpanel/

Verhagen, A. A. E. (2013). The Groningen Protocol for newborn euthanasia: Which way did the slippery slope tilt? *Journal of Medical Ethics, 39,* 293-295. doi: 10.1136/medethics-2013-101402

Weisstub, D. N. (1998). *Research on human subjects: Ethics, law and social policy.* Kidlington, Oxford, England: Pergamon Press.

White, B. P., Becker-Blease, K. A., & Grace-Bishop, K. (2006). Stimulant medication use, misuse, and abuse in an undergraduate and graduate student sample. *Journal of American College Health, 54*(5), 261–268

Wijdicks, E. F. M., Varelas, P. N., Gronseth, G. S., & Freer, D. M. (2010). Evidence-based guideline update: Determination brain death in adults. *Neurology, 74,* 1911–1918.

Williams, T. (2002). Patient empowerment and ethical decision making: The patient/partner and the right to act. *Dimensions of Critical Care Nursing, 21*(3), 100–104.

Zayek, M. M., Trimm, R. F., Hamm, C. R., Peevy, K. J., Benjamin, J. T., & Eyal, F. G. (2011). The limit of viability: A single regional unit's experience. *Archives of Pediatric and Adolescent Medicine, 165*(2), 126–133.

12

Relationships in Children's Health-Care Settings

Judy A. Rollins

Objectives

At the conclusion of this chapter, the reader will be able to:

1. Discuss what relationships are, how they vary, and how and why they have changed in health-care settings over the past three decades.

2. Determine the special issues of relationships in working with children in health-care settings and encounters, and draw implications for healthy relationships.

3. Outline relationships among professionals that are critical to optimal health care for children with special needs, and describe optimal relationships for today's health-care system and children's needs.

4. Determine the effects of caring and quality of relationships on children's psychosocial development as well as physical health. Summarize the major relationship factors that influence children's recovery.

Regardless of health-care setting, meeting the psychosocial needs of children and families occurs not in isolation but within the structure of relationships. Involvement, caring, and interpersonal connection form the basis from which care is delivered (Totka, 1996). Over the years, messages in the literature regarding professionalism and patient–provider relationships have changed in value from detachment and distancing to intimacy, commitment, and involvement (Williams, 2001). Discussions have addressed which types of relationships are most effective and which are most likely to result in harm, as well as the effects of under- or overinvolvement on children, families, and health-care professionals.

Before delving into the topic of relationships, it is important to acknowledge that fundamental differences exist between caring for children and caring for adults. For example, with children, physical boundaries are not the same. Health-care providers hold, kiss, and nurture children (see Figure 12.1). However, although physical boundaries of care are taken away, it is expected that emotional boundaries remain clear (Totka, 1996). Additionally, when children are ill, their parents are in crisis, making them vulnerable to the health-care provider's words and actions. Further, when parents are either physically or emotionally unavailable to their children, the struggle intensifies as the health-care provider tries to fill the gaps of care and advocacy. These issues add to the complexity of relationships in pediatric health-care settings.

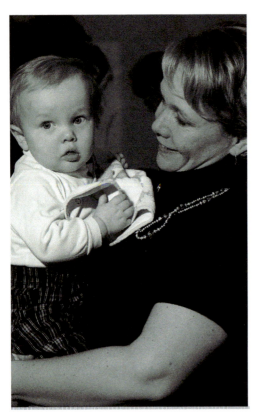

Figure 12.1. In pediatrics, although the physical boundaries of care are taken away, it is expected that emotional boundaries remain clear.

We now know that there is no "one kind" of relationship that meets all needs and purposes of children, families, and health-care professionals in health-care settings. This chapter explores the types of relationships that develop between health-care professionals and the children and families they serve, as well as the relationships that develop among members of the health-care team.

A Historical Perspective in Nursing

Nurses as a group typically have more contact with the child than any other members of the health-care team. Historically, the role of the nurse has been to provide physical care under the control of the doctor, while at the same time remaining professionally detached from the patient (Pearson, Vaughan, & Fitzgerald, 1996). Within this biomedical model, the patient was perceived as a biologic body to be attended by the nurse, and emotional detachment and distancing were valued ideals (Williams, 2001). Gow (1982) offered the following account of a nurse that illustrates the confusing messages regarding professionalism that she experienced as a student:

> E. M. Jones tells us that when she was a student there seemed to be a motto, "Don't Become Involved with Your Patients." She felt that this was a protective device to spare the nurse from emotional breakdown as a result of "painful, disturbing, and depressing problems of their patients." I agree that this attitude was supposed to protect the nurses, but it seems to me that as a result, both the nurse and the patient ended up suffering. A nurse who felt distressed over a patient's predicament would use defense mechanisms (such as avoidance of the patient) to keep herself from getting emotionally involved. However, by the mere fact that she was having these feelings she was already emotionally involved. Instead of admitting this, a process of denial went on, and the nurse never came to grips with her emotions; the patient suffered from loneliness and the feeling that the nurse was uncaring and coldhearted. The nurse was also useless in providing supportive care, since she required support herself, which she never received. (p. 12)

To control interaction with patients, nurses used distancing tactics, such as closed questions, leading questions, a rapid succession of questions, and direct statements (Williams, 2001). Macleod Clark's (1982) comprehensive study of nurse–patient interaction in surgical settings found the average duration of contact to be 1.1 minutes; further, this contact was superficial in nature and focused on the completion of physical tasks.

The introduction of the nursing process and later the focus on Primary Nursing challenged the notion of detachment (May, 1991). Both initiatives facilitate the provision of individualized care and focus on the nurses' personal relationships and commitment to patients. From this, a new definition of nurse–patient relationship emerges, one characterized by commitment, closeness, and involvement (Williams, 2001). These innovations, collectively referred to as "The New Nursing" (Savage, 1990), involve a clear redefinition of nursing care to include administering to the sick body and addressing wider, related psychological, emotional, social, and spiritual needs of the patient (May, 1991). Current perspectives lead to a broader interpretation of caring, which includes both "caring for" and "caring about" (Savage, 1995). Research findings indicate that "caring about" necessitates emotional involvement and commitment to the patient (Swanson, 1991).

Today, in place of distancing, the presence of the nurse has emerged as a key theme. Activities include giving time to and being with the patient and demonstrating an appreciation for the patient's experience. In exploring patients' and nurses' views on the beneficial effects of nursing care, Ersser (1991, 1998) found the potential for physical closeness and a psychological or existential closeness, which were considered valued and important. Further, communication that is patient-centered has been shown to facilitate a positive nurse–patient relationship (McCabe, 2004). It is clear that a fundamental change in perspective has taken place, whereby close, intimate nurse–patient relationships are increasingly prescribed rather than discouraged (Williams, 2001).

The Doctor–Patient Relationship

Dramatic changes have occurred in doctor–patient relationships during the past century. In the early 1900s, patients expected little from doctors and did not hold them in high esteem. The 1910 Flexner report revealed that diploma mills were churning out MD degrees, which served to further this attitude (Holoweiko, 1998). The flu epidemic and other infectious diseases were killing off entire families; doctors could do little to help. Family and friends provided most health care; asking a doctor to visit was a last resort.

Advances in medical science and technology changed the public's opinion of doctors. For example, pharmaceutical research post–World War II led to hundreds of potent compounds, dramatically expanding doctors' abilities to combat disease. Holoweiko (1998) also credited the media's portrayal of physicians—Ben Casey, Dr. Kildare, Marcus Welby—as almost god-like captains of the ship, not only curing patients' illnesses but resolving their emotional and relationship problems as well. Physicians were put on a pedestal, from which flowed a doctor-knows-best philosophy accepted with little question by patients.

With the movements for civil rights, peace in Vietnam, consumer rights, and women's equality during the 1960s and 1970s, most institutions were questioned. Paternalism was brought under fire, including the doctor–patient relationship (Holoweiko, 1998). Protestors of yesterday are now in their 60s or 70s, and, better educated than previous generations, they are accustomed to challenging authority. Furthermore, the world of health information is available to anyone with Internet access.

Managed Care

Managed care also is changing the doctor–patient relationship and, as a result, medical ethics. Most physicians were schooled in relationships that were convenantal, continuous, confidential, supportive, and personal. La Puma (1996) contrasted these relationships with the type more commonly seen today (see Table 12.1).

Forster (1998) offered examples of doctors who are unhappy with this depersonalization of doctors and patients and the accompanying shift in language—for example, *gatekeepers* and *clients*—that characterizes the changed relationship. He deemed this unhappiness with language a symptom that masks depression over the loss of the traditional doctor–patient relationship, or, at the very least, a reflection of a fear that the idealized doctor–patient relationship is no longer attainable. However, Forster concluded that if doctors are competent and treat patients with compassion and concern, it matters little what someone chooses to call them.

Diversity

Diversity in the medical profession in America has increased dramatically over the years. In addition to more female physicians, many racial and ethnic groups are represented. Reynolds, Cowden, Brosco, and Lantos (2015) pointed out ethical concerns that sometimes arise when parents ask that a doctor of a particular race or ethnic group not care for their child. They commented that such requests sometimes seem legitimate and other times seem offensive, with the difference reflecting a clash of fundamental values. Although generally physicians try to respect patient or parental preferences, the authors state that "requests based on racist attitudes . . . do not seem worthy of respect" (p. 381). The authors presented a situation in which parents requested a White doctor and analyze the ways doctors might think about and respond to such a request. Through an ethics round, each author offers thoughtful comments about where they would draw the line. Concludes Lantos:

> Reasons and motives matter. Some patient preferences are more ethically justifiable than others. A parental request for a different physician that is based only on the color of their doctor's skin needn't be honored. Such parents may be informed that such requests will not be honored. They should be informed that they are free to seek care elsewhere. When offered such a choice, as in this case [described in the article], most parents will gratefully accept good medical care for their child. The parents, the child, and the doctors will all be better off as a result. (p. 385)

Types of Professional–Patient Relationships

"When a child is the patient, the patient is the family." This is one of the first lessons we learn when we enter the world of pediatrics. Therefore, professionals must ensure that the therapeutic relationship extends to parents and the wider family, thus embracing the principles of family-centered care (Roberts, Fenton, & Barnard, 2015).

The quality of a professional–patient relationship can have significant implications. To investigate hospitalized children's views of their relationships with nurses and doctors, Corsano and colleagues (2012) asked 27 children (6 to 15 years old) in a pediatric oncol-

Table 12.1

A Comparison of Characteristics of Doctor–Patient Relationships of the Past and Today	
The Past	**Today**
Covenant • Fidelity and altruism governed relationship. • Doctors put patients' interests before their own. • Relationship typically began through recommendation from a trusted source.	**Contract** • Neither doctor nor patient truly has free choice. • Patients as a whole are increasingly wary of physicians as a group. • Relationship typically begins with selection from a list.
Continuous • Physician sometimes cared for several generations of the same family.	**Episodic** • Physicians couple and uncouple in group arrangements. • Physicians are selected and deselected by managed-care plans. • Patients change doctors because of change in insurance.
Confidential • In 1976, approximately 70 physicians, nurses, managers, trainees, and students had access to a hospitalized patient's chart.	**Wide Open** • By 1996, approximately 210 physicians, nurses, managers, trainees, and students had access to a hospitalized patient's chart.
Collegial • Trying to define patient's disease, gaining the wisdom of another colleague provided incentives for referrals; also financially rewarding.	**Solitary** • Physicians face financial disincentives to refer patients or prescribe an off-formulary medication.
Personal • Focus was on the individual.	**Population-based** • Focus is on health of the population.

Note. Adapted from "Does the Doctor-Patient Relationship Mean More to Doctors than Patients?" by J. La Puma, 1996 [Electronic version], *Managed Care.* Retrieved from www.managedcaremag.com /archives/1996/1/does-doctor-patient-relationship-mean-more-doctors-patients

ogy unit to draw him- or herself with a doctor or nurse from the unit while they were doing something. The researchers analyzed the drawings using the *Pictorial Assessment of Interpersonal Relationships* (PAIR) (Bombi, Pinto, & Cannoni, 2007) and a qualitative analysis. They reported that the children viewed their relationships with health professionals positively, in particular with the nurses. The children perceived the relationship as close, intimate, cohesive, and without conflict, and, in some cases, becoming an emotional bond. Findings indicated that this relationship helped the children cope with painful and uncomfortable medical procedures, which gradually became familiar and accepted.

In researching and defining the nurse–patient relationship, Morse (1991) found that relationships can be either mutual or unilateral, according to the outcome of covert interactive negotiations or implicit interplay between the two persons. Mutual relationships fall into four broad types and depend on certain circumstances (e.g., length of time the nurse and patient have together), the needs and desires of the nurse and the patient, and personality factors. In a unilateral relationship, one person is unwilling or unable to develop the relationship to the level desired by the other. For example, a nurse who is "burned out" may not have the emotional energy to invest in the relationship when a patient clearly desires or needs a relationship with greater involvement.

The four broad types of mutual relationships, listed in order of involvement and intensity, are *clinical, therapeutic, connected*, and *overinvolved*. The characteristics of each type are summarized in Table 12.2 and listed below (Morse, 1991; Stein-Parbury, 1993).

Clinical Relationship

Because of limited personal emotional involvement, the professional may not remember the patient, and the patient may not remember the professional. In a clinical relationship,

- professionals and families interact in a routine or standard manner;
- technical care is provided;
- the health situation involved typically is perceived by both parties as being minor and routine;
- the patient's vulnerability and dependence is almost nonexistent;

Table 12.2

Types and Characteristics of Nurse–Patient Relationships				
	Types of Relationships			
Characteristics	**Clinical**	**Therapeutic**	**Connected**	**Overinvolved**
Time	Short/transitory	Short/average	Lengthy	Long-term
Interaction	Perfunctory/rote	Professional	Intensive/close	Intensive/intimate
Patient's needs	Minor Treatment-oriented	Needs met Minor/moderate	Extensive/crisis "Goes the extra mile"	Enormous needs
Nurse's perspective of the patient; patient's perspective of own role	Only in patient role	First: in patient role Second: as a person	First: as a person Second: in patient role	Only as a person
Nursing commitment	Professional commitment	Professional commitment Patient's concerns secondary	Patient's concerns primary Treatment concerns secondary	Committed to patient only as a person Treatment goals discarded

Note. From "Negotiating Commitment and Involvement in the Nurse–Patient Relationship," by J. Morse, 1991, *Journal of Advanced Nursing, 16*, p. 457. Copyright 1991 by Blackwell. Reprinted with permission.

- little negotiation is involved;
- there is implicit agreement between both parties to keep the relationship at this level; and
- the relationship is short in duration. (Morse, 1991; Stein-Parbury, 1993)

Therapeutic Relationship

A therapeutic relationship is the most common type formed and is considered the "ideal" by most administrators and educators. At Rainbow Babies and Children's Hospital, for example, a therapeutic relationship is defined as one that reflects the philosophy and values of the health-care institution, the department of nursing, child life, and the individual nurse, while respecting patient–family values (McAliley, Lambert, Ashenberg, & Dull, 1996). In a therapeutic relationship,

- the patient typically is facing a situation that he or she perceives as neither life-threatening nor serious;
- care is given quickly and effectively;
- the patient's internal and external resources for meeting the demands of the situation are adequate and available;
- although the professional perceives the patient as a patient, there is also recognition and understanding of the patient as a person;
- the professional serves as support mobilizer and enhancer; and
- the relationship is usually of short or average duration. (Morse, 1991; Stein-Parbury, 1993)

Connected Relationship

A connected relationship may develop when the patient and professional have been together long enough for the relationship to have evolved beyond a clinical and a therapeutic relationship, or when the process is accelerated because of the patient's extreme need. Many children with cancer have identified this kind of relationship as being the single most important thing that has helped them to cope with the cancer experience (Rollins, 2009). Research findings indicate that developing reciprocal trust is the basic social process that enables professionals and children to reach the goal of becoming connected (Wilson, Morse, & Penrod, 1998). In connected relationships,

- the professional and patient perceive each other as people first and their roles as patient and professional become secondary;
- both the professional and patient choose to enter this level of relationship;
- trust and commitment are deep and complete;
- the professional will "bend and break the rules" and "go the extra mile" on the patient's behalf;
- the patient actively seeks the professional's advice and opinion;
- the professional functions as a source of support;
- self-disclosure is high; and
- both the professional and the patient experience change as a result of their relationship. (Morse, 1991; Stein-Parbury, 1993)

Overinvolved Relationship

This type of relationship usually develops when the patient has extraordinary needs and the professional chooses to meet them, or when the patient and the professional have spent an extensive length of time together and mutually respect, trust, and care for each other. In an overinvolved relationship,

- the professional is committed to the patient as a person, and this overrides the professional's commitment to the treatment regime, other professionals, the institution and its need, and the professional's responsibilities toward other patients;
- the professional is a complete confidant of the patient and is treated as a member of the patient's family;
- the relationship continues beyond the professional's work hours and the professional remains a key figure in the patient's life;
- the professional may become territorial and believe that he or she is the only one who can give proper and appropriate care to the patient; and
- the professional views the patient as a person, the patient relinquishes the patient role, and the professional relinquishes the impersonal professional relationship. (Morse, 1991; Stein-Parbury, 1993).

Special Considerations in Patient–Professional Relationships

Most researchers and clinicians agree that certain circumstances influence the type of relationship that is likely to develop between patients and professionals. The type of illness is a significant factor in the characteristics of the roles and resulting relationships. For example, patient passivity and professional assertiveness are the most common reactions to acute illness; patient cooperation and professional guidance are common characteristics in less acute illness; and professionals participating in a treatment plan where patients have the bulk of the responsibility to help themselves is common in chronic illness (Hughes, 1994).

Chronic Illness

With chronic illness, the opportunity exists for professionals and patients to come to know each other over a long period of time, and therefore for the possibility of a connected relationship to develop. Both parties come to understand and appreciate each other as people, and often share on a personal level the pain of loss and the joy of successful adaptation that accompanies living with chronic illness.

Although the average length of hospital stay for children remains short, the increase in the number of children undergoing organ transplantation means very long stays for a growing number of children (see Figure 12.2). Allenbach and Steinmiller (2004) found that inconsistent nursing practices created nurse–patient boundary issues in a cardiac step-down unit related to confidentiality, limit setting, and professionalism with children awaiting organ transplantation and their families. Nursing staff worked

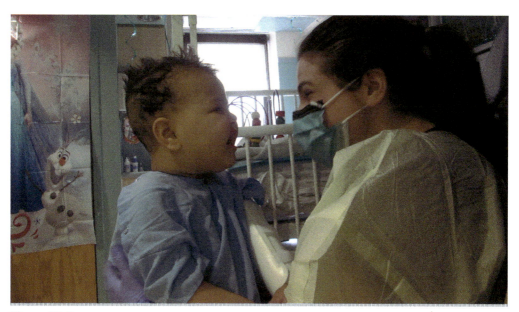

Figure 12.2. Long hospital stays provide time for warm relationships to develop. *Note.* Photo courtesy of Jessica Uze.

together to design and implement a plan to translate the principles of therapeutic relationships into daily practice. The plan outlined concrete solutions and resources available within the hospital to empower staff in the ongoing effort to manage relationships with children with chronic diseases and their families.

Life-Threatening Illness and Death

More involved and intense relationships tend to develop when a child has a life-threatening condition or is dying. Davies et al. (1996) conducted interviews with 25 nurses who had cared for at least one chronically ill child who had died. Findings indicated that nurses struggled with both grief distress and moral distress within the context of a mutually caring relationship between the nurse and child wherein both the patient and the nurse made a difference in each other's lives. These relationships evolved as nurses shared special times with children by sitting, listening, or being present during the child's vulnerable moments.

Totka (1996) also reported intense relationships between nurses and children who were dying. This theme represented some of the most significant stories in pediatric nurses' practices. She found that a child's death did more than affect the nurse emotionally; it actually transformed that nurse's practice. "Establishing a relationship with one who is dying is a privileged experience" (Stanley, 2000, p. 36). Talking about hopes and fears requires trust, and trust develops through getting to know each other. The connected relationship affords this important opportunity.

Home Care

Although a team of professionals is involved when a child receives home health-care services, families report that the single most important part of successful home care is the nursing staff (Creasser, 1996). Nurses come into the home as strangers and intrude into intimate family relationships that have been cultivated over years (Coffman, 1997; Petit de Mange, 1998). It is often difficult for the family and the nurse to set and maintain boundaries. In the words of a mother who has had home care services for her medically fragile child at home for over 10 years:

> Nurses can be in the home for long periods of time. This makes it difficult to remember they are not family or personal friends. They are professionals paid to take care of the child. It is not her role to baby sit with other children, clean the house, do laundry, pay bills, or criticize the family's lifestyle—unless that lifestyle affects the child's care. (Creasser, 1996, p. 42)

The home care nurse is exposed to private family conversations and interactions (Baptiste, 1996). Sometimes a nurse may be with the family for years. He or she may become the family's confidante or vice versa. The nurse may feel like both a "guest" and a "professional." Families, justifiably, may feel ambivalent about the nurse, for although they need the service the nurse provides, they also see the nurse as the cause of their loss of privacy.

Not only boundary but also authority issues can become a source of tension between parents and professionals. Wegener (1996) recommended that families establish "house rules" or guidelines with which they are comfortable: "These rules would then frame, from the beginning, the working relationship between the family, nurses, and nursing agency" (p. 21).

Negotiating Relationships

Morse (1991) described the process patients and nurses use to negotiate a relationship. The degree of intensity in the negotiation depends upon the patient's perception of the seriousness of the situation and his or her feeling of vulnerability and dependence. The patient first evaluates whether the nurse is a good person, asking questions such as "Are you from around here?" "Are you married?" and "Do you have children?" From there, he or she tries to determine whether the nurse is a good nurse by asking, "Do you like nursing?" "Have you been a nurse long?" and asking other patients for references ("Is she good?"). When satisfied with the answers, the patient may then make some overtures toward the nurse (e.g., waving as the nurse passes; calling the nurse by name) so that he or she will willingly become involved.

While the patient is assessing the nurse, the nurse is assessing the patient, looking for a "personality click." Different from the nursing assessment, the nurse evaluates the patient's personal needs and support system, assesses the patient as a person, and consciously chooses whether to make an emotional investment in the patient or just do his or her job (Morse, 1991).

Power

Within the relationship, both the professional and the patient have power (see Table 12.3; Sully, 1996). The way in which professionals and patients interact depends in part on how they use their power. For example, professionals can assert their superior knowl-

Table 12.3

Issues of Powerfulness and Powerlessness of Patients and Professionals		
Variable	**Patients**	**Professionals**
Powerful	Are central figures and focus in health-care system	Have specialist knowledge
	Can be more or less cooperative	Speak a specialist jargon that patients may not understand
	Can have crises that demand immediate attention	Control access to tests and treatments
	Have rights and can complain if rights are violated	Often require appointments
	Professionals' sense of success or failure tied to condition of patients	Familiar with the health-care system
		Can close ranks to protect one another in the face of a patient's complaint
Powerless	Access to health-care professionals is often controlled	Must obey protocols and may feel they have little personal discretion
	May not understand the health-care system and have difficulty using it	Usually cannot choose whether to treat a particular patient
	May be in a weakened state because of medical condition	Cannot relax vigilance because mistakes can have fatal consequences
	May fear serious illness or death	Constantly exposed to suffering and distress

Note. Adapted from "The Impact of Power in Therapeutic Relationships," by P. Sully, 1996, *Nursing Times, 92*(41), pp. 40–41.

edge by using jargon, or they can attempt to use language patients can understand. Patients can be constantly demanding, or they can limit their requests to only the most urgent ones at busy times.

Professionals can examine their motives about their involvement with patients and families and determine whether these behaviors are empowering or paternalistic. Table 12.4 provides a guide. Once individuals have insight into their behavioral tendencies, they can be helped in making changes in their interactions with children and families (Rushton, Armstrong, & McEnhill, 1996).

Power also can be asserted subtly (Ray, 1997). For example, *time* is a power issue. In any relationship, the person who controls the clock has more power. In a job interview, for instance, it is permissible for the employer to be late but not the job applicant. Parents, not children, ultimately are the ones to decide how family time is spent (e.g., bedtimes, holidays, doctors' appointments). Bosses determine the time of the meeting, not the employees. Time has special meaning for people who are dying. One moment, time seemed more or less infinite; suddenly, this is no longer the case, which can result in intense feelings of powerlessness.

Health-care professionals who demonstrate that they respect and value the child's and family's time can do much to equalize this balance of power and improve patient–family–professional relationships. Some methods include offering appointment times that are convenient for families, continually updating the family and offering apologies when there are unexpected delays, and providing pagers or noting mobile phone

Table 12.4

Characteristics of Paternalistic and Empowering Behaviors	
Paternalistic Behavior	**Empowering Behavior**
• Assumes needs of the patient and family without verification or mutual goal setting • Replaces or subverts primary relationships • Fosters dependency; projects own needs onto the patient and family • Undermines confidence by conveying that parents are incapable of acting on their child's behalf • Limits choices and opportunities for autonomous decision-making • Sabotages efforts of treatment team	• Provides specific caregiving interventions based on a plan of care that is developed with the patient and family • Supports and recognizes primary relationships • Supports the autonomy of parents; assumes that parents have the capacity to act as their child's primary advocate • Supports parents and patients to act on their own behalf; conveys support and affirms abilities • Helps reveal and explore the full range of options and choices pertinent to decisions • Collaborates with the treatment team to achieve goals

Note. From "Establishing Therapeutic Boundaries as Patient Advocates," by C. Rushton, L. Armstrong, and M. McEnhill, 1996, *Pediatric Nursing, 22*(3), p. 188. Copyright 1996 by Jannetti. Adapted with permission.

numbers for families to allow them the freedom to move about while waiting for appointments, treatments, tests, or doctors to make hospital rounds. Health-care professionals can be flexible with regard to changing plans. When a child is dying, the features of a connected relationship—breaking the rules, going the extra mile—can be put into play to accommodate the child's and family's wishes about how they wish to spend their time.

Touch also has power implications. The person with more power touches the other person more often (Ray, 1997). For example, teachers pat their students on the shoulder, yet a student returning this gesture likely would be considered disrespectful. A manager may congratulate an employee with a hearty pat on the back, but the employee patting the boss on the back likely would be considered forward. In an effective parent–professional partnership, both partners are equals. The professional who overuses touch in this manner may be perceived as condescending and may threaten this balance.

Height, or looking down on someone, has power implications. Although much that professionals do in health-care settings must be done from above, there are still opportunities to get down on the child's level or sit by a parent with one's face looking up rather than down at the individual. The *chin* is the most powerful part of the body (Ray, 1997). When the chin is in the air, the person appears superior, condescending, or confrontational.

The use of *space* is another power consideration. Individuals who take up a lot of space are more powerful. Using big gestures, wide movements, arms akimbo or on the hips all send messages of power. Also, any sort of *pointer* or extension held in the hand, such as a pen or eyeglasses, operates as a symbol of authority. This reflects back to the days when parents or teachers shook their fingers at us (Ray, 1997).

Power shifts somewhat when the health-care setting is the home. In a study on negotiating lay and professional roles in the care of children with complex health-care needs, Kirk (2001) found that being on home territory, and in possession of expertise in caregiving and in managing encounters with professionals, provided parents with a sense of control with which to enter negotiations with professionals. Kirk issued a caution regarding the importance of not letting changes in the balance of power lead to the development of parent–professional relationships that are characterized by conflict rather than partnership.

Boundaries

Within every relationship there are boundaries. Boundaries serve to help people take care of themselves and prevent abuses. The intense nature of relationships that professionals develop with children and their families may result in unclear boundaries. When professionals are either overinvolved or underinvolved, boundaries are ambiguous. Sheldon and Foust (2014) point out that a shared understanding between the professional, child, and family of expectations ensures that the role of each remains clear. Responsibility for implementing and maintaining professional boundaries belongs explicitly to the professional (Roberts et al., 2015)

Boundary Violations

Professionals typically enter relationships with children and families with professional boundaries intact. However, in time, the relationship may begin to meet the professional's need for love, acceptance, meaningful relationships, affiliation, and regard by others (Pennington, Gafner, Schilit, & Bechtel, 1993). Because boundary violations often begin subtly, professionals frequently do not know that they have "crossed the line" until after the fact (Totka, 1996). The following behaviors can alert the professional to boundary problems (Willis-Brandon, 1990):

- Exaggerated feelings of shame, guilt, or inadequacy;
- Seeing oneself as a victim;
- An exaggerated sense of responsibility for things beyond one's control;
- Setting unrealistic expectations of oneself or others;
- Inability to tolerate differences in approach or human error;
- Avoiding conflict and confrontation;
- Giving help when it is not needed or requested; and
- Putting the needs of others above personal needs.

Rushton and colleagues (1996) recommended using mechanisms such as personal inventory questionnaires regarding professional boundaries, simulations of common clinical situations where boundary violations are possible, role-playings, and team strategy sessions.

Policy Statement for Pediatricians

In 2009, the American Academy of Pediatrics (AAP) issued a policy statement on appropriate boundaries in the pediatrician–family–patient relationship (AAP, 2009). Topics the document addresses include romantic and sexual relationships, inadvertent sexuality in the physician–patient relationship, and gifts or other expressions of affection or gratitude. Although the policy statement was intended for pediatricians, most of the issues discussed are faced by other health-care professionals as well.

Reliable data on the prevalence of sexual contact between physicians and their patients or their patients' family members is difficult to find. The AAP (2009) pointed out that interpersonal entanglements raise at least two serious questions: (a) Can a patient or family member make clear and free choices to accept or reject affections, especially sexual, in the context of the unavoidably unequal physician–patient–family relationship? and (b) Once such intimacy develops, can the parties maintain a proper and effective therapeutic relationship?

Some professionals may feel sexually attracted to children, which may put children at risk of sexual abuse or exploitation. But the more likely situation is a misunderstanding during routine discussions and examinations (Silber, 1994). For example, pediatricians, nurses, and other professionals may be misunderstood when they first discuss sexual maturation and sexuality with patients. Similarly, examining an adolescent's maturing genitals or breasts may be distressing or misunderstood, especially without the presence of a parent or other adult. Some kinds of touching may be confusing or offensive to children, depending on their stage of physical and emotional maturation. Words, body language, and other aspects of professional conduct may inadvertently offend or insult patients and family members, such as the use of endearments like *honey* or *dear* (AAP, 2009).

Conducting anticipatory discussions before a physical examination is performed can reduce fears and misunderstandings and lead to enhanced professional, child, and family comfort. Issues of concern can be clarified. For example, children may have a strong preference regarding whether a male or female performs their exam, and whether they would like someone else present.

Needless to say, romantic or sexual relationships with children and youth are always inappropriate. However, romantic or sexual relationships with adult family members of patients should also be avoided given the potential for adverse effects on professional judgment and family member behavior concerning the patient's health (AAP, 2009). Further, children should not have to be concerned about confidentiality or have anxiety over the potential for the professional to have a conflict of loyalty because of his or her involvement with a parent.

Gifts or other expressions of gratitude can be a concern. The AAP recommendations state that it may be appropriate to accept modest gifts from patients and their families. However, when the physician feels uncomfortable accepting a gift, he or she may want to suggest alternatives such as a charitable donation in the physician's name.

Models

Today, most institutions have rules and policies that establish clear boundaries in certain areas about what professionals can and cannot do. However, many boundary issues are not simply black and white but fall into the gray zone. Perhaps what is more helpful is a process to help professionals sort out boundary issues. The Rainbow Babies and Children's Hospital in Cleveland, Ohio, developed a therapeutic relations decision-making framework to (a) foster a proactive process of conscious deliberation regarding nurse–patient interactions and (b) afford a nonthreatening mechanism for retrospective review of apparently nontherapeutic relationships (McAliley et al., 1996). The framework is based on an "act utilitarian" approach to moral reasoning and promotes the clarification of personal philosophy and values.

The model encourages the nurse to contemplate the potential negative and positive outcomes of the interaction being examined within each of five contexts (McAliley et al., 1996):

- Philosophy and policy of the organization
- Impact on desired patient–family outcomes
- Developmental stage of the relationship
- Potential impact on other patients, family, and staff
- The nurse's philosophy and values regarding role and the nature of a therapeutic relationship

The Rainbow Therapeutic Relations Decision-Making Model has been used successfully in a variety of situations, some fairly complex. See Text Box 12.1: Overinvolvement?, and Text Box 12.2: Underinvolvement?, for examples.

The Department of Health (2012) in the United Kingdom offers the 6Cs (care, compassion, competence, communication, courage, and commitment) as a framework of values and behaviors to guide nurses in developing therapeutic relationship. The professional demonstrates consideration and respect for the child and family; provides information to ensure the child and family are empowered; empathizes; shows courage through advocacy by raising concerns when necessary; delivers competent, evidence-based care; and communicates with consideration of different needs relative to children's ages, development, and ability (Roberts et al., 2015).

Relationships Among Professionals

In recent years, under the constraints of cost-containment and with the rise of new technologies, shifts in division of labor have occurred among health-care professions. For example, nurse technicians are performing certain tasks that in the past only registered nurses were permitted to do. Physician Assistants and Nurse Practitioners are prescribing medications and assuming other functions previously performed only by physicians.

Among physicians, questions are being raised about which tasks actually require the knowledge of a physician, much less a specialist physician, and which could be delegated to less skilled, but far more manageable, paraprofessionals. Shifts in "who does what" can lead to confusion, turf issues, and tension. These factors must be considered alongside the normal conflicts that arise among professionals caring for children in health-care settings. Regarding the advent of Primary Care Groups in England, Richards, Carley, Jenkins-Clarke, and Richards (2000) believe that the most successful approach to address these anxieties is to establish more equitable and less hierarchical models of multiprofessional teamwork.

When speaking of relationships between professionals in health-care settings, usually the first relationship to come to mind is the nurse–doctor relationship. Less common in clinical practice in recent years is the "doctor–nurse game," a stereotypical

Text Box 12.1
Overinvolvement?

Co-primary nurses were contemplating becoming Big Sisters for a 10-year-old foster child who would continue to have periodic admissions to their unit. The head nurse manager (HNM) and clinical nurse specialist (CNS) had strong reservations about this. They were concerned that this interaction would interfere with the bonding process between the patient and her newly assigned (third) foster family. There was the potential that the nurses would not stick with the commitment very long (given that their work and family/social lives were already very full) and that this already traumatized child would experience their withdrawal as yet another rejection. It was also likely that other patients and families would hear about some of their adventures together. Although some might find the relationship laudable, others could view it as discriminatory. The nurses were not told that developing such a relationship was prohibited, but the Rainbow Framework was used to identify potential consequences and to help them examine their motives. The nurses chose to pursue the relationship. However, they reframed it for themselves and restructured it for the child involved, thus preventing most of the complications that had concerned the HNM and CNS.

Note. From "Therapeutic Relations Decision Making: The Rainbow Framework," by L. McAliley, S. Lambert, M. Ashenberg, and S. Dull, 1996, *Pediatric Nursing, 22*(3), p. 203. Copyright 1996 by Jannetti. Reprinted with permission.

Text Box 12.2
Underinvolvement?

A generally sensitive and skilled nurse made the comment to the CNS that she really enjoyed working with the failure-to-thrive patients when their parents were not present (as was frequently the case). She viewed the parents as uninvested and antagonistic and felt they just complicated care. Although she was adept at implementing behavioral feeding plans and getting the children to grow while in the hospital, she had lost sight of the fact that failure-to-thrive is usually a family problem. Hospital gains would not be maintained if parents were not made partners in care and if nothing changed for them. The most helpful domains in the Rainbow Framework for discussion with this nurse were "patient–family outcome goals" and "philosophy and values of the nurse." She could be helped to see that the greater need and professional challenge lay with the family rather than the child. Engaging and empowering the family would result in long-term effects and reflect more positively on the nurse and institution.

Note. From "Therapeutic Relations Decision Making: The Rainbow Framework," by L. McAliley, S. Lambert, M. Ashenberg, and S. Dull, 1996, *Pediatric Nursing, 22*(3), p. 203. Copyright 1996 by Jannetti. Reprinted with permission.

pattern of interactions, first described in the 1960s, in which (female) nurses showed initiative and offered advice while appearing to defer passively to the doctor's authority (Sweet & Norman, 1995). What remains, however, is each profession continuing to have ideal expectations of the other, which inevitably fall short as a result of differing views about the qualities to be valued.

The doctor–nurse relationship traditionally has been a man–woman relationship. The relationship often has been described as a dominant–subservient relationship with a clear understanding that the doctor is a man and the nurse is a woman. However, in recent years the number of women studying medicine has increased. Gjerberg and Kjolsrod (2001) investigated what happens to the doctor–nurse relationship when both the doctor and the nurse are women. They reported that female doctors often find that they are met with less respect and confidence and are given less help than their male colleagues. The female doctors attribute this behavior in part to the nurse's desire to reduce status differences between the two groups. In response to this difference in treatment, female doctors in this study indicated that they do as much as possible themselves and attempt to make friends with the nurses.

English (1997) reported an increased emphasis for the team approach in which doctors, nurses, and other health workers adapt and develop new skills. Although the team approach to the delivery of health care has always been important, it has become more so as the boundaries between professional groups have become blurred:

> Doctors and nurses are becoming managers; nurses are taking on jobs previously done by doctors; support workers are taking over jobs done by nurses; and similarly, technicians, physiotherapists, and radiographers are all taking on tasks previously done by others . . . unless there is dialogue and trust between the groups, one or more of them are likely to feel threatened as their roles are changed. (English, 1997)

The way in which team members interact has implication for quality of care. Riskin et al. (2015) explored the impact of rudeness on medical team performance, pointing out that hospital-based medical teams routinely experience rudeness. In a randomized trial with 24 NICU teams participating in a training simulation, they found that rudeness had adverse consequences on diagnostic and procedural performance by team members. They also reported that information-sharing mediated the adverse effect of rudeness on diagnostic performance, and help-seeking mediated the effect of rudeness on procedural performance.

The call throughout health care is the need for collaboration. Lockhart-Wood (2000) proposed that a number of characteristics are significant in influencing the collaborative process: (a) excellent communication skills, (b) respect for the value of colleagues' roles, (c) the ability to share points of view, and (d) trust.

Mutual respect for a profession's unique perspective and for an individual's unique strengths provide the basis for the trust needed for effective and rewarding working relationships between members of the child's health-care team (see Figure 12.3). Finding ways to better understand each other is the path to mutual respect. One way in which professionals may come to understand each other is through receiving some of their training together and understanding more of each others' roles from the start of professional training.

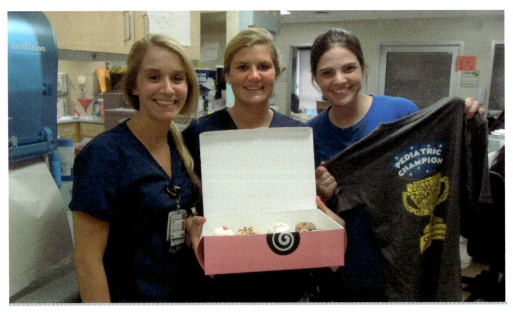

Figure 12.3. Each month, child life specialists honor the Nurse of the Month, a nurse who has gone above and beyond in providing psychosocial support for children. *Note.* Photo courtesy of Jessica Uze.

Little can be achieved in isolation. To make a significant difference in improving the quality of health care for children, members of the health care team and their representative organizations must learn to work together. Too much is at stake to do otherwise.

Conclusion

Caring, in terms of health care, is something special. It is a process, a way of relating to someone; it needs to develop in the same way that a friendship emerges over time (Castledine, 1998). Quality health care for children depends on caring individuals working well together. Establishing and maintaining effective relationships between professionals and the children and families they serve, as well as between the professionals themselves, are key.

Study Guide

1. Discuss what relationships are, how they vary, and how and why they have changed in health-care settings.

2. How do nurses' relationships with children in the health-care system differ from those of doctors, child life specialists, and other health-care providers? What factors have influenced changes in these relationships?

3. Compare and contrast the four types of mutual relationships.

4. How does nature of the illness or type of care required affect the type of relationship?

5. What are some of the sources of tension between parents and health-care providers, and how might they be addressed?

6. Describe power and empowerment in human relationships and their importance for children and their families in health care.

7. Boundaries exist in human relationships; explain boundaries, and describe healthy boundaries in child health-care relationships.

8. Are there professional and institutional policies that affect professional relationships? Describe.

9. Relationships *among* professionals also are critical to optimal health care for children with special needs. Describe *optimal* relationships for today's health-care system and children's needs.

10. Caring affects children's psychosocial development as well as their physical health. Summarize the major relationship factors that influence children's recovery, maintenance, and quality of life.

#14266

References

Allenbach, A., & Steinmiller, E. (2004). Waiting together: Translating the principles of therapeutic relationships one step further. *Journal for Specialists in Pediatric Nursing, 9*(1), 24–31.

American Academy of Pediatrics (AAP). (2009). Pediatrician–family–patient relationships: Managing the boundaries. *Pediatrics, 124*(6), 1685–1688.

Baptiste, G. (1996). A nursing perspective. In K. Gunter & R. Manago (Eds.), *Beyond discharge: Interdisciplinary perspectives for transitioning children with complex medical needs from hospital to home* (pp. 15–18). Bethesda, MD: Association for the Care of Children's Health.

Bombi, A., Pinto, G., & Cannoni, E. (2007). *Pictorial Assessment of Interpersonal Relationships (PAIR).* Firenze, Italy: Firenze University Press.

Castledine, G. (1998). The relationship between caring and nursing. *British Journal of Nursing, 7*(14), 866.

Coffman, S. (1997). Home-care nurses as strangers in the family. *Western Journal of Nursing Research, 19*(1), 82–96.

Corsano, P., Majorano, M., Vignola, V., Cardinale, E., Izzi, G.., & Nuzzo, M. (2012). Hospitalized children's representations of their relationship with nurse and doctors. *Journal of Child Health Care, 17*(3), 1–11.

Creasser, C. (1996). A family perspective. In K. Gunter & R. Manago (Eds.), *Beyond discharge: Interdisciplinary perspectives for transitioning children with complex medical needs from hospital to home* (pp. 39–44). Bethesda, MD: Association for the Care of Children's Health.

Davies, B., Clarke, D., Connaughty, S., Cook, K., MacKenzie, B., McCormick, J., ... Stutzer, C. (1996). Caring for dying children: Nurses' experiences. *Pediatric Nursing, 22*(6), 500–507.

Department of Health. (2012). *Compassion in practice: Nursing midwifery and care staff, our vision and strategy.* London, UK: Department of Health.

English, T. (1997). Personal paper: Medicine in the 1990s needs a team approach. *British Medical Journal, 314*(7081), 661–663.

Ersser, S. (1991). A search for the therapeutic dimensions of nurse–patient interaction. In R. McMahon & A. Pearson (Eds.), *Nursing as therapy* (pp. 43–84). London, UK: Chapman & Hall.

Ersser, S. (1998). The presentation of the nurse: A neglected dimension of therapeutic nurse–patient interaction? In R. McMahon, & A. Pearson (Eds.), *Nursing as therapy* (2nd ed., pp. 37–63). London, UK: Thornes.

Forster, J. (1998). Remember when . . . doctors were doctors, not "providers"? *Medical Economics, 75*(13), 125–126. Retrieved July 31, 2001, from www.findarticles.com

Gjerberg, E., & Kjolsrod, L. (2001). The doctor–nurse relationship: How easy is it to be a female doctor cooperating with a female nurse? *Social Science Medicine, 52*(2), 189–202.

Gow, K. (1982). *How nurses' emotions affect patient care.* New York, NY: Springer Publishing.

Holoweiko, M. (1998). Here's looking at: doctor–patient relations. Good news—the pedestal is gone. *Medical Economics, 75*(20), 54–56, 63, 67.

Hughes, J. (1994). *Organization and information at the bedside.* Unpublished doctoral dissertation, University of Chicago.

Kirk, S. (2001). Negotiating lay and professional roles in the care of children with complex health care needs. *Journal of Advanced Nursing, 34*(5), 593–602.

La Puma, J. (1996, January). Does the doctor–patient relationship mean more to doctors than patients? [Electronic version]. *Managed Care.* Retrieved March 2003, from www.managed caremag.com/archives/9601/MC9601.ethics.shtml

Lockhart-Wood, K. (2000). Collaboration between nurses and doctors in clinical practice. *British Journal of Nursing, 9*(5), 276–280.

Macleod Clark, J. (1982). *Nurse–patient verbal interaction: An analysis of recorded conversations on selected surgical wards.* Unpublished PhD thesis, University of London.

May, C. (1991). Affective neutrality and involvement in nurse–patient relationship: Perceptions of appropriate behaviour among nurses in acute medical and surgical wards. *Journal of Advanced Nursing, 16,* 555–558.

McAliley, L., Lambert, S., Ashenberg, M., & Dull, S. (1996). Therapeutic relations decision making: The rainbow framework. *Pediatric Nursing, 22*(3), 199–203, 210.

McCabe, C. (2004). Nurse–patient communication: An exploration of patients' experiences. *Journal of Clinical Nursing, 13*(1), 41–49.

Morse, J. M. (1991). Negotiating commitment and involvement in the nurse–patient relationship. *Journal of Advanced Nursing, 16,* 455–468.

Pearson, A., Vaughan, B., & Fitzgerald, M. (1996). *Nursing models for practice* (2nd ed.). Oxford, England: Butterworth Heinemann.

Pennington, S., Gafner, G., Schilit, R., & Bechtel, B. (1993). Addressing ethical boundaries among nurses. *Nursing Management, 24*(6), 36–39.

Petit de Mange, E. (1998). Pediatric considerations in homecare. *Critical Care Nursing Clinics of North America, 10*(3), 3339–3346.

Ray, M. (1997). *I'm here to help.* New York, NY: Bantam Books.

Reynolds, K., Cowden, J., Brosco, J., & Lantos, J. (2015). When a family requests a white doctor. *Pediatrics, 136*(2), 381–386.

Richards, A., Carley, J., Jenkins-Clarke, S., & Richards, D. (2000). Skill mix between nurses and doctors working in primary care—delegation or allocation: A review of the literature. *International Journal of Nursing Studies, 37*(3), 185–197.

Riskin, A., Erez, A., Foulk, T., Kugelman, A., Gover, A., Shoris, I., . . . Bamberger, P. (2015). The impact of rudeness on medical team performance: A randomized trial. *Pediatrics, 136*(3), 487–495.

Roberts, J., Fenton, G., & Barnard, M. (2015). Developing effective therapeutic relationships with children, young people and their families. *Nursing Children and Young People, 27*(4), 30–35.

Rollins, J. (2009). What a hospital should be. In W. Turgeon (Ed.), *Creativity and the child: Interdisciplinary perspectives* (pp. 201–211). Oxford, England: Inter-Disciplinary Press.

Rushton, C., Armstrong, L., & McEnhill, M. (1996). Establishing therapeutic boundaries as patient advocates. *Pediatric Nursing, 22*(3), 185–189.

Savage, J. (1990). The theory and practice of the "New Nursing." *Nursing Times, 86,* 42–45.

Savage, J. (1995). *Nursing intimacy: An ethnographic approach to nurse patient interaction.* London, UK: Scutari Press.

Sheldon, L., & Foust, J. (2014). *Communication for nurses, talking with patients* (3rd ed.). Boston, MA: Jones Bartlett Education.

Silber, T. (1994). False allegations of sexual touching by physicians in the practice of pediatrics. *Pediatrics, 94,* 742–745.

Stanley, K. (2000). Silence is not golden: Conversations with the dying. *Clinical Journal of Oncology Nursing, 4*(1), 34–40.

Stein-Parbury, J. (1993). *Patient and person.* Melbourne, Australia: Churchill Livingstone.

Sully, P. (1996). The impact of power in therapeutic relationships. *Nursing Times, 92*(41), 40–41.

Swanson, K. (1991). Empirical development of a middle range theory of caring. *Nursing Research, 40,* 161–166.

Sweet, S., & Norman, I. (1995). The nurse–doctor relationship: A selective literature review. *Journal of Advanced Nursing, 22*(1), 165–170.

Totka, J. (1996). Exploring the boundaries of pediatric practice: Nurse stories related to relationships. *Pediatric Nursing, 22*(3), 191–196.

Wegener, D. (1996). A social work perspective. In K. Gunter & R. Manago (Eds.), *Beyond discharge: Interdisciplinary perspectives for transitioning children with complex medical needs from hospital to home* (pp. 19–24). Bethesda, MD: Association for the Care of Children's Health.

Williams, A. (2001). A literature review on the concept of intimacy in nursing. *Journal of Advanced Nursing, 33*(5), 660–667.

Willis-Brandon, C. (1990). *Learning to say no: Establishing healthy boundaries.* Deerfield Beach, FL: Health Communications.

Wilson, S., Morse, J., & Penrod, J. (1998). Developing reciprocal trust in the caregiving relationship. *Qualitative Health Research, 8*(4), 446–465.

13

Promoting Children's Well-Being in the Community

Judy A. Rollins and Carmel C. Mahan

Objectives

At the conclusion of this chapter, the reader will be able to:
1. Define the concept of well-being.
2. Analyze four theoretical perspectives related to well-being.
3. List three advantages of home health care for children.
4. Discuss the role of education services in meeting children's psychosocial and developmental needs.
5. Describe the role of a change agent.

With the Healthy People 2020 initiative came a new conceptual framework: health-related quality of life and well-being (HRQoL), a multidimensional measure that encompasses physical, mental, emotional, and social functioning (HealthyPeople.gov, 2016). HRQoL goes beyond statistical measures to focus on how health status affects quality of life.

Related to quality of life is the concept of well-being, which assesses the positive aspects of a person's life, such as positive emotions and life satisfaction. Kobau, Sniezek, Zack, Lucas, and Burns (2010) define well-being as a relative state where one maximizes his or her physical, mental, and social functioning in the context of supportive environments to live a full, satisfying, and productive life. People generally agree that at minimum, well-being includes the presence of positive emotions and moods (e.g., contentment, happiness), the absence of negative emotions (e.g., depression, anxiety), satisfaction with life, fulfillment, and positive functioning (Centers for Disease Control and Prevention [CDC], 2013a). In simpler terms, well-being is thought to have three aspects: physical, social, and mental.

This chapter explores children's well-being within the context of community. With few exceptions, children—even those with complex medical needs—live their lives within the broader community, not within health-care institutions. During the past several decades, changes in pediatric health-care policy, practice, and reimbursement have caused a shift away from inpatient care toward more accessible community-based care. Although there will always be a place for specialized inpatient care for critically ill or injured children, community-based services have proliferated to meet these changing needs. This has led to the development and expansion of a variety of community-based health-care settings, such as outpatient surgery centers, freestanding urgent-care centers, urgent clinics in pharmacies, and other options. Home-care options have expanded, and the role of school nursing offices has likewise expanded to meet the increasingly complex health-care needs of children at school and at home.

This chapter begins with an overview of theoretical perspectives on well-being. We next review home health care and then describe the role of educational services in children's health care. A discussion of selected family circumstances and other issues that have implications for children's well-being follows.

Health encompasses more than a child's physical health. Good mental health is a vital part of good health. In fact, all health is tied to emotional and behavioral health: Emotional and behavioral problems directly predict or influence the course of major nonpsychiatric medical conditions (Hudziak & Ivanova, 2016). Because nearly 20% of American children have some form of mental disorder (CDC, 2013b), a separate section on mental illness and substance abuse prevention is presented. The chapter concludes with information about the role of a change agent.

Theoretical Perspectives

Four theoretical perspectives that examine the factors affecting child and family well-being are (1) the bioecological systems model, (2) social determinants of health, (3) adverse childhood experiences, and (4) trauma-informed care.

Bioecological Systems Model

A family does not exist in isolation. Families are situated in larger contexts, such as the community and the broader societal network. White and Klein (2008) explained that a bioecological model focuses on these contexts, placing emphasis on how individuals and families adapt to changing conditions. Key assumptions include the following (Hanson, 2013, p. 50):

1. Individuals and groups are both biological and social in nature.
2. Humans depend on their environment for survival.
3. Humans are social in nature and depend on others.
4. Human life is finite and time can be seen as both a constraint and a resource.
5. Interactions are spatially organized.
6. Human interaction can be understood at different levels—both at the population level and at the level of the individual.

Bronfenbrenner (1979) viewed the family as one component or ecosystem within the ecological systems. Bronfenbrenner's framework places families in the broader context of the ecosystems and social environment within which they must interact. This concept is especially relevant for understanding families with children with disabilities by describing the range of influences and the interaction of systems over time (Hanson, 2013).

The ecological environment can be pictured as a nested set of structures or systems that interact with each other (see Figure 13.1) (Bronfenbrenner, 1979). Bronfenbrenner

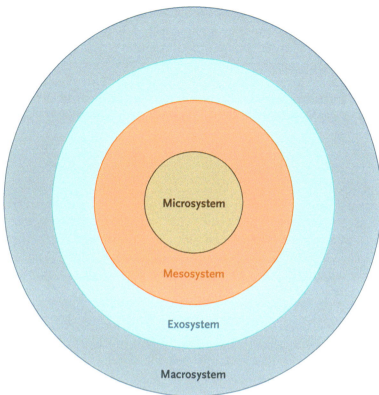

Microsystem
Pattern of activities, roles, and interpersonal relations the developing person experiences in a given setting with particular physical andmaterial characteristic
- Family
- Child care environments
- Early education programs

Mesosystem
Interrelationships among the microsystems; the immediate systems with which families and children may interact
- Between home and child care program
- Between home and school
- Between home and hospital

Exosystem
One or more settings in which the developing person is not an active participant, but in which events occur that affect or are affected by what happens in that developing person's setting
- Policies of the child care and education programs and institutions
- Neighborhoods
- Families' social networks
- Parents' employers and employment policies

Macrosystem
Societal and cultural beliefs and values that serve to shape and influence the lower order systems
- Societal and cultural views on childrearing patterns, early education, the meaning of disability
- Health and education intervention philosophies and policies

Figure 13.1. Ecological systems framework. *Note.* Adapted from *The Ecology of Human Development,* by U. Bronfenbrenner, 1979, Cambridge, MA: Harvard University Press; "Families in Context: Conceptual Frameworks for Understanding and Supporting Families," by M. Hanson, 2013, in M. Hanson and E. Lynch (Eds.), *Understanding Families: Supportive Approaches to Diversity, Disability, and Risk* (2nd ed., pp. 43–71), Baltimore, MD: Paul H. Brookes.

expanded the model (1999) to describe the effect of the individual's personal characteristics and the influence of time on development. The time variable considers both the timing of an event and the cumulative effects of an event over time on development. Although the family remains the prime context of development, viewing families through the lens of the bioecological systems framework allows for an examination of the multiple and interconnected influences on the family (Hanson, 2013). Thinking of families as systems embedded in larger ecological systems may yield critical intervention points and opportunities to reinforce and enhance clinical treatment.

Social Determinants of Health

For the past two decades, the health-care community has increasingly recognized that health is not just a medical problem and today formally acknowledges and addresses the social determinants of health: the factors apart from medical care that can be influenced by social policies and can shape health in powerful ways. Social determinants of health are the conditions in which people are born, grow, live, work, and age (World Health Organization, 2011).

Braveman and Gottlieb (2014) spoke of the causal relationships that have been established between social and socioeconomic factors and many health outcomes. For example, we know that asthma can be exacerbated by exposure to pollution and allergens, which are more common in disadvantaged neighborhoods. Rosenberg (2014) explains how social determinants may apply:

> A medical mystery: A child lands in the hospital with asthma. The doctor prescribes medicines. The child uses them properly. Yet, 2 months later, she is back in the hospital. Maybe the problem is that the child lives alongside mold, insects, and rats. That child doesn't need a doctor—she needs a lawyer, who can persuade, or threaten, the landlord to clean it up.

Medical–Legal Partnerships

As with the case of the child with asthma described above, many social determinants are legal in nature. A legal need is an adverse social condition with legal remedies that reside in regulations, laws, or policies. According to Sandel et al. (2010), low-income households on average have 1 to 3 unmet civil legal needs related to income, housing problems, employment, and family issues, and fewer than 1 in 5 legal problems of low-income households are addressed with help from a private or legal aid lawyer. When families do not receive the benefit of laws intended to address social determinants of health, such as income supports and insurance, housing and utilities, employment and education, legal status, and family stability, health care is undermined.

To meet this need, a growing number of health-care institutions are forming medical–legal partnerships, bringing legal resources on board to help families. According to the National Center for Medical-Legal Partnership (2016) (see Appendix 13.1: Resources), medical-legal partnerships have been established in 294 health institutions in 41 states. Core components of the partnerships designed to improve health include providing legal advice and assistance, improving health-care systems, and promoting change outside the system (Sandel et al., 2010). For an example of a medical–legal partnership success story, see Case Study 13.1.

🐻 Case Study 13.1

Child HeLP: A Successful Medical–Legal Partnership

The actions of medical–legal partnerships have made differences in the lives of children and their health. For example, the Cincinnati Child Health-Law Partnership (Child HeLP) in Cincinnati, Ohio, identified a pattern of referrals for poor-quality housing from patients living within 19 building complexes owned by a common firm (Beck et al., 2012). The first case in the fall of 2009 involved a mother with two children who were cared for at a Cincinnati Children's Hospital pediatric primary-care center. Both children had a previous diagnosis of asthma, and one was newly diagnosed with an elevated lead level. During a well-child care visit, the family reported a pest infestation, peeling paint, and water leakages, and was referred to Child HeLP.

In May of the following year, a physician referred the family of another child with asthma to Child HeLP:

> The child's mother described the presence of mold. She also presented a letter from her landlord stating that she would be evicted if she installed an air-conditioning unit in her child's bedroom. Three similar referrals were made in the 6 weeks that followed. Early in July 2010, Child HeLP staff recognized that these and other recent referrals all originated from families living in buildings owned and managed by a single out-of-town developer. (Beck et al., 2012, p. 833)

Attorneys worked with families to pursue a legal strategy appropriate to their social and environmental situation. As a result of Child HeLP's efforts, of the 14 case units for which outcome data were available, repairs and abatements were completed in 10, and six families were relocated to a safer code-compliant apartment. Four building complexes received complex-wide mold removal, pest abatement, and window repairs. The Legal Aid Society of Greater Cincinnati helped families form tenant associations, and as a result, 11 of the 19 complexes received significant systemic repairs (e.g., installation of new roofs, ceilings, and drywall; integrated pest management; replacement of sewage systems; refurbishment of air-conditioning and ventilation systems; replacement of hallway lights; repair of playground equipment).

Note. From "Medical-Legal Partnerships: Making a Difference in Children's Healthcare," by J. Rollins, 2015, *Pediatric Nursing, 41*(1), p. 8.

Adverse Childhood Experiences

Childhood experiences, whether positive or negative, can have a tremendous impact on whether an individual becomes a victim or a perpetrator of violence as well as on lifelong health and opportunity. Adverse childhood experiences (ACEs) have been linked to risky health behaviors, chronic health conditions, low life potential, poor learning capacity, and early death. The risk for these outcomes increases as the number of ACEs increases (CDC, 2016).

In a landmark study, 9,508 adults who had completed a standardized medical evaluation at a large health maintenance organization (HMO) responded to a survey about

ACE. Seven categories were explored: psychological, physical, or sexual abuse; violence against mother; or living with household members who were substance abusers, mentally ill or suicidal, or ever imprisoned (Felitti et al., 1998). The number of these experiences was then compared to measures of adult risk behavior, health status, and disease. Compared with respondents who had no exposure to adverse childhood experiences, those who had experienced four or more categories of ACE, had a

- 4- to 12-fold increase in risk for alcoholism, drug abuse, depression, and suicide attempts;
- 2- to 4-fold increase in smoking, poor self-rated health, 50 or more sexual-intercourse partners, and sexually transmitted disease; and
- 1.4- to 1.6-fold increase in physical inactivity and severe obesity.

As children, 52% of respondents had experienced at least one ACE, 27% had experienced at least two, 14% had experienced three, and 7% had experienced four or more. There was also a graded relationship to the presence of adult disease, including ischemic heart disease, cancer, chronic lung disease, skeletal fractures, and liver disease.

In 2011, the American Academy of Pediatrics (AAP) issued a position statement referring to the impact of this "toxic stress" on children's brain development and called on the entire pediatric community to reduce external threats to healthy brain growth (AAP Committee on Psychosocial Aspects of Child and Family Health, 2012). Explained Jack P. Shonkoff, a physician and professor of child health and development, "When bad things happen early in life, the brain and other parts of the body don't forget" (Shonkoff in Kuehn, 2014, p. 585).

A growing number of promising strategies exist for preventing or reducing ACE by helping parents deal with the stress in their own lives so that they can deal with the stress in their children's lives. One strategy is working with a medical–legal partnership to recruit lawyers and law students to help families get access to resources (see example above). Another successful program is Health Leads, which puts college students and other volunteers into pediatric practices to help create compendiums of community-based resources for participant families. And a third, Nurse-Family Partnership, involves a visiting nurse program for vulnerable first-time mothers. For more information about these programs, see Appendix 13.1: Resources.

Trauma-Informed Care

Increasingly, health-care providers are recognizing that children and families with experiences of trauma are found in multiple service sectors, not just behavioral health. For example, the juvenile justice and child welfare systems reveal high rates of personal histories of trauma. Children frequently bring their experiences of trauma into the school systems, which often interferes with their school success. And regarding health care, many patients have significant trauma histories that can have adverse effects on their health and responsiveness to health interventions.

Further, often the systems intended to help are themselves trauma-inducing. Consider the following practices, for example:

- use of isolation and restraints in the behavioral health system,
- abrupt removal of a child from an abusing family in the child welfare system,

- use of invasive procedures in the medical system,
- harsh disciplinary practices in educational system/schools, and
- intimidating practices in the criminal justice system (Substance Abuse and Mental Health Services Administration [SAMHSA], 2014a).

SAMSA designed a framework that helps systems "talk" to each other, to understand better the connection between trauma and behavioral health issues and to guide systems to become trauma-informed (SAMHSA, 2014a). The framework is built on a concept of trauma that can be shared among practitioners, researchers, and trauma survivors:

> Individual trauma results from an event, series of events, or set of circumstances that is experienced by an individual as physically or emotionally harmful or life threatening and that has lasting adverse effects on the individual's functioning and mental, physical, social, emotional, or spiritual well-being. (SAMHSA, 2014a, p. 7)

Events and circumstances may be an actual or extreme threat of physical or psychological harm (e.g., natural disasters, violence) or severe life-threatening neglect of a child that imperils healthy development. This event or circumstance could be a single event or reoccurring. The individual's perception of the experience, which helps determine whether it is a traumatic event, may be linked to factors such as cultural beliefs, availability of social supports, or the individual's developmental stage. Adverse effects may occur immediately or have a delayed onset. Duration can be short to long term, and sometimes the individual does not connect the traumatic events and the effects. Examples of such effects include the inability to (a) cope with the normal stresses and strains of daily living, (b) form trusting relationships and benefit from them, (c) manage cognitive processes, (c) regulate behavior, or (d) control the expression of emotions.

A program, organization, or system that is trauma informed:

- realizes the widespread impact of trauma and understands potential paths for recovery;
- recognizes the signs and symptoms of trauma in clients, families, staff, and others involved in the system;
- responds by fully integrating knowledge about trauma into policies, procedures, and practices; and
- seeks to actively resist re-traumatization.

There are six key principles fundamental to a trauma-informed approach (see Text Box 13.1). Changes in multiple levels of an organization are required. Even for organizations where tending to trauma is not an aspect of how they do business, understanding the role of trauma and a trauma-informed approach may help in reaching the organization's goals and objectives. See Appendix 13.1: Resources for additional information on recognizing childhood trauma and implementing a trauma-informed approach.

Home Health Care

As the health-care environment changes, children with complex medical needs are frequently returning home to be cared for by in-home nursing staff, with increasing parental responsibility for care. Families who hope to return to some measure of normalcy after weeks or months in the hospital often welcome this trend. Yet it is not a trend without risks, as factors that affect both parents and siblings within the hospital may be exacerbated in the home environment. The ongoing responsibility of understanding the operation and functions of medical equipment without the backup of readily available professionals creates additional stress. Siblings may feel less recognized or supported because of the additional time devoted to the care of the ill child at home. They may also feel more conspicuous or different in the community and may be reluctant to have their peers visit.

For all of these reasons, planning for the transition from hospital to home is essential for every member of the family. While parents learn the responsibilities of home health care, attention needs to be given to sibling involvement and adjustment. The opportunity to anticipate changes and develop positive coping styles may be facilitated by child life specialists or other members of the health-care team. Ongoing opportunities to express feelings and concerns through creative activities, journaling, art, and music should be provided. Specific interventions may include a school visit by a health-care professional or peer preparation for the return of a child with complex medical needs. Creating a role for siblings in these specific interventions may be helpful, both in assessing siblings' understanding of the situation and in helping them master

---

Text Box 13.1
Six Key Principles Fundamental to a Trauma-Informed Approach

Safety—Staff and the people they serve feel physically and psychologically safe.

Trustworthiness and transparency—Operations and decisions are conducted with transparency with the goal of building and maintaining trust with clients, family members, and staff.

Peer support—Peers refers to individuals with lived experiences of trauma, or in the case of children, family members of children who have experienced traumatic events and are key caregivers in their recovery.

Collaboration and mutuality—Importance is placed on partnering and leveling power differences between staff and clients and among organizational staff, from housekeeping personnel to administrators.

Empowerment, voice, and choice—Individuals' strengths and experiences are recognized and built upon. Staff are facilitators of recovery rather than controllers of recovery.

Cultural, historical, and gender issues—The organization actively moves past cultural stereotypes and biases; offers access to gender responsive services; leverages the healing value of traditional cultural connections; incorporates policies, protocols, and processes that are responsive to individuals' racial, ethnic, and cultural needs; and recognizes and addresses historical trauma.

Note. From "SAMHSA's Concept of Trauma and Guidance for a Trauma-informed Approach" by Substance Abuse and Mental Health Services Administration, 2014. Rockville, MD: Author. Retrieved from http://store.samhsa.gov/shin/content//SMA14-4884/SMA14-4884.pdf

a challenging experience. As in most other aspects of the health-care experience, the inclusion of siblings as active participants rather than observers will facilitate positive coping. Special attention may be required over time, as the developmental needs and concerns of both the ill child and his or her healthy siblings may change significantly through each new developmental stage. Additional support for well siblings of a chronically ill child may include professional counseling and support-group involvement with peers in similar situations.

Recent programming developed for children with complex medical needs includes medical day-care settings where children's medical needs, therapies, and socialization are provided in a group setting. Staffed by a variety of health-care professionals, including developmental teachers; speech, physical, and occupational therapists; and child life specialists, these centers fill a unique role in allowing parents to work and maintain activities of daily living. Centers provide the children with an environment that emphasizes individual growth and development within an appropriate social setting rather than in the isolated environment of home. Outdoor play, field trips, and special events are possible with a staff of trained health-care professionals. Many children make extraordinary psychosocial and physical progress within this developmentally appropriate and engaging day-care setting. Because these facilities are most often located within or near hospitals, the challenges of frequent hospitalizations for these children may be more easily managed because of familiar staff and smoother transitions from one setting to another.

Education and Health Care

In 1975, the Education for All Handicapped Children Act (PL-94-142) was passed, mandating federal programs to provide special education services for children ages 5 to 21 years. In 1986, PL-99-457 expanded coverage to include services for infants, toddlers, and preschoolers, so that services could be provided from birth until age 21. Refinements continued over time that were eventually incorporated into the Individuals with Disabilities Education Act, reauthorized as PL-108-446 in 2004.

Each state was tasked with identifying a lead agency, such as the health department or school system, to manage coordination of services and ensure public awareness of the referral and eligibility criteria and processes, which differ from state to state. This has bearing on the current subject of community-based health care because nursing and related service providers, such as occupational and physical therapists and speech–language pathologists, are provided through the program. Pediatricians, hospitals, family members, day-care providers or social-service workers, or anyone who has a concern about a child's development, can make referrals to early intervention services. With the rising numbers of premature infants surviving at earlier postconceptional ages, many referrals come from NICUs or NICU follow-up clinics. Children may also be referred for genetic conditions, chronic illnesses, or physically disabling conditions. Children remain eligible until age 3 years, or until they meet the outcomes on their Individualized Family Service Plan. In Maryland and New Mexico, services have been expanded so that at age 3, parents can choose to remain with the Infant/Toddler Program or to transition to school-based services.

Child Find referral services are available if a child between the ages of 3 and 5 years is suspected of having a developmental delay or a need for habilitative services. Children found eligible for Child Find services receive school-based services through an Individualized Education Program, or IEP, as do children between the ages of 5 and 21 years.

Referring children who may have or be at risk for developmental delays can be one way to improve coordination of care among health care and other providers. Parents can consent for early intervention providers to communicate with a child's health-care providers, while the program provides families with local, sometimes home-based services that improve access, availability, and convenience of service provision for their children. Without the early intervention program, a pediatrician might refer a child for physical therapy, which would require the parents to transport the child to a facility, possibly pay for parking, wait for services, and then travel home. Through the Infant/Toddler Program, a physical therapist can come to the home to teach parents a variety of ways to support their child's development within the home environment. The families may also identify community settings at which to meet for services, depending on the goals. This approach allows greater flexibility and control for family members trying to manage a number of appointments for a child with medical and/or developmental needs. See Case Study 13.2 for an example of how the process might work.

As children reach school age, there is a transition from home-based to school-based educational and related services. The nursing office at school may now offer gastrostomy tube feedings, dressing changes, and flu shots in addition to administering daily medications and bandaging small injuries. The nurses, teachers, and aides see the children every day at school and get to know them very well. They can offer supports needed by individual children because of their familiarity with them and their parents. In addition, nurses are usually the school personnel with training for the automated external defibrillator (AED), and they are responsible for providing emergency care until an ambulance arrives in the event of sudden serious illness or injury.

Child life specialists, nurses, and others with knowledge of the child can often smooth the way for children's entry or re-entry into the school setting. A presentation to the child's class explaining the child's condition, what to expect, and how to help can demystify the experience for everyone. Children themselves are sometimes comfortable participating in the presentation. Presentations to siblings' classrooms may also prove helpful.

Selected Family Circumstances With Psychosocial Implications for Children's Well-Being

Circumstances for families can be positive or negative, usual or unusual, chosen or unwelcome. Family circumstances can change gradually or unexpectedly, and can have psychosocial implications for children and their families.

Military Families

There is a saying in the military community: When one member of a family serves, everyone serves. The military culture includes solid, sustaining values such as duty,

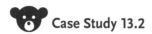 **Case Study 13.2**

Charles

Charles was referred to the Infant/Toddler (I/T) Program at the recommendation of his oncologist. He had been diagnosed with a glioblastoma of the posterior fossa at the age of 14 months, and had been treated with chemotherapy and surgery. The tumor had compressed his right auditory nerve, leaving him deaf in that ear. At age 21 months, Charles was evaluated and found to have delays in cognitive, receptive, and expressive language and fine and gross motor skills. His hearing loss had already been documented, and he soon had a hearing aid for the ear that still had some hearing. While waiting for his aid to come in, he was able to borrow one from the Maryland Hearing Aid Bank. He began to receive weekly therapy by a special educator, occupational therapist (OT), and physical therapist (PT). Speech and language therapy (SLT) was soon added. Charles progressed slowly, interrupted by frequent hospitalizations. His teacher, a child life specialist, helped Charles and his family develop positive coping strategies for his hospitalizations, and prepared them for surgeries and procedures. She also added medical play to his interventions to help him process his feelings about these encounters, and about his illness.

As he approached age 3, an audiologist and a teacher for the deaf met with the family, along with the I/T team in preparation for transition. At that time, he still received OT and SLT services, in addition to special instruction services. His immune system was still compromised, and his family was reluctant to place him in a school setting. For the sake of continuity, his I/T teacher applied to work for the Home and Hospital Instruction department and continued to see Charles at home, where he continued to received OT and SLT services. At age 4, Charles transitioned to a local school that had a high level of services for children with hearing impairment, including classes conducted in American Sign Language (ASL) and frequency modulation (FM) services that allowed him to hear the teacher without the interference of other sounds in the room. Throughout his participation in the program, Charles's pediatrician, neurosurgeon, and oncologist were regularly updated on his progress, with parental consent. The oncologist, in particular, maintained active communication with Charles's providers and family.

Charles had a sister born when he was 2.5 years old who was diagnosed with a moderate to severe hearing loss at age 4 months. Marie was immediately referred to the I/T Program. By the time services began, she had received her hearing aids. She received special instruction, picked up by Charles's provider at the family's request. The teacher did medical play and teaching around the issues of Marie's hearing aids as she began to resist using them. When Charles and Marie began to notice differences between themselves and other children, the teacher worked with the family, to help them understand that Charles and Marie were more like other children than they were different. When SLT services were added, Charles's provider again picked up services. One reason the I/T providers were allowed to stay with Charles after age 3 was because his sister was receiving services in the home. This was before extended eligibility rules went into effect. This family's story illustrates how different parts of complex systems can work together for the good of children and their families. Charles's mother was a strong advocate for her children throughout the process and was able to get the placement, services, and equipment they needed to succeed.

personal courage, service before self, honor, fortitude in facing adversity, optimism, love of and loyalty to country, community support, and a commitment to excellence (Blaisure, 2012).

We know many facts about military families. For example, today approximately 45% of active-duty service members are parents, compared to 15% during the Vietnam War (Boberiene & Hornback, 2014). The two-parent married family is the norm (Department of Defense, 2010). Members of the armed forces are more likely to be married than their civilian peers. A small percentage of these marriages, about 7%, are dual military, with both husband and wife serving. The average military family has two or three children; over half of these children are 7 years of age or younger.

Military children are part of a unique culture with distinct characteristics, which means that the children

- are typically geographically dislocated from extended family,
- are prone to frequent and prolonged separation from one or both parents because of military deployments,
- move every 2 to 4 years,
- will attend six to nine different schools before they are 18, and
- will move at least twice during their high school years (National Military Family Association, 2012).

Frequent moves disrupt social support networks, continuity of care, and established resources, which can cause disorder and the potential for family or child instability (Lester et al., 2010). The stress and constant change associated with deployments and repeated moves shape the culture of military family life. Relocating every 2 to 4 years might seem detrimental to military children. However, research indicates that frequent relocation is associated with improved coping, resilience, and fewer school problems (Weber & Weber, 2005). Also, Klein and Adelman (2008) reported that, overall, military adolescents are less prone to risky sexual and substance use behaviors than their civilian peers. Johnson and Ling (2013) cite possible reasons for this aversion to risk-taking to include access to (a) confidential services, (b) physical community shared by military families on and off military bases, (c) resilient peers, and (d) families with job security. Relocation has another benefit: Children have the opportunity to start over and re-create themselves while limiting the influence of destructive peer groups.

Military children may sometimes seem reserved or difficult to get to know because of the frequent moves and also because the reduction in military forces has led to smaller military communities and fewer military-based peer groups. Children living on or near base are immersed in the military culture and have immediate access to support systems and services. Children of parents in the National Guard and Reserves are often less fortunate: "They may be the only child in their school system to have a military parent and therefore lack an understanding support network" (Johnson & Ling, 2013, p. 196).

Circumstances of Extreme Stress

Military families are amazingly resilient despite the many changes associated with military life. Although most families are able to handle the everyday stresses associated with being a part of the military, three circumstances bring extreme stress and test the coping ability of even the most resilient families: *deployment*, *combat injury*, and *death*.

Deployment. Flake, Davis, Johnson, and Middleton (2009) reported that by 5 years of age, 40% of military children have been affected by deployment, the movement of an individual or a military group to accomplish a task or mission. Since 2002, more than 2 million children have been separated from their deployed mother or father (Boberiene & Hornback, 2014).

There are several models describing the deployment cycle, ranging from three to seven phases (Johnson & Ling, 2014). According to a basic model, deployment can be divided into three distinct phases:

1. *Predeployment:* Readying to deploy—training, preparation, packing
2. *Deployment:* Time away from home—actual movement to and time at the duty location
3. *Postdeployment:* Return from deployment—reintegrating with family and military unit, resting, recuperating to prepare for the next predeployment phase

Families have tasks to accomplish at each phase. In predeployment, families prepare for detachment and reorganization. Daily living, division of labor, and anticipation of reunion are the tasks of the deployment phase. Homecoming begins the postdeployment stage, with the important tasks of reunion, reintegration, and reorganization (Johnson & Ling, 2013).

During deployment, families with school-age children tend to stay in their current home, while 30%–50% of families relocate to the hometown of one of the parents for extended family support (Flake et al., 2009). The spouse or partner left behind may face myriad challenges, such as rumors, discrimination based on deployed spouse's rank, difficulty maintaining friendships, difficulty communicating with the deployed spouse, parenting difficulties, trouble with job or schooling, financial problems, meeting personal needs, asking for help when needed, jealousy, and trust problems (Easterling & Knox, 2010). Children of deployed parents have higher rates of anxiety symptoms than their same-age peers (Chandra, Martin, Hawkins, & Richardson, 2010). They experience significantly greater challenges during pre- and postdeployment, including more school, family, and peer-related difficulties. Particularly troubling are findings from a study of the effects of deployment on early childhood development that suggest that parental deployment is related to adverse risk for developmental delays in children (Nguyen, Ee, Berry-Caban, & Hoedebeck, 2014). The researchers call for early detection and aggressive screening techniques in military communities to possibly mitigate these outcomes.

See Table 13.1 for children's common age-related feelings and responses during deployment. Although deployment is extremely stressful, most children in military families are resilient to the effects and are thriving. Parents who respond sensitively, parents with strong and stable relationships, and siblings who provide emotional support help children develop the most effective coping strategies (Boberiene & Hornback, 2014). High-quality family communication, which involves empathy between parents and children, is also cited as a condition that promotes better emotional well-being during and after deployment.

During predeployment, many families prepare videos or DVDs of the parent and child together or an audiotape of the parent reading or singing to the child, to use once the parent is deployed. Internet access, while often spotty, is typically available at overseas deployment sites. Thus, Skype, and FaceTime are popular ways for children and parents to keep in touch, although younger children are sometimes confused when they see their parent. Low-tech methods can be successful as well (see Case Study 13.3).

Combat injury. More than 50,000 service members have been physically injured in combat since the current conflicts began in 2002, and even more have been later diagnosed with post-traumatic stress disorder (PTSD) or traumatic brain injury (TBI) (Fischer, 2014). No literature exists that systematically examines the effect of parental combat injury on children. However, research indicates that sudden health-altering events, such as a combat injury, may have more profound effects on children than parental illness (Cozza, Chun, & Miller, 2011). When the service member first returns home with a combat injury, in most cases it is unclear how much things have changed or will change; thus, adjusting to these changes may be delayed. Children typically experience sudden changes in living arrangements, schedules, parenting practices, and the amount of time spent with their parents. Noninjured parents often must make rapid decisions with little time for preparation. Because the injured partner's needs are overwhelming, children's needs may go unaddressed. The child's developmental stage is a good guide to how he or she might respond. (For details, see Rollins and King, 2015.)

If the injuries are visible, children may worry that their injured parent will no longer be able to take care of or play with them. Some children might think that the injury is punishment for something bad that they or the service member wished for, thought, or did. Others may worry that they can "catch it" and be afraid to go near the injured parent.

Injuries produce difficult feelings for spouses as well, especially if they are called on to play an active role in caregiving. Spouses may experience grief at the loss of their mate's good health, and the loss of their own expectations of what the future might have been like—the death of a dream. They can feel anxious about being up to the task of caregiving and have other worries, such as losing the emotional bond they once enjoyed. Practical matters, such as financial worries about keeping up with medical and household expenses, may also be part of the picture. Unanswered questions can produce fear: "Is this situation temporary or permanent, and, if permanent, can I handle it?" Finally, some caregivers experience anger at being in the caregiving role, which is quite normal for people being handed a role they didn't expect or prepare for. Other caregivers in the family, such as the service member's mother, father, partner, or friend, will likely experience many of these feelings as well.

Invisible combat injuries, such as PTSD, TBI, and depression, create other troublesome issues for families (Price, 2013). For example, PTSD symptoms such as re-experiencing traumatic events through vivid daytime memories or dreams are typically accompanied by intense emotions (e.g., grief, guilt, fear, anger). These symptoms are frightening both to the individual experiencing them and to their family members. Children may not understand what is going on or why and may worry about their parent's well-being. Again, as with physical injuries, they may wonder whether their parent will be able to properly take care of them. Further, out of fear of re-experiencing traumatic events, service members with PTSD might try to avoid places and experiences that could trigger upsetting memories or even withdraw from the family. Children

Table 13.1

Children's Feelings and Responses to Deployment by Age		
Age	**Possible Feelings**	**Possible Responses**
Infants and toddlers	Sense increased stress in home Confusion	Irritability Difficulty with transitions More frequent bouts of crying Night waking
Preschoolers	Confusion Surprise (everything feels so different) Guilt (about causing parent to go away) Anger	More defiant Easily frustrated Difficult to comfort Alternate between resorting to younger patterns of behavior and becoming controlling and demanding Clinginess Irritability Trouble separating from parent Aggression and angry outbursts Attention-seeking behaviors (positive and negative) Sleep disturbances Acting out scary events Feeding issues (more picky)
School age	Confusion Anger Guilt Increased sadness (lack of family normalcy and loss of deployed parent's presence) Worry about deployed parent's return Worry whether remaining parent will leave or die	New behavior problems or intensification of already existing ones Regression Changes in eating and sleeping Rapid mood swings (e.g., angry outbursts followed by clinging behavior) Displays anger at parent for missing important events Displays anger at both parents for disrupting their normal way of life and sense of security Need to be and do "normal things" (e.g., parties)
Adolescents	Anger Sadness Depression Anxiety Fear	Misdirected or acting-out behavior toward others or themselves School problems (e.g., sudden and/or unusual changes) Apathy, loss of interest, uncommunicative, denial of feelings) Significant weight loss Drug or alcohol abuse Regression Increased importance of friends to the detriment of reasonable family life Trying to take charge of the family.

Note. From "The 'So Far' Guide for Helping Children and Youth Cope with the Deployment of a Parent in the Military Reserves," by D. Levin and C. Daynard, 2005, Needham, MA; "Infants and Young Children in Military Families: A Conceptual Model for Intervention," by A. Lieberman and P. Van Horn, 2013, *Clinical Child and Family Psychology Review, 16,* 282–293; "Health and Mental Health Needs of Children in US Military Families," by B. Siegel and B. Davis, and The Committee on Psychosocial Aspects of Child and Family Health and Section on Uniformed Services, 2013, *Pediatrics, 131*(6), e2002–2015.

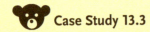 **Case Study 13.3**

Unwashed T-shirts

A father, deployed when his son was 8 months old, left behind several un-washed T-shirts that his wife put on the child's crib. The father continued sending home worn T-shirts that his wife exchanged for freshly laundered ones while continuing to give the worn ones to the child and showing the child videos and photos of his father. When the father returned 10 months later, the child instantly recognized him and reached out to him. Loving links can work wonders in bridging the painful separation of deployment.

Note. From "Infants and Young Children in Military Families: A Conceptual Model for Intervention," by A. Lieberman & P. Van Horn, 2013, *Clinical Child and Family Psychology Review, 16,* p. 288.

might misunderstand and think that their parent isn't interested in or doesn't care about them.

Children need information about their parent's invisible wounds. They need to know that the symptoms are not related to them and that they are not to blame. But according to Price (2013, p. 4), "The most important thing is to help each member of the family, including the children, have a voice in expressing what he or she needs." Play and other creative activities can provide that voice.

Death. Some military children are faced with the death of a parent or sibling who is either killed while deployed or commits suicide during or following deployment. Suicide rates among veterans are about triple that of the general public, with dramatic increases among veterans ages 18–29, an age where many individuals are parents (McCarthy et al., 2015). (For recommendations for helping children cope with a family member's death, see below and Chapter 6: The Child Who Is Dying.)

Caring for Military Families

Many families have been affected by over a decade at war, and ongoing activities in the Middle East and elsewhere suggest that U.S. military involvement will continue. Although military facilities provide health-care services for many military children, civilian professionals provide approximately two-thirds of health-care services (Gorman, Eide, & Hisle-Gorman, 2010). Johnson and Ling (2013) developed a strategy to support the unique needs of military children and their families using the acronym I CARE. The acronym stands for

- *Identify* military children and where they are in relation to deployment and move to recognize those children who are at risk for neglect, abuse, and inadequate coping, as well as previous patterns of coping and potentially mitigating factors.

- *Correlate* refers to considering the developmental stage, presenting complaints, and treatments in the current holistic context of the military family.

- *Ask* the child and caregiver about changes in household composition and coping, perhaps using scales that identify children who are at risk for psychosocial dysfunction; inquire about plans for a smooth deployment, reunion, and reintegration.
- *Ready* resources of a variety of local and national services can be suggested to families, with help offered to access appropriate ones. (See Appendix 13.1: Resources.)
- *Encourage* strong families and healthy problem-solving through a variety of prevention strategies and early involvement with local and national support services; encourage and normalize expectations of the entire family through the deployment cycle.

To help children cope with trauma and grief, Sories, Maier, Beer, and Thomas (2015) suggested systemic family-based play therapy. Although typical approaches to play therapy primarily focus on the child and involve the parents only tangentially, family-based play therapy considers the family as the treatment unit and expands the application of play-therapy techniques to the entire family. Filial therapy, a child-centered approach in which the therapist trains and coaches the parent to apply nondirective play therapy techniques to the parent–child relationship, helps both child and parent by using play to work through traumatic events in a validating and empathic way. This evidence-based approach is highly applicable to military families in which children and/or parents have PTSD, grief, and other sequelae of deployment-related traumatic events.

Recognizing the need to better understand the effects of war on military families, the Department of Defense initiated the Millennium Cohort Family Study, the largest study of military families in U.S. military history. This study will follow U.S. military families around the world for 21+ years to evaluate the impact of military experiences during and after military service (Crum-Cianflone, Fairbank, Marmar, & Schlenger, 2014).

Homeless Families

The number of homeless families with children has steadily increased since the mid-1980s. Based on U.S. Census data and the U.S. Department of Education's count of homeless children in public schools, approximately 2.5 million children experienced homelessness in the United States in 2013, which represents 1 in every 30 children (Bassuk, DeCamdoa, Beach, & Berman, 2014). See Text Box 13.2 for a summary of the major causes of homelessness for children.

Homelessness is also tracked by the U.S. Department of Housing and Urban Development (HUD), which reported a decrease in unsheltered family homelessness in 2014 and an increase in sheltered families (HUD, 2014). A typical sheltered family is composed of a single mother in her late 20s with two or three children, often younger than 6 years. In general,

the mothers do not have high school diplomas and have poor job skills and limited work opportunities that pay a livable wage. Many are victims of domestic violence. They have many more medical, mental health, and substance use problems compared to their housed counterparts. (Bassuk, 2010, p. 497)

HUD's narrow definition of homelessness and its single-night point-in-time (PIT) counting method does not include homeless families and children living in "doubled-up" situations with relatives or friends—a number estimated at 75% of homeless children nationally (United States Interagency Council on Homelessness, 2014). Doubled-up families often have strong incentive to not disclose their status because it might put the primary tenant of the apartment at risk of eviction for lease violation. Also not accurately reflected in the count are homeless children living in motels, hotels, trailer parks, campgrounds, or similar settings.

The passage of the federal McKinney-Vento Homeless Assistance Act of 1987 led to an expanded definition of the homeless child. The definition included doubled-up families as well as children in other homeless circumstances. See Text Box 13.3 for examples of children defined as homeless.

The Impact of Homelessness on Children

Homeless can be devastating for children, especially young children, and may lead to changes in brain architecture that can interfere with learning, emotional self-regulation, cognitive skills, and social relationships (Bassuk et al., 2014). Virtually no aspect of their lives is unaffected.

Physical health. According to The National Center on Family Homelessness (2015), children experiencing homelessness are sick 4 times as often other children, with 4 times as many respiratory infections, 2 times as many ear infections, and 5 times as many gastrointestinal problems. They are 4 times as likely to have asthma. Regarding food, they go hungry at 2 times the rate of other children and have high rates of obesity resulting from nutritional deficiencies.

Mental health. Children who are homeless have 3 times the rate of emotional and behavioral problems compared with housed children (National Child Traumatic Stress Network, 2005). In a systematic review and meta-analysis, Bassuk, Richard,

---

Text Box 13.2

Major Causes of Homelessness for Children in the United States

1. Persistently high rates of poverty for families
2. A lack of affordable housing
3. Continuing effects of the Great Recession
4. Racial disparities
5. Challenges of single parenting
6. Traumatic experiences, especially domestic violence, whose effects prolong homelessness for families

Note. Adapted from "Ending Child Homelessness in America" by E. Bassuk, 2010, *American Journal of Orthopsychiatry, 80,* 496–504.

and Tsertsvadze (2015) found that, overall, 10% to 26% of homeless preschoolers had mental health problems requiring clinical evaluation, a proportion that increased to 24% to 40% among homeless school-age children. This rate for homeless school-age children is 2 to 4 times the rate reported for poor children (Howell, 2004).

By 12 years of age, over 80% of homeless children have been exposed to at least one serious violent event, and almost 25% have witnessed acts of violence within their families (Buckner, Beardslee, & Bussuk, 2004). The effect of witnessing violence and other traumatic events on all children is well documented. However, with residential instability and often resultant separation from their primary caregiver, children who are homeless face additional risks. Without their caregiver's comfort, responsiveness, support, structure, and guidance during stressful times, children may feel less safe and manifest more symptoms than children exposed to violence who are not homeless. Herbers, Cutuli, Monn, Narayan, and Masten (2014) emphasized that positive parenting has the potential to reduce the number of trauma symptoms and behavioral problems.

Developmental milestones and academic performance. Homeless children are 4 times as likely to show delayed development and have 2 times the rate of learning disabilities as non-homeless children (The National Center on Family Homelessness, 2010). Mobility disrupts children's learning routines, their relationships with teachers and peers, and the curriculum that they previously followed. School attendance is often erratic. The McKinney-Vento Homeless Assistance Act of 1987 helps ensure that children have the opportunity to continue their education. Even if families lack normally required

Text Box 13.3
Examples of Children Defined as Homeless by the McKinney-Vento Act

Homeless children are "individuals who lack a fixed, regular, and adequate nighttime residence." The following are examples of children who would fall under this definition:

- Children and youth sharing housing resulting from loss of housing, economic hardship, or a similar reason
- Children and youth living in motels, hotels, trailer parks, or campgrounds because of a lack of alternative accommodations
- Children and youth living in emergency or transitional shelters
- Children and youth abandoned in hospitals
- Children and youth awaiting foster-care placement
- Children and youth whose primary nighttime residence is not ordinarily used as a regular sleeping accommodation (e.g., a park bench)
- Children and youth living in cars, parks, public spaces, abandoned buildings, substandard housing, or bus or train stations
- Migratory children and youth living in any of the above situations

Note. From "McKinney-Vento Homeless Assistance Act of 1987," by U.S. Department of Education, 2015. Retrieved from http://www2.ed.gov/programs/homeless/legislation.html

documents, such as immunization records or proof of residence, schools are required to enroll homeless children and youth immediately (U.S. Department of Education, 2015). Even transportation will be provided for children to attend their school of origin if it is in the child's or youth's best interest.

Responding to Child Homelessness

Examining the domains of adaptive functioning, academic achievement, and emotional and behavioral health within each child using cluster analysis, Huntington, Buckner, and Bassuk (2008) found that homeless children are not homogeneous. Children clustered into two main subgroups with different needs and functioning levels. Despite their adverse circumstances, children in the higher functioning group did well in all three domains; those in the lower functioning group did poorly in all three domains. The researchers found that in the lower functioning group, mothers experienced more intense mental health symptoms, and more children in this group had been exposed to physical and/or sexual violence. Thus, the researchers emphasized using a person-centered approach: targeting children who are lower functioning for intensive and often scarce resources while continuing to support children who are higher functioning.

Parenting is a challenging task made increasingly so by homelessness. Along with higher-than-average rates of chronic medical conditions, histories of untreated trauma, mental health conditions, and limited role models for positive parenting, homeless parents are further stressed by the multiple demands of the shelter system, the loss of predictable routines, and fragmented social supports. Although significant adversity during childhood can result in negative lifelong developmental difficulties for children, strategies focused on improving parenting capacities can mitigate some of these outcomes (Kim-Spoon, Haskett, Longo, & Nice, 2012). Three promising programs include

- *Parenting Through Change (PTC)*—A 14-week program that targets five parenting practices: (1) skill encouragement, (2) problem-solving, (3) limit setting, (4) monitoring, and (5) positive involvement (Forgatch & DeGarmo, 1999).
- *Family Care Curriculum*—A strengths-based 6-week program that integrates best practice from four frameworks: (1) Effective Black Parenting, (2) trauma-informed care, (3) attachment theory, and (4) self-care (Sheller & Hudson, 2010).
- *Family Talk*—A 6- to 11-session program designed for families with parental depression to improve parental responsiveness and skills. Core elements include (1) conducting assessments on all family members, (2) teaching about depression as well as risks and resilience in children, (3) linking information to the family's experiences, (4) decreasing feelings of guilt and blame in children, and (5) helping children to develop relationships within and outside the family to encourage their independent functioning in school and in activities outside the home (Beardslee, Gladstone, Wright, & Cooper, 2003).

Foster Care

About a half million children are living in foster care in the United States on any given day (Council of Foster Care, Adoption, and Kinship Care, Committee on Adolescence, and Council on Early Childhood, 2015). There are several different types of foster care (see Text Box 13.4).

According to the American Academy of Pediatrics (2016), prior to entering foster care, children and teens typically have received only fragmentary and sporadic health care. There is a high prevalence of undiagnosed or undertreated chronic medical problems, often as a result of going without necessary medications or equipment. Fractures, infections, burns, and bruises are common and frequently a result of abuse. For example, of children and teens entering foster care,

- about 50% have chronic physical problems (e.g., asthma, anemia, visual loss, hearing loss, neurological disorders).
- about 10% are medically fragile or complex.
- many have a history of prenatal (maternal) substance exposure and/or premature birth.

Text Box 13.4
Types of Foster Care

- **Straight or family foster care:** The state or local government places a child with certified foster parents who are not related to the child.
- **Kinship foster care:** Children are placed with a relative (or in some areas, close family friends), often without going through the court system. Thus, this kind of foster care is not always reported to an agency for oversight.
- **Pre-adoptive foster care:** Children are placed with families who will adopt them.
- **Treatment foster care** (therapeutic foster care): Children are placed with foster families with special training to care for children with certain medical or behavioral needs (e.g., medically fragile children, children with emotional or behavioral disorders, HIV-positive children).
- **Residential or group settings** (congregate care, institutional care): Children are placed in community-based group homes, campus-style residential facilities, and secure facilities. Programs and staff training are designed for working with children with certain special needs (e.g., adolescent males who are involved in the juvenile justice system, children and youth with serious mental health problems).
- **Emergency-care setting:** Children are temporarily placed in a shelter/group facility or a family setting designed to keep them safe while assessing their needs and finding a more appropriate placement to meet their needs.
- **Shared family care (SFC):** Parent(s) and children are placed together in the home of a host family that mentors and supports the parents as they develop the skills and supports necessary to care for their children independently. SFC is used (1) to prevent out-of-home placement, (2) to provide a safe environment for the reunification of a family that has been separated, or (3) to help parents consider other permanency options, including relinquishment of parental rights.
- **Another planned permanent living arrangement (APPLA):** A case plan designation for children in out-of-home care when there is no goal for placement with a legal permanent family. There must be sufficient reason to exclude all possible legal permanent family goals, and designations are required to include plans for permanent placements that meet children's developmental, educational, and other needs.

Note. Adapted from "Foster Parents: FAQs" by American Academy of Pediatrics, 2013. Retrieved from https://www.healthychildren.org/English/family-life/family-dynamics/adoption-and-foster-care/Pages/Foster-Parents-FAQs.aspx

The distress of the transition to foster care may worsen some physical issues. Children with asthma, for example, may experience more frequent flare-ups.

However, mental and behavioral health is the largest unmet health need for children and teens in foster care (AAP, 2016). "Children and teens entering foster care are at high risk of having experienced considerable early adversity and demonstrate high levels of psychopathology, educational difficulties, and neurodevelopmental disorders compared to peers reared at home" (Pritchett et al., 2016, p. 1). An environment becomes very stressful when parents are chronically or frequently unresponsive, unpredictably responsive, or harsh. Frequent or unremitting adversity, especially if not tempered by care from a responsive, attuned, nurturing caregiver, can affect the neurobiology of the developing brain (AAP Committee on Psychosocial Aspects of Child and Family Health, 2012). Toxic stress alters genetic expression in ways that alter the architecture of the brain, especially the amygdala, hippocampus, and right prefrontal cortex, those areas involved in stress response, emotional regulation, attention, cognition, executive function, and memory.

The potential outcomes are predictable: insecure attachment behaviors, hyperactivity, impulsivity, difficulty with transitions, limited cognitive development, dissociation between affect and emotions, easy frustration, and so on (AAP, 2016). Further, pre–foster care educational factors such as frequent school absences and poor academic achievement add up to high rates of educational difficulties. For example, kindergartners in foster care have half the vocabulary of their peers, and almost half of school-aged children and teens in foster care are involved in special education (AAP, 2016).

Minnis (2013) describes a new concept, maltreatment-associated psychiatric problems (MAPP), which seeks to explain the experience of children who have experienced abuse or neglect in early life. MAPP is a syndrome of overlapping complex neurodevelopmental problems. The early life events of many children in foster care face place them at an increased risk of developing problems, and when problems do arise in the context of maltreatment, they are likely to be complex and overlapping.

Caring for Children in Foster Care

Critically important is the presence of a competent, caring, nurturing, stable foster or kinship parent who will support and advocate for the child's health and well-being. Foster care can be a life-changing event for children, an opportunity for intervention and healing. Studies show significant improvements in health status, development, intelligence, school attendance, and academic achievement as a consequence of foster care placement (Hahn et al., 2005). However, vulnerability for continuing mental health issues can continue into adulthood. In a study of young adults who lived in foster care during adolescence, Pecora and colleagues (2005) found a prevalence of post-traumatic stress disorder twice that of combat veterans.

Community interventions have been used successfully with children in foster care. Child Directed Interaction Training (CDIT) for young children in kinship care was piloted with 14 grandmothers and great-grandmothers with their 2- to 7-year old children. Participants attended a twice-weekly, 8-session CDIT program at a local community library. Post-training, kinship caregivers in the CDIT condition demonstrated more positive relationships with their children and reported clinically and statistically significant decreases in parenting stress and caregiver depression, as well as fewer externalizing child behavior problems than waitlist controls (N'zi, Stevens, & Eyberg, 2016). The Fostering Healthy Futures Program is a preventive intervention for children age 9–11 years who have recently been placed in foster care because of maltreatment. The 9-month program aims to promote well-being by identifying and addressing mental health issues, preventing adolescent risk behavior, and promoting competence. The program includes group skills training and mentoring. Among the positive findings: The intervention youth had 44% fewer placement changes and were 5 times as likely, 1 year postintervention, to have permanency, a greater rate of reunification, and higher rates of adoption when compared with a treatment-as-usual control group (Taussig, Culhane, Garrrido, & Knudtson, 2012).

Foster Care Goals

Reunification is usually the ultimate goal, but practical steps must be followed to support families both before and after reunification (Monroe & Harris, 2013). One of the most common reasons reunification fails is neglect. Parents need to know and understand that children have specific needs that must be met if they are to achieve healthy growth and development. The parent–child relationship should be reestablished before the child reenters the home. Parents need to know what support services (e.g., medical, financial, housing, child care, substance abuse/mental health) are available and how to access them. They can be helped in identifying external and internal support systems. Some parents, especially those overwhelmed with managing a house and caring for children, may benefit from instruction in time management.

In 1997, Congress enacted the Adoption and Safe Families Act (ASFA [Pub L No. 105-89]), which dramatically shifted the focus of foster care from the rights of birth parents and reunification to children's need for health, safety, and permanency (Szilagyi et al., 2015). Legislators increased adoption incentives and mandated that states begin proceedings to terminate parental rights when a child or adolescent has spent 15 of the previous 22 months in foster care, unless a compelling reason exists not to, such as impending family reunification. Of those children discharged from foster care in 2013, almost 60% were reunited with their families and over 21% were adopted (U.S. Department of Health and Human Services, 2016). The remaining children went under legal guardianship, were emancipated, or aged out of foster care.

Adoption

Approximately 2% of the U.S. child population is adopted, either from foster care or through private, domestic, or international adoption (Child Trends, 2012). Open adoptions have been increasingly common since the 1970s, when research began to suggest that adoptees in open adoptions have better psychosocial outcomes than adoptees in semi-open and closed adoptions (Crea & Barth, 2009; Siegel, 2008). With open adoption, the biological and adoptive families have access to varying degrees of each other's personal information and have an option of contact. The adoptive parents are the legal parents and hold all rights; however, the biological and adoptive families may have various levels of contact, from sharing photos to face-to-face contact.

Adopted children are less likely to live below the poverty level than the general population of children (Child Trends, 2012). Compared with children overall, young adopted children are more likely to be read to every day, be sung to or told stories every day, and eat meals with their families six or more days per week. Adopted school-age children and teens are more likely than older children in general to participate in organized activities outside of school. Younger adopted children read for pleasure at about the same rate as the general population, but older adopted children are less likely to do so. Regarding school engagement (i.e., caring about doing well, doing required homework), adopted children as a group are less likely to be doing well than are all children.

Although most parents report that their adopted children are in excellent or very good health, the prevalence of special health-care needs (39%) is twice as high as is reported in the overall population of children. Behavior and conduct problems, attention-deficit disorder, and attention-deficit/hyperactivity disorder are reported more frequently for adopted children than for children overall (Child Trends, 2012).

There are two views about when children should be told that they are adopted (American Academy of Child & Adolescent Psychiatry [AACAP], 2015). Some experts believe it should happen at the youngest possible age so that they can begin to accept and integrate the concept of being adopted. Others say that telling children early may just confuse them, thus advising to wait until the child is older. However, everyone agrees that adoptive parents should be the ones to tell the children. To hear the news from someone else either intentionally or accidentally can result in anger and mistrust toward the parents. The child may view the adoption as bad or shameful because it was kept a secret.

All children go through a stage of struggling with their identity during adolescence; this may be more intense for adopted children, particularly those from other countries or cultures. Although some adopted children develop emotional or behavioral problems, they may not be the results of issues related to being adopted (AACAP, 2015).

Refugee and Migrant Families and Unaccompanied Children

Migration refers to the movement of people from one place to another either within a country or to another country; thus a migrant is a person who has gone through migration. The United States remains the principal destination of international migrants in the world and one of the leading countries for granting asylum and resettling refugees. Push and pull factors provide reasons for migration. Individuals are fleeing from push factors, such as intersectional discrimination resulting from various forms of violence, poverty, gender, and economic inequality, and also the effects of natural disasters in their countries of origin. Pull factors include family reunification, better job and educational opportunities, higher levels of human security, and the chance for a better standard of living (Inter-American Commission on Human Rights, 2015).

If families with children apprehended at the U.S. border express fear of persecution, they are transferred to a family immigration detention center, or if centers are full, they are sent to live with a family member or sponsor in the United States for the duration of the proceedings. The second step is an interview to determine whether the family members have a fear of persecution in case of being returned to their home country; if there is a significant possibility, the family could be eligible for asylum. If this is the case, some families remain detained and others may obtain conditional release during the next step, the deportation proceeding, where the immigration judge decides to deny or grant asylum. If asylum is denied, families may appeal to the Board of Immigration Appeals, then to a federal circuit court, and even to the U.S. Supreme Court if a constitutional issue is implicated.

Regarding unaccompanied children, prior to the enactment of the 2008 Trafficking Victims Protection Reauthorization Act (TVPRA) and as a "matter of practice," Mexican unaccompanied children arriving in the United States were automatically "turned back" to Mexico through the nearest port of entry during daylight hours and within 24 hours of arrival. Now U.S. border officials are required to determine whether an unaccompanied child from Mexico may present certain protection needs prior to initiating his/her return to Mexico. Concretely, officials must determine within 48 hours of apprehension that the child:

- has not been a victim of a severe form of trafficking and there is no credible evidence that the child will be at risk of being trafficked upon return to Mexico;
- does not have a fear of returning to Mexico owing to a credible fear of persecution; and
- is able to make a voluntary, independent decision to withdraw his or her application for admission to the United States. (Cavendish & Cortazar, 2011, p. 23)

Unaccompanied children from countries other than Mexico and Canada are also handled in accordance with the TVPRA, which provides that unaccompanied children from noncontiguous countries must be treated with more protections to ensure that they are not victims of human trafficking and/or do not have "credible fears" of persecution in their home countries, before any attempt to deport them. According to federal law, unaccompanied minors must be moved out of detention centers within 72 hours. Most children are released to family members; those without family in the United States are placed in foster care (Wiltz, 2015).

The term *migrant* also refers to families who move across the country seeking seasonal or temporary work in the agricultural, dairy, or fishery industry. This diverse population includes Southeast Asians, African Americans, Anglos, and other ethnic groups, with Latinos being the largest ethnic group represented. When parents are working, children are often required to work with them or to care for their siblings. Children in migrant families may not speak English, and language skills in their own language may be poor. Their constant mobility and academic interruption, social and cultural isolation, hard work outside school, poor health, and poverty all contribute to low academic achievement, which likely leads to dropping out of school. Other common problems include low health expectations, overcrowded living conditions, and poor sanitation. Migrant children are at increased risk for respiratory and ear infections, bacterial and viral gastroenteritis, intestinal parasites, skin infections, scabies and head lice, pesticide exposure, tuberculosis, poor nutrition, anemia, short stature, undiagnosed congenital anomalies, undiagnosed delayed development, intentional and unintentional injuries, substance use, and teenage pregnancy (Migrant Clinicians Network, 2014). See Appendix 13.1: Resources for information about projects and programs serving migrant children and their families.

Immigrant Families

Immigrants are people who come into a country from another country. While the word *migration* denotes the act of *moving from* one place to another, *immigration* denotes the act of an individual or family *moving to* a new country from another country.

Children and teens living in immigrant families represent the fastest-growing group of American children, with the largest share from Mexico (Child Trends, 2014). They often face risks for healthy development. For example, poverty is more likely an issue for immigrant children than nonimmigrant children. They are more likely to have parents with very low educational attainment and to have three or more siblings (Hernandez, Denton, & Macartney, 2008). They are far less likely to have health insurance. Perhaps in part because many immigrant children have undocumented parents, they are more likely than native children to use public benefits. Compared with nonimmigrant children, their health is more likely to be poor or only fair, yet researchers have remarked that the health status of young immigrant children is better than expected, given their level of socioeconomic disadvantage. However, Hamilton, Cardoso, Hummer, and Padilla (2011) report that rates of adverse health conditions, such as asthma, allergies, developmental delays, and learning disabilities, increase with successive generations of residence in the United States.

On the other hand, although findings differ by country of origin and racial-ethnic status, youth in immigrant families do not differ significantly from those in native-born families in terms of their self-esteem, psychological well-being, and psychological distress (Harris, 1999). However, academic achievement differs, with adolescents in immigrant families having somewhat higher math test scores and somewhat lower reading scores, again differing by country of origin (Kao, 1999).

Selected Issues With Psychosocial Implications for Children's Well-Being

Health promotion and illness/injury prevention efforts are also major components of community health care. Problems addressed early reduce health-care costs and needless suffering. Historically, the U.S. health-care system has been crisis oriented (i.e., we wait until a health problem arises before intervening) rather than prevention oriented. However, through its *Healthy People* initiative, the U.S. Department of Health and Human Services announced a bold shift in its approach from a disease-care system to a health-care system (U.S. Department of Health and Human Services, 2003). The initiative provides science-based national objectives for improving the health of all Americans. See Appendix 13.1: Resources for information about Healthy People 2020 leading health indicators.

Whether it is at home or school, in the neighborhood, church, clubs, or other places where people gather, there are many sources of predictable stress for children. For example, younger children become anxious when separated from parents. Social and academic pressures create stress for older children. And, unlike in the not-so-distant past, many children today are overscheduled and have little time to play creatively or relax after school.

We will focus on a selection of issues with strong psychosocial implications for children, families, and health-care professionals in the community. Left unaddressed, some of these issues may have effects on a child's well-being that last a lifetime.

School Violence and Bullying

Americans have become increasingly concerned about horrific events of violence, such as school shootings, and the reasons behind them. Reasons often cited include mental illness, the availability of guns, or some fundamental difference in children and the stresses they endure today.

We know that there are links between school violence and bullying. In a survey of more than 15,000 students, Grades 6 through 10, victims of bullying were more likely than children who had never been bullied to believe that violence was a solution to their problems (Nansel, Overpeck, Haynie, Ruan, & Scheidt, 2003). A child who bullies or is bullied is more likely to be involved in one or more of four violence-related behaviors: (1) carrying a weapon in the last 30 days, (2) carrying a weapon in school in the last 30 days, (3) frequent fighting during the last year, and (4) sustaining an injury during the last year from a fight that required medical treatment.

Further, the students most likely to carry a weapon said they bullied others in or away from school or were being bullied away from school. Bullies, both boys and girls, are more likely to be engaged in frequent fighting and injured in a fight, which is also true for boys who are bullied away from school.

Increased awareness and effective interventions have led to a decrease in bullying in schools (Zuckerman, Bushman, & Pedersen, 2012). The percentage of students who report being bullied decreases steadily with age, with a high of 22% in Grades 3 and 4, to a low of 9% by Grade 12 (Limber, Olweus, & Luxenberg, 2013). However, particularly disturbing is the finding that for 24% of students who are bullied, the bullying continues for several years or longer.

Empathy

Lack of empathy has been cited as a reason that children bully (Rollins, 2014). In fact, an effective bullying prevention program was built on the notion that developing empathy is the key to prevention. Roots of Empathy, an innovative evidence-based classroom program, increases young children's empathy through visits by a neighborhood infant and parent every 3 weeks over the school year (Roots of Empathy, n.d.).

However, brain research suggests that some children who bully do not lack empathy but that their brains empathize differently. Decety, Michaliska, Akitsuki, and Lahey (2009) compared the fMRI scans of 8 boys 16–18 years of age with aggressive conduct disorder to those of a control group of adolescent boys with no unusual signs of aggression. Both groups viewed video scenes of people accidentally hurting themselves, such as when a heavy bowl was dropped on their hands, and intentionally, such as when a person stepped on another's foot. With the nonaggressive boys, the expected parts of the brain signaled that the boys felt empathy for the people in pain. However, the aggressive boys' scans who had signaled empathy toward pain associated that pain empathy with pleasure in the reward centers of the brain.

Decety and colleagues concluded that children who bully do not lack empathy, but instead associate the pain of their victims as a positive feeling. They suggested that bullies' abusive behavior feeds their brains with a feeling of reward. Therefore, although they are empathetic, they are not empathetic in a way that causes remorse.

Research has found that children in general are less empathetic today than in the past. Konrath, O'Brien, and Hsing (2011) conducted a meta-analysis of American college students ($N = 13,737$) and found a 48% decrease in empathic concern and a 34% decrease in perspective-taking since 1979. This finding held true across gender, race, and educational backgrounds. This decline was marked by a rise in self-esteem, individualism, and narcissism (Twenge, Konrath, Foster, Campbell, & Bushman, 2008). High school and college students' values have shifted toward extrinsic (money, fame, and image) concerns and away from intrinsic (community, affiliation) concerns. Negative consequences include lower empathy, less concern for others, and less civic engagement (e.g., interest in social issues, government, and politics) (Twenge, 2013).

We see the potential downside—lack of empathy, sense of entitlement—of an emphasis on self-esteem above all else. Anticipatory guidance for parents, as well as sound guidance when problems arise, can stress the need for balance when promoting self-esteem.

Cyberbullying

Extensive use of technology has engendered a new form of bullying. Bullying is now divided into two separate categories: traditional bullying and cyberbullying, or electronic bullying. Cyberbullying is much like other types of bullying, except that it takes place online and through text messages. According to the National Crime Prevention Council (NCPC), cyberbullies can be classmates, online acquaintances, and even anonymous users, but most often they do know their victims (NCPC, n.d.). Some examples of ways children bully online include the following:

- Sending someone mean or threatening e-mails, instant messages, or text messages
- Excluding someone from an instant messenger buddy list or blocking their e-mail for no reason
- Tricking someone into revealing personal or embarrassing information and sending it to others
- Breaking into someone's e-mail or instant-message account to send cruel or untrue messages while posing as that person
- Creating websites to make fun of another person, such as a classmate or teacher
- Using websites to rate peers as prettiest, ugliest, etc. (NCPC, n.d.)

Although both boys and girls sometimes bully online, just as in face-to-face bullying, they tend to do so in different ways. Boys may send messages of a sexual nature or threaten to fight or hurt someone. Girls tend to bully by spreading rumors and by sending messages that make fun of someone or exclude others. They also tell secrets (NCPC, n.d.).

Many of the effects of cyberbullying on children are the same as with bullying in person, such as a drop in grades, low self-esteem, a change in interests, or depression.

Yet cyberbullying can seem more extreme to its victims for the following reasons (NCPC, n.d.):

- It often occurs in the child's home. Being bullied at home can take away the place children feel safest.
- It can be harsher. Often children say things online that they wouldn't say in person, mainly because they can't see the other person's reaction.
- It can be far reaching. Children can send e-mails making fun of someone to their entire class or school with a few clicks or post them on a website for the whole world to see.
- It can be anonymous. Cyberbullies often hide behind screen names and e-mail addresses that don't identify who they are. Not knowing who is responsible for bullying messages can add to a victim's insecurity.
- It may seem inescapable. Although it may seem easy to get away from a cyberbully by just getting offline, for some children this would take away one of the major places they socialize.

The National Crime Prevention Council has a wealth of resources for traditional bullying and cyberbullying. See Appendix 13.1: Resources.

Tobacco, Alcohol, and Other Drug Use

The 2015 Monitoring the Future (MTF) survey of drug use and attitudes among American 8th, 10th, and 12th graders shows encouraging news, with decreasing use of alcohol, cigarettes, and many illicit drugs over the preceding 5 years (National Institute on Drug Abuse, 2015a). The report shows no increase in the use of marijuana among teens, decreasing use of synthetic drugs, and decreasing misuse of prescription drugs. However, the findings highlighted continuing concerns over the high rate of electronic cigarette (e-cigarette) use and softening of attitudes around some types of drug use, particularly a continued decrease in the perceived harm of marijuana use.

Substance use among adolescents is a major social problem associated with academic underachievement, emotional/psychiatric symptoms, family conflict, and legal difficulties (Kamininer & Winters, 2011). High dropout rates in treatment programs reflect the fact that treating adolescent substance use can be difficult. In one study, of 160 admissions to residential treatment, only 30% of male adolescents completed treatment (Neumann et al., 2010). Furthermore, the fact that adolescent substance users frequently have co-occurring disorders (e.g., depression) adds another layer of complexity to treatment.

Substance use sometimes results in the teen's entry into the correctional system. Research suggests that juvenile drug courts designed especially to address low treatment completion rates, frequent relapse, and recidivism can be more effective than other treatments for adolescents (Konecky, Cellucci, & Mochrie, 2016).

Opioids and Heroin

In 2014, heroin use in the general population increased from 373,000 in 2007 to 914,000 (SAMHSA, 2015). For youth ages 12–17, the percentage of lifetime use of heroin decreased from 0.2% in 2013 to 0.1% in 2014, but past-year use increased from 0.1% to 0.8% (National Institute on Drug Abuse, 2015b).

This increase may in part be driven by the transition to heroin use among the growing population of youth with a history of nonmedical use of prescription opioids (Mars, Bourgois, Karandinos, Montero, & Cicarone, 2014). Heroin is cheaper than prescription opioids and is readily available.

Deaths from prescription painkillers have reached epidemic levels in the past decade, with 46 people dying per day from an overdose (CDC, 2015). For youth ages 12–25 years, opioid-related deaths have either doubled, tripled, or quadrupled in 35 states (Levi, Segal, Martin, Biasi, & May, 2015).

In response, the National Association of School Nurses (2015) has issued a position statement that calls for safe and effective management of opioid pain reliever (OPR)-related overdose to be incorporated into the school emergency preparedness and response plan. The plan states that school nurses should facilitate access to naloxone for management of OPR-related overdose in the school setting.

In March 2016, the U.S. House of Representatives Committee on Oversight & Government Reform (COGR) held a hearing on America's Heroin and Opioid Abuse Epidemic (COGR, 2016). The hearing had two purposes: (1) to highlight the alarming increase in abuse of illegal opioids, such as heroin, as well as controlled prescription opioids, such as hydrocodone and oxycodone, and (2) to examine the strategies of the Office of National Drug Control Policy and SAMHSA to address opioid abuse (Full House Committee on Oversight and Government Reform, 2016). Among actions taken, President Obama's FY Budget called for $1 billion in new mandatory funding over 2 years to expand access to treatment for prescription drug abuse and heroin use and $500 million to continue and build on current efforts across the Departments of Justice (DOJ) and Health and Human Services (HHS) (Office of the Press Secretary, The White House, 2016).

The CDC's main strategies for responding to the heroin epidemic are to prevent people from starting heroin use, reducing heroin addiction, and reversing heroin overdose (CDC, 2015). Federal funds or federal pass-through money to states should be available to develop and implement evidence-based prevention and treatment programs.

Stress

Stress is an individual's response to any situation or factor that creates a negative emotional or physical change or both (Kaneshiro, 2014). (For more details about stress and coping, see Chapter 2: Preparing Children's for Health-Care Encounters.) In small doses, stress can be good, for example motivating; however, excessive stress can interfere with the way people think, act, and feel.

There are three levels of stress seen in children (Middlebrooks & Audage, 2008):

1. *Positive stress* is necessary and promotes resilience, the ability to function competently under threat. Examples: first day of school, family wedding, making new friends, or short-lived adverse experiences such as being punished or going to the doctor for immunizations. With adult support, children can learn to control and triumph over positive stress.

2. *Tolerable stress* results from adverse experiences that are more intense in nature but short-lived and can usually be overcome. Examples: family disruptions, accidents, or a death of a loved one. With appropriate adult support, children can easily cope and turn it into positive stress. If children do not receive support, tolerable stress can become detrimental.
3. *Toxic stress* results when experiences are long in duration and intensity. Examples: abuse, neglect, violence, and overall hardships without adult support (see Adverse Childhood Experiences, above). Toxic stress can lead to permanent changes in brain development if children do not receive sufficient support.

High school students' answers to the CDC Youth Risk Behavior Surveillance System (YRBSS) reflect one area of the impact of stress in their lives. Students were asked questions concerning depression and its extent. See the responses in Table 13.2. In all areas, a higher percentage of girls than boys responded affirmatively to the five questions. The percentage of students feeling sad or hopeless did not change significantly from 2011, while the percentage who were seriously considering attempting suicide or making a suicide plan, who attempted suicide, and who had a suicide attempt treated by a doctor or nurse all decreased from the previous survey (CDC, 2013b).

Classrooms can be a setting for addressing children's stress. An intervention offered by familiar, trusted professionals in a school setting may feel less invasive to the students, and that might increase participation rates. One study of urban middle school students looked at mindfulness-based stress reduction (MBSR) as a possible method for reducing the effects of stress and trauma among low-income middle school students in a city public school system. Sibinga, Webb, Ghazaarian, and Ellen (2016) studied the effects of mindfulness instruction on middle school students in two Baltimore City Public Schools. Students ($N = 300$) were randomly assigned to the mindfulness program or a health education "Healthy Topics" (HT) program. The groups were comparable at baseline. Post-program, the MBSR students had significantly lower

Table 13.2

Percentage of Students Grades 9–12 Over the Past 12 Months, by Behavioral Characteristic			
Behavior	Total Nationwide	Females	Males
Felt sad or hopeless	29.9%	39.1%	20.8%
Seriously considered attempting suicide	17.0%	22.4%	11.6%
Made a suicide plan	13.6%	16.9%	10.3%
Attempted suicide	8.0%	10.6%	5.4%
Suicide attempt treated by a doctor or nurse	2.7%	3.6%	1.8%

Source. "Mental health surveillance among children—United States, 2005–2011," by Centers for Disease Control and Prevention, 2013bb, *Morbidity and Mortality Weekly Report, 62,* 2, 1–40.

levels of somatization, depression, negative affect, negative coping, self-hostility, and post-traumatic symptom severity than the HT group. See Appendix 13.1: Resources for information about using MBSR with youths. Suggested apps are also listed.

University of California–San Francisco Benioff Children's Hospital Oakland and East Bay Regional Park District partnered in a project where nature is used as treatment for young people to combat stress and build resilience (Razani, Meade, Schudel, Johnson, & Long, 2015). Health-care professionals at a primary-care clinic recruit children to join monthly excursions to local parks. Children are encouraged to bring family members along. The excursions, facilitated by a naturalist and physician, include unstructured exploration, physical activity, and a group picnic. Razani and colleagues report that nature has served as a tool to treat some of the stress associated with poverty, and each child's response to nature is unique. They conclude that nature is about friends, family, community, and the security of place.

Corporal Punishment

Corporal punishment has been an issue of debate for many years. About 80% of children around the world are spanked or otherwise physically punished by their parents (UNICEF, 2014). Many adults will say that their parents hit them, and they turned out just fine. However, a recent review of data from 75 studies—a total of 50 years of data from more than 160,000 children—concluded that being spanked as a child appears to be linked to a host of long-term behavioral and mental health issues (Gershoff & Grogan-Kaylor, 2016). Through their analysis, the researchers examined the relationship between childhood spanking and 17 outcomes and found that 13 out of these 17 outcomes were significantly associated with spanking. Outcomes included more aggression, more antisocial behavior, more externalizing problems, more internalizing problems, more mental health problems, and more negative relationships with parents. Spanking also was significantly associated with lower moral internalization, lower cognitive ability, and lower self-esteem. Researchers stopped short of saying that the data could conclusively say that spanking as punishment causes these problems, or vice versa. They note, for example, that children with behavior problems tend to elicit more spankings from their parents in general. Their study also revealed that the more children are spanked, the greater the risk that they will be physically abused by their parents.

A history of spanking from parents was associated with adult antisocial behavior, adult mental health problems, and adult support for physical punishment. Gershoff and Grogan-Kaylor (2016) stated that although these findings suggest that there may be lasting effects of spanking that reach into adulthood, they are only suggestive, because adults who engage in antisocial behavior or who are experiencing mental health problems may focus on negative memories of their childhoods and report more spanking than they received. Support for spanking of children as an adult may be an example of intergenerational transmission of spanking or an example of selectively remembering their past as a way of rationalizing their current beliefs.

Gershoff and Grogan-Kaylor (2016) questioned whether spanking would be associated with detrimental child outcomes when studies relying on harsh and potentially abusive methods were removed. Study findings show that the answer to this question is yes. Spanking is a risk factor, and the more the child is hit and the longer he or she is hit, the greater the risk will be.

At the 2015 annual meeting of the American Academy of Pediatrics, Victor Vieth, founder and senior director of the Gundersen National Child Protection Training Center in La Crosse, Wisconsin, stated that religion is a top reason—if not the number one reason—for the use of corporal punishment. He stressed the importance of understanding religion's influence on discipline and developing culturally sensitive responses to parents who object for religious reasons to alternative approaches (Vieth, as cited in Kilgore, 2015).

We know that corporal punishment sends a message to children that violence is an acceptable way to solve problems, which is very sad when safe, effective, evidence-based strategies are available for disciplining children (Rollins, 2012). See Appendix 13.1: Resources for information about *Play Nicely*, a multimedia program and handbook for parents and health-care professionals.

Corporal Punishment in Schools

Most developed countries have abolished the use of use of corporal punishment in schools, with the exception of some parts of the United States (primarily the South and West), Australia, and Singapore. Today, 19 states continue to permit the practice. According to the legislation to end corporal punishment currently under consideration in the U.S. House of Representatives, every 30 seconds during the school year, a public school student is corporally punished (H.R. 2268, 2015). The bill was sent to the House subcommittee on Early Childhood, Elementary, and Secondary Education in 2015; it has yet to move forward.

Approximately 20,000 children sustain serious physical injuries from corporal punishment imposed by teachers or other school personnel each year (DeNies, 2012). Even in the absence of physical injury, as discussed above, corporal punishment can have adverse effects. The AAP reaffirmed its policy statement in 2012, pointing out that corporal punishment may adversely affect a student's self-image and school achievement and may also contribute to disruptive and violent student behavior. Corporal punishment can have a severe impact on social skills development, leading to aggressive behaviors.

Disparities exist in the practice of corporal punishment in schools. For example, although they make up only 17.1% of the national student population, African American students make up over 35% of all students subject to physical punishment at school. Further, children with disabilities are subjected to corporal punishment at disproportionately high rates, approximately twice the rate of the general student population in some states (U.S. Department of Education, 2009).

Children's Use of TV, Internet, and Video Games

In the past, children's media use was basically limited to watching television or listening to music. Few parents complained about children listening to too much music. However, today the idea of children watching too much television has become a real concern to parents, along with newer technologies such as the Internet, smartphones, iPods and iPads, and video games (Conrad, 2016a). Table 13.3 presents the results of a survey conducted by the nonprofit organization Common Sense Media related to technology use in U.S. households with children age 8 years or younger.

Children consume a little over 3 hours of media in a typical day, which includes computer use, cell phone use, tablet use, music, and reading (see Figure 13.2). The bulk of the time (two-thirds) is with screen media, with reading comprising only 20 minutes per day. Screen media time dramatically increases from 53 minutes per day for children under 2 years to almost 3 hours per day for children ages 5 to 8 years (Conrad, 2016b).

TV viewing remains the type of media children spend the most time with, with 65% of children under 8 years watching TV daily, usually about 100 minutes per day. By 8 years of age, 96% of children surveyed had watched TV, 90% had used a computer, 81% had played console video games, and 60% had played games or used apps on a portable device (cell phone, handheld gaming system, iPod, or tablet) (Conrad, 2016b).

Aside from the obvious physical implications of heavy media use (e.g., inactivity, obesity), there are other concerns. One concern is that young people whose communication with friends, family members, and other individuals occurs primarily via electronics are losing vital social skills for interacting with others in person. There is also talk of media addiction. In the 2013 edition of the American Psychiatric Association's *Diagnostic and Statistical Manual of Mental Disorders* (DSM-5), Internet Gaming Disorder is identified as a condition warranting more clinical research. Pew Research Center's Internet, Science & Tech division is active in research on the implications of

Table 13.3

Media in U.S. Households With Children Age 8 Years or Younger	
Percentage of households that	
Have a TV	98
Have cable TV	68
Have a video player	80
Have high-speed Internet	68
Have an e-reader	9
Percentage of children who	
Have access to a computer at home	72
Own a video-game system	67
Own an educational gaming system	29
Have a TV in their bedroom	42
Own a cell phone	2
Have a video player in their bedroom	29
Have a video-game system in their bedroom	11
Have a computer in their bedroom	4
Live in a home in which the TV is left on all the time	10
Live in a home in which the TV is left on most of the time	29

Note. Adapted from "Children and Technology—Stats for Technology in the Home," by B. Conrad, 2016. Retrieved from http://www.techaddiction.ca/children-and-technology.html

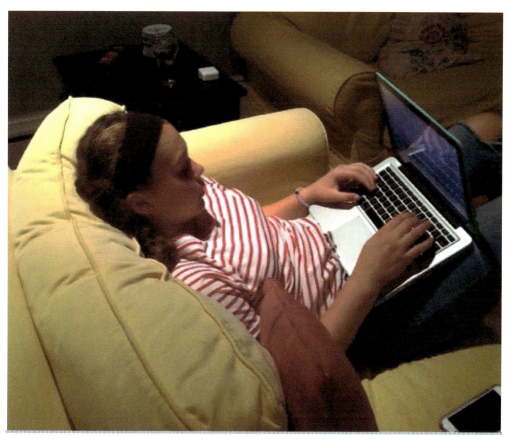

Figure 13.2. Children consume more than 3 hours of media in a typical day.

media use, including child and teen use. Much of the research on and even treatment of media addiction is taking place in Asia, where children's addiction to smartphones has become a serious problem (Hwang & Jeong, 2015).

Disasters

Natural disasters have always occurred. In the distant past, they might have affected small villages, and stories of the disaster might have taken months to travel to other communities. As people began living in larger groups, and more closely together than those who lived more agrarian lives, the impact of disasters, natural or man-made, was amplified by the larger population affected. Today, we live through disasters in our own communities as well as those affecting others around the world. They begin to feel inescapable. If adults feel this way, imagine how confusing it must be for young children to be exposed to disaster imagery over and over again.

Even in a disaster situation, children need some sense of normalcy; play, the work of children, offers that. Play can offer adults a window into the minds of children, as they talk over artwork, a board game, or medical play. Parents and health-care providers who listen to children can address their questions and concerns in a nonthreatening way, as questions or issues arise. This often elicits underlying issues sooner than a more structured intervention would do.

Social, emotional, and mental health issues loom large in any disaster situation. The disaster, whether natural or man-made, raises concerns about personal safety and survival, the safety and survival of family members and loved ones, and the danger of the disaster continuing or reoccurring. This is in addition to the pain of physical injuries. Reeves (2015) reviewed the literature on trauma-informed care and found that health-care encounters can retraumatize patients who have experienced traumatic life events, including disasters. Pediatric illness and injury potentially are among the most common emotionally traumatic experiences for children and families. Millions of children who present for medical care have been exposed to prior traumatic events, such as violence or natural disasters. (Marsac et al., 2016). In addition, health-care providers can experience symptoms of trauma related to their work. Trauma-informed care has the potential to mitigate these negative consequences as well:

> Trauma-informed care minimizes the potential for medical care to become traumatic or trigger trauma reactions, addresses distress, provides emotional support for the entire family, encourages positive coping, and provides anticipatory guidance regarding the recovery process. When used in conjunction with family-centered practices, trauma-informed approaches enhance the quality of care for patients and their families and the well-being of medical professionals and support staff. (Marsac et al., 2016, p. 70)

After the 2008 earthquake in Sichuan, China, Jia et al. (2013) conducted research on the possible association between traumatic experiences and longitudinal development of mental health for children and adolescents. They looked at symptoms of PTSD and depression in children 8–16 years of age at 15 and 36 months after the earthquake. Their results suggested that a substantial proportion of children who had family members or friends seriously injured, had lost family members, or had lost significant others were still suffering symptoms of PTSD and depression even 3 years after the earthquake. They also found that the earthquake might have a delayed impact on the psychosocial functioning of the children and adolescents who were not directly affected by the earthquake. They reported that use of mental health-care services dropped substantially from the 15th month to the 36th month, raising concerns about the unmet psychological needs of children and adolescents who survive or are exposed to disasters. One unexpected finding was that children who were not directly affected by the earthquake had symptoms that grew worse over the study period. Jai and colleagues speculate that these children had less access to mental health-care services, as access was focused on those most severely affected by the quake.

Some studies that look at measures of PTSD and depression symptoms have concluded that young children are not as severely affected as older children and adolescents. However, one study following the 2011 East Japan earthquake and tsunami looked at behavior problems and found a different result. Fujiwara et al. (2014) studied children who were preschool age (2–5 years) at the time of the earthquake. They identified target communities that were affected by the quake and an unaffected community as a comparison and found clinically significant behavior problems in 26% of young children 2 years after the Great East Japan Earthquake. The rate of internalizing problems (28%) was higher than the rate of externalizing problems. Because internalized problems are less likely to be recognized, these behavior problems may have been underestimated during the 2 years following the earthquake. They also found, as have previous studies, that a disaster's long-term impact on mental health is influenced by a variety of other factors, including trauma experiences before the disaster and trauma related directly to the disaster. Losing one's home, being separated from family, or seeing a close friend or family member killed or injured were among the experiences that increased the incidence of behavior problems. Fujiwara and colleagues call for further interventions for young children exposed to disasters, such as psychoeducational programs to provide information on traumatic symptoms and coping strategies and recovery, in collaboration with school and preschool principals, teachers, and school counselors.

Wars, bombings, terrorist attacks, and mass shootings are all recent events that have had an impact on children and families. After the Boston bombings in April 2013, Guerriero et al (2014) found a 3-fold increase in functional neurological symptom disorders in children over a baseline of 2.6 cases per week in the emergency room at Boston Children's Hospital. According to Thomson (2014), functional neurological symptom disorders are physical complaints that are not primarily explained by physiological or structural abnormalities. Examples include weakness, paresthesia, nonepileptic seizures, and headaches, to name a few. The stress and coping model developed by Lazarus and Folkman (1984) is one that is frequently used to explain functional neurological symptoms. Briefly, the model seeks to explain the reactions to stressors as coping strategies that may be adaptive or maladaptive (see Chapter 2: Preparing Children for Health-Care Encounters).

The International Center to Heal Our Children: Building Healthy Minds and Futures was created at Children's National Medical Center (CNMC) in Washington, DC, shortly after the terrorist events that occurred on September 11, 2001 in New York City, Washington, DC, and Pennsylvania. The Center's vision is to help foster, promote, and maintain the emotional health of children who are psychologically traumatized secondary to acts of violence, disasters, and terrorism. The National Center for Disaster Medicine & Public Health (NCDMPH) has developed several resources for health-care professionals to help children in disasters (see Appendix 13.1: Resources).

Mental Illness and Substance Abuse Prevention

The behavioral and physical health of Americans relies on preventing mental and/or substance-use disorders in children, adolescents, and young adults. An individual's mental or substance-use disorder can have a powerful effect on the health of other individuals, their families, and communities. In some instances, such as a mass school shooting in even a very small community, the impact can be felt throughout the nation.

Symptoms signaling the development of a behavioral disorder are often manifested 2 to 4 years before a disorder is present (SAMHSA, 2016). Also, according to the 2014 National Survey on Drug Use and Health Report, of adults with any mental illness, 18.2% had a substance use disorder, while those adults with no mental illness had only a 6.3% rate of substance use disorder in the past year (SAMHSA, 2014b). Thus, if communities and families can intervene early, behavioral health disorders might be prevented, or symptoms can be mitigated.

Tackling the issue of behavioral health requires a comprehensive approach that sees prevention as part of an overall continuum of care. The behavioral health continuum of care model recognizes multiple opportunities for addressing behavioral health problems and disorders (see Figure 13.3). The model includes the following components (SAMHSA, 2016):

- *Promotion*—These strategies are designed to create environments and conditions that support behavioral health and the ability of individuals to withstand challenges. Promotion strategies also reinforce the entire continuum of behavioral health services.
- *Prevention*—Delivered prior to the onset of a disorder, these interventions are intended to prevent or reduce the risk of developing a behavioral health problem, such as underage alcohol use, prescription drug misuse and abuse, and illicit drug use.
- *Treatment*—These services are for people diagnosed with a substance use or other behavioral health disorders.
- *Recovery*—These services support individuals' abilities to live productive lives in the community and can often help with abstinence.

About 1 in 10 children live with a *serious* mental or emotional disorder (USDH-HS, 1999). About one-half of all lifetime cases of mental illness begin by age 14 (Kessler et al., 2005). Effective treatments exist; however, there are long delays—sometimes decades—between the first onset of symptoms and when people seek and receive treatment (Wang et al., 2005). Even when parents seek help for their children, with a shortage of psychiatric beds, there is often nowhere for them to go. Families often live

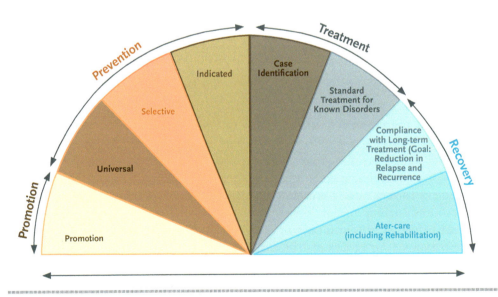

Figure 13.3. Continuum of care. *Source:* "Prevention of Substance Abuse and Mental Illness," by Substance Abuse and Mental Health Services Administration, 2016. Retrieved from www.samhsa.gov /prevention

in isolation, having little interaction with or support from their communities. A mother of a child with mental illness shares her experience:

> I live with a son who is mentally ill. I love my son. But he terrifies me. A few weeks ago, Michael pulled a knife and threatened to kill me and then himself after I asked him to return his overdue library books. His 7- and 9-year-old siblings knew the safety plan—they ran to the car and locked the doors before I even asked them to. I managed to get the knife from Michael, then methodically collected all the sharp objects in the house into a single Tupperware container that now travels with me. Through it all, he continued to scream insults at me and threaten to kill or hurt me.
>
> That conflict ended with three burly police officers and a paramedic wrestling my son onto a gurney for an expensive ambulance ride to the local emergency room. The mental hospital didn't have any beds that day, and Michael calmed down nicely in the ER, so they sent us home with a prescription for Zyprexa and a follow-up visit with a local pediatric psychiatrist. (Long, 2012)

Reducing the stigma that surrounds mental illness is a first step in helping families feel safe in speaking out. We can encourage families to tell their stories, and, applying an important concept of family-centered care, ask them for suggestions on what they think might be helpful to them as a family. Working in partnership with families, we can let them know that we are in this together and will make every effort to ensure the best possible outcomes for their child and family (Rollins, 2013).

The Health-Care Professional as an Agent of Change

Health-care professionals can address issues that affect children and family's well-being by assuming the role of a change agent. As described in Chapter 7: Families in Children's Health-Care Settings, to be a change agent is to facilitate or aid the process of change in a deliberate manner. Change can occur at various levels, such as with individuals or with systems.

The Role of Change Agent at the Individual Level

Several models are available to assist health-care professionals in advocating for change at the individual level. The transtheoretical model of behavior change (TTM) developed by James Prochaska and his colleagues is a particularly effective tool (Prochaska, Norcross, & DiClemente, 1994). In the TTM model, behavior change is conceptualized in terms of movement through a series of five discrete stages: (1) precontemplation, (2) contemplation, (3) preparation, (4) action, and (5) maintenance.

Individuals in the *precontemplation* stage are characterized by resistance to recognizing and modifying problem behaviors. They have no intention of changing their behavior in the next 6 months. *Contemplators* recognize a problem and are seriously considering changing their behavior. At the *preparation* stage, individuals intend to take action to change their behavior in the next 30 days. At the *action* stage, individuals are performing the desired behavior change at the designated criterion level. The *maintenance* stage represents continuous long-term change wherein the person works to consolidate behavioral and cognitive/experiential gains made while transitioning through the previous stages to avoid relapse.

Smoking cessation is an example that illustrates the effectiveness of the TTM model. Consider a family consisting of a father, a mother, and a preschooler with asthma. The father frequently smokes at home and in the presence of his son. The father is at the precontemplative stage in the TTM model (he has no intention of changing his behavior). An effective intervention might include education about the harmful relationship between smoking and asthma. As the father begins to consider changing his behavior (the contemplation and preparation stages), an effective intervention might focus on developing a plan to limit smoking to outside of the home. As the plan is put into place (action stage), the health-care provider might praise the father for his effort and point out the benefits for his son. In the maintenance stage, an effective intervention might involve periodic assessment of the extent to which the plan is working to reduce asthma symptoms in the son.

The Role of Change Agent at the System Level

At the system level, strategies to effect change are just as complex as those at the individual level. Situational factors such as goals, resources, and urgency help to determine an appropriate strategy to use for system-level change. Some strategies to effect change at the system level include (a) political action; (b) planning, need analysis, and evaluation; and (c) grassroots movements.

Political Action

Political action and policy development can be thought of as "decision-making through both private and public mechanisms occurring in city councils, hospitals, small businesses, community organizations, universities, courts and state legislatures" (Phillips, 2000). In a more comprehensive sense, political action and social policy might also be thought to encompass neighborhood advocacy, media campaigns, and judicial policy making (Phillips, 2000). Political action and policy making are usually directed toward changing social conditions through a variety of tactics. Social planners and community organizers have developed a wide variety of strategies to effect social change that range from formal planning with community representatives to highly confrontational tactics designed to disrupt social activities.

Porter (1991) described several situations wherein political action and policy development resulted in significant changes in health-related issues. In one situation, an obstetrician organized members of a community and succeeded in placing adolescent health-care services in a local school. His motivation was based on high teen pregnancy rates and the inability of teens to access prenatal health care. In a second example, a minister's wife and public health nurse were successful in convincing the local medical community to open a free clinic in a migrant labor camp. The free clinic eventually became the basis for a formal arrangement at the county level to provide needed medical services to migrant workers.

Planned Change, Needs Analysis, and Evaluation

A variety of theorists, including Julian and Lyons (1992) and Green and Kreuter (1991), have defined specific models that are applicable to health planning. Two of the more prevalent approaches include rational and strategic planning. Rational planning is characterized by a comprehensive review of possible solutions and the selection of the best possible alternative. Strategic planning is more focused on defining two or three critical success factors and implementing strategies to achieve specific objectives.

In addition to defining a particular course of action, the planning function should address needs assessment and evaluation of progress toward desired outcomes. A needs analysis is a tool for decision-making. A critical question addressed by needs analyses focuses on whether health-care services are available to a specific population and, if so, whether the services are adequate. If inadequate, it must be determined what specific actions are needed to correct the inadequacy.

For example, Schable et al. (1995) interviewed 541 women with HIV or AIDS. At the time of the interviews, 478 women were part of family units (mother and children) and 234 of those family units consisted of two or more children. The most common caretaker was the mother alone (46%). Grandparents were caretakers in 16% of the families; in 15% of the families, both mother and father were caretakers. Of the children of mothers who used injection drugs or lived alone, in a shelter, or with friends, almost one-quarter were cared for by their grandparents. Only 30% of the mothers knew about childcare assistance services, and only 8% had used these services. This information led planners to conclude that increased provisions for childcare assistance and planning for future permanent placement of orphaned children were urgently needed. These researchers identified the gaps in services and projected future needs of HIV-infected women.

Evaluation is an essential part of the planning process and in many cases leads to improved services for children and their families. For example, if health-care professionals conducted lead poisoning screenings at a public library or local shopping mall, several evaluation questions such as the following would be particularly relevant:

- Did the intervention make a difference?
- Were children referred appropriately?
- Did families whose children had high levels of lead seek treatment for their children?
- Was the treatment effective?

Evaluation procedures provide a structured means to answer such questions, which provide a basis for changing interventions in ways that more effectively address identified needs.

Grassroots Movements

A grassroots movement represents an alternative approach to system-level change. One model for using grassroots strategies is Freire's train-the-trainer program (Hope & Timmel, 1990). It is an effective, culturally sensitive, health-care strategy that works well to empower diverse individuals, families, and local communities. The train-the-trainer program has been used in less-developed countries to provide outreach and health care to underserved families.

In central Ohio, a team successfully implemented Freire's program to meet the needs of medically underserved families (Julian, Strayer, & Arnold, 1998). The train-the-trainer program presents practical methods for:

- group process and team building to build a sense of community,
- breaking through apathy with empowerment strategies, and
- developing critical awareness of the causes of various problems and determining true needs.

An important philosophy of this model is having the participants themselves choose the content of their education rather than having experts develop curricula for them (i.e., development must rise from the community served). Besides providing care to those who have minimal access to health-care delivery systems, the train-the-trainer model helps families transcend themselves and their limitations by drawing from their internal capacities as well as referencing a reality that is greater, outside of, and beyond themselves (Farley, 1993).

Miller (1997) documented a successful grassroots program called the Birthing Project. The Birthing Project provides pregnant women with a role model who acts as an advocate to help them navigate the maze of health-care options and determine where to receive necessary prenatal care during their pregnancies. These advocates are with the pregnant women prenatally, for the birth of their child, and during the first year of the neonate's life. In the first 3 years of the program, there was a 30% decline in the African American infant mortality rate and a decline in drug-exposed babies in the Sacramento area (Miller, 1997).

Volunteers provide a critical resource for many grassroots initiatives. It is important to follow a policy of inclusion—not exclusion—and to enable all who wish to and are able to be volunteers. In such situations, health-care professionals or other responsible parties will need to train and retrain volunteers until they feel competent and confident. Health-care providers also will need to assist in the development of leadership to sustain participation and address issues related to power and barriers. Volunteer coalitions are a wonderful way to reach out to those who have difficulty accessing health care.

Conclusion

Promoting well-being goes beyond the traditional view of prevention as only avoiding or minimizing illness and risk factors. Promoting well-being emphasizes the individual's physical, mental, and social resources, and enhances protective factors and conditions that foster health. Children and families exist within various contexts, and within these contexts are factors that either promote or discourage individual or family well-being. Adopting the role of change agent may lead to fundamental alterations in attitudes and behaviors. Such change often has the capacity to dramatically alter health-care practices and promote optimal child and family health. Political action, planning, needs analysis and evaluation, and grassroots movements represent a variety of tools that might be used to produce change at the system or community level. Such change has the potential to dramatically benefit large numbers of people and to prevent suffering.

Study Guide

1. What is well-being?

2. Provide an example that illustrates Bronfenbrenner's concept of multiple and interconnected influences on the family.

3. Analyze three social determinants and describe how they might influence a child's health.

4. Discuss the relationship between Adverse Childhood Experiences (ACE) and a selection of negative health outcomes.

5. List and describe the six key principles of a trauma-informed approach.

6. What home health-care services are available for children in your community?

7. Discuss the role of education services in children's health care.

8. Discuss the concept of empathy and how it relates to children today.

9. What are the similarities and differences between traditional bullying and cyberbullying?

10. What steps are being taken to address homelessness or other unfortunate family circumstances in your community?

11. List and explain the three levels of stress seen in children.

12. What is your attitude toward corporal punishment and why?

13. What services does your community have to support families of children and teens with mental health or substance use disorders?

14. Describe the role of the change agent.

Appendix 13.1

Resources

Publications

Healthy People 2020
https://www.healthypeople.gov/sites/default
/files/HP2020_brochure_with_LHI_508
_FNL.pdf
Healthy People 2020 brochure updated with
the leading health indicators

Integrating Behavioral Health Across the Continuum of Care
American Hospital Association. (2014). *Integrating behavioral health across the continuum of care*. Chicago, IL: Health Research & Education Trust. Retrieved from http://www.hpoe
.org/Reports-HPOE/Behavioral%20
health%20FINAL.pdf
The purpose of this guide is to help hospitals
and care systems consider the impact of better
integrating behavioral health across multiple
health care delivery settings—and provide the
tools to do so.

The Handbook of Frequently Asked Questions Following Traumatic Events: Violence, Disasters, or Terrorism
Joshi, P., Lewin, S., & O'Donnell, D. (2005).
The handbook of frequently asked questions following traumatic events: Violence, disasters, or terrorism. Washington, DC: International Center to
Heal Our Children: Building Healthy Minds
and Futures, Children's National Health System. Retrieved from https://childrensnational
.org/~/media/cnhs-site/files/resources/ichoc
/handbook.ashx?la=en
Focuses on the psychological impact of trauma,
violence, and disasters on children. Designed
to help parents and other caregivers enhance
their understanding of how to talk with
children when faced with such tragedies, in
addition to providing some answers to tough
questions.

Understanding Childhood Trauma
http://www.samhsa.gov/child-trauma/under
standing-child-trauma
An infographic developed by SAMHSA's
National Child Traumatic Stress Initiative to
help people learn to recognize the signs and
symptoms of child traumatic stress.

What Child Advocates Can Do for Unaccompanied Youth
http://center.serve.org/nche/downloads/child_
wel_uy.pdf
A question and answer sheet regarding facts
about unaccompanied youth.

Organizations/Websites

Healthy Foster Care America
https://www.aap.org/en-us/advocacy-and
-policy/aap-health-initiatives/healthy
-foster-care-america/Pages/default.aspx
Healthy Foster Care America (HFCA) is an
initiative of the American Academy of Pediatrics and its partners to improve the health
and well-being of children and teens in foster
care. Partners have included representatives
from child welfare, family practice, social
work, nursing, government, the legislative and
judicial fields, child psychiatry and psychology,
education, advocacy organizations, alumni, and
families.
See more at: https://www.aap.org/en-us
/advocacy-and-policy/aap-health-initiatives
/healthy-foster-care-america/Pages/About-Us
.aspx#sthash.ZIPkNlL4.dpuf

Health Leads
http://www.healthleadsusa.org/
A social enterprise that envisions a health-
care system that addresses all patients' basic
resource needs as a standard part of quality
care. Works with leading health-care organizations to tackle social co-morbidities by
connecting patients to the community-based
resources they need to be healthy—from food
to transportation to health-care benefits.

Migrant Clinicians Network
http://www.migrantclinician.org/about
/our-story
Migrant Clinicians Network is a 501(c)3 nonprofit organization that creates practical solutions at the intersection of poverty, migration,
and health. The organization provide bridge
case management, support, technical assistance,
and professional development to clinicians in
Federally Qualified Health Centers (FQHCs)
and other health-care delivery sites with the

ultimate purpose of providing quality health care that increases access and reduces disparities for migrant farmworkers and other mobile underserved populations. The website presents many excellent examples of successful programs for working with migrant families.

National Center for Disaster Medicine & Public Health
http://ncdmph.usuhs.edu/
Serves as the academic center of excellence for education, training, and educational research in disaster medicine and public health preparedness in the United States

National Center for Medical-Legal Partnership
http://medical-legalpartnership.org/
A national organization with the mission to improve the health and well-being of people and communities by leading the health, public health, and legal sectors in an integrated, upstream approach to combating health-harming social conditions

The National Center on Family Homelessness
http://www.familyhomelessness.org
The National Center on Family Homelessness is the nation's foremost authority on family homelessness. The Center conducts state-of-the-art research and develops innovative solutions to end family homelessness in America and give every child a chance.

stopbullying.gov
http://www.stopbullying.gov/prevention/at-school/
A website that provides information from various government agencies on what bullying is, what cyberbullying is, who is at risk, and how you can prevent and respond to bullying

Mindfulness Meditation

Beach, S. (2014, October 21). Teaching mindfulness to teenagers: 5 ways to get started. [Web log post]. Retrieved from http://www.huffingtonpost.com/sarah-rudell-beach-/teaching-mindfulness-to-teenagers_b_5696247.html

Apps
Stop, Breathe, and Think.
http://www.stopbreathethink.org/?
Opens with a short "interview" where the user selects several words to describe how he or she is feeling, and then the app recommends guided meditations for the person's current state

Smiling Mind
https://itunes.apple.com/au/app/smiling-mind/id560442518?mt=8&ign-mpt=uo%3D4
Designed especially for adolescents

Take a Break!
https://itunes.apple.com/us/app/take-break!-guided-meditations/id453857236?mt=8
Provides short guided meditations for stress relief.

Policy Statements

American Academy of Pediatrics Policy Statement on Corporal Punishment
http://www.aacap.org/AACAP/Policy_Statements/2012/Policy_Statement_on_Corporal_Punishment.aspx

American Psychological Association Resolution on Corporal Punishment
http://apa.org/about/policy/corporal-punishment.aspx

Programs

Nurse–Family Partnership
http://www.nursefamilypartnership.org/
A free maternal-health visiting program that introduces vulnerable first-time parents to caring maternal and child health nurses. Allows nurses to deliver the support first-time mothers need to have a healthy pregnancy, become knowledgeable and responsible parents, and provide their babies with the best possible start in life.

Play Nicely
http://www.childrenshospital.vanderbilt.org/interior.php?mid=1998
Play Nicely is a 40-minute multimedia program that teaches how to manage aggression in young children. Developed at Vanderbilt University, program content is based on material from many sources including the American Academy of Pediatrics, the National Association for the Education of Young Children, and the American Psychological Association. The program was improved by comments from people of different backgrounds, including preschool teachers, parents, psychologists, and health-care professionals. In published research, *Play Nicely* has been found to increase comfort level and knowledge of how to

manage childhood aggression. One year after receiving the program, parents reported that the program helped them manage aggression in their young child. Research documents that the program is embraced by those of different socio-demographic backgrounds.

References

American Academy of Child & Adolescent Psychiatry. (2015). Adopted children. *Facts for families guide.* Retrieved from http://www.aacap.org/AACAP/Families_and_youth/Facts_for_Families/FFF-Guide/The-Adopted-Child-015.aspx

American Academy of Pediatrics (AAP). (2012). Policy statement: Corporal punishment in schools. *Pediatrics, 130*(1), w248.

American Academy of Pediatrics. (2016). *Healthy Foster Care America.* Retrieved from https://www.aap.org/en-us/advocacy-and-policy/aap-health-initiatives/healthy-foster-care-america/Pages/Health-Issues.aspx

American Academy of Pediatrics Committee on Psychosocial Aspects of Child and Family Health; Committee on Early Childhood, Adoption, and Dependent Care; Section on Developmental and Behavioral Pediatrics, Garner, A. S., Shonkoff, J. P., Siegel, B., … Wood, D. (2012). Early childhood adversity, toxic stress, and the role of the pediatrician: Translating developmental science into lifelong health. *Pediatrics, 129*(1), e224–e231.

Bassuk, E. (2010). Ending child homelessness in America. *American Journal of Orthopsychiatry, 80,* 496–504. doi:10.1111/j.1939-0025.2010.01052.x

Bassuk, E., DeCamdoa. C., Beach, C., & Berman, F. (2014). *America's youngest outcasts: A report card on child homelessness.* Washington, DC: American Institutes for Research, The National Center on Family Homelessness. Retrieved from http://www.homelesschildrenamerica.org/media-docs/282.pdfna

Bassuk, E., Richard, M., & Tsertsvadze, A. (2015). The prevalence of mental illness in homeless children: A systematic review and meta-analysis. *Journal of the American Academy of Child & Adolescent Psychiatry, 54*(2), 86–96.

Beardslee, W. R., Gladstone, T. R., Wright, E. J., & Cooper, A. B. (2003). A family-based approach to the prevention of depressive symptoms in children at risk: Evidence of parental and child change. *Pediatrics, 112,*119–131.

Blaisure, K. (2012). *Serving military families in the 21st century.* New York, NY: Routledge.

Boberiene, L., & Hornback, B. (2014). How can policy strengthen community support for children in military families. *American Journal of Orthopsychiatry, 84*(5), 439–446.

Braveman, P., & Gottlieb, L. (2014). The social determinants of health: It's time to consider the causes of the causes. *Public Health Reports, 2*(129), 19–31.

Bronfenbrenner, U. (1979). *Understanding family process: Basics of family systems theory.* Thousand Oaks, CA: Sage Publications.

Bronfenbrenner, U. (1999). Environments in developmental perspective: Theoretical and operational models. In S. L. Friedman, & T. D Wachs (Eds.), *Measuring environment across the life span: Emerging methods and concepts* (pp. 3–28). Washington, DC: American Psychological Association Press.

Buckner, J., Beardslee, W., & Bassuk, E. (2004). Exposure to violence and low-income children's mental health: Direct, moderated, and mediated relations. *American Journal of Orthopsychiatry, 74*(4), 413–423.

Cavendish, B., & Cortazar, M. (2011). *Children at the border: The screening, protection and repatriation of unaccompanied Mexican minors.* Washington, DC: Appleseed Foundation.

Centers for Disease Control and Prevention. (2013a). *Well-being concepts.* Retrieved from http://www.cdc.gov/hrqol/wellbeing.htm#three

Centers for Disease Control and Prevention. (2013b). Mental health surveillance among children—United States, 2005–2011. *Morbidity and Mortality Weekly Report, 62,* 2, 1–40.

Centers for Disease Control and Prevention. (2015). *Vital signs: Today's heroin epidemic.* Retrieved from http://www.cdc.gov/vitalsigns/heroin/index.html

Centers for Disease Control and Prevention. (2016). Postpartum depression. *Reproductive health.* Retrieved from http://www.cdc.gov/reproductivehealth/Depression/index.htm

Chandra, A., Martin, L., Hawkins, S., & Richardson, A. (2010). The impact of parental deployment on child social and emotional functioning: Perspectives of school staff. *Journal of Adolescent Health*, *46*(3), 218–223.

Child Trends. (2012). *Adopted children*. Available at: http://www.childtrends.org/?indicators=-adopted-children

Child Trends. (2014). *Immigrant children*. Retrieved from http://www.childtrends.org/?indicators=immigrant-children

Conrad, B. (2016a). *Media Statistics—Children's use of TV, Internet, and video games*. Retrieved from http://www.techaddiction.ca/media-statistics.html

Conrad, B. (2016b). *Children and technology—Stats for technology in the home*. Retrieved from http://www.techaddiction.ca/children-and-technology.html

Council on Foster Care, Adoption, and Kinship Care, Committee on Adolescence, and Council on Early Childhood. (2015). Health care issues for children and adolescents in foster care and kinship care. *Pediatrics*, *136*(4), e1131–e1140.

Cozza, S., Chun, R. S., & Miller, C. (2011). The children and families of combat injured service members. In E. C. Richie (Ed.), *War psychiatry* (pp. 503–533). Washington, DC: Borden Institute.

Crea, T. M, & Barth, R. P. (2009). Patterns and predictors of adoption openness and contact: 14 years postadoption. *Family Relations: Interdisciplinary Journal of Applied Family Studies*, *58*, 607–620.

Crum-Cianflone, N., Fairbank, J., Marmar, C., & Schlenger, W. (2014). The Millennium Cohort Family Study: A prospective evaluation of the health and well-being of military service members and their families. *International Journal of Methods in Psychiatric Research*, *23*(3), 320–330.

Decety, J., Michalska, K., Akitsuki, Y., & Lahey, B. (2009). Atypical empathic responses in adolescents with aggressive conduct disorder: A functional MRI investigation. *Biological Psychology*, *80*(2), 203. doi:10.1016/j.biopsych. 2008.09.004

DeNies, Y. (2012). *Should your child be spanked at school? In 19 states, it's legal*. Retrieved from http://abcnews.go.com/US/spanking school-19-states-corporal-punishmentlegal/story?id=15932135#.UFsIdY5gIqY

Department of Defense. (2010, October). *Report on the impact of deployment of members of the armed forces on their dependent children*. Retrieved from http://www.militaryonesource.mil/12038/MOS/Reports/Report_to_Congress_on_Impact_of_Deployment_on_Military_Children.pdf

Easterling, B., & Knox, D. (2010). Left behind: The deployment experience of military wives. *Journal of Family Life*. Retrieved from www.journaloffamilylife.org/militarywives

Farley, S. (1993). The community as partner in primary health care nursing and health care. *Nursing & Health Care*, *14*(5), 224–229.

Felitti, V., Anda, R., Nordenberg, D., Williamson, D., Spritz, A. Edwards, V., . . . Marks, J. (1998). Relationship of childhood abuse and household dysfunction to many of the leading causes of death in adults: The Adverse Childhood Experiences (ACE) Study. *American Journal of Preventive Medicine*, *14*(4), 245–258.

Fischer, H. (2014). *A guide to U.S. military casualty statistics: Operation Inherent Resolve, Operation New Dawn, Operation Iraqi Freedom, and Operation Enduring Freedom*. Washington, DC: Congressional Research Service.

Flake, E., Davis, B., Johnson, P., & Middleton, L. (2009). The psychosocial effects of deployment on military children. *Journal of Developmental and Behavioral Pediatrics*, *30*(4), 271–278.

Forgatch, M., & DeGarmo, D. (1999). Parenting through change: An effective prevention program for single mothers. *Journal of Consulting and Clinical Psychology*, *67*(5), 711–724.

Fujiwara, T., Yagi, J., Homma, H., Mashiko, H., Nagao, K., Okuyama, M., & Great East Japan Earthquake Follow-up for Children Study Team. (2014). Clinically significant behavior problems among young children 2 years after the Great East Japan Earthquake. *PLOS ONE*, *9*(10) e109342.

Full House Committee on Oversight and Government Reform. (2016, March 22). *America's heroin and opioid abuse epidemic.* Retrieved from https://oversight.house.gov/hearing/americas-heroin -and-opioid-abuse-epidemic/

Gershoff, E. T., & Grogan-Kaylor, A. (2016, April 7). Spanking and child outcomes: Old controversies and new meta-analyses. *Journal of Family Psychology, 30*(4), 453–469. doi.org/10.1037 /fam0000191

Gorman, G., Eide, M., & Hisle-Gorman, E. (2010). Wartime military deployment and increased pediatric mental and behavioral health complaint. *Pediatrics, 126*(6), 1058–1056.

Green, L. W., & Kreuter, M. W. (1991). *Health promotion planning: An educational and environmental approach.* Mountain View, CA: Mayfield.

Guerriero, R. M., Pier, D. B., deGusmao, C. M., Bernson-Leung, M. E., Maski, K. P., Urion, D. K., & Waugh, J. L. (2014). Increased pediatric functional neurological symptom disorders after the Boston Marathon bombings: A case series. *Pediatric Neurology, 51*(5), 619–623.

H.R. 2268, 114th Cong. (2015–2016)—Ending Corporal Punishment in Schools Act of 2015. Retrieved from https://www.congress.gov/bill/114th-congress/house-bill/2268

Hahn, R. A., Bilukha, O., Lowy, J., Crosby, A. Fullilove, M., Liverman, A., … Task Force on Community Preventive Services. (2005). The effectiveness of therapeutic foster care for the prevention of violence: A systematic review. *American Journal of Preventive Medicine, 28* (2 suppl 1), 72–90.

Hamilton, E. R., Cardoso, J. B., Hummer, R. A., & Padilla, Y. C. (2011). Assimilation and emerging health disparities among new generations of U.S. children. *Demographic Research, 25,* 783–818.

Hanson, M. (2013). Families in context: Conceptual frameworks for understanding and supporting families. In M. Hanson, & E. Lynch (Eds.), *Understanding families: Supportive approaches to diversity, disability, and risk* (2nd ed., pp. 43–71). Baltimore, MD: Paul H. Brookes.

Harris, K. M. (1999). The health status and risk behaviors of adolescents in immigrant families. In National Research Council and Institute of Medicine, *Children of immigrants: Health adjustment and public assistance* (pp. 286–347). Washington, DC: The National Academies Press. Retrieved from http://www.nap.edu/books/0309065453/html/

HealthyPeople.gov. (2016). *Health-related quality of life & well-being.* Retrieved from https://www .healthypeople.gov/2020/topics-objectives/topic/health-related-quality-of-life-well-being

Herbers, J. E., Cutuli, J. J., Monn, A. R., Narayan, A. J., & Masten, A. S. (2014). Trauma, adversity, and parent-child relationships among young children experiencing homelessness. *Journal of Abnormal Child Psychology, 42*(7), 1167–1174. doi: 10.1007/s10802-014-9868-7

Hernandez, D. J., Denton, N. A., & Macartney, S. E. (2008). Children in immigrant families: Looking to America's future. *Social Policy Report, 22*(3). See more at http://www.childtrends .org/?indicators=immigrant-children#sthash.j0TqOEVR.dpuf

Hope, A., & Timmel, S. (1990). *Training for transformation.* Gwerw, Zimbabwe: Mambo Press.

Howell E. (2004). Access to children's mental health services under Medicaid and SCHIP. *New Federalism, National Survey of America's Families* (NASF), the Urban Institute (Series B, No. B-60). Retrieved from http://www.urban.org/research/publication/access-childrens-mental -health-services-under-medicaid-and-schip

Hudziak, J., & Ivanova, M. (2016). The Vermont family based approach. *Child and Adolescent Psychiatric Clinics of North America, 25,* 167–178.

Huntington, N., Buckner, J. C., & Bassuk, E. L. (2008). Adaptation in homeless children: An empirical examination using cluster analysis. *American Behavioral Scientist, 51,* 737–755.

Hwang, R., & Jeong, S. (2015). Predictors of parental mediation regarding children's smartphone use. *Cyberpsychology, Behavior, and Social Networking, 18*(12), 737–743.

Inter-American Commission on Human Rights. (2015). *Human rights situation of refugee and migrant families and unaccompanied children in the United States of America.* Washington, DC: Author.

Jia, Z., Shi, L., Duan, G., Liu, W., Pan, X., Chen, Y., . . . Tian, W. (2013). Traumatic experiences and mental health consequences among child survivors of the 2008 Sichuan earthquake: A community-based follow-up study. *BMC Public Health, 13*, 104.

Johnson, H., & Ling, C. (2013). Caring for military children in the 21st century. *Journal of the American Association of Nurse Practitioners, 25*, 195–201.

Julian, D., & Lyons, T. (1992). A strategic planning model for human services: Problem solving at the local level. *Evaluation and program planning, 15*, 247–254.

Julian, T., Strayer, J., & Arnold, R. (1998). Project Community CARE: A neighborhood health intervention. *Community Psychologist, 31*, 18–20.

Kaminiener, Y., & Winters, K. (2011). *Clinical manual of adolescent substance abuse treatment.* Washington, DC: American Psychiatric Publishing.

Kaneshiro, N. K. (2014). Stress in childhood. *The University of Maryland Medical Center.* Retrieved from http://umm.edu/health/medical/ency/articles/stress-in-childhood

Kao, G. (1999). Psychological well-being and educational achievement among immigrant youth. In National Research Council and Institute of Medicine, *Children of immigrants: Health adjustment and public assistance* (pp. 410–447). Washington, DC: The National Academies Press. Retrieved from http://www.nap.edu/books/0309065453/html/

Kessler, R. Berglund, P., Demier, O., Jin, R., Merikangas, K., & Walters, E. (2005). Lifetime prevalence and age-of-onset distributions of DSM-IV disorder in the National Co-morbidity Survey Replication (NCSR). *General Psychiatry, 62*, 593–602

Kilgore, C. (2015, November 2). AAAP: Treat corporal punishment as a risk factor. *Family Practice News.* Retrieved from http://www.familypracticenews.com/specialty-focus/child-adolescent-medicine/single-article-page/aap-treat-corporal-punishment-as-a-risk-factor/110db91ad45907de1d25170537a644ad.html

Kim-Spoon, J., Haskett, M. E., Longo, G. S., & Nice, R. (2012). Longitudinal study of self-regulation, positive parenting, and adjustment problems among physically abused children. *Child Abuse & Neglect, 36*(2), 95–107.

Klein, D., & Adelman, W. (2008). Adolescent pregnancy in the U.S. military: What we know and what we need to know. *Military Medicine, 173*(7), 658–665.

Kobau, R., Sniezek, J., Zack, M. M., Lucas, R. E., & Burns, A. (2010). Well-being assessment: An evaluation of well-being scales for public health and population estimates of well-being among U.S. adults. *Health and Well Being, 2*(3), 272–297.

Konecky, B., Cellucci, T., & Mochrie, K. (2016). Predictors of program failure in a juvenile drug court program. *Addictive Behaviors, 59*, 80–83.

Konrath, S., O'Brien, E., & Hsing, C. (2011). Changes in dispositional empathy in American college students over time: A meta-analysis. *Personality and Social Psychology Review, 15*(2), 180–198.

Kuehn, B. (2014). AAP: Toxic stress threatens kids' long-term health. *JAMA, 312*(6), 585–586.

Lester, P., Peterson, K., Reeves, J., Knauss, L., Glover, D., Mogil, C., & Beardslee, W. (2010). The long war and parental combat deployment: Effects on military children and at-home spouses. *Journal of the American Academy of Child and Adolescent Psychiatry, 49*, 310–320.

Levi, J. Segal, L., Martin, A., Biasi, A., & May, K. (2015). *Reducing teen substance misuse: What really works.* Washington, DC: Trust for America's Health. Retrieved from http://www.healthyamericans.org/assets/files/TFAH-2015-TeenSubstAbuse-FnlRv.pdf

Limber, S., Olweus, D., & Luxenberg, H. (2013). *Bullying in U.S. schools.* Retrieved from http://www.violencepreventionworks.org/public/index.page

Long, L. (2012, December 16). 'I am Adam Lanza's mother': A mom's perspective on the mental illness conversation in America. Retrieved from http://www.huffingtonpost.com/2012/12/16/i-am-adam-lanzas-mother-mental-illnessconversation_n_2311009.html

Mars, S. G., Bourgois, P., Karandinos, G., Montero, F., & Ciccarone, D. (2014). "Every 'never' I ever said came true": Transitions from opioid pills to heroin injecting. *International Journal of Drug Policy, 25*, 257–266.

Marsac, M. L., Kassam-Adams, N., Hildenbrand, A. K., Nicholls, E., Winston, F. K., Leff, S. S., & Fein, J. (2016). Implementing a trauma-informed approach in pediatric health care networks. *Pediatrics, 170*(1), 70–77.

McCarthy J., Bossarte, R., Katz, R., Thompson, C., Kemp, J., Hannemann, C., . . . Schoenbaum, M. (2015). Predictive modeling and concentration of the risk of suicide: Implications for preventive interventions in the US Department of Veterans Affairs. *American Journal of Public Health, 105*(9), 1935–1942.

Middlebrooks, J. S., & Audage, N. C. (2008). *The effects of childhood stress on health across the lifespan.* Atlanta, GA: National Center for Injury Prevention and Control of the Centers for Disease Control and Prevention.

Migrant Clinicians Network. (2014). *Children's health.* Retrieved from http://www.migrantclinician.org/issues/childrenshealth

Miller, C. (1997, November/December). Sisterly support, healthy babies: With one-on-one mentoring for moms. The Birthing Project boosts babies' health. *Children's Advocate,* 1–12.

Minnis, H. (2013). Maltreatment-associated psychiatric problems: An example of environmentally triggered ESSENCE? *The Scientific World Journal, 2013,* Article ID 148468. Retrieved from http://dx.doi.org/10.1155/2013/148468

Monroe, R., & Harris, V. (2013). *Family reunification following foster care.* Department of Family, Youth and Community Sciences, Florida Cooperative Extension Service, Institute of Food and Agricultural Sciences, University of Florida. Retrieved from http://edis.ifas.ufl.edu/fy1366

N'zi, A., Steens, M., & Eyberg, S. (2016). Child directed interaction training for young children in kinship care: A pilot study. *Child Abuse & Neglect, 55,* 81–91.

Nansel, T., Overpeck, M., Haynie, D., Ruan, W., & Scheidt, P. (2003). Relationships between bullying and violence among U.S. youth. *Archives of Pediatric and Adolescent Medicine, 157,* 348–353.

National Association of School Nurses. (2015). *Naloxone use in the school setting: The role of the school nurse. Position statement.* Retrieved from http://www.nasn.org/portals/0/positions/2015psnaloxone.pdf

National Center for Medical-Legal Partnership (NCMLP). (2016). *Main page.* Retrieved from http://medical-legalpartnership.org

National Center on Family Homelessness. (2010). *Homeless children stats.* Retrieved from http://rcaa.org/division/family-services/news/homeless-children-stats

National Child Traumatic Stress Network. (2005). *Facts on trauma and homeless children.* Retrieved from http://nctsnet.org/nctsn_assets/pdfs/promising_practices/Facts_on_Trauma_and_Homeless_Children.pdf

National Crime Prevention Council. (n.d.). *Cyberbullying.* Retrieved from http://www.ncpc.org/topics/cyberbullying

National Institute on Drug Abuse. (2015a). *Monitoring the Future Survey, overview of findings 2015.* Retrieved from https://www.drugabuse.gov/related-topics/trends-statistics/monitoring-future/monitoring-future-survey-overview-findings-2015

National Institute on Drug Abuse. (2015b). *National Survey of Drug Use and Health: Trends in prevalence of various drugs for ages 12 or older, ages 12 to 17, Ages 18 to 25, and ages 26 or older; 2012–2014 (in percent).* Retrieved from https://www.drugabuse.gov/national-survey-drug-use-health

National Military Family Association. (2012). Military deployment: The impact on children and family adjustment and the need for care. *Current Opinion in Psychiatry, 22*(3), 369–373.

Nguyen, D., Ee, J., Berry-Caban, C., & Hoedebecke, K. (2014, October–December). The effects of military deployment on early child development. *United States Army Medical Department Journal,* 81–86.

Office of the Press Secretary, The White House. (2016, February 2). *FACT SHEET: President Obama proposes $1.1 billion in new funding to address the prescription opioid abuse and heroin use epidemic.* Retrieved from https://www.whitehouse.gov/the-press-office/2016/02/02/president-obama-proposes-11-billion-new-funding-address-prescription

Pecora P. J., Kessler R. C., Williams, J, O'Brien, K., Downs, A. D., & English, D. Holmes, K. E. (2005). *Improving family foster care: Findings from the Northwest Foster Care Alumni Study.* Seattle, WA: Casey Family Programs.

Phillips, D. A. (2000). Social policy and community pssychoogy. In J. Rappaport, & E. Seidman (Eds.), *Handbook of community psychology* (pp. 397–421). New York, NY: Kluwer Academic /Plemum.

Price, J. (2013). When a child's parent has PTSD. *National Center for PTSD.* Retrieved from http://www.ptsd.va.gov/professional/pages/pro_child_parent_ptsd.asp

Pritchett, R., Hockaday, H., Anderson, B., Davidson, C., Gillberg, C., & Minnis, H. (2016). Challenges of assessing maltreated children coming into foster care. *The Scientific World Journal, 2016,* Article ID 5986835. Retrieved from http://www.hindawi.com/journals /tswj/2016/5986835/

Prochaska, J., Norcross, J., & DiClemente, C. (1994). *Changing for good.* New York, NY: Morrow.

Razani, N., Meade, K., Scjiudel, C. Johnson, C., & Long, D. (2015). Healing through nature: A park-based health intervention for young people in Oakland, California. *Children, Youth and Environments, 25*(1), 147–159.

Reeves, E. (2015) A synthesis of the literature on trauma-informed care. *Issues in Mental Health Nursing, 36*(9), 698–709.

Rollins, J. (2012). 2012: Revisiting the issue of corporal punishment in our nation's schools. *Pediatric Nursing, 38*(5), 248, 269.

Rollins, J. (2013). The aftermath of December 14, 2012. *Pediatric Nursing, 39*(1), 10–11.

Rollins, J. (2014). Some thoughts about empathy. *Pediatric Nursing, 40*(4), 162–163.

Rollins, J., & King, E. (2015). Promoting coping for children of hospitalized service members with combat injuries through creative arts engagement. *Arts & Health: An International Journal for Research, Policy and Practice, 7*(2), 109–122.

Roots of Empathy. (n.d.). *About our program.* Retrieved from http://www.rootsofempathy.org/en /what-we-do.html

Rosenberg, T. (2014, December 11). Big ideas in social change, 2014. *The New York Times.* Retrieved from http://opinionator.blogs.nytimes.com/2014/12/11/big-ideas-in-social-change-2014/?_r=0

Sandel, M., Hansen, M., Kahn, R., Lawton, E., Paul, E., Parker, V., … Zuckerman, B. (2010). Medical-legal partnerships: Transforming primary care by addressing the legal needs of vulnerable populations. *Health Affairs, 29*(9), 1697–1705.

Schable, B., Diaz, T., Chu, S., Caldwell, M., Conti, L., Alston, O. M., … Davidson, A. J. (1995). Who are the primary caretakers of children born to HIV infected mothers? Results from a multi-state surveillance project. *Pediatrics, 95*(4), 511–515.

Sheller, S., & Hudson, K. (2010). *The family care curriculum.* Philadelphia, PA: Author.

Sibinga, E. M., Webb, L., Ghazarian, S. R., & Ellen, J. M. (2016) School-based mindfulness instruction: A RCT. *Pediatrics, 137*(1). doi: 10.1542/peds.2015-2532. Epub 2015 Dec 18.

Siegel, D. H. (2008). Open adoption and adolescence. *Families in Society: The Journal of Contemporary Social Services, 89*(3). 366–374. doi: 10.1606/1044-3894.3762

Sories, G., Mair, C., Beer, A., & Volker, T. (2015). Addressing the needs of military children through family-based play therapy. *Contemporary Family Therapy, 37*(3), 209–220.

Substance Abuse and Mental Health Services Administration. (2014a). *SAMHSA's concept of trauma and guidance for a trauma-informed approach.* Rockville, MD: Author. Retrieved from http://store.samhsa.gov/shin/content//SMA14-4884/SMA14-4884.pdf

Substance Abuse and Mental Health Services Administration. (2014b). *National Survey on Drug Use and Health.* Retrieved from http://store.samhsa.gov/shin/content/NSDUH14-0904/NS DUH14-0904.pdf

Substance Abuse and Mental Health Services Administration (SAMHSA). (2015). *Results from the 2014 National Survey on Drug Use and Health: Detailed tables.* Retrieved from http://www.samh sa.gov/data/sites/default/files/NSDUH-DetTabs2014/NSDUH-DetTabs2014.htm#tab7-2a

Substance Abuse and Mental Health Services Administration. (2016). *Prevention of substance abuse and mental illness*. Retrieved from http://www.samhsa.gov/prevention

Szilagyi, M., Rosen, D., Rubin, D., Zlotnik, Council of Foster Care, Adoption, and Kinship Care, Committee on Adolescence, and Council on Early Childhood. (2015). Health care issues for children and adolescents in foster care and kinship care. *Pediatrics, 136*(4), e1142–e1166.

Taussig, H., Culhane, S., Garrido, E., & Knudtson, M. (2012). RCT of a mentoring and skills group program: Placement and permanency outcomes for foster youth. *Pediatrics, 130*(1), e33-e39.

Thomson, L. (2014). Functional neurological disorders: It is all in the head. In R. D. Anbar (Ed.), *Functional symptoms in pediatric disease: A clinical guide* (pp. 15–25). New York, NY: Springer Science + Business Media.

Twenge, J. (2013). The evidence for Generation Me and against Generation We. *Emerging Adulthood, 1*(1), 11–16.

Twenge, J., Konrath, S., Foster, J., Campbell, W., & Bushman, B. (2008). Egos inflating over time: A cross-temporal Metaanalysis of the narcissistic personality inventory. *Journal of Personality, 76*, 875–902.

UNICEF. (2014). *Hidden in plain sight: A statistical analysis of violence against children*. New York, NY: UNICEF.

U.S. Department of Education. (2009). *Anniversary of Title VI marks progress and reminds us that every child has the right to an education*. Retrieved from http://www.ed.gov/news/press-releases /anniversary-title-vi-marks-progress-and-reminds-us-every-childhas-right-education

U.S. Department of Education. (2015). *McKinney-Vento Homeless Assistance Act of 1987*. Retrieved from http://www2.ed.gov/programs/homeless/legislation.html

U.S. Department of Health and Human Services. (1999). *Mental health: A report of the Surgeon General*. Rockville, MD: U.S. Department of Health and Human Services, Substance Abuse and Mental Health Services Administration, Center for Mental Health Services.

U.S. Department of Health and Human Services. (2003). *Steps to a healthier US: A program and policy perspective—The power of prevention*. Washington, DC: Author.

U.S. Department of Health and Human Services, Administration for Children and Families, Administration of Children, Youth and Families, Children's Bureau. (2016). *Child welfare outcomes 2010–2013: Report to Congress*. Washington, DC: Author. Retrieved from https://www.acf.hhs .gov/sites/default/files/cb/cwo10_13.pdf#page=7

U.S. Department of Housing and Urban Development (HUD). (2014). The 2014 point-in-time estimates of homelessness. *The 2014 Annual Homeless Assessment Report to Congress, Vol 1*. Washington, DC: Author.

U.S. Interagency Council on Homelessness (USICH). (2014). *Opening doors: Federal strategic plan to prevent and end homelessness*. Washington, DC: Author.

Wang, P., Berglund, P., Olfson, M., Pincus, H., Wells, K., & Kessler, R. (2005). Failure and delay in initial treatment contact after first onset of mental disorders in the National Co-morbidity Survey Replication (NCSR). *General Psychiatry, 62*, 603–613.

Weber, D., & Weber, D. (2005). Geographic relocation frequency, resilience, and military adolescent behavior. *Military Medicine, 170*(7), 638–642.

White, J., & Klein, D. (2008). *Family theories* (3rd ed.). Thousand Oaks, CA: Sage Publications.

Wiltz, T. (2015, August 24). Unaccompanied children from Central America, one year later. *HuffPost Latino Voices*. Retrieved from http://www.huffingtonpost.com/entry/unaccompanied -children-from-central-america-one-year-later_us_55db88b4e4b04ae497041d10

World Health Organization. (2011). *What are the social determinants of health?* Retrieved from http:// www.who.int/social_determinants/sdh_definition/en/

Zuckerman, D., Bushman, S., & Pedersen, S. (2012). *Bullying and violence*. Retrieved from http:// center4research.org/violencerisky-behavior/z-other-violence/bullying-and-violence

Epilogue

Judy A. Rollins

As we imagine the future of children's health care and its psychosocial implications, those who advocate for children and their families will face ongoing as well as new challenges. We look at what some of these challenges might be, within the context of some of the more prominent trends of today.

Hospitals

We continue to see the hospital being reinvented to conform to the forces that are replacing the acute, inpatient-oriented illness model of health care with a disease-prevention, health-promotion, primary-care model. Hospitals are merging to form regional health-care systems with names that sound more like businesses than health-care institutions. Growing numbers of religious hospitals are finding it difficult to survive.

What does the future hold for hospitals? Hospitals will no longer conduct the "core business" of U.S. health care; however, they can play a key role by empowering others and facilitating the integration of health services across the continuum of care. For example, with the overwhelming trend toward vertical integration of health-care organizations, hospital-based case-management programs have taken the lead in considering how existing case-management models can expand to meet patient and provider needs along a continuum of care. Parents, particularly parents of children with special health-care needs, need to have a voice in the creation of these management models to ensure that psychosocial care and other important elements of comprehensive family-centered care are included.

Expansion of the Hospitalist

In an era of cost containment, only very sick children are hospitalized and as quickly as possible are sent home or to a less costly medical setting. Shorter hospital stays mean that inpatient conditions are more acute and require more of the attending physician's time and personal attention—time that many ambulatory physicians no longer have. Today's pediatricians and other primary care physicians spend the bulk of their time in an office or clinic where the skills a physician needs and the illnesses seen are fundamentally different from the skills needed in the hospital setting.

Inpatient and outpatient medicine have become so dissimilar in recent years that a new medical specialist emerged in 1996 called a hospitalist (Wachter & Goldman, 1996). Sometimes called inpatient specialists, hospitalists are physicians who spend 25% or more of their time in the hospital setting working as the physician-on-record of hospitalized patients. Although variations exist, the basic concept is that the hospitalist accepts patients from community physicians and manages their in-hospital care, keeps the primary physicians up to date on their patients' progress, and transfers care back to those physicians upon a patient's discharge. The profession has exploded in popularity, from 11,000 hospitalists in 2003 to over 40,000 in 2013 (Scheurer, 2013).

The goals of the hospitalist approach are to increase the efficiency of inpatient care while decreasing its costs. Proponents of this approach argue that inpatient specialists can give more personalized care to hospitalized patients because they spend most of their time in the hospital rather than in the office. Being "in-house" allows them to see patients several times a day, adjust therapies more efficiently, better coordinate care among consulting specialists, and quickly respond to patient problems or complications. They believe that this intensive care shortens hospital stays, decreases medical costs, and improves the quality of care (Wachter & Goldman, 1996). Others cite benefits such as patient satisfaction and physicians enjoying having more time to see patients in the office without the often-competing demands of hospital work (Brandner, 1995; Henry, 1997).

Opponents argue that decreased cost of inpatient care does not necessarily equal more cost-effective or high-value care. The hospitalist is likely to be unfamiliar with the patient's history and current psychosocial milieu, and might order more aggressive workups and intervention than would the patient's personal physician, thus increasing the cost of care in both the short and long term (Epstein, 1997). Further, with shorter hospital stays and more complex problems, some opponents of the hospitalist approach point out that the physician–patient relationship and continuity of care are more important than ever before. For children with special health-care needs and the variety and number of coordinated services they often require, the hospitalist approach may result in less favorable outcomes. Ryan (1997) noted the inconsistency of preaching continuity of care but "abandoning it at the hospital door as an unnecessary burden."

In a review of research on hospitalist performance from 1996 through 2010, the majority of articles demonstrated that hospitalists are efficient providers of inpatient care on the basis of reductions in their patients' average length of stay (69%) and total hospital costs (70%); however, the clinical quality of hospitalist care appears to be comparable to that provided by their colleagues (White & Glazier, 2011).

Hospitalists and the Outpatient Clinic

Although the hospitalist movement has grown and evolved in hospitals across North America, the role of hospitalists in the clinic has received little attention. Children's hospitalists Mahant and Weinstein (2016) believe there is benefit for working in both settings. When hospitalists follow children who have had complicated hospitalizations after discharge, they can see firsthand the downstream effects of the clinical decisions they made during the inpatient stay, providing feedback on the quality of their clinical management. They also find that seeing what can be accomplished in the outpatient setting informs their practice on the inpatient unit so that care is efficient and value added:

> For example, two ways of approaching a diagnostic dilemma are a "shot gun" approach, wherein all potential diagnoses are investigated at once, or a "serial"

approach, wherein likely or most serious causes are investigated first and then the patient's clinical course dictates which direction to pursue next. We have often observed that inpatient care can be impatient, resulting in the shotgun approach because of an underappreciation of what can be accomplished in the ambulatory setting and the benefits of careful observation over time. (p. 3)

Mahand and Weinstein (2016) also cited advantages to seeing frequently hospitalized children with complex conditions when they are not in crisis, which allows them an appreciation of the children's lives at their baseline health status. The calm environment makes it easier to discuss care preferences and long-term goals. This continuity of care has been shown to reduce length of hospital stay and keep the child and family in the comfort and safety of their home (Cohen et al., 2010). Mahand and Weinstein have also found that this broader insight into the care of patients and an understanding of who they are have enriched their experiences as physicians. They found that this insight is richer when they travel the course with children through the inpatient unit and the clinic over time. It provides additional meaning to their work balance and offers protection from career burnout.

Professionals

What is ahead for professionals? At this writing, perhaps the one of the most crucial issues is the nursing shortage. Research indicates a relationship between the work environment of a hospital and the quality of care it provides. In a study of 488 hospitals in 12 European countries and 617 hospitals in 4 U.S. states, features of the hospital work environment (e.g., better staffing ratios of patients to nurses, nurse involvement in decision-making, and positive doctor–nurse relations) were associated with improved patient outcomes, including mortality and patient satisfaction (Aiken et al., 2012). A lower likelihood of burnout was also associated with a better work environment.

An aging workforce makes this shortage different from previous ones. Today, about one-third of the nursing workforce is over 50 years of age (Health Resources and Services Administration, 2013). With many older nurses leaving acute-care settings due a the requirement to work 12-hour shifts (Rollins, 2015a), patient care delivery models may need to be redesigned to support an older workforce, using new technology and offering flexibility in scheduling, increased time off, and sabbaticals.

Will the nursing shortage and other changes affect psychosocial care for children in health-care settings? We already see that faced with less time for each patient, nurses often are forced to abbreviate, but hopefully never eliminate, preparation or other essential elements of psychosocial support. Nursing technicians already have assumed some tasks that were commonly performed by nurses (e.g., checking vital signs). Such tasks provide opportunities to conduct psychosocial assessments and deliver psychosocial support. As this trend is predicted to continue, how can we ensure that critical elements of psychosocial care will not be neglected? Perhaps future training for such personnel will place a greater emphasis on psychosocial content.

The shortage of pediatric subspecialists also will have an impact on children's psychosocial care. According to the American Academy of Pediatrics (AAP), a shortage of pediatric medical subspecialists and pediatric surgical specialists currently exists in the United States (AAP, 2016). Because of the growing numbers of children with chronic health problems and special health-care needs, this shortage is likely to intensify. Children may have to travel far from home to receive the services of a pediatric subspecialist, resulting in an increase in separation from family members and friends. Health care at a distance also can mean greater disruption for other family members, especially siblings. The AAP believes an appropriately financed graduate medical education system is critical to ensuring that sufficient numbers of trained pediatricians are available to provide optimal health care to all children.

In an effort to keep health-care costs down, many health-care services that were traditionally provided by physicians are increasingly being pushed down to less expensive providers. For example, hospitals may use a certified registered nurse anesthetist rather than an anesthesiologist. Physician assistants and nurse practitioners are stepping into other areas in which physicians traditionally have had a monopoly. We must ensure that psychosocial knowledge and skills are essential elements of the education for all health-care professionals who assume these roles.

We are hopeful that more hospitals and other pediatric and community settings will employ child life specialists. The position statement on child life by the AAP concludes that child life services make a difference in pediatric care. The statement recommends the following (AAP, Committee on Hospital Care, 2014, pp. e1475–e1476):

1. Child life services should be delivered as part of an integrated patient-and family-centered model of care and included as a quality indicator in the delivery of services for children and families in health-care settings.

2. Child life services should be provided directly by certified child life specialists in pediatric inpatient units, emergency departments, chronic care centers, and other diagnostic/ treatment areas to the extent appropriate for the population served. In hospitals with a small number of inpatient or outpatient pediatric visits, ongoing consultation with a certified child life specialist is recommended to educate health-care team members and support developmentally appropriate, patient- and family-centered practice.

3. Child life services staffing should be individualized to address the needs of specific inpatient and outpatient areas. Child life specialist-to-patient ratios should be adjusted as needed for the medical complexity of patients served, including psychosocial and developmental vulnerability as well as family needs and preferences.

4. Child life services should be included in the hospital operating budget as an essential part of hospital-based pediatric care. Advocacy for financing of child life services should occur at the facility, community, state, and federal levels.

5. Additional research should be conducted to evaluate the effects of child life services on patient care outcomes, including patient and family experience/ satisfaction, staffing ratios, throughput, and cost-effectiveness.

Children in all health-care settings will benefit if these recommendations are followed. However, because of cost implications, this expansion is only likely to occur if families as consumers understand the importance of psychosocial support for their children and the child life specialist's ability to provide such support. Greater efforts must be undertaken to educate families and health-care professionals about the role of the child life specialist as an essential member of the child's health-care team.

Workforce Diversity

The increasing percentage of children from racial and ethnic minority groups will influence recruitment efforts for diversity among pediatricians, pediatric nurses, and others in the pediatric health-care workforce. It is projected that by 2020, 44.5% of American children ages 0 to 19 years will belong to a racial or ethnic minority group (U.S. Census Bureau, 2000). Considering cultural attributes in addition to race and ethnicity (e.g., lesbian, gay, bisexual, transgender) would greatly increase this projection of diversity. Thornton, Powe, Roter, and Cooper (2011) examined patient–physician social concordance using four social characteristics: race, gender, age, and education. Results showed that lower patient–physician social correspondence was associated with less favorable patient perceptions of care and lower global satisfaction ratings; conversely, stepwise patient–physician similarities were show to improve patient perceptions of care in an additive fashion. Does this "sameness" foster trust, which is essential in any caring relationship between children and professionals? More research is needed on the relationship between pediatric workforce diversity and satisfaction, access, quality, and outcomes of pediatric care.

Care for the Caregiver

A family-centered approach to care embraces caring for caregivers as well as the patient. Although progress has been made in addressing some of the many needs of family caregivers, initiatives for professional caregivers have not kept pace. Institutions must apply the principles of family-centered care to their own "family."

Berwick, Nolan, and Whittington (2008) described a set of organizing principles for health-care delivery—the Triple Aim—which is widely accepted as a compass to optimize health-system performance. Principles include improving the patient experience of care, improving population health, and reducing costs. Bodenheimer and Sinsky (2014) pointed out that burnout is associated with lower patient satisfaction, reduced health outcomes, and may even increase costs, the opposite of intended outcomes of the Triple Aim. Physicians and other members of the health-care workforce report widespread burnout and dissatisfaction (Sakallaris, Miller, Saper, Kreitzer, & Jonas, 2016). Among physicians, burnout is especially prevalent among ED physicians, general internists, neurologists, and family physicians (Shanafelt et al, 2012). In a 2014 survey, 68% of family physicians and 73% of general internists said they would not choose the same specialty if they could start their careers over again (Kane & Peckham, 2014). Thus, Bodenheimer and Sinsky recommended adding a fourth aim: improving the work life of health-care providers, including clinicians and staff. In other words, practice joy, because a healthy population requires a healthy workforce. They offer several practical steps (e.g., implementing team documentation, locating physicians with their team members) so that unnecessary work is reengineered out of practice. Such steps can bring joy back to practice. Bodenheimer and Sinsky remind us that health care is a relationship between those who provide care and those who seek care, "a relationship that can only thrive if it is symbiotic, benefiting both parties" (p. 575).

Hospitals are increasingly developing interventions to help staff cope with working in a stressful environment. Whether it is a 5-minute stretch break when a dancer appears on the unit, or restorative events off-site, such the Days of Renewal program for caregivers at Shands Hospital in Gainesville, Florida (Graham-Pole, Sonke, & Henderson, 2004), such interventions have tremendous potential to prevent burnout and retain valuable staff. Greater dissemination of information about successful programs can provide a starting point for others to develop model programs for caregivers in their institutions.

Complementary, Alternative, and Integrative Health

Although the term *complementary and alternative medicine* (CAM) is in common use, many health-care professionals use the term *integrative medicine* to designate practices that are not alternative but instead integrated into traditional ones. Also, the most recent name for the National Institutes of Health's CAM center—National Center for Complementary and Integrative Health (NCCIH)—uses the word *health* instead of *medicine*. The NCCIH points out that there are many definitions for *integrative health care* but that all involve bringing conventional and complementary approaches together in a coordinated way (NCCIH, 2016).

The 2012 National Health Interview Survey of almost 45,000 Americans, including 10,000 children ages 4 to 17, found that 11.6% of the children had used or been given some form of complementary health product or practice (e.g., yoga, dietary supplements, mindfulness) during the past year (Black, Clarke, Barnes, Stussman, & Nahin, 2012). Among children, the highest rates of use are often found among those with a chronic, recurrent, or incurable illness (Adams et al., 2014). For example, in a survey of 129 families with children with cancer, 60.5% reported their child's current or previous use of CAM products or practices (Valji et al., 2013).

As the use of CAM approaches in the United States grows, especially among children with chronic illness or disability, distinctions among unproven therapies, CAM, and biomedicine may become blurred (AAP, Committee on Children with Disabilities, 2001). The AAP stresses the importance of providing balanced advice about therapeutic options, guarding against bias, and establishing and maintaining a trusting relationship with families.

One form of CAM gaining popularity among children is mindfulness—a mental training that develops sustained attention that can change the ways people think, act, and feel. Mindfulness is easy to learn and implement with individuals and groups of children, and is basically cost free. Studies indicate that mindfulness can reduce symptoms of stress and depression and promote wellbeing among children (University of Exeter, 2013).

A growing number of individuals consider the use of the arts to be a form of CAM, and, in fact, music was one of the therapies funded for research by the Office of Alternative Medicine (now the NCCIH) at the National Institutes of Health. Each year, more artists join children's health-care teams at hospitals, hospices, and in the home (Rollins & Riccio, 2002). Academic undergraduate and graduate arts and health programs are springing up nationally and internationally. More artists will be prepared to plan, implement, and evaluate effective arts services in patient-care settings, and also to facilitate arts-based health promotion interventions in schools and community settings.

Mental Health

According to the C. S. Mott Children's Hospital National Poll on Children's Health, 55% of adults ($N = 2,648$) polled believe children's mental and emotional health is worse today than when they were children (Davis et al., 2016). The researchers cite possible explanations as less quality family time, lower quality of personal friendships, less coping and staying positive, and the perception of more stress than in the past.

A total of 13% to 20% of children in the United States experience a mental disorder in a given year; surveillance during 1994–2011 showed an increase in prevalence (Perou et al., 2013). Further, mental health hospitalizations among children and adolescents increased by 24% between 2007 and 2010 (Bardach et al., 2014).

Mental health disorders are an important public health issue in the United States because of their prevalence, early onset, and impact on the child, family, and community. Unfortunately, there is a shortage of placements for children who need acute psychiatric care or intensive residential care. Providers are reluctant to add additional inpatient psychiatric beds for children because Medicaid reimbursement rates are low.

While awaiting placement, children and teens may stay multiple nights in an emergency department (ED). For example, at Connecticut Children's Medical Center, the total number of patients who spent two or more nights in the ED quadrupled from 40 in 2010 to 161 in 2012 (Chedekel, 2014). When placement is unavailable, children return home to their families, but frequently visit the emergency department five or six times per year.

The mental health community is exploring childhood development in terms of what is normal and abnormal, trying to understand how factors affecting development can have an effect on mental health (Goldberg, 2014). The aim is to try to predict, and ultimately prevent, developmental problems that could lead to mental illness. They hope to identify risk factors that increase a child's chances of developing a mental disorder and research medications used to treat them.

The Affordable Care Act (ACA) is providing one of the largest expansions of mental health and substance-use disorder coverage in a generation, and may stop the cycle of poverty associated with mental illness. We have seen an increase in the use of collaborative care models that include access to medical and behavioral health services, social work services, housing and employment services, and case management, all at one site (Rollins, 2015b).

Technology

Technology abounds across the health-care continuum. Some hospitals have become nearly paperless in this digital age. Nurses are using handheld computers—small personal computers weighing about 14 ounces—to facilitate real-time documentation.

The device stores the majority of the patients' medical record information, including current orders, recent laboratory results, scheduled nursing interventions, and history, which all remain secure through individual security passwords. The nurse downloads information to the hospital information system throughout the shift through connection ports located throughout the unit. This system is designed to give the nurse more time at the bedside by eliminating the need for one-time charting at the end of shift in the nurses' station. Ideally, for pediatric nurses, a portion of this "saved time" will be devoted to addressing psychosocial issues for children in their care.

Telemedicine—the use of electronic communication and information technologies to provide or support clinical care at a distance (Office for the Advancement of Telehealth, 2001)—is gaining popularity, especially in rural or remote settings. Dhamar et al. (2013) reported significant improvements in the quality of care for seriously ill and injured children treated in remote rural EDs by using telemedicine consultations with pediatric critical-care medicine physicians at the University of California, Davis Children's Hospital. Creative strategies will be needed to meet challenges in some areas of practice, such as appropriate criteria for supervision of nonphysician clinicians, reimbursement for telemedicine services, privacy of patient information, universal standards for telemedicine technologies, professional and medical liability, regulatory and jurisdictional issues related to multistate licensure of clinicians, and high costs of transmission of medical information (AAP, Committee on Pediatric Workforce, 2003). To date, most telemedicine has addressed emergency or critical care. Health-care professionals that recognize the importance of psychosocial care for children must advocate for also addressing psychosocial issues as telemedicine networks are established and expanded.

Although often used interchangeably with the term telemedicine, the term telehealth is typically used to refer to a broader scope of health-care services, including nonclinical services such as distance training and education. Telehealth is rapidly becoming mainstream. In 2013, 52% of hospitals used telehealth and an additional 10% were beginning the process of implementing telehealth service (American Hospital Association, 2013). Consumer acceptance of and confidence in telemedicine is growing as well. In a survey of 1,547 consumers and 403 practitioners in the United States, 76% of patients said they would choose telehealth over human contact (Pennic, 2013). Seventy percent reported that they are comfortable communicating with doctors via texting, email, or video instead of seeing them in person.

E-mail transactions between families and providers are becoming more common. E-mail is more spontaneous than letter writing and offers more permanence than oral conversations. Follow-up e-mail allows retention and clarification of advice provided in the health-care setting when parents and children under duress may forget to ask important questions. Educational handouts can be attached to e-mails. Further, e-mail messages are less likely to accidentally fall through the cracks of a busy practice. Several medical groups, including the American Medical Association, have developed guidelines for e-mail use that address topics such as when e-mail should and should not be used, expected response time, who else in the office will have access to messages, and so on.

Families also are accessing the Internet for health-related research through websites, newsgroups, chat rooms, and Listservs. Ahmann (2000) pointed out that although the use of the Internet can empower consumers, encourage both collaboration and a family-centered approach to care, and could contribute to improved outcomes and cost savings, at the same time, care and caution are needed regarding interpretation of health-related information from this source. The questions in the Text Box E.1 can be used by both professionals and families for evaluating a health-related website.

Research

Advances in medical research should continue at an accelerated rate, with an emphasis on genetic research. When the Human Genome Project formally began in 1990, its

---

Text Box E.1.
Questions to Consider in Evaluating a Health-Related Website

1. Is it clear who has written the information on the website? Are his or her credentials listed? Is the author qualified to write on the given topic?

2. Is the site maintained by a credible, reputable, medical organization, government agency, or university?

3. What is the purpose of the website? To inform? To persuade? To sell?

4. Is there any potential conflict of interest involved? Does the site sell products? Have commercial advertising? Can you tell who sponsored or paid for this site?

5. What is the source of information on the website? Is the information based on clinical or scientific studies? Testimonials? Opinion? Are references provided for information cited on the website?

6. Does the website seem to provide a balanced, unbiased view? Is a range of reference sources identified? If treatment options are described, how much information and detail are offered regarding options? Are claims of benefits of specific treatments substantiated?

7. How current is the information? When was the site produced? Updated?

8. Does the website provide a means of contacting its webmaster?

Note. From "Supporting Families' Savvy Use of the Internet for Health Research," by E. Ahmann, 2000, *Pediatric Nursing, 26*(4), p. 421. Copyright 2000 by Jannetti. Reprinted with permission.

Sources
DISCERN Instrument
www.discern.org.uk/
Click on "Discern"; click on "discern instrument."

HONCode Site-Checker
www.hon.ch/HONcode_check.html

Information Quality (IQ) Tool
www.hitiweb.mitretek.org/iq

Siwek, J. (April 25, 2000). One last piece of advice. *The Washington Post*, Health Section, p. 23.

The Quality Information Checklist (QUICK)
www.quick.org.uk/menu.htm

original goal was to map and sequence the complete set of human genes by 2005. This goal, quite remarkably, was achieved in early 2000. Genetic research holds promise for great strides in the diagnosis and treatment of many childhood diseases. However, emerging genetic technology often enables testing and screening before the development of definitive treatment or preventive measures, opening the door to ethical questions about whether use of such technology promotes the best interests of the child (AAP, Committee on Bioethics, 2001). Chandler and Smith (1998) also pointed out that through striving to eradicate congenital disability, a community risks promoting a cult of perfectionism that may have discriminatory effects on people—whether children or adults—with disabilities.

We are seeing an increase in research with children in general due to federal funding requirements. In 1996, the National Institutes of Health (NIH) and the American Academy of Pediatrics held a joint workshop concerning the participation of children in clinical research. There was a valid concern that treatment modalities developed based on research conducted on adults, without adequate data from children, were being used to treat children for many diseases and disorders. From this workshop came the recommendation that the NIH develop a policy for including children in clinical research.

> The NIH concluded that when there is a sound scientific rationale for including children in research, investigators should be expected to do so unless there is a strong overriding reason that justifies their exclusion from the studies. Although this is the same scientific rationale that is the basis for the policy requiring the inclusion of women and minorities in clinical research, this policy does not mandate the inclusion of children in all clinical research. Because the issues and sensitivities surrounding children's participation in research are significantly different from those regarding women and minorities, such a mandate would be inappropriate. Nonetheless, even though the inclusion of children is not an absolute requirement, applicants for NIH funding will be expected to address this issue in their proposals. (NIH, 1997, p. 34)

With the likelihood of more children participating in research, researchers will have a greater obligation than ever before to help assure that children have adequate understanding of a research project before assenting or consenting to participation. Creative methods also will need to be devised to help children express their wishes and understanding in nontraditional ways. And, of course, attention to risk factors specific to children's developmental levels will remain a priority. For example, a developmental concern of school-age children is rule conformity. Thus, school-age children are vulnerable to coercion to participate due to respect for authority (Conrad & Horner, 1997). Researchers may need reminders to avoid using authority figures to recruit subjects, to approach a child with his or her parent present, and to reinforce the right to decline to participate.

Future decades likely will see an increase in African American and Latino children's participation in research. A dramatic increase in childhood obesity, especially among African American and Latino children, has stirred the research community. Additionally, ethnic and racial differences have surfaced in other areas. For example, researchers at the Children's Hospital of Pittsburgh in Pennsylvania have released findings that suggest that a significant number of children, mainly African American, may have "double diabetes," Type 1 and Type 2 (National Association of Children's Hospitals and Related Institutions [NACHRI], 2003).

Although race, or ethnicity, and gender often are viewed as variables that exert their effects through innate or genetically determined biological mechanisms, a growing body of research suggests that these variables have strong—and in many areas, predominately—sociological and psychological dimensions (AAP, Committee on Pediatric Research, 2000). Studies that do not address the importance of social determinants as fundamental causes or contributors to disease and unfulfilled potential limit the scope and impact of research conclusions.

The American Academy of Pediatrics points out that community-based research with children raises ethical issues not normally encountered in research conducted in academic settings (AAP, Committee on Native American Child Health and Committee on Community Health Services, 2004). Conventional risk–benefit assessments often fail to recognize harms that can occur in socially identifiable populations as a result of research participation. Many such communities will require more stringent measures of beneficence that must be applied directly to the participating communities. In its recommendations, the AAP emphasizes the need for community involvement in the research process.

Outcomes research is of critical importance in exploring the efficacy of interventions. The move from episodic care to a continuum of care emphasizes the need for continued research across all organizational boundaries. The family—"as the constant in a child's life, while the service systems and support personnel within those systems fluctuate" (Shelton & Stepanek, 1994)—likely will be called on to play a more collaborative role in outcomes research. Health status measures—functional outcome, well-being, or quality of life—are more likely to be used than reliance on medical information alone. A multidimensional definition of health encompasses physical, psychological, and social aspects, as well as asking meaningful questions, such as "Can the child participate in normal school activities? Can the child play with friends? Can the child live a life free of painful symptoms?"

Looking Forward

What will health care look like in the coming decades? Two primary factors will be the drivers of the changes we will see.

The first factor is the system for payment for health-care costs. The Affordable Care Act has made an incredible difference in the health and lives of many American children and their families. Yet many view the ACA as a first step in universal coverage. What other steps will take place in between depends in part on our nation's leaders but also on advocacy efforts from health-care professionals, families, and concerned citizens.

Technology is the second driver. According to health entrepreneur Sean Mehra (2013), the opportunities at the intersection of health and technology will enable humanity to create health and wealth on a global scale, seizing major business opportunities while generating tremendous positive social effects for everyone, everywhere. He concludes, "Health is ripe for technological disruption and worthy of the world's best resources."

Both of these driving factors have the potential for monumental changes, some of which we are unable to even imagine. The implications of such changes on children's psychosocial care remain to be seen. Advocates for this essential element of children's health care must be part of the conversation as this exciting future unfolds.

References

Adams, D., Whidden, A., Honkanen, M., Dagenais, S., Clifford, T., Baydala, L., . . . Vohra, S. (2014). Complementary and alternative medicine: A survey of its use in pediatric cardiology. *Canadian Medical Association Journal, 2*(4), e217–e224.

Ahmann, E. (2000). Supporting families' savvy use of the Internet for health research. *Pediatric Nursing, 26*(4), 419–423.

Aiken, L., Sermeus, W., Van den Heed, K., Sloane, D., Busse, R., McKee, M., . . . Kutney-Lee, A. (2012). Patient safety, satisfaction and quality of hospital care: Cross sectional surveys of nurses and patients in 12 countries in Europe and the United States. *British Medical Journal, 344*, e1717. doi: http://dx.doi.org/10.1136/bmj.e1717

American Academy of Pediatrics, Committee on Bioethics. (2001). Ethical issues with genetic testing in pediatrics. *Pediatrics, 107*(6), 1451–1455.

American Academy of Pediatrics, Committee on Children with Disabilities. (2001). Counseling families who choose complementary and alternative medicine for their child with chronic illness or disability. *Pediatrics, 107*(3), 598–601.

American Academy of Pediatrics, Committee on Hospital Care. (2014). Child life services. *Pediatrics, 133*(5), e1471–e1478.

American Academy of Pediatrics, Committee on Native American Child Health and Committee on Community Health Services. (2004). Ethical considerations in research with socially identifiable populations. *Pediatrics, 113*(1), 148–151.

American Academy of Pediatrics, Committee on Pediatric Research. (2000). Race/ethnicity, gender, socioeconomic status—Research exploring their effects on child health: A subject review. *Pediatrics, 105*(6), 1349–1351.

American Academy of Pediatrics, Committee on Pediatric Workforce. (2003). Scope of practice issues in the delivery of pediatric health care. *Pediatrics, 111*(2), 426–435.

American Academy of Pediatrics, Committee on Pediatric Workforce. (2016). Financing graduated medical education to meet the needs of children and the future pediatrician workforce. *Pediatrics, 137*(4). doi:10.1542/peds.2016-0211. Retrieved from http://pediatrics.aappublications.org/content/pediatrics/137/4/e20160211.full.pdf

American Hospital Association. (2013). *2013 AHAA Annual Survey Information Technology Supplement*. Retrieved from http://www.ahadataviewer.com/Global/IT%20surveys/2013%20AHA%20Annual%20Survey%20%20IT%20Supplement%20Survey.pdf

Bardach, N. S., Coker, T. R., Zima, B. T., Murphy, J. M., Knapp, P., Richardson, L. P., . . . Mangione-Smith, R. (2014). Common and costly hospitalizations for pediatric mental health disorders. *Pediatrics, 133*(4), 602-609.

Berwick, D., Nolan, T., & Whittington, J. (2008). The triple aim: Care health, and cost. *Health Aff (Millwood), 27*(3), 759–769.

Black, L., Clarke, T., Barnes, P., Stussman, B., & Nahin, R. (2012). Use of complementary health approaches among children aged 4–17 years in the United States. National Health Interview Survey, 2007–2012. *National health statistics reports, no 78*. Hyattsville, MD: National Center for Health Statistics.

Bodenheimer, T., & Sinsky, C. (2014). From triple to quadruple aim: Care of the patient requires care of the provider. *Annals of Family Medicine, 12*(6), 573–576.

Brandner, J. (1995). Will hospital rounds go the way of the house call? *Managed Care, 4*(7), 25–28.

Chandler, M., & Smith, A. (1998). Prenatal screening and women's perception of infant disability: A Sophie's choice for every mother. *Nursing Inquiry, 5*, 71–76.

Chedekel, L. (2014). Long ER stays for kids in crisis on the rise. *Connecticut Health I-Team*. Retrieved from http://c-hit.org/2014/07/10/long-er-stays-for-kids-in-crisis-on-the-rise/

Cohen, E., Friedman, J., Mahant, S., Adams S., Jovcevska, V., & Rosenbaum, P. (2010). The impact of a complex care clinic in a children's hospital. *Child: Care, Health and Development, 36*(4), 574–582.

Conrad, B., & Horner, S. (1997). Issue in pediatric research: Safeguarding the children. *Journal of the Society of Pediatric Nurses, 2*(4), 163–171.

Davis, M., Wietecha, M., Clark, S., Singer, D., Matos-Moreno, A., Kauffman, A., & Shhultz, S. (2016). *C.S. Mott Children's Hospital National Poll on Children's Health.* Ann Arbor, MI: University of Michigan. Retrieved from http://www.mottnpch.org/reports-surveys/today-versus-back-day-kids-health-getting-worse

Dharmar, M., Romano, P., Kuppermann, N., Nesbitt, T., Cole, S., Andrada, E., … Marcin, J. (2013). Impact of critical care telemedicine consultations on children in rural emergency departments. *Critical Care Medicine, 41*(10), 2388–2395.

Epstein, D. (1997). The role of "hospitalists" in the health care system. *New England Journal of Medicine, 336*, 444.

Goldberg, J. (2014). Mental illness in children. *WebMD.* Retrieved from http://www.webmd.com/mental-health/mental-illness-children?page=4#3

Graham-Pole, J., Sonke, J., & Henderson, J. (2004). The University of Florida Center for the Arts and Health Research and Education "Days of Renewal" program, a case study. In L. Kable (Ed.), *Caring for caregivers: A grassroots USA–Japan initiative* (pp. 21–28). Washington, DC: Society for the Arts in Healthcare.

Health Resources and Services Administration. (2013). *The U.S. nursing workforce: Trends in supply and education.* Washington, DC: HRSA.

Henry, L. (1997). Will hospitalists assume family physicians' inpatient care roles? *Family Practice Management, 4*(7), 54–60, 65–66, 69.

Kane, L., & Peckham, C. (2014). *Medscape Physician Compensation Report 2014.* Retrieved from http://www.medscape.com/features/slideshow/compensation/2014/public/overview#24.

Mahant, S., & Weinstein, M. (2016). Hospitalists and the outpatient clinic: Time to reconsider. *The Journal of Pediatrics, 168*, 3–4.

Mehra, S. (2013, June 23). *7 predictions for the future of health care technology* [Blog]. Retrieved from http://venturebeat.com/2013/06/23/7-predictions-for-the-future-of-health-care-technology/

National Association of Children's Hospitals and Related Institutions (NACHRI). (2003). Children's hospitals on cutting-edge of pediatric research. *Child Health Trends Update, 2*(3). Retrieved July 25, 2004, from http://www.childrenshospitals.net/Content/ContentGroups/Media_Center1/Child_Health_Trends_Update1/2003/Child_Health_Trends_Update_-_Pediatric_Research_and_Obesity.htm

National Center for Complementary and Integrative Health. (2016). *Complementary, alternative, or integrative health. What's in a name?* Retrieved from https://nccih.nih.gov/health/integrative-health

National Institutes of Health (NIH). (1997). Policy on the inclusion of children as subjects in clinical research. *NIH Guide, 26*(3), 34.

Office for the Advancement of Telehealth. (2001). *2001 Report to Congress on telemedicine.* Rockville, MD: Author.

Pennic, F. (2013). Survey: 76% of patients would choose telehealth over human contact. *HIT Consultant.* Retrieved from http://hitconsultant.net/2013/03/08/survey-patients-would-choose-telehealth-over-human-contact/

Perou, R., Bitsko, R., Blumberg, S., Pastor, P., Ghandour, R., Cfroerer, J., … Huang, L., (2013). Mental health surveillance among children—United States, 2005–2011. *Morbidity and Mortality Weekly Report, 62*(02), 1–35.

Rollins, J. (2015a). The 12-hour shift. *Pediatric Nursing, 41*(4), 162–164.

Rollins, J. (2015b). Arts & America: Arts, health, & wellness. In C. Lord (Ed.), *Arts & America: Arts culture, and the future of America's communities* (pp. 79–91). Washington, DC: Americans for the Arts.

Rollins, J., & Riccio, L. (2002). ART is the heART: A palette of possibilities for hospice care. *Pediatric Nursing, 28*(4), 355–362.

Ryan, C. (1997). Writer questions the inevitability of FPs' declining role in inpatient care. *Family Medicine, 29*, 382–383.

Sakallaris, B., Miller, W., Saper, R., Kreitzer, M., & Jonas, W. (2016). Meeting the challenge of a more person-centered future for US healthcare. *Global Advances in Health and Medicine Journal, 5*(1), 51–60.

Scheurer, D. (2013). Thousands of hospitalists set their sites on HM 13. *The Hospitalist.* Retrieved from http://www.the-hospitalist.org/article/danielle-scheurer-thousands-of-hospitalists-set-their- sights-on-hm13/

Shanafelt, T. D., Boone, S., Tan, L., Dyrbye, L, Sotile, W., Satele, D., … Oreskovich, M. (2012). Burnout and satisfaction with work-life balance among US physicians relative to the general U.S. population. *Archives of Internal Medicine, 172*(18): 1377–1385.

Shelton, T., & Stepanek, J. (1994). *Family-centered care for children needing specialized health and developmental services.* Bethesda, MD: Association for the Care of Children's Health.

Shortell, S., Gillies, R., & Devers, K. (1995). Reinventing the American hospital. *Milbank Quarterly, 73*(2), 131–160.

Thornton, R. L., Powe, N. R., Roter, D., & Cooper, L. A. (2011). Patient-physician social concordance, medical visit communication and patients' perceptions of health care quality. *Patient Education and Counseling, 85*(3), e201–e208.

University of Exeter. (2013, June 19). Mindfulness can increase wellbeing and reduce stress in school children. *ScienceDaily.* Retrieved from www.sciencedaily.com/releases/2013/06/130619195139.htm

U.S. Census Bureau. (2000). *Projections of the total resident population by 5-year age groups, race, and Hispanic origin with special age categories: Middle series, 2016 to 2020.* Washington, DC: U.S. Census Bureau; 2000. Retrieved from www.census.gov/population/projections/files/natproj/summary/np-t4-e.pdf

Valji, R., Adams, D., Dagenais, S., Clifford, T., Baydala, L., King, W. J., & Vohra, S. (2013). Complementary and alternative medicine: A survey of its use in pediatric oncology. *Evidence-Based Complementary and Alternative Medicine, 2013*, Article ID 527163. http://dx.doi.org/10.1155/2013/527163

Wachter, R., & Goldman, L. (1996). The emerging role of "hospitalists" in the American healthcare system. *New England Journal of Medicine, 335*, 514–517.

White, K., & Glazier, R. (2011). Do hospitalist physicians improve the quality of inpatient care delivery? A systematic review of process, efficiency and outcome measures. *BMC Medicine, 9*, 58. DOI: 10.1186/1741-7015-9-58. Retrieved from http://bmcmedicine.biomedcentral.com/articles/10.1186/1741-7015-9-58

Index

In this index, *b* denotes box, *f* denotes figure, and *t* denotes table.

A

AAP. *See* American Academy of Pediatrics (AAP)
Abdel-Khalek, A., 351
ACA. *See* Affordable Care Act (ACA)
Acceptance of condition, 196–197, 201
Acebo, C., 337
ACEs (adverse childhood experiences), 491–492
    See also Foster care; Homeless families; Trauma-informed care
ACMG (American College of Medical Genetics), 442, 443
Active listening, 374–375
Activity rooms, 17–18
Acute stress disorder (ASD), 274–275
Adaptations. See Family adaptive tasks; Physical limitations
Adelman, W., 498
ADHD (attention-deficit/hyperactivity disorder), 454–455
Admission Assessment Tool for Child with ASD, 24f
Adolescents
    about, 17–19
    the arts and, 141, 143, 144
    blended families and, 281
    confidentiality and, 439
    developmental aspects of chronic illnesses, 179t
    digital grieving, 255–256
    grief of, 226, 230, 231t
    informed decision-making, 439–440, 457
    leadership skills support in, 185t
    parental illness and effects on, 277
    personal space and, 317
    preparation for health-care encounters, 64–66, 67
    sources of stress for, 34, 44
    spiritual care interventions for, 368t, 371–372
    spiritual distress in, 363t
    tobacco, alcohol, and other drug use and, 515–516

transition to adulthood and, 180–181, 194–195
    understanding of death, 218t, 219
    who are dying, 242
    See also Adulthood, transition to; LGBT children
Adoption, 509–510
Adoption and Safe Families Act (ASFA), 509
Adulthood, transition to, 180–181, 194–195
Adverse childhood experiences (ACEs), 491–492
    See also Foster care; Homeless families; Trauma-informed care
Aesthetic chills, 128–129
Affordable Care Act (ACA), xxiv, xxvi–xxvii, 191, 192, 322, 433
Ahmann, E., 548
Akard, T., 138
Akitsuki, Y., 513
Allen, N., 293
Allenbach, A., 472
Alsop, P., 131
Altman, I., 314
Ambulatory care experiences, 35–37
See also Outpatient treatment
American Academy of Pediatrics (AAP)
    accepting gifts, 478
ADHD, 454
    Baby Doe regulations, 445
    on child life specialists, 544
    culturally effective care, 425
    ethics committees, 445
    family-centered care, 189–190
    foster care, 507
    genetic screenings, 442, 443
    informed consent and parent permission, 436, 437
    medical home, 193
    palliative care, 244–245, 441
    play, 90, 91, 93
    relationship boundaries, 477–478
    research on children, 456, 550, 551
    sudden death in emergency department, 234
    toxic stress, 492, 508
    vaccines, 435
    workforce shortages, 543–544
American College of Medical Genetics (ACMG), 442, 443

About the Editors and Contributors

Editors

Judy A. Rollins, PhD, RN, Rollins & Associates, Inc., Washington, DC, is a nurse with a fine arts degree in the visual arts, an MS in child development and family studies, and a PhD in health and community studies. She is adjunct assistant professor in the Department of Family Medicine and the Department of Pediatrics at Georgetown University School of Medicine in Washington, DC; adjunct instructor at the Center for Arts in Medicine at the University of Florida, Gainesville, Florida; Scholar at The Institute for Integrated Health, Baltimore, Maryland; and editor of *Pediatric Nursing.* Dr. Rollins consults, writes, and researches on children's issues, with a special interest in the use of the arts for children in health-care settings and a focus on children with cancer and their families.

Rosemary Bolig, PhD, retired from almost 50 years of teaching, research, and service in 2016. She served on the faculties of the Johns Hopkins Medical Center, The Ohio State University, Mount Vernon College, and the University of the District of Columbia as well as online Walden University as a professor of early childhood education. Dr. Bolig has published many articles on children in health care, children under stress (and especially play's ameliorative influences), and child life programs' theoretical bases and professional development. She has been an advocate for change in children's health care and a recipient of the Child Life Council's Outstanding Contributor award.

Carmel C. Mahan, MSEd, CCLS, is currently an early intervention specialist with the Baltimore County Public School System in Baltimore, Maryland. She has a BS in Human Development and Family Relations from the University of Connecticut and a MSEd in Special Education from Fordham University. She has over 20 years' experience as a child life specialist in a variety of acute-care settings and 12 years' early intervention experience. She has published articles and a chapter for a nursing textbook as well as co-authoring a book with Dr. Rollins on training for artist-in-residence programs. She and Dr. Rollins have collaborated on a number of projects to benefit children and families in health-care settings and to educate the professionals who care for them about their psychosocial needs. This is her first collaboration with Dr. Bolig.

Contributors

Elizabeth Ahmann, ScD, RN, ACC has a background in nursing, public health, and both ADHD and health and wellness coaching. She has written many articles and multiple chapters on family-centered care and about families of children with illness and disability; authored two editions of the book *Home Care for the High Risk Infant;* and is co-editor of the "Family Matters" section in Pediatric Nursing. She is a coach in private practice in Cheverly, Maryland, and adjunct faculty at Maryland University of Integrative Health.

Jessika C. Boles, PhD, CCLS is a child life specialist in the pediatric intensive care unit at the Monroe Carell, Jr. Children's Hospital at Vanderbilt in Nashville, Tennessee. She has also previously worked as a child life specialist in pediatric oncology, serving adolescents and young adults at St. Jude Children's Research Hospital. She earned her doctorate from the University of Memphis in educational psychology, and her research agenda addresses child development and learning processes specifically in culturally charged sites of learning such as the hospital, outpatient clinic, community, and family. She is a regular contributor for *Pediatric Nursing* and serves on the board of directors for the Child Life Council. She also teaches undergraduate and graduate level courses in child life and play-based interventions at Lipscomb University and Vanderbilt University.

Lynn B. Clutter, PhD, APRN, CNS, CNE, IBCLC has worked extensively in nursing care of the family. She is a full-time assistant professor in the BSN nursing program at The University of Tulsa in Tulsa, Oklahoma, where she enjoys mentoring nursing students. She is a part-time Lactation Consultant at Saint Francis Hospital. Lynn's teaching and clinical education encompass areas of pediatrics and perinatal nursing, community health, mental health, genetics, ethics, and research. Her research experience is qualitative and quantitative with publication topics of adolescent parenting, unintended pregnancy, and open adoption, use of the peanut ball in labor and delivery, test anxiety and cortisol levels, nursing student clinical experiences, attachment, children's pain, and spiritual care. She is professionally active serving on the Wong-Baker FACES Foundation board and serves in leadership in several professional organizations. She has practiced as a Clinical Nurse Specialist and as a nurse educator receiving awards in leadership, scholarship, research, and practice. Lynn has been married for 37 years, has five children, and two grandsons.

Lois J. Pearson, MEd, CCLS, has been providing psychosocial care for children and families for more than 30 years as a certified child life specialist. She has had a role in starting and implementing three child life programs: in a community hospital, in a large children's hospital, and, most recently, in an adult hospital providing psychosocial support for children of adult patients. Her interests in children's trauma and grief work have led her to develop programming and extensive writing in these areas. In addition to clinical work, she has been a faculty member of the School of Education at Edgewood College within the child life program for many years.

Teresa A. Savage, PhD, RN, has over 40 years of experience in the nursing of children. Her interest in ethics grew from the issues she encountered in neonatal care and follow-up, but expanded to include all aspects of bioethics. She served as an ethics consultant at a major academic medical center, a rehabilitation hospital, and a residential facility for children and adults with intellectual and developmental disabilities. Her ethics work also involved serving on two ethics committees and three institutional review boards. Recent research includes exploring life support decisions for extremely premature infants and another study on end-of-life care for adults with intellectual and developmental disabilities. She is a board member of the American Society for

Bioethics and Humanities and has faculty appointments at the University of Illinois at Chicago College of Nursing and in the Department of Disability and Human Development, and at Northwestern University Feinberg School of Medicine Department of Physical Medicine and Rehabilitation and in the Center for Bioethics and Humanities.

Mardelle McCuskey Shepley, B.A., M.Arch., M.A., D.Arch., LEED, EDAC, is a professor in the Department of Design and Environmental Analysis and associate director of the Institute for Healthy Futures at Cornell University. Dr. Shepley is a fellow in the American Institute of Architects and the American College of Healthcare Architects. She has authored/co-authored five books, including *Healthcare Environments for Children and their Families* (1998), A *Practitioner's Guide to Evidence-Based Design* (2008), *Design for Critical Care* (2009), *Health Facility Evaluation for Design Practitioners* (2010), and *Design for Pediatric and Neonatal Critical Care* (2014). Mardelle has worked in professional practice for 25 years. She is founder of ART+Science design research consultants.